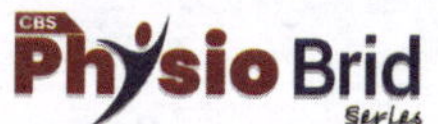

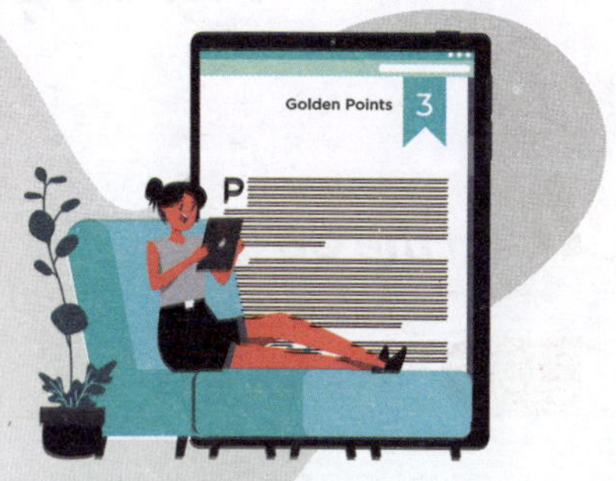

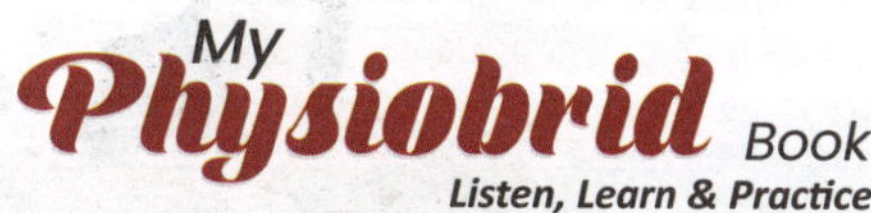

Reading is not enough, Now *Listen, Learn & Practice* Every Chapter

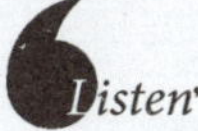

'Listen'

i. Golden Points

Get Chapter-wise One Liners in **PODCAST form** (audio) for quick revision of chapters

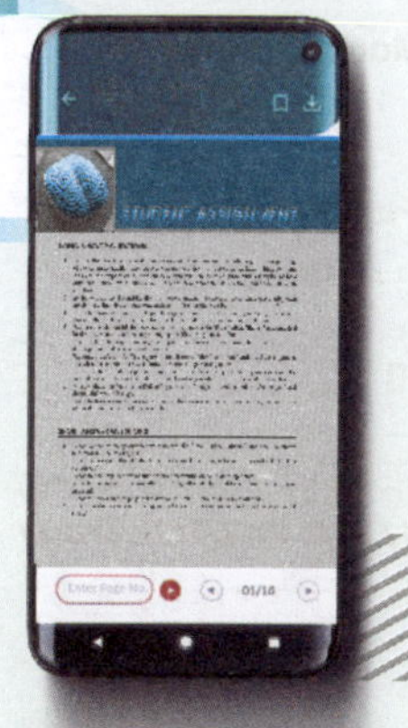

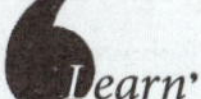

'Learn'

ii. Solved Exercises

Subjective and Objective exercises of the book have been given with their solution (in PDF) to evaluate and assess the complete chapter knowledge

- **40+** Long Answer Questions
- **80+** Short Answer Questions
- **150+** Multiple Choice Questions

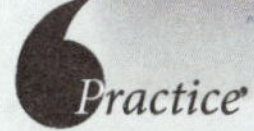

'Practice'

iii. MCQs

200+ Chapter-wise Multiple Choice Questions in Practice and Review mode to provide in-depth concept clarity

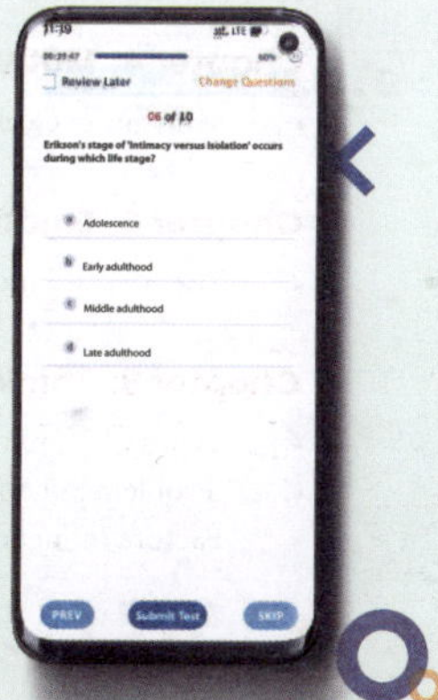

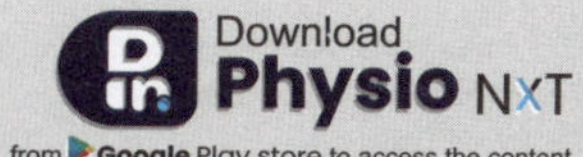

Download
Physio NxT

from ▶ **Google** Play store to access the content

CBS Physiobrid Books >
Textbook of Psychology
The Hybrid Edition

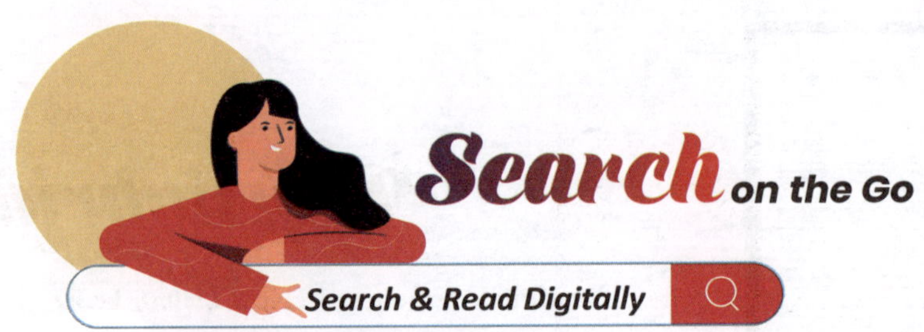

Mapping of the most important topics from the Book at one place with one click search
Get **50+** Important topics of the book at one click

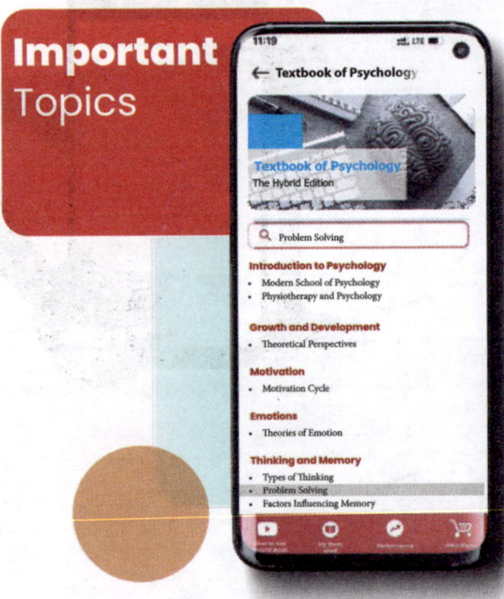

Chapter 1: Introduction to Psychology

- Modern School of Psychology
- Physiotherapy and Psychology

Chapter 2: Growth and Development

- Theoretical Perspectives

Chapter 4: Motivation

- Motivation Cycle

Chapter 6: Emotions

- Theories of Emotion

Chapter 8: Thinking and Memory

- Types of Thinking
- Problem Solving
- Factors Influencing Memory

Chapter 9: Learning

- Learning Disability

Chapter 10: Personality

- Factors Influencing Development of Personality

Chapter 12: Substance Abuse

- Consequences of Substance Use

Chapter 13: Behavior Modification

- Behavior Modification

Chapter 14: Pediatric Psychology

- Models of Development Psychology

Chapter 18: Counseling

- Aims of Counseling

Chapter 19: Psychology and Physiotherapy

- Biopsychosocial Model
- Stress

and Many more...

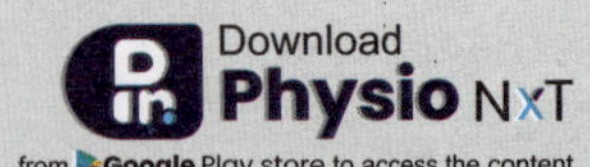

CBS Physiobrid Books >
Textbook of Psychology
The Hybrid Edition

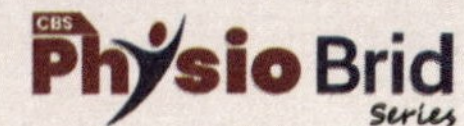

High Yield Topics
Revise on the Go

Get **50+** Topic-wise Selective Images & Tables with their descriptions
for LMR and Quick reference, based on the topics of University examination

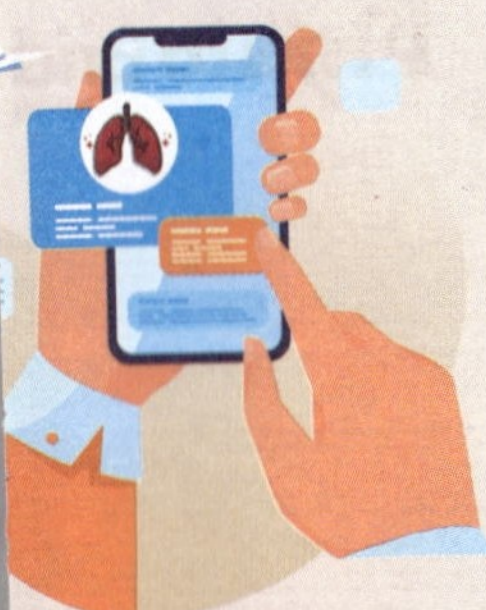

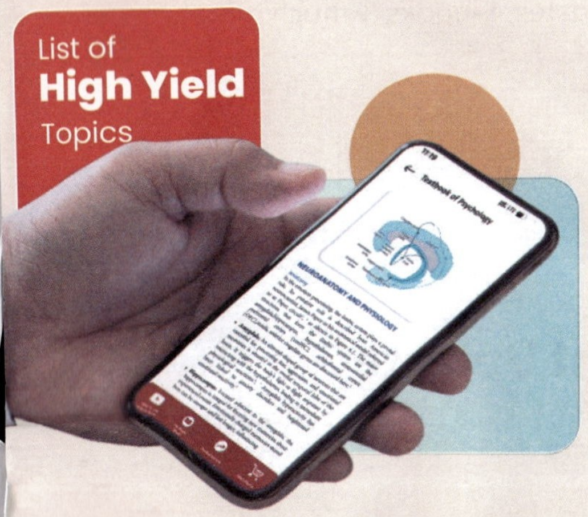

and Many more...

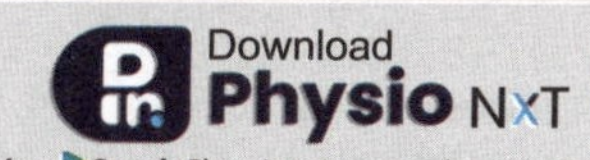

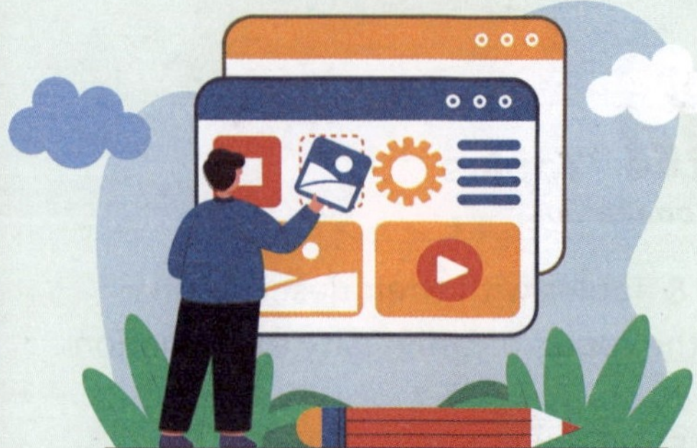

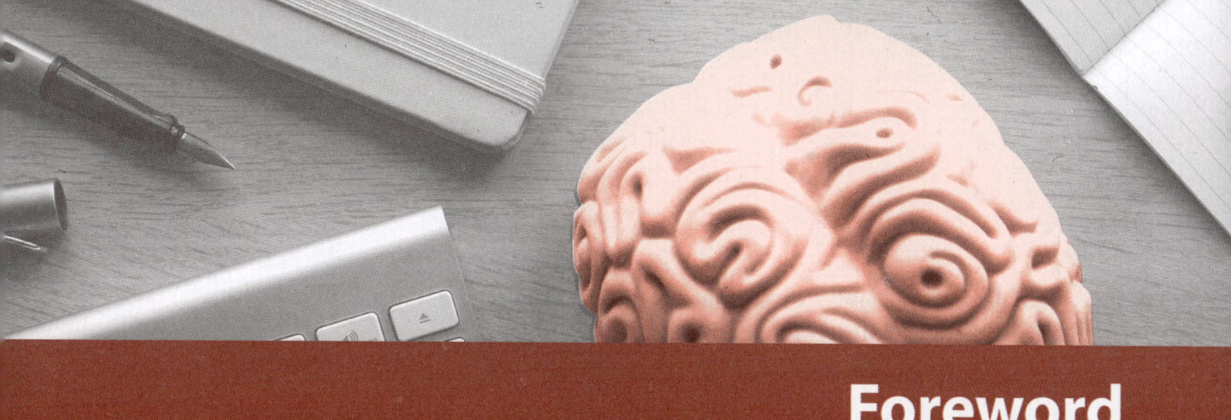

*"Where the mind goes, the body will follow.
Stay strong mentally, and the physical strength will follow."*
—Dr John Rusin

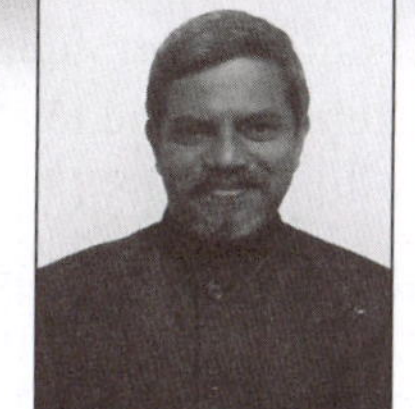

Psychology is the study of how our minds work and why we behave the way we do. It helps us understand our thoughts, feelings, and actions, as well as how our life experiences shape who we are. Physiotherapy is not just about fixing the body; it is also about helping people take charge of their lives, improve their well-being, and overcome both physical and mental challenges. To be a good physiotherapist, you need to understand how pain, motivation, mental strength, and patient involvement affect recovery. Psychology and physiotherapy work together, showing how our minds and bodies influence our overall health. As physiotherapy students, you not only learn how to treat physical problems but also how to consider the mental and emotional parts of a patient's healing process.

As I have three decades of association with psychology and physiotherapy, and have also been an expert member in framing physiotherapy curriculum at national level, I am excited to introduce this special book entitled, *Textbook of Psychology for Physiotherapy Students*, written by Dr Manu Goyal and Dr Kanu Goyal, both well-respected educators in the field of physiotherapy. This book shows the authors' hard work and expertise in making a resource that is both informative and practical.

This book offers a way of looking at how psychology connects to physiotherapy. It is different from other textbooks because it matches what students learn as per university syllabus and Ministry of Health and Family Welfare prescribed national physiotherapy curriculum, and it also focuses on what future physiotherapists need in their work.

Dr Goyal's knowledge and passion for improving physiotherapy education is evident throughout the book. This book goes beyond just teaching theories; it gives clear steps on how to use psychological ideas in real-life clinical situations through case studies, so that students can connect with patients in a caring and effective way.

"Alone, we can do so little; together, we can do so much."
—Helen Keller

The book also includes important inputs from experts who have shared their knowledge and research, making it even better. Each chapter includes different viewpoints from top professionals in psychology, physiotherapy, and similar fields. I have no doubt that their collective contributions will inspire, challenge, and support your journey toward becoming not just a skilled physiotherapist, but also an empathetic and insightful practitioner.

"Words are capable of arousing the strongest emotions and prompting all men's actions."
—*Sigmund Freud*

Whether you are just beginning your studies in physiotherapy or are already a practicing professional, the chapters provide a well-structured path to understanding how mental and emotional factors play a crucial role in physical recovery. Dr Goyal's writing is clear and accessible, making complex topics easy to understand and apply. There are questions at the end of chapters to prepare for university examination. Student Assignment introduced in the chapters helps in self-motivation and progress. References aid further reading and clarification to have evidence-based learning.

I would also like to extend my heartfelt congratulations to the CBS Publishers & Distributors for recognizing the importance of this work and for making it accessible to a wide audience. The experts in the advisory committee elevate the standard of your publications. The commitment of CBS Publishers to publish books in the PhysioBrid Series that contribute meaningfully to both education and practice is truly commendable. The effort put into ensuring this book reaches the hands of those who need it most will undoubtedly make a significant impact on the future of physiotherapy education.

"When you want to know how things really work, study them when they're coming apart."
—*William Gibson, Zero History*

Wish the readers all the best. May God bless the authors and contributors. My prayer for their future endeavors.

Professor Dr L Gladson Jose
BPT, MPT (Cardiopulmonary), MSc (Psychology), MPhil (Psychology), PhD, PGDSM, PGDGC, DTEd.
Principal
Dr M V Shetty College of Physiotherapy, Mangalore, Karnataka
Former Principal
Nandha College of Physiotherapy, Erode, Tamil Nadu
Former Principal
Sandhya Institute of Physiotherapy, Kakinada, Andhra Pradesh
Task Force Member
National Model Curriculum for Physiotherapy
Ministry of Health and Family Welfare, Government of India

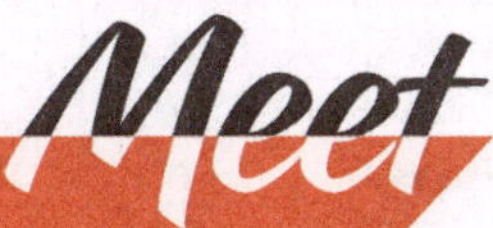

Meet

The Advisory Board

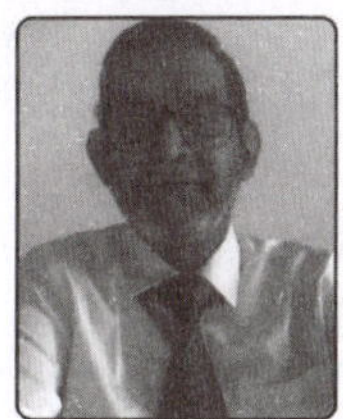

S Srinivas Rau
Dip. PT, BPT, MPT (Rehabilitation)
Professor and Head of Department
Institute of Health Sciences
Bhubaneswar, Odisha

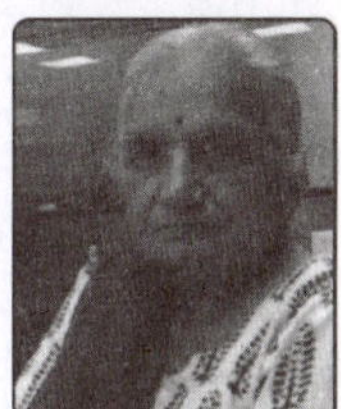

Krishna Garg
MBBS, MS, PhD, FAMS, FASI
Ex-Professor & HOD Anatomy
LHMC, Delhi
Faculty Kalka Dental College, Meerut and
Bakson Homeopathic Medical College-
Greater Noida, Uttar Pradesh

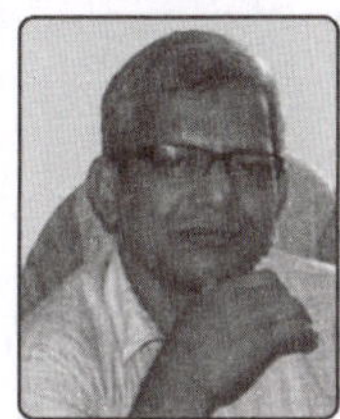

Patitapaban Mohanty
BPT, MPT (Musculoskeletal), PhD
Professor
Swami Vivekananda National Institute of
Rehabilitation Training and Research
Cuttack, Odisha

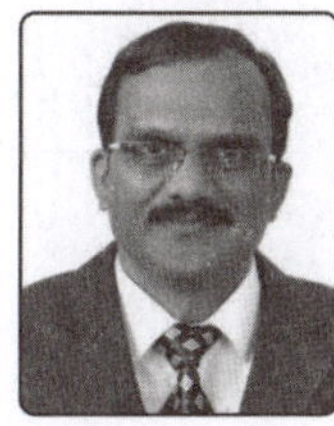

Purusotham Chippala
BPT, MPT (Neurology), PhD
Professor
Nitte Institute of Physiotherapy
Mangalore, Karnataka

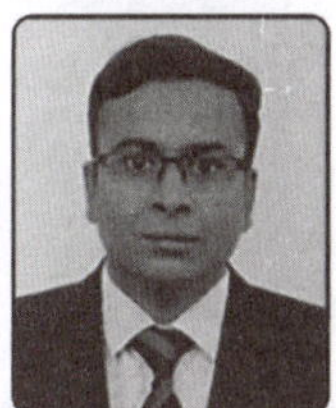

Rajeev Aggarwal
BPT, MPT (Neurology), PhD
Senior Physiotherapist and In-charge
Neurophysiotherapy Unit
AIIMS, New Delhi

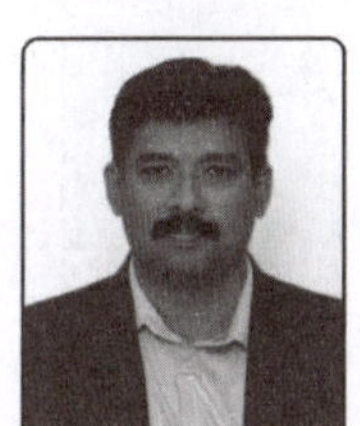

Narkeesh Arumugam
BPT, MPT (Neurology) PhD, DO (Spain),
DOMTP (OCO Canada), PG Master Diploma in
Osteopathy (UK)
Diploma in Master Chiropractor (Sweden)
Professor and HOD
Punjabi University, Patiala, Punjab

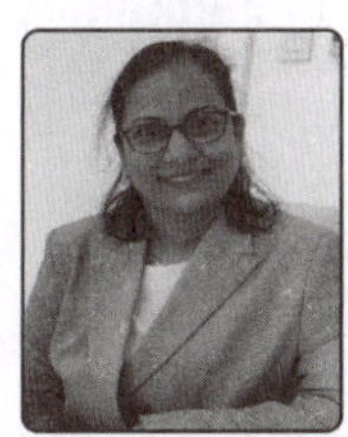

Manisha A Rathi
BPT, MPT (CBR), PhD
Principal
Khyati College of Physiotherapy
Ahmedabad, Gujarat
Adjunct Professor
Dr D Y Patil College of Physiotherapy
Pimpri, Pune, Maharashtra

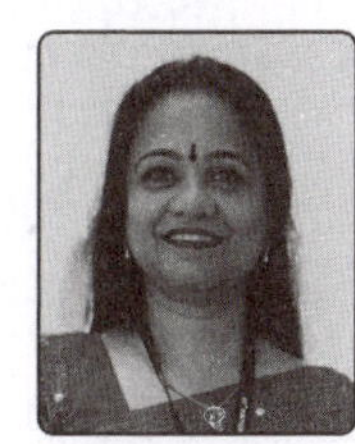

Zubia Veqar
BPT, MPT (Musculoskeletal), PhD
Professor and Honorary Director
Centre for Physiotherapy and
Rehabilitation Sciences, Jamia Millia Islamia
New Delhi

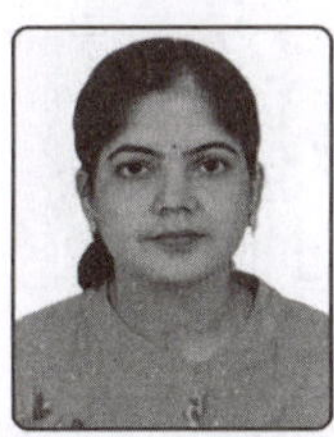

Harshita Sharma
BPT, MPT (Cardiopulmonary), PhD
Ex-Deputy Director
Amity Institute of Physiotherapy
Noida, Uttar Pradesh

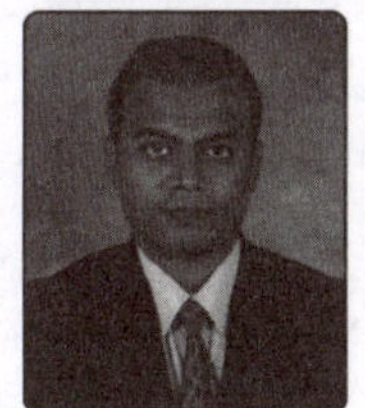

P Senthil Selvam
BPT, MPT (Orthopedics), PhD, PGDHA, MBA
Professor & HOD
Vels Institute of Science, Technology &
Advanced Studies (VISTAS)
Chennai, Tamil Nadu

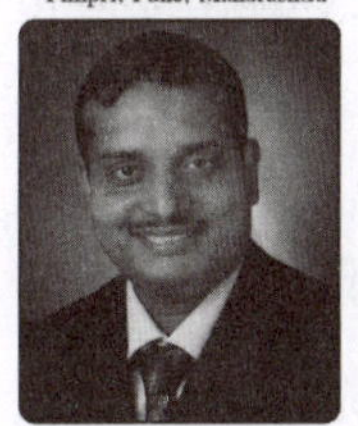

Umasankar Mohanty
BPT, MPT (Manual Therapy), MISEP
MIASP, FAGE, PhD
President
Manual Therapy Foundation of India
Managing Director
Vedanta Educational and Charitable Trust
Mangaluru, Karnataka

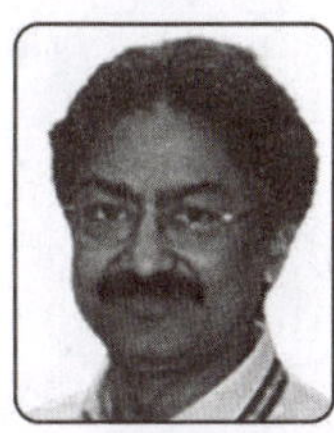

Vishwa Prakash Gupta
BSc, DPT, MPT (Cardiopulmonary)
Ex-Chief Physiotherapist
AIIMS, New Delhi
Adjunct Professor
Jamia Hamdard, New Delhi

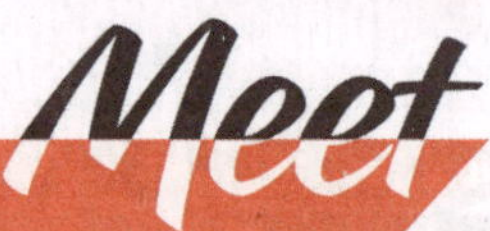

Meet

The Advisory Board

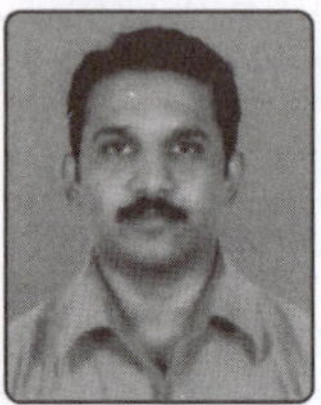

K S Sharad
BPT, MPT (Orthopedics) MSc (Yoga Therapy)
Principal
BCF College of Physiotherapy
Indo-American Hospital Vaikom
Kottayam, Kerala

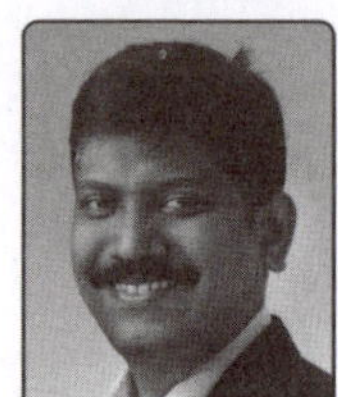

John Solomon M
BPT, MPT (Neurosciences), PhD
Additional Professor & HOD
Manipal College of Health Professionals
MAHE, Manipal, Karnataka

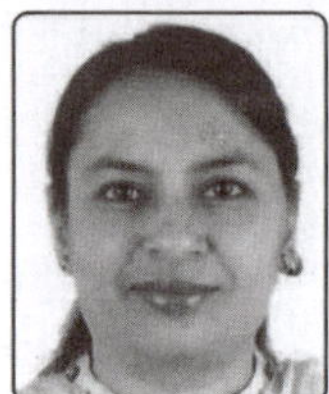

Chitra Kataria
BPT, MPT (Orthopedics), PhD
Principal
Indian Spinal Injuries Centre
Institute of Rehabilitation Sciences
New Delhi

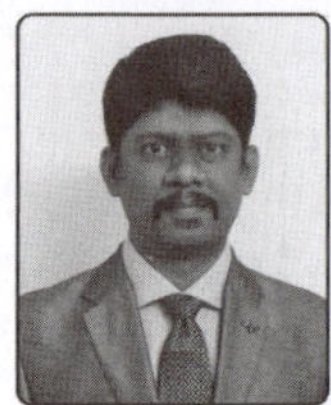

P Mohankumar
BPT, MPT (Biomechanics), PhD
Head I/c - Physiotherapy
School of Allied Health Sciences
Hindustan Institute of Technology & Science
Chennai, Tamil Nadu

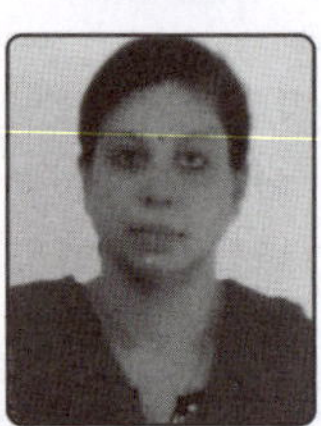

Sumeeta Khaund
BPT, MPT (Cardiopulmonary)
Associate Professor
Department of Physiotherapy
Rajasthan Vidyapeeth, Deemed to be University
Udaipur, Rajasthan

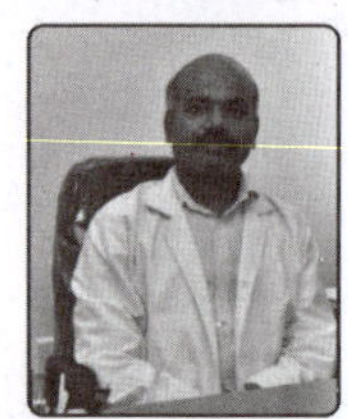

V Kiran
BPT, MPT (Cardiorespiratory), PhD
Professor and Vice Principal
Apollo College of Physiotherapy
Chittoor, Andhra Pradesh

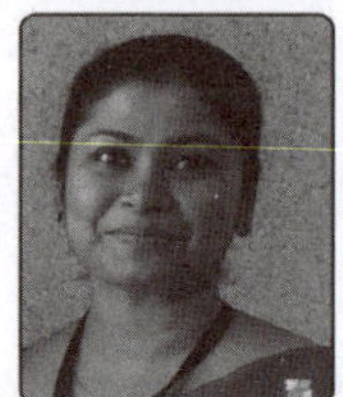

Anila Paul
BPT, MPT (Orthopedics), PhD Scholar
Professor & HOD
Medical Trust Institute of Medical Sciences
College of Physiotherapy
Irumpanam, Kochi, Kerala

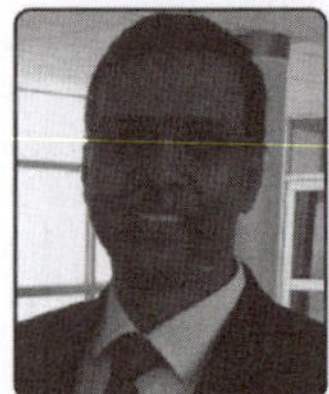

Sanjeev Gupta
BPT, MPT (Orthopedics), PhD
Professor - Physiotherapy
School of Allied Health Sciences
Manav Rachna International Institute of
Research and Studies
Faridabad, Haryana

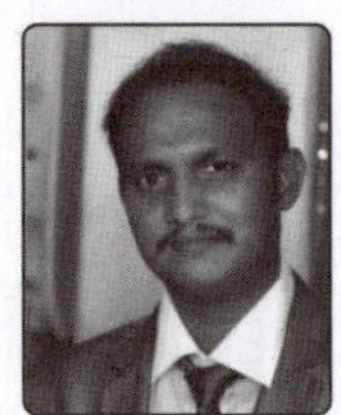

Vincent Jeyaraj
BPT, MPT (Orthopedics), MSW, FRCPT,
PGDOSIM, PG Dip. (Geriatric Care), PhD
Professor cum Vice Principal
Madha College of Physiotherapy
Chennai, Tamil Nadu

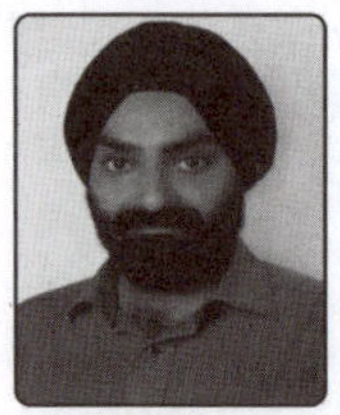

Navinder Pal Singh
BPT, MPT (Sports)
Professor & Principal
Jammu College of Physiotherapy
Nardani, Raipur, Bantalab Road
Jammu, J&K

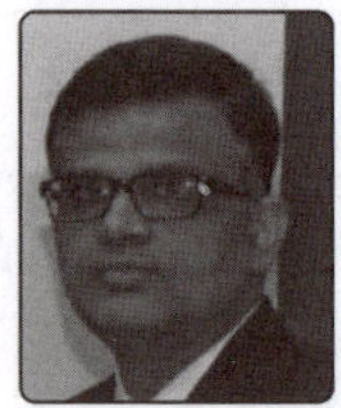

C S Ram
BPT, MPT (Sports), PhD
Director & Principal
Banarasidas Chandiwala
Institute of Physiotherapy
New Delhi

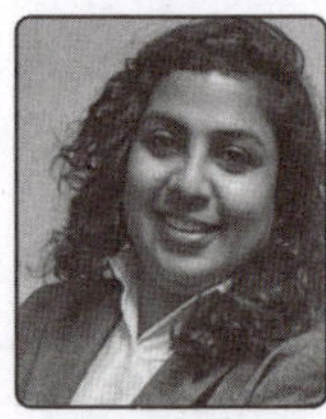

Divya Gupta
BPT, MPT (Pediatrics),
MPH, PG Diploma (Yoga)
Project Manager & Editorial Head – Physiotherapy
CBS Publishers & Distributors Pvt. Ltd.
New Delhi

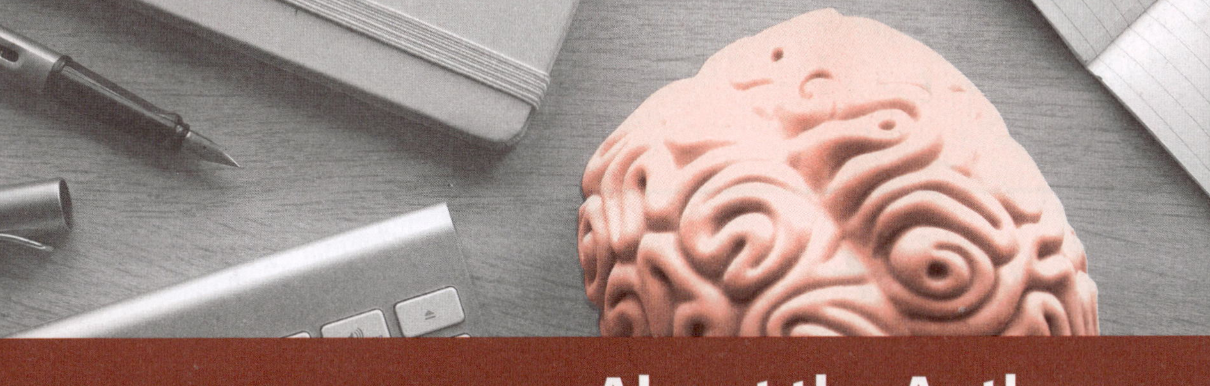

About the Authors

Manu Goyal *BPT, MPT (Orthopedics), MSc (Applied Musculoskeletal Physiotherapy), PhD (Physiotherapy)*, is a Professor and Principal at Maharishi Markandeshwar Institute of Physiotherapy and Rehabilitation, a constituent institute of Maharishi Markandeshwar (Deemed to be University), Mullana, Ambala, Haryana, India. He holds PhD degree in Physiotherapy, Masters of Physiotherapy in the specialization of Orthopedics, Master of Science in Applied Musculoskeletal Physiotherapy, Diplomate in Osteopathic Manipulative Theory and Practice, Postgraduate Certificate in Diabetes Education. His research interests are focused on various domains including fitness, balance and stability, musculoskeletal, neurological, diabetes, osteopathy. Nearly 35 copyrights are registered and 5 patents are published under his name under Intellectual Property Rights, under Government of India. He has nearly 110 publications in peer-reviewed national and international journals with total citations of approximately 494. He has contributed to several books as a writer and editor.

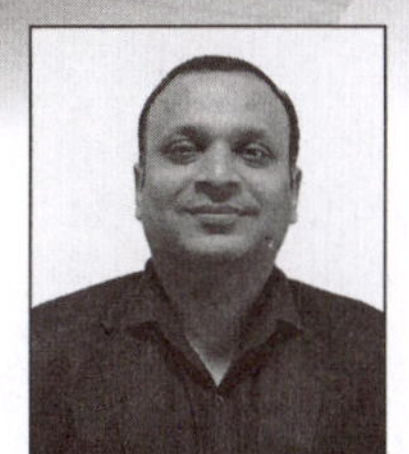

Kanu Goyal *BPT, MPT (Pediatrics), PhD (Pursuing)*, is an Assistant Professor at Maharishi Markandeshwar Institute of Physiotherapy and Rehabilitation, a constituent institute of Maharishi Markandeshwar (Deemed to be University), Mullana, Ambala, Haryana, India. She holds degree in Masters of Physiotherapy in the specialization of Pediatrics, Diplomate in Osteopathic Manipulative Theory and Practice and is currently pursuing PhD in Physiotherapy. Her research interests are focused on various domains including fitness, balance and stability, musculoskeletal, neurological, pediatrics among others. Nearly 30 copyrights are registered and 5 patents are published under her name under Intellectual Property Rights, under Government of India. She has nearly 53 publications in peer-reviewed national and international journals with total citations of approximately 201. She has contributed to several books as a writer and editor.

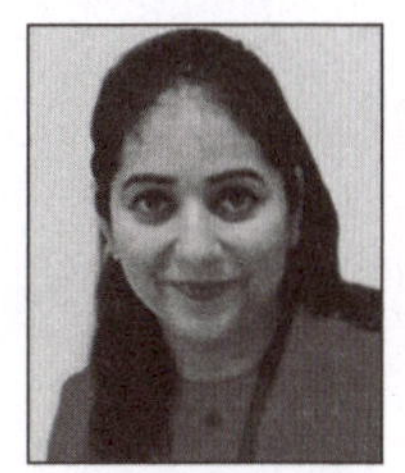

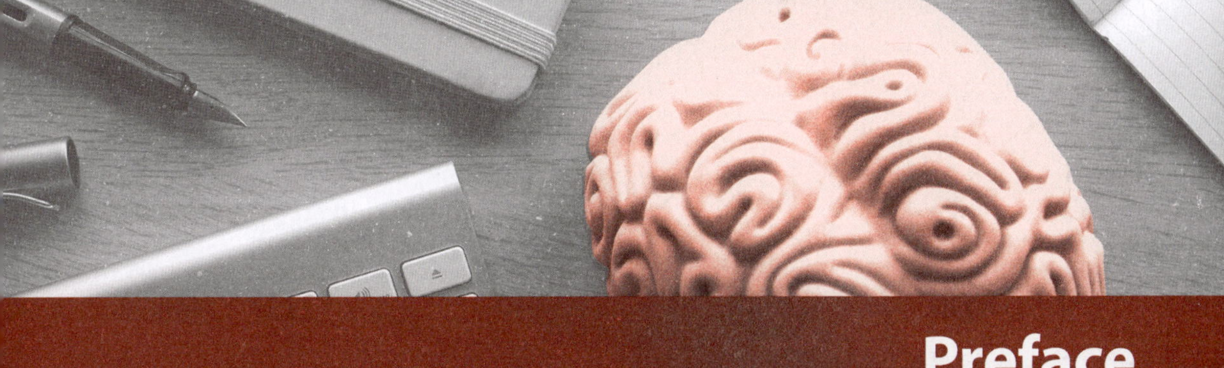

Preface

There is a necessity of having a systematized and thorough book on psychology for aspiring physiotherapists. This attempt has been made to meet the requirements of the students according to the prescribed curriculum for psychology.

The *Textbook of Psychology for Physiotherapy Students* has been written to bridge the gap between physiotherapy and psychology, emphasizing the importance of psychological understanding in the treatment of patients. Understanding the emotional and psychological behavior of the patients during the framework of the rehabilitation care is of utmost importance for every physiotherapist.

This book has been designed to provide a lucid and succinct overview of the psychological concepts pertaining to physiotherapy. This book is a collaborative effort by reputed healthcare professionals to improve the knowledge of students and enable them to develop interest and positive attitude toward the subject and its implications in the clinical practice.

The textbook consists of 19 chapters that cover a wide range of topics. Each chapter has been structured to cater to the syllabi of various universities offering Bachelor of Physiotherapy (BPT) programs, ensuring that students receive pertinent knowledge. It is quite possible that there might be a need to enhance the content. The authors would be grateful to the students for their valuable inputs to enhance the quality of the book in future editions.

This book may be useful as a reference material for learning, training and research purposes. The sole aim has been to provide a platform where the students can enhance their knowledge up to the maximum.

We wish that all the students enjoy reading this book and it will certainly help in enriching their thought process by incorporating the psychology aspects during patient care.

Manu Goyal

Kanu Goyal

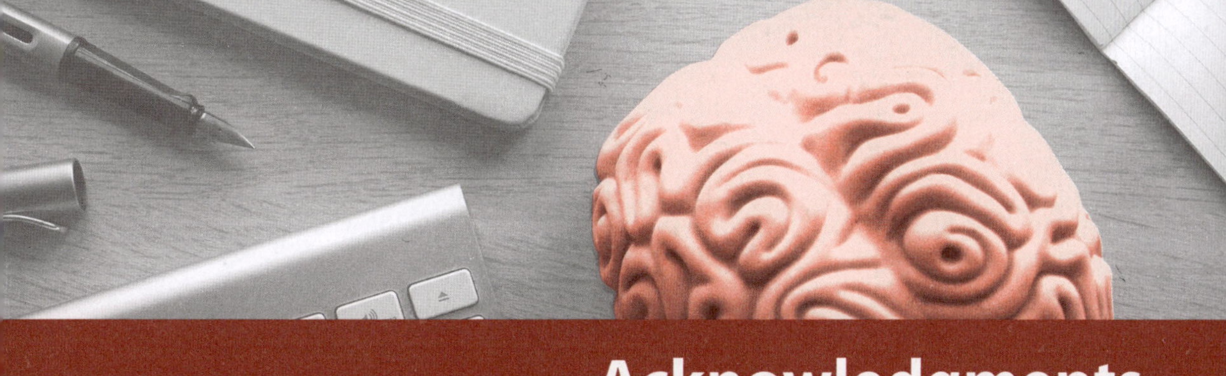

Acknowledgments

The *Textbook of Psychology for Physiotherapy Students*, would not have been possible without the blessings of the Almighty God. A heartfelt gratitude to our parents for their constant support, blessings and entrusting us always for our work. We are thankful to our adorable daughter for allowing us to spare some time every day to complete the book. We are thankful to the worthy management of Maharishi Markandeshwar Trust, Ambala for providing us with the professional recognition. We are extremely thankful to all the esteemed contributors for their significant contribution, devotion of time, hard work and knowledge to this book. Each chapter is written so well that it reflects the deep understanding and extensive knowledge of each contributor making this book easily understandable for the readers.

We extend our special thanks to **Mr Satish Kumar Jain** (Chairman) and **Mr Varun Jain** (Managing Director), M/s CBS Publishers and Distributors Pvt Ltd for their wholehearted support in publication of this book. We have no words to describe the role, efforts, inputs and initiatives undertaken by **Mr Bhupesh Aarora** (Sr. Vice President – Publishing & Marketing (Health Sciences Division)] for helping and motivating us.

Our special thanks are due to Dr Divya Gupta, PT (Project Manager & Editorial [Scientific] Head – Physiotherapy) and Dr Apurva Chatterjee, PT (Content Strategist – Physiotherapy) for their valuable support, suggestions and advice that have helped us in refining the text and making it more comprehensive.

We sincerely thank the entire CBS team for bringing out the book with utmost care and attractive presentation. We would like to thank Ms Nitasha Arora (Assistant General Manager Publishing – Medical and Nursing), Ms Daljeet Kaur (Assistant Publishing Manager) and Dr Anju Dhir (Product Manager and Medical Development Editor) for their publishing support. We would also extend our thanks to Ms Surbhi Gupta (Sr. English Editor), Mr Ashutosh Pathak (Sr. Proofreader cum Team Coordinator) and all the production team members for devoting laborious hours in designing and typesetting the book.

Last but not least, we are thankful to our colleagues, peers, family and friends without whose support this book would not have been possible.

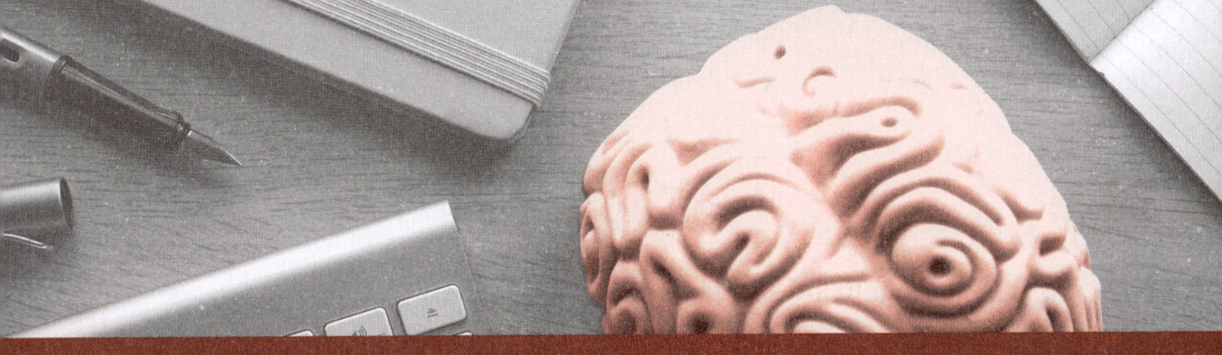

Contributors and Reviewers

CONTRIBUTORS

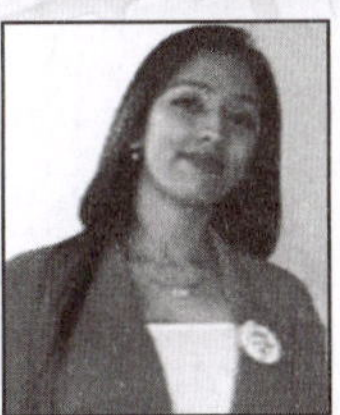

Aditi Popli
BPT, MPT (Orthopedics), PhD Scholar

Assistant Professor
Maharishi Markandeshwar Institute of Physiotherapy and Rehabilitation
Maharishi Markandeshwar (Deemed to be University)
Ambala, Haryana

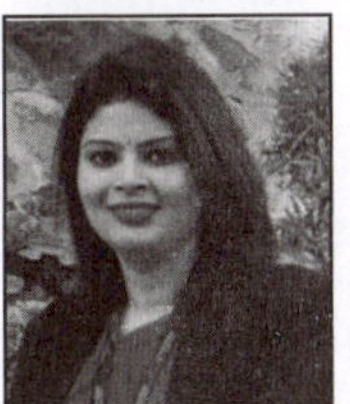

Ankita Sharma
BPT, MPT (Musculoskeletal), PhD

Associate Professor
Amity Institute of Physiotherapy
Amity University
Noida, Uttar Pradesh

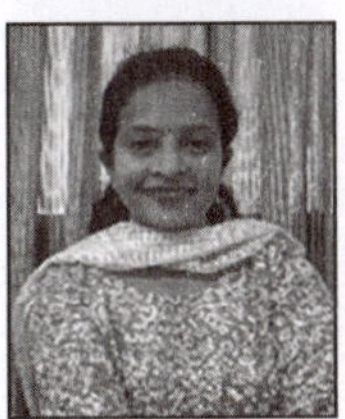

Chandani Pandey
MA (Psychology), MPhil (Clinical Psychology), PhD Scholar

Assistant Professor
Department of Clinical Psychology
Amity University
Mohali, Punjab

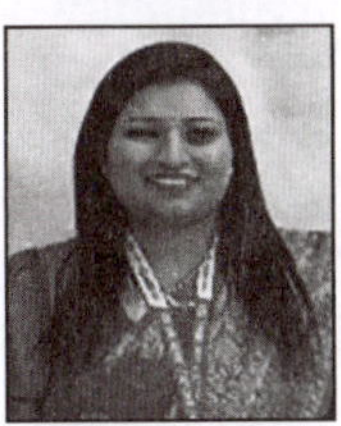

Divya Aggarwal
BPT, MPT (Neurology), PhD

Assistant Professor
Department of Physiotherapy, School of Allied Health Sciences
Manav Rachna International Institute of Research and Studies
Faridabad, Haryana

The names of the contributors and reviewers are arranged in alphabetical order.

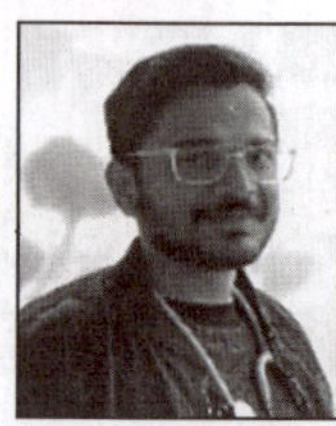

Hem Jivani

MBBS, MD (General Medicine)

Assistant Professor
Maharishi Markandeshwar Institute of Medical Sciences and Research
Maharishi Markandeshwar (Deemed to be University)
Ambala, Haryana

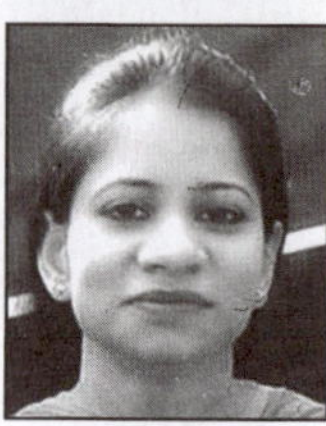

Hina Vaish

BPT, MPT (Cardiopulmonary), PhD (Pursuing)

Assistant Professor
Department of Physiotherapy, School of Health Sciences
Chhatrapati Shahu Ji Maharaj University
Kanpur, Uttar Pradesh

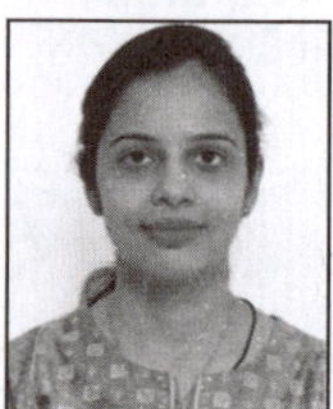

Kajal Taneja

MBBS, MD (Psychiatry), DNB, (Child and Adolescent Psychiatry)

Assistant Professor
Maharishi Markandeshwar Institute of Physiotherapy and Rehabilitation
Maharishi Markandeshwar (Deemed to be University)
Ambala, Haryana

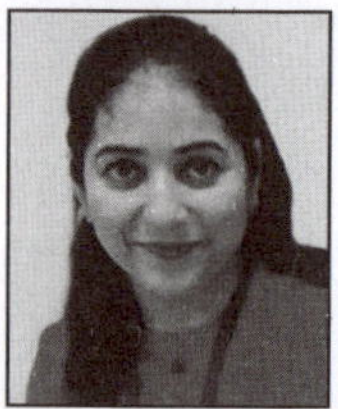

Kanu Goyal

BPT, MPT (Pediatrics), PhD (Pursuing)

Assistant Professor
Maharishi Markandeshwar Institute of Physiotherapy and Rehabilitation
Maharishi Markandeshwar (Deemed to be University)
Ambala, Haryana

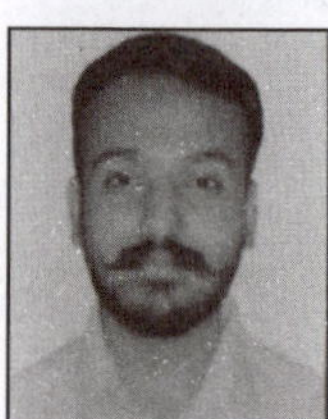

Lakshay Panchal

BPT, PhD (Pursuing)

Demonstrator
Maharishi Markandeshwar Institute of Physiotherapy and Rehabilitation
Maharishi Markandeshwar (Deemed to be University)
Ambala, Haryana

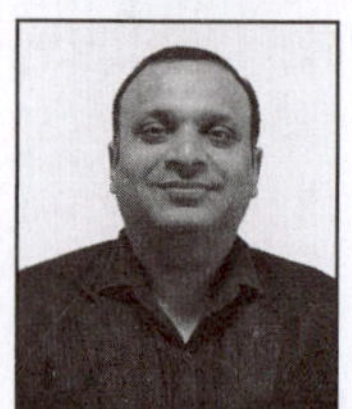

Manu Goyal

BPT, MPT (Orthopedics), MSc (Applied Musculoskeletal Physiotherapy), PhD (Physiotherapy)

Professor and Principal
Maharishi Markandeshwar Institute of Physiotherapy and Rehabilitation
Maharishi Markandeshwar (Deemed to be University)
Ambala, Haryana

The names of the contributors and reviewers are arranged in alphabetical order.

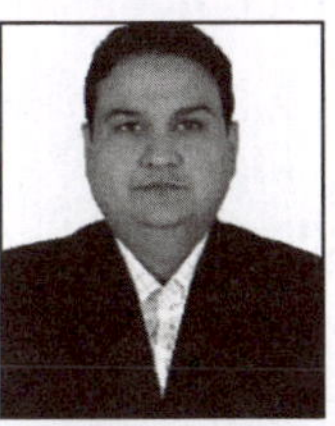

Moattar Raza Rizvi
BSc, MSc (Animal Physiology), PhD (Medical Physiology)

Professor and Dean
College of Healthcare Professions (CoHP), DIT University
Dehradun, Uttarakhand

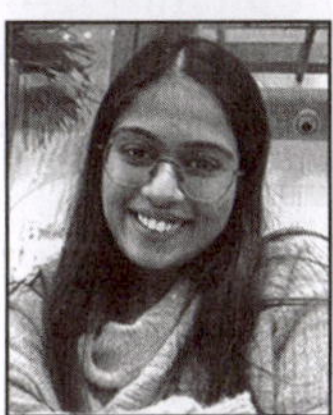

Muskan Gupta
BPT

Student
SGT University
Gurugram, Haryana

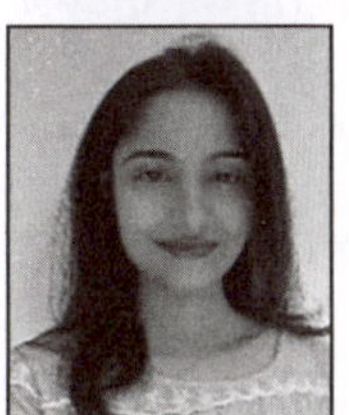

Neha Sharma
BPT, MPT (Pediatrics), PhD

Assistant Professor
Maharishi Markandeshwar Institute of Physiotherapy and Rehabilitation
Maharishi Markandeshwar (Deemed to be University)
Ambala, Haryana

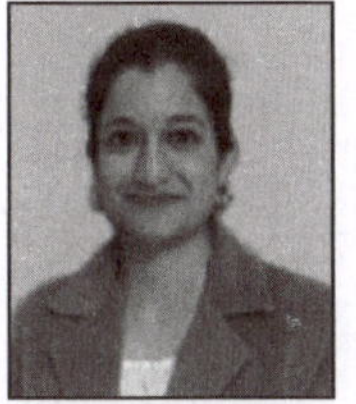

Nishchint Banga
BPT, MPT (Neurology)

Assistant Professor
Noida International University
Gautam Budh Nagar, Uttar Pradesh

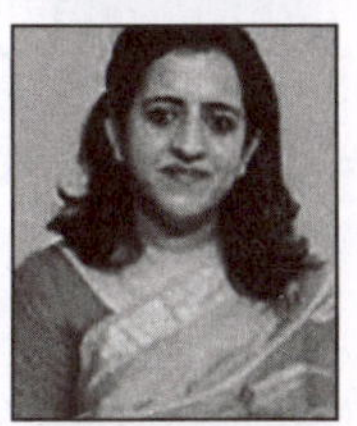

Parul Sharma
BPT, MPT (Neurology), PhD Scholar

Assistant Professor
School of Physiotherapy
Delhi Pharmaceutical Sciences & Research University
New Delhi

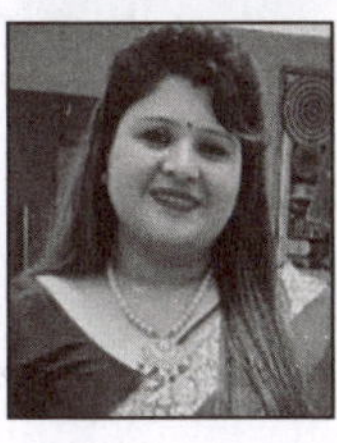

Pooja Sharma
BPT, MPT (Musculoskeletal), PhD

Associate Professor
Department of Physiotherapy, School of Allied Health Sciences
Manav Rachna International Institute of Research and Studies
Faridabad, Haryana

The names of the contributors and reviewers are arranged in alphabetical order.

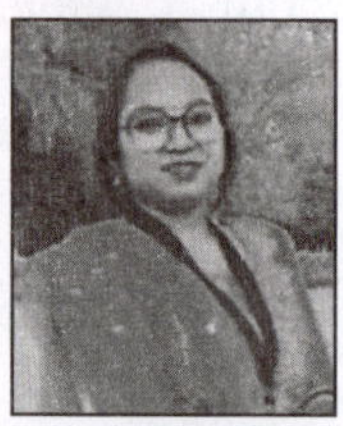

Pragya Mitra
MPhil (Clinical Psychology)

Assistant Professor
Department of Clinical Psychology
Nai Subah Institute of Mental Health & Behavioral Sciences
Varanasi, Uttar Pradesh

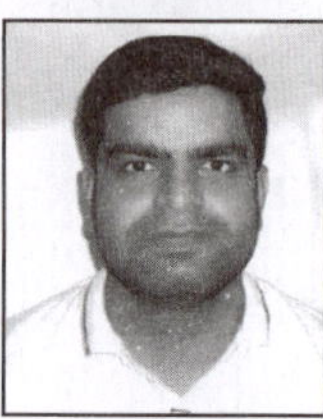

Prateek Sharda
MBBS, MS (General Surgery), FMAS

Consultant
Sharda Hospital
Rohtak, Haryana

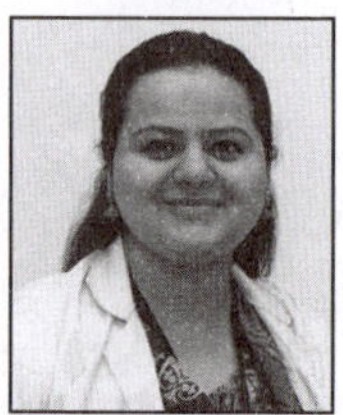

Priyanka Sethi
BPT, MPT (Neurology), PhD

Assistant Professor
Department of Physiotherapy, School of Allied Health Sciences
Manav Rachna International Institute of Research and Studies
Faridabad, Haryana

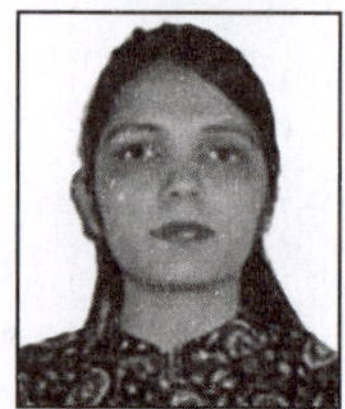

Rittu Sharma
BPT, MPT (Neurology), PhD Scholar

Assistant Professor
Maharishi Markandeshwar Institute of Physiotherapy and Rehabilitation
Maharishi Markandeshwar (Deemed to be University)
Ambala, Haryana

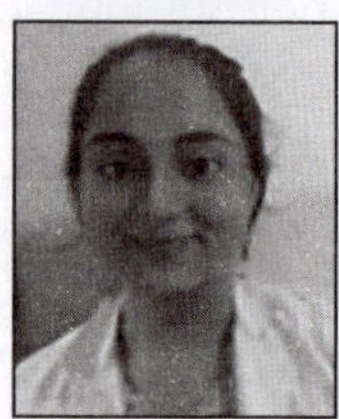

Riya Kalra
BPT, MPT (Orthopedics)

Student
Maharishi Markandeshwar Institute of Physiotherapy and Rehabilitation
Maharishi Markandeshwar (Deemed to be University)
Ambala, Haryana

The names of the contributors and reviewers are arranged in alphabetical order.

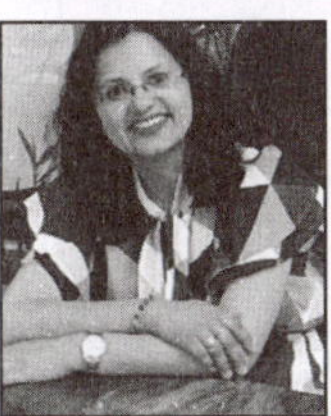

Shweta Sharma

BPT, MPT (Pediatrics), PhD

Assistant Professor
Maharishi Markandeshwar Institute of Physiotherapy and Rehabilitation
Maharishi Markandeshwar (Deemed to be University)
Ambala, Haryana

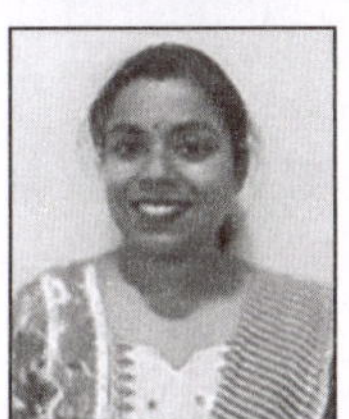

Sunanda Bhowmik

BPT, MPT (Pediatrics)

Assistant Professor
Maharishi Markandeshwar Institute of Physiotherapy and Rehabilitation
Maharishi Markandeshwar (Deemed to be University)
Ambala, Haryana

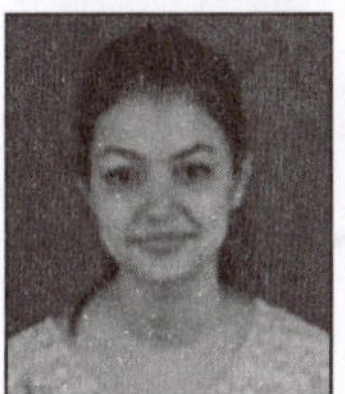

Sushma K C

BPT, MPT (Pediatrics), PhD (Pursuing)

Physiotherapist
Maharishi Markandeshwar Institute of Physiotherapy and Rehabilitation
Maharishi Markandeshwar (Deemed to be University)
Ambala, Haryana

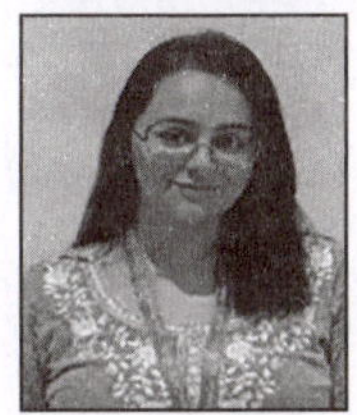

Urvi

BPT

Consultant (Medico Marketing)
Ozone Pharmaceuticals Ltd.
New Delhi

REVIEWERS

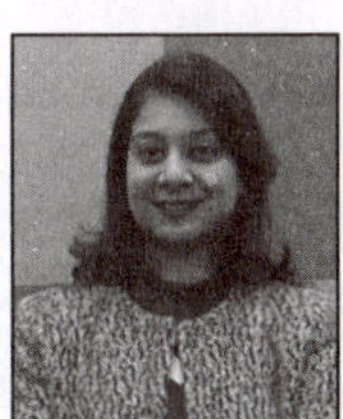

Apurva Chatterjee

BPT, MPT (Neurology), PhD Scholar

Content Strategist (Physiotherapy)
Nursing Next Exam Prep Pvt Ltd.
Noida, Uttar Pradesh

The names of the contributors and reviewers are arranged in alphabetical order.

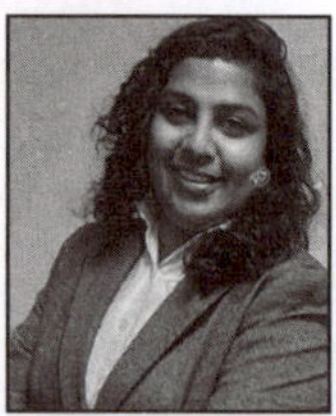

Divya Gupta
BPT, MPT (Pediatrics), MPH, PG Dip (Yoga)

Project Manager & Editorial (Scientific) Head – Physiotherapy
CBS Publishers & Distributors Pvt. Ltd
New Delhi

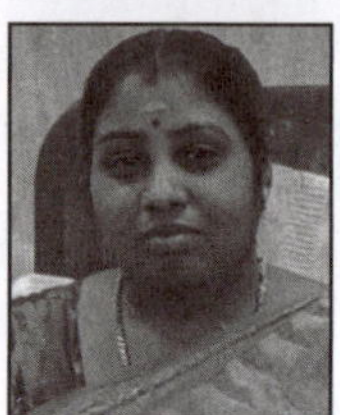

G Dhanalakshmi Arumugam
BSc (N), MSc (Medical Surgical Nursing), MSc (Psychology), PhD

Principal
Vijaya College of Nursing
Chennai, Tamil Nadu

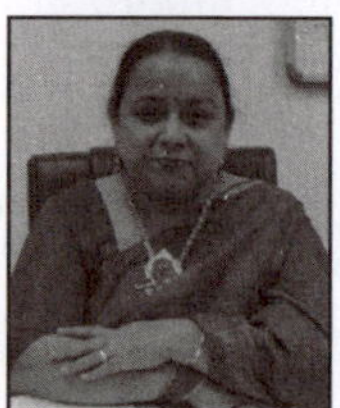

Kavita Kaushal
BPT, MPT (Neurology)

Professor and Principal
College of Physiotherapy, Adesh Institute of Medical Sciences & Research
Adesh University
Bathinda, Punjab

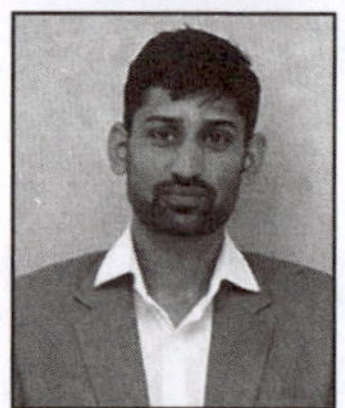

Keshar Choudhary
BPT, MPT (Orthopedics), PhD

Head of Department
Department of Physiotherapy
University of Technology
Jaipur, Rajasthan

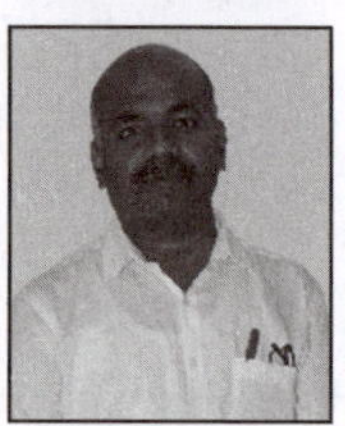

Kiran V
BPT, MPT (Cardiorespiratory), PhD

Professor
Apollo College of Physiotherapy
Dr N T R University of Health Sciences
Chittoor, Andhra Pradesh

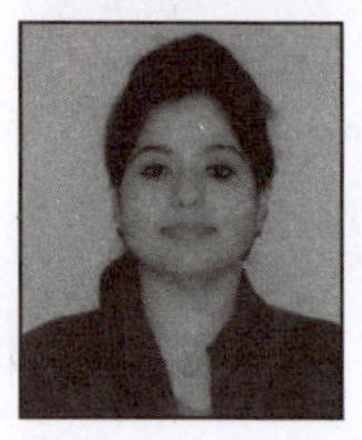

Namrata Suri
BPT, MPT (Musculoskeletal), PhD Scholar

Assistant Professor
Integral Institute of Allied Health Sciences and Research
Integral University
Lucknow, Uttar Pradesh

The names of the contributors and reviewers are arranged in alphabetical order.

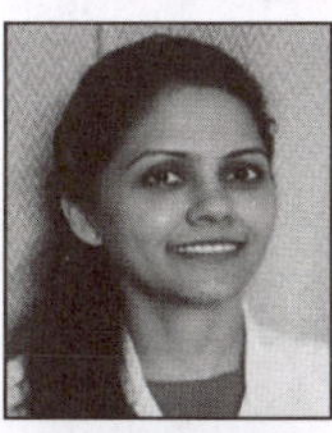

Preeti Gazbare
BSc (PT), MPT (Neuroscience), PhD

Professor
Dr D Y Patil College of Physiotherapy
Dr D Y Patil Vidyapeeth (Deemed to be University)
Pune, Maharashtra

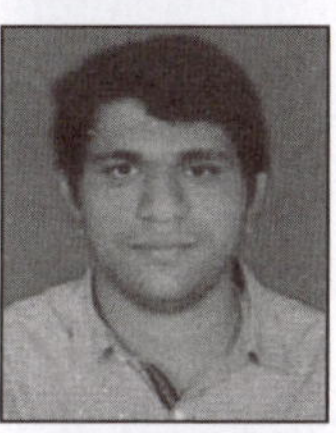

Pritesh Yeole
BPTh, MPTh (Neurosciences)

Professor
MVP Samaj's College of Physiotherapy
Maharashtra University of Health Sciences
Nashik, Maharashtra

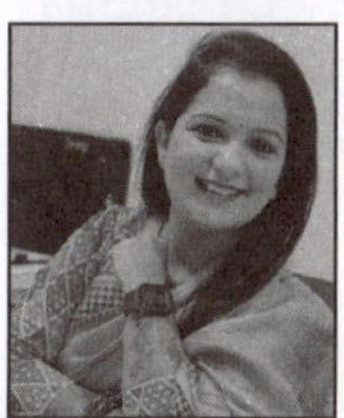

Priyanka Rishi
BPT, MPT (Orthopaedics), PhD

Associate Professor
Faculty of Physiotherapy
SGT University
Gurugram, Haryana

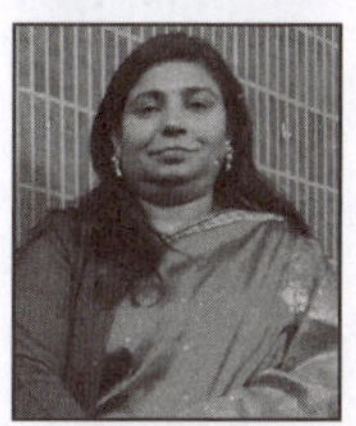

Richa Agrawal
BPT, MPT (Sports), PGDHA, PGDFM, COMP

Assistant Professor
Dolphin Institute of Biomedical & Natural Sciences
Dehradun, Uttarakhand

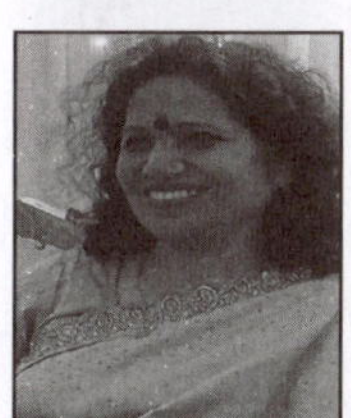

Shama Lohumi
BSc (N), MA (English), MSc (Community Health Nursing), PhD (Psychology)

Principal
Shivalik Institute of Nursing
Shimla, Himachal Pradesh

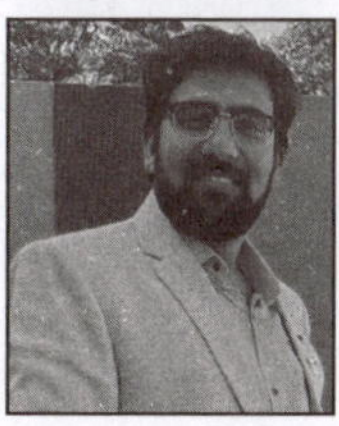

Shashank Apte
BPT, MPT (Neurology)

Assistant Professor
Department of Physiotherapy
College of Life Science Center Hospital and Research Institute
Gwalior, Madhya Pradesh

The names of the contributors and reviewers are arranged in alphabetical order.

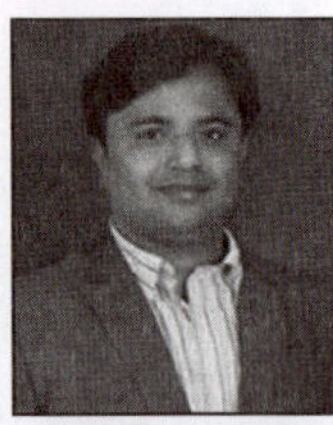

Sudeep Hiralal Kale
BPT, MPT (Cardiorespiratory), PhD

Professor & HOD
Terna Physiotherapy College
Navi Mumbai, Maharashtra

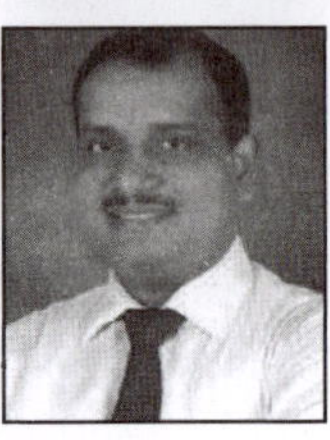

Umasankar Mohanty
BPT (Hons.), MPT (Manual Therapy), PhD

President
Manual Therapy Foundation of India
Mangalore, Karnataka

The names of the contributors and reviewers are arranged in alphabetical order.

Special Features of the Book

Learning Objectives in the beginning of every Chapter help readers understand the purpose of the chapter.

LEARNING OBJECTIVES

After the completion of the chapter, the readers will be able to:
- Define psychology and its core areas of practice, research, and applications.
- Explain the historical development of the field, including major theoretical perspectives.
- Describe the relationship between mental health and physical health.
- Identify the biological, psychological, and social factors that contribute to mental health problems.

CHAPTER OUTLINE

- Introduction
- Definition of Psychology
- Enigmatic Journey of Understanding Ourselves: A Historical Background to Psychology

Chapter Outline gives a glimpse of the content covered in the chapter.

KEY TERMS

Cognitive psychology: It focuses on the study of the higher mental processes.
Counseling psychology: It focuses primarily on educational, social and career adjustment problems.
Environmental psychology: It considers the relationship between people and their physical environment including how our physical environment affects our emotions and the amount of stress we experience in a particular setting.

Key Terms are added in each chapter to help understand difficult scientific terms in easy language.

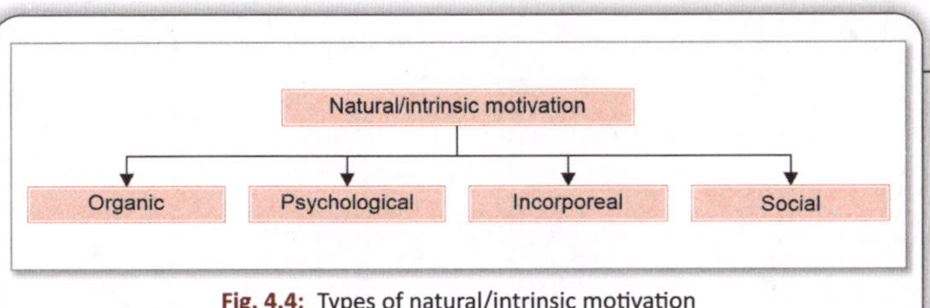

Fig. 4.4: Types of natural/intrinsic motivation

The book is well illustrated with relevant **Figures**.

Table 1.1: Major landmarks in the development of psychology

Years	Developmental landmarks of psychology
1879	1st Psychological lab, Germany
1890	William James published psychology principles
1895	Functionalism
1900	Sigmund Freud established psychodynamics
1924	Behaviorism
1951	Client-centered humanistic psychology
1954	Establishment of motivation and personality
1957	Social psychology
1985	Cognitive psychology
2000	Neuropsychology, evolutionary psychology

Numerous **Tables** have been used in the chapters to facilitate learning in a quick way.

MUST KNOW

- **Structuralism (Wundt):** Breaking down the mind into its basic structures.
- **Functionalism (James):** Emphasizes the function of mental processes and how they help us adapt to the environment.
- **Behaviorism (Watson, Skinner):** Focuses on observable behavior and how it is shaped by learning through conditioning.
- **Psychoanalysis (Freud):** Explores the unconscious mind and the role of early childhood experiences in shaping personality.
- **Humanism (Maslow, Rogers):** Highlights human potential, self-actualization, and the importance of free will and subjective experience.

Must Know boxes give an overview of important facts about the concerned topic.

CASE STUDY

Patient Profile
Name: Michael Smith
Age: 2 years
Gender: Male
Medical history: Premature birth at 32 weeks, neonatal jaundice, and mild respiratory distress syndrome
Family history: No known neurological disorders

Presenting Symptoms
- Delayed motor milestones (not sitting independently, not crawling, not walking)
- Muscle stiffness (spasticity) in the legs
- Poor trunk control and balance
- Difficulty using hands for fine motor tasks (grasping toys, self-feeding)
- Limited speech and communication skills

Case Study demonstrates example(s) of specific clinical scenarios that are often encountered by Physiotherapists.

Physio CORNER

Developmental delays in autism spectrum disorder (ASD) can vary widely, as ASD is a complex neurodevelopmental condition characterized by challenges in social interaction, communication, and repetitive behaviors. Understanding these developmental delays is crucial for early identification, intervention, and support. Here are the key areas where developmental delays are often observed in children with autism:

Social and Emotional Development

- **Social interaction:**
  - **Limited eye contact:** Difficulty making or maintaining eye contact.
  - **Difficulty with social cues:** Challenges in understanding and responding to social cues, such as facial expressions and body language.
  - **Lack of interest in peers:** Limited interest in playing or interacting with other children, preferring solitary activities.

Physiotherapy correlation of the topics under study is mentioned as **Physio Corner**.

SUMMARY

- Psychology, a discipline that delves into the intricacies of human thought and behavior, has evolved significantly over time, transitioning from philosophical musings to a robust scientific field. This chapter offers a comprehensive introduction to psychology, outlining its historical development, theoretical frameworks, and practical applications.
- **Historical development:** The journey of psychology is a fascinating one, beginning with early inquiries in ancient Greece and progressing through various stages of scientific evolution. Philosophers like Plato and Aristotle laid the groundwork by exploring the essence of the soul and perception.

Important takeaway points of respective chapters have been highlighted under **Summary** boxes.

REFERENCES

1. Cherniak, Christopher, Nisbett, Richard & Ross, Lee. Human Inference: Strategies and Shortcomings of Social Judgment. Philosophical Review. 1983; 92 (3):462
2. Cutler BL, Wells GL. Psychological science in the courtroom: Consensus and controversy. Expert testimony regarding eyewitness identification. 2009:100–23.
3. Seedat S, Scott KM, Angermeyer MC, Berglund P, Bromet EJ, Brugha TS, Demyttenaere K, De Girolamo G, Haro JM, Jin R, Karam EG. Cross-national associations between gender and mental disorders in the World Health Organization World Mental Health Surveys. Archives of general psychiatry. 2009 Jul 1;66(7):785–95.

Giving extra edge to the study, **References** have been included at the last of every chapter.

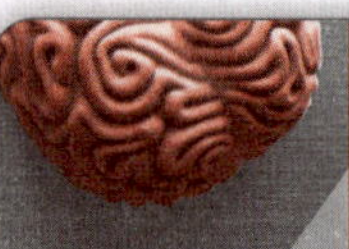

STUDENT ASSIGNMENT

LONG ANSWER QUESTIONS

1. What is psychology, and how does it contribute to our understanding of human behavior and mental processes? Explain various aspects of human cognition and behavior.
2. Write an overview of the historical development of psychology as a scientific discipline.

SHORT ANSWER QUESTIONS

1. What is psychology, and how does it contribute to our understanding of human behavior and mental processes?
2. What are the various aspects of human cognition and behavior that psychology explores?

MULTIPLE CHOICE QUESTIONS

1. The scientific study of both the mind and observable behaviors is the definition of:
   a. Sociology
   b. Psychology
   c. Anthropology
   d. Neuroscience
2. John B Watson, a prominent figure in psychology, is most associated with which school of thought?
   a. Psychoanalysis
   b. Behaviorism
   c. Humanism
   d. Cognitive psychology

At the end of chapters, **Student Assignment** section is given which contains practice questions and multiple choice questions to help students attain mastery over the subject.

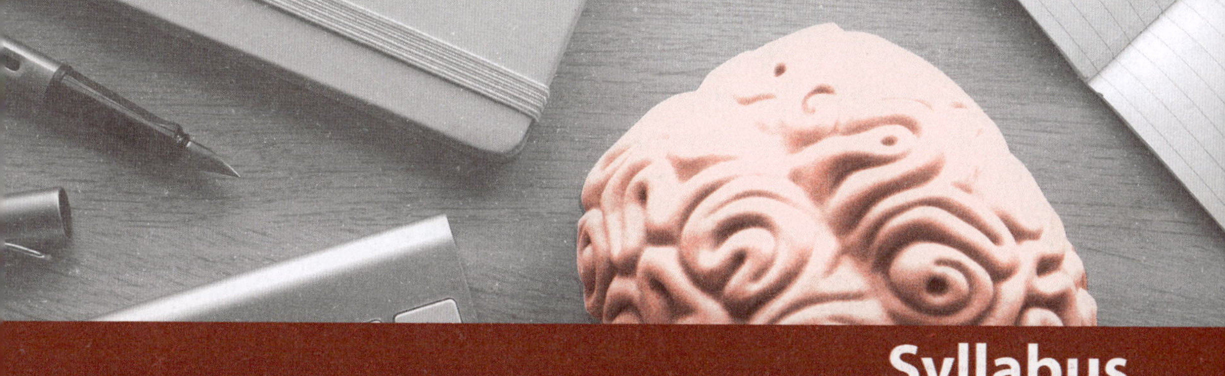

Unit 1 Introduction to Psychology

- **Describe schools:** Structuralism, functionalism, behaviorism, psychoanalysis.
- **Describe methods:** Introspection, observation, inventory and experimental method.
- **Describe branches in brief:** Pure psychology and applied psychology.
- Describe importance of study of psychology in physiotherapy.

Unit 2 Developmental Psychology

- **Describe growth and development:** Nature of growth and development, characteristics of growth and development, developmental periods of infancy.
- Describe childhood, adolescence, adulthood and old age, factors affecting growth and development.
- Describe role of heredity and environment and their relative importance in physical, psychological and social development.

Unit 3 Emotions and Perception

- Describe concept and definition of emotions, theories of emotions, physiological changes due to emotional state, nature and control of anger, fear and anxiety.
- **Describe sensation, attention and perception:** Meaning and definition.
- Describe types of sensation and perception.
- Describe principles of perception, illusion and hallucination and concept of attention and factors determining attention.

Unit 4 Motivation and Learning

- Definition of motivation, needs, drives and motives, primary motives and secondary motives, and achievement motivation.
- Discuss the theories of motivation.
- Describe theories of learning.

- Describe concepts, characteristics, types, laws of leaning, theories of learning, trial and error theory.
- Describe conditioning—classical and operant, insight theory of learning, factors influencing learning.
- **Describe the effective ways to learn:** Massed/spaced, whole/part, recitation/reading, serial/free recall, incidental/intentional learning, knowledge of results, association, organization, and mnemonic methods.
- Describe intelligence; discuss characteristics, types, IQ, Mental age.
- Describe assessment of intelligence, intelligence tests—verbal and performance test.

Unit 5 Psychology of Frustration and Stress

- **Describe frustration and stress under the following headings:** Definition, causes, sources of frustration, conflict, different types of conflicts, adjustment and maladjustment, defense mechanism.
- Describe different types of anxiety, tension, physiological symptoms, causes, reactions to stress, psychosomatic problems, coping strategies.
- Discuss the management of stress.

Unit 6 Personality

- Define personality and describe factors in personality development.
- **Describe tools of measurement of personality:** Observation, situational test, questionnaire, rating scale, interview, and projective techniques.
- **Describe defense mechanisms:** Denial of reality, rationalization, projection, reaction formation, identification, repression, regression, intellectualization, undoing, introjection, acting out.
- Describe psychological reactions of a patient during admission and treatment in terms of possible anxiety, shock denial, suspicion. Loneliness, shame, guilt, rejection, fear, withdrawal, depression, egocentric, justify and loss of hope.

Unit 7 Social Psychology

- Describe different types of leaders and different theoretical approaches to leadership.
- Describe development of attitude and change of attitude.

Unit 8 Clinical Psychology

- Describe models of training, abnormal behavior assessment, clinical judgment, psychotherapy, self-management methods, physiotherapist-patient interaction, aggression.
- **Discuss the following:** Self-imaging, stress management, assertive training, group therapy, body awareness, pediatric, child and geriatric clinical psychology.

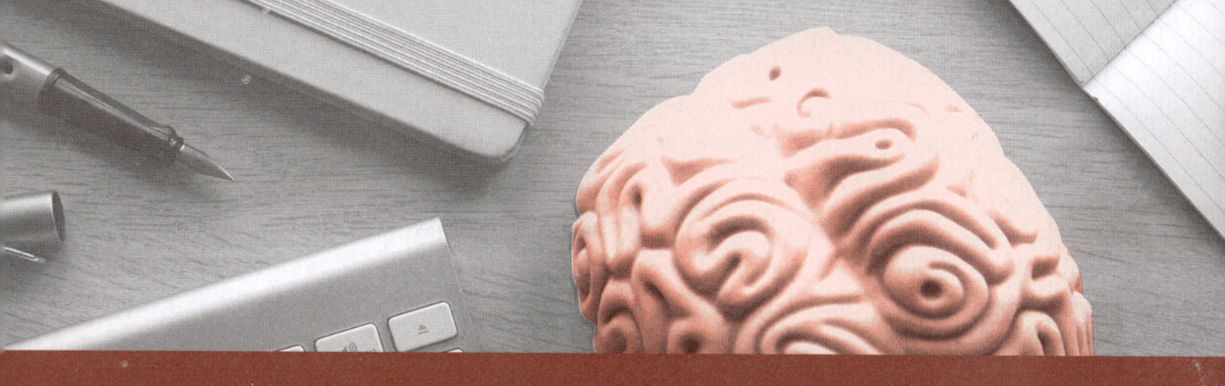

Contents

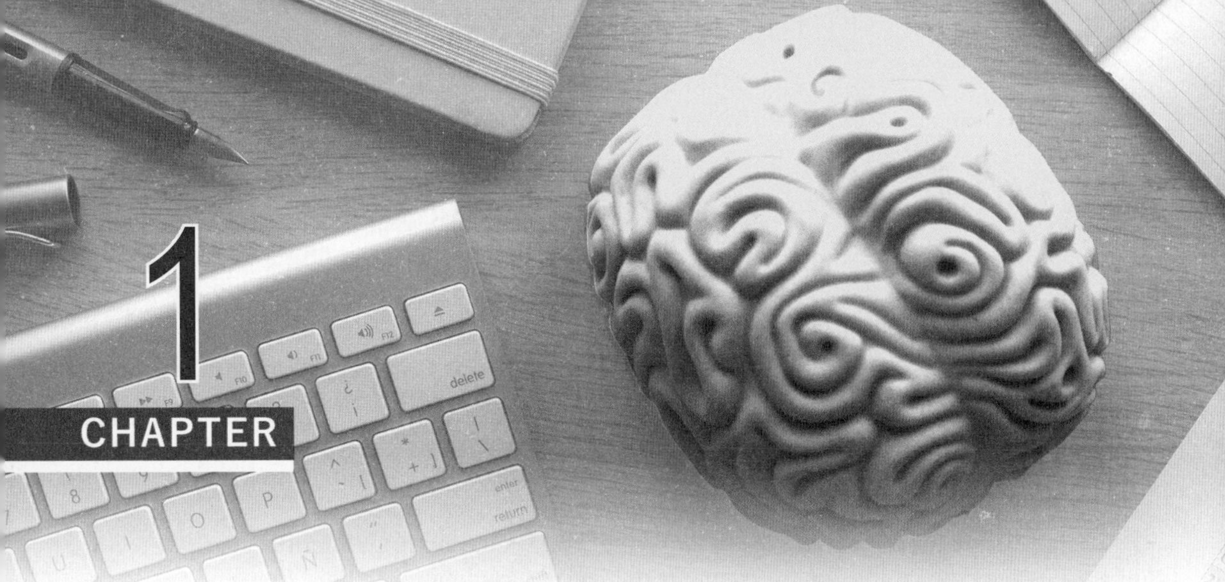

CHAPTER 1

Introduction to Psychology

Aditi Popli, Hem Jivani, Sunanda Bhowmik

LEARNING OBJECTIVES

After the completion of the chapter, the readers will be able to:
- Define psychology and its core areas of practice, research, and applications.
- Explain the historical development of the field, including major theoretical perspectives.
- Describe the relationship between mental health and physical health.
- Identify the biological, psychological, and social factors that contribute to mental health problems.

CHAPTER OUTLINE

- Introduction
- Definition of Psychology
- Enigmatic Journey of Understanding Ourselves: A Historical Background to Psychology
- Branches of Psychology
- Modern School of Psychology
- Levels of Explanation in Psychology
- Underlying Questions Addressed by Psychology
- Unveiling the Vast Landscape: A Deep Dive into the Scope of Psychology
- Psychology in Clinical Practice
- Physiotherapy and Psychology
- A Glimpse into the Future: Recent Advances in Psychology

KEY TERMS

Cognitive psychology: It focuses on the study of the higher mental processes.

Counseling psychology: It focuses primarily on educational, social and career adjustment problems.

Environmental psychology: It considers the relationship between people and their physical environment including how our physical environment affects our emotions and the amount of stress we experience in a particular setting.

> **Geopsychology:** The study of the psychological connections to physical environments such as weather conditions, climatic change, soil conditions, and behavior.
>
> **Parapsychology:** The scientific study of phenomena that is beyond the scope of conventional psychology, including telepathy, extrasensory perception, birth and death, and associated issues.

INTRODUCTION

Psychology is the scientific study of human thought and behavior. It explores the cognitive as well as unconscious dimensions of the human experience, including everything from memories and emotions to motivations and actions. This chapter will give students a foundation on the topics like theories of psychology and the biological basis of behavior, allowing them to:

- Connect the dots between the brain and mental processes.
- Examine how we change and grow throughout our lives.
- Use cognitive processes to understand how we perceive, learn, remember, and make conscious decisions.
- Employ social psychology to discover how relationships and social situations affect our thoughts, feelings, and behaviors.

By studying this chapter on introduction to psychology, readers may obtain an important understanding of the complexity of the human experience.

DEFINITION OF PSYCHOLOGY

Psychology is defined as a method of studying the mind and behavior. The English word "*psychology*" is derived from the Greek words "*psyche*", which means life, and "*logos*", which means explanation. Furthermore, psychology is "the scientific exploration of the human experience", which goes beyond the study of thoughts and actions. It incorporates the influence of emotions, social interactions,[1] and biological factors on our overall experience of being human.[3] Psychology model is shown in Figure 1.1.

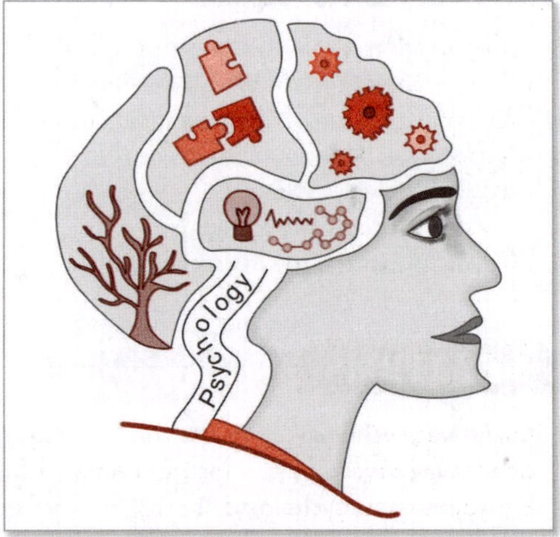

Fig. 1.1: Psychology model

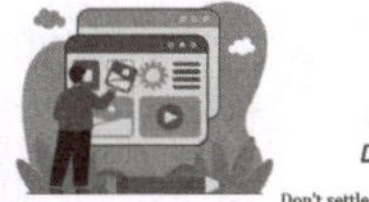 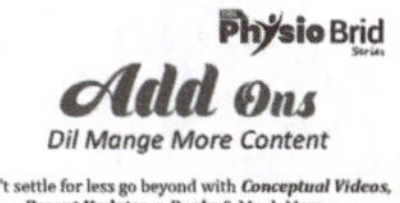

> ### MUST KNOW
>
> **Other definitions:**
> - William James (1890): Psychology is "the science of mental life, both of its conscious and unconscious phenomena".
> - John B Watson (1913): Psychology is "the study of behavior".
> - Carl Jung (1920): Psychology is "the science of the psyche", where psyche refers to the totality of the human mind and soul, including both conscious and unconscious aspects.
> - American Psychological Association (APA, 2017): Psychology is "the scientific study of mind and behavior".

As a kind of science, psychology is practiced by all people. There is a curiosity about our reality that we all want to explore and answer. The reasons behind events, their likelihood of reoccurring, and methods for replicating or altering them are all questions that we seek answers to. With this kind of knowledge, we can forecast both our own and other people's actions. We might even gather data—that is, any information collected by formal measurement or observation—to help us with our project.[3] Psychological aspects are shown in Figure 1.2.

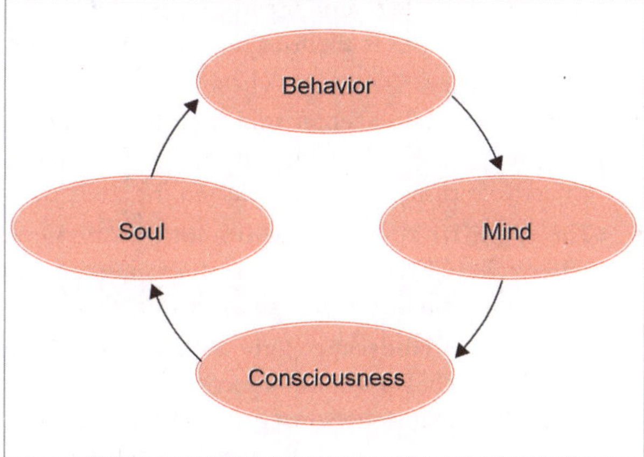

Fig. 1.2: Different aspects in Psychology

It has been argued that people are "everyday scientists", conducting research to unravel the mysteries of behavior.[2] When a person scores miserably in an important test, he tries to explore his shortcomings which he could not understand or retain that was necessary. Also, he explores the methods that can make things easier for him and can be beneficial for subsequent attempts.

ENIGMATIC JOURNEY OF UNDERSTANDING OURSELVES: A HISTORICAL BACKGROUND TO PSYCHOLOGY

The human mind has captivated thinkers for millennia. Although psychology is a relatively new scientific field, its roots are found in past in mythology, philosophy, and medicine. Let us take a quick peek at this intriguing history:

- **Early inquiries (Ancient Greece and beyond):** Philosophers such as Plato and Aristotle contemplated the essence of the soul, awareness, and perception.[22] Their preliminary investigations into the mind prepared the way for later psychological research.[10]

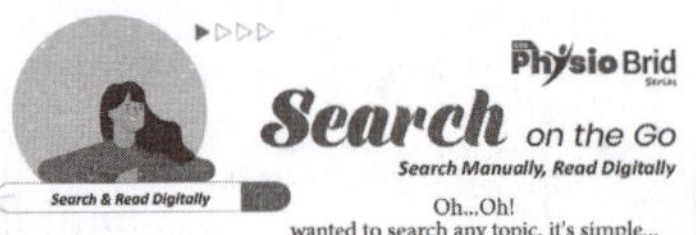

- **The shift toward science (19th century):** A pivot shift in orientation toward a more scientific approach took place during the nineteenth century. In 1879, Wilhelm Wundt, who is often referred to as the father of psychology, established the first laboratory for experimental psychology. This was the first time that methodologies from science were applied to the study of mental and behavioral processes.[22]

- **The battle of the schools (Late 19th and early 20th centuries):** As many different schools of thought arose, each vied to define the heart of psychology. Wundt promoted structuralism that aimed to fragment the mind into basic elements. William James, the founder of functionalism, placed a strong emphasis on how mental processes help us adapt to our surroundings.[22]

- **The rise of psychoanalysis (Early 20th century):** With his groundbreaking theory of psychoanalysis, Sigmund Freud elevated the unconscious mind to an essential component. Even though many of his theories regarding the nature of the psyche and the significance of early experiences are still up for debate, they had a significant influence on psychology.[22]

- **Behaviorism takes center stage (Mid-20th century):** John B Watson's behaviorism shifted the focus to observable behavior and the environment's role in shaping it. This approach emphasized objective measurement and rejected the study of unobservable mental processes.[4]

- **The cognitive revolution (Mid-20th century):** A shift occurred, acknowledging the mind's active role in processing information, memory, and learning. This led to the rise of cognitive psychology, exploring how an individual thinks, reasons, and solves problems.[21]

- **The modern landscape (Late 20th century—present):** Psychology has become much more diverse. Psychologists today incorporate multiple viewpoints, such as humanistic, biological, cognitive, and interpersonal perspectives. A greater emphasis is being paid to things like positive psychology, emotions, cultural effects, actions, and thoughts.[4]

Major landmarks in the development of psychology are enlisted in Table 1.1.

Table 1.1: Major landmarks in the development of psychology

Years	Developmental landmarks of psychology
1879	1st Psychological lab, Germany
1890	William James published psychology principles
1895	Functionalism
1900	Sigmund Freud established psychodynamics
1924	Behaviorism
1951	Client-centered humanistic psychology
1954	Establishment of motivation and personality
1957	Social psychology
1985	Cognitive psychology
2000	Neuropsychology, evolutionary psychology

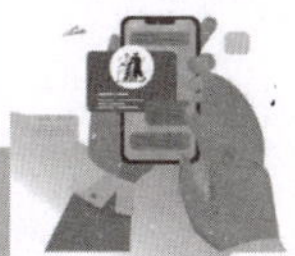
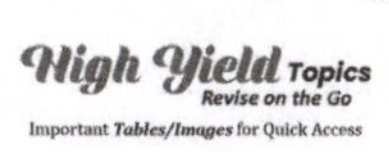

BRANCHES OF PSYCHOLOGY

The field of psychology is very vast. To make it understandable to the readers, psychology has been broadly classified into pure and applied psychology (Fig. 1.3). Differences in objectives and methodologies of pure and applied psychology are enlisted in Table 1.2.

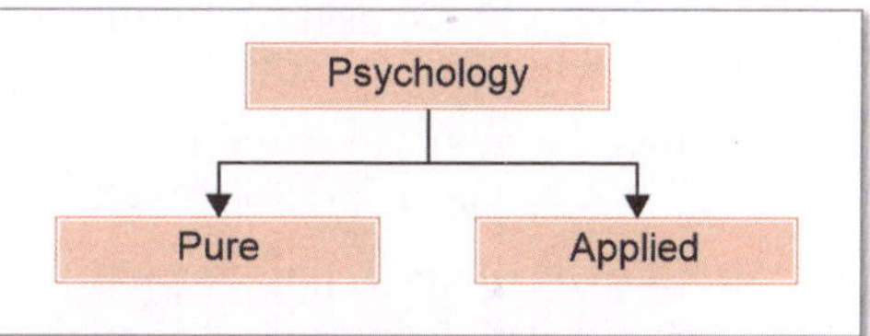

Fig. 1.3: Broad classification of psychology

Table 1.2: Differences in objectives and methodologies of pure and applied psychology

Aspects	Pure psychology	Applied psychology
Focus	Emphasizes theoretical research and knowledge advancement.	Emphasizes practical application of psychological principles.
Goal	Seeks to understand fundamental psychological processes.	Aims to address specific issues or solve practical problems.
Research	Often conducted in controlled laboratory settings.	Often involves real-world settings and applied research methods.
Outcome	Generates theories and models to explain human behavior.	Produces interventions and strategies for real-life problems.
Examples	Cognitive psychology, developmental psychology.	Clinical psychology, industrial-organizational psychology.
Application	Less direct application in practical settings.	Directly applicable in various fields.
Time frame	Long-term focus on accumulating knowledge.	Immediate focus on addressing current issues.
Funding	May rely more on academic or government funding.	May receive funding from private organizations or industries.
Collaboration	Collaboration with other scientists and researchers is common.	Collaborations with professionals from diverse fields is common.
Contribution to field	Contributes to the theoretical foundation of psychology.	Contributes to the development and growth of applied practices.

Pure Psychology

Pure psychology is a theoretical science. It is based on research-oriented approach and focuses on understanding fundamental principles and theories of human behavior and cognition. Branches of pure psychology include:

- **General psychology:** It deals with the basic psychological principles, rules, and theory that govern an individual's behavior.[34]

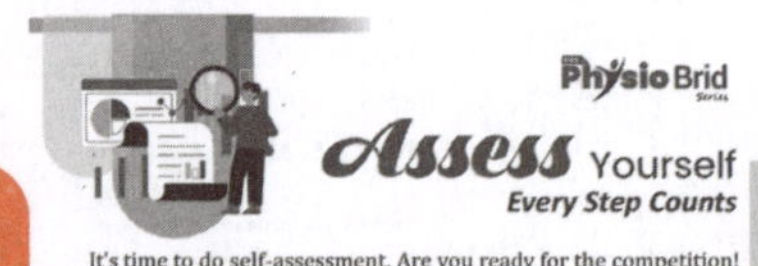

- **Geopsychology:** Geo refers to a term "*Geography*" which deals with the psychological connections to physical environment like weather conditions, climatic change, soil conditions and behavior.[34]
- **Parapsychology:** It tackles issues concerning telepathy, extrasensory perception, birth and death, and associated issues.[34]
- **Social psychology:** It puts emphasis on group phenomena like social beliefs, attitude, opinions, behavior which help to build good interpersonal relationships.[34]
- **Physiological psychology:** This branch of pure psychology is more concerned with physiological and biological basis of behavior. All glands, muscles, sense organs, nervous system are all linked to behavioral aspects.[34]
- **Developmental psychology:** Developmental psychology studies the human's behavioral relationship between growth and development, i.e., from birth to death.[34]

Applied Psychology

Applied psychology is a practical science that refers to the study and ability to solve problems within human behavior such as health issues, workplace issues or education. It improves the quality of life for individuals, organizations, and communities. Branches of applied psychology include:

- **Educational psychology:** Within the field of applied psychology, educational psychology aims to apply psychological theories, concepts, and methods to human behavior in educational settings. This branch includes psychological strategies for enhancing every facet of the teaching and learning process. By applying psychological understanding regarding motivation and learning, educational psychologists are most frequently involved in improving the effectiveness of instruction in schools.[34]
- **Medical psychology:** The biggest subfield in psychology is medical psychology.[5] This area of applied psychology explains the origins of mental diseases, atypical patient interactions, and offers recommendations for both beneficial therapy and successful reintegration of the affected individual into society.[34]
  - **Clinical psychology:** Assesses, diagnoses, and treats mental health disorders.[35]
  - **Health psychology:** Examines the mind-body connection, focusing on how psychological factors influence health and illness.
  - **Forensic psychology:** Applies psychological principles to legal matters, including criminal behavior, risk assessment, and competency evaluations.
- **Industrial-organizational psychology:** Focuses on workplace behavior, improving employee well-being, productivity, and organizational effectiveness.[35]
  - **Workplace psychology:** This area of applied psychology looks for ways to apply psychological theories, concepts, and methods to the study of how people behave in industrial settings. Industrial psychologists use psychological concepts to help public and

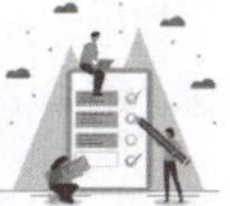
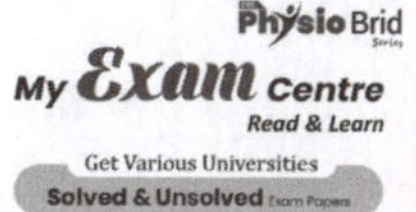

commercial businesses with staff training and supervision, hiring and placement processes, and internal communication enhancements.

- **Official psychology:** Using psychological concepts and methods, forensic psychology is a subfield of applied psychology that examines how people behave, including clients, offenders, witnesses, and so on. This area of psychology can be used to properly understand the underlying causes of any crime, offense, conflict or legal issue.

- **Defense psychology:** This area of psychology focuses on the application of psychological theories and methods to the field of military science. This area of psychology addresses a wide range of issues, including how to maintain a positive morale among residents and soldiers during times of conflict, how to better recruit people for positions involving handling capacities, organizational climate, and leadership, etc.

- **Counseling psychology:** Provides guidance and support on personal, social, and emotional issues.[35]

- **Sports psychology:** Enhances athletic performance and mental well-being of athletes and coaches.

- **Political psychology:** This area of psychology is concerned with the application of psychological concepts and methods to the study of politics and the pursuit of political objectives.[34]

MODERN SCHOOL OF PSYCHOLOGY

There were discussions over terminology and methods of explanation for the human mind and behavior when psychology first emerged as a separate scientific discipline from biology and philosophy. The core theories in the field of psychological research are represented by several schools of psychology. The main schools of psychology are as follows—Gestalt psychology, psychoanalytic psychology, behavioral psychology, structuralism, functionalism, and humanistic psychology.[6]

> **MUST KNOW**
>
> - **Structuralism (Wundt):** Breaking down the mind into its basic structures.
> - **Functionalism (James):** Emphasizes the function of mental processes and how they help us adapt to the environment.
> - **Behaviorism (Watson, Skinner):** Focuses on observable behavior and how it is shaped by learning through conditioning.
> - **Psychoanalysis (Freud):** Explores the unconscious mind and the role of early childhood experiences in shaping personality.
> - **Humanism (Maslow, Rogers):** Highlights human potential, self-actualization, and the importance of free will and subjective experience.
> - **Cognitive psychology:** Examines mental processes like thinking, memory, attention, and language.
> - **Evolutionary psychology:** Views behavior and mental processes through the lens of natural selection and adaptation.

Structuralism

Structuralism is widely regarded as the founding school of thought in psychology. Key figures in this movement includes Oswald Külpe, Edward B Titchener, and Wilhelm Wundt. The primary aim of structuralism was to dissect mental processes into their basic components. Researchers employed techniques like introspection to delve into the inner workings of the human mind. Through introspective experiments, trained observers evaluated their own experiences. This method, also termed experimental self-observation, aimed to teach individuals how to objectively analyze their thoughts. While the empirical validity of structuralist methods may be questioned, their impact on the development of experimental psychology was significant.

Functionalism

Functionalism emerged as a counterpoint to structuralism, deeply shaped by the philosophies of William James. It delves into the functions and adaptability of the mind, rather than its underlying mechanisms. The functionalist perspective underscores the significance of discerning the purposes served by mental states, positing that such understanding enriches the comprehension of how the mind facilitates individuals in responding to and acclimating to their environment. In contrast to structuralism's analysis of consciousness components, functionalism aimed to uncover the underlying causes of thoughts and behaviors. While functionalism's distinct prominence diminished, its influence permeated into behaviorism, applied psychology, and educational psychology. Unlike certain psychological paradigms, functionalism lacks a singular dominant theory or progenitor; instead, it is affiliated with a diverse array of scholars and intellectuals such as Harvey Carr, James Rowland Angell, and John Dewey. Some historians raise doubts about whether functionalism qualifies as a formal psychological school due to its absence of a central figure or well-established doctrines.

Gestalt Psychology

The foundational premise of Gestalt psychology lies in perceiving the world as unified whole rather than fragmented parts. Originating in Germany and Austria during the late 1800s as a reaction against the atomistic approach of structuralism, this psychological school was championed by intellectuals such as Kurt Koffka, Wolfgang Köhler, and Max Wertheimer. Gestalt psychologists championed the notion of viewing concepts and behaviors holistically, preferring to perceive them as unified whole rather than breaking them down into discrete elements. They embraced the principle of holism, asserting that the entire entity transcends the mere aggregation of its constituent parts, a foundational tenet of Gestalt theory. Often applied to elucidate optical illusions, Gestalt principles elucidate phenomena like apparent motion, as described by Wertheimer in his analysis of train lights. This principle elucidates how a rapid succession of images can create the illusion of movement.

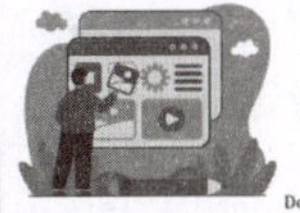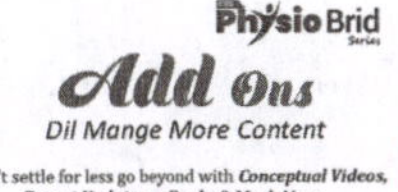

Behavioral Psychology

Behaviorism rose to prominence as a significant psychological paradigm during the 1950s, founded on the principles espoused by leading theorists like John B Watson, Ivan Pavlov, and BF Skinner. This school of thought posits that external factors, rather than internal ones, are the primary determinants of behavior.[20] Central to behaviorism is the emphasis on observable behaviors, leading to the development of influential theories such as operant conditioning and classical conditioning. The impact of behaviorism on the field of psychology has been profound, with many

of its concepts and methodologies still widely utilized today. Techniques such as aversion therapy, token economies, and behavioral training, which originated from behaviorist principles, are frequently employed in psychotherapeutic and behavior modification interventions. Aspects of behaviorism are shown in Figure 1.4.

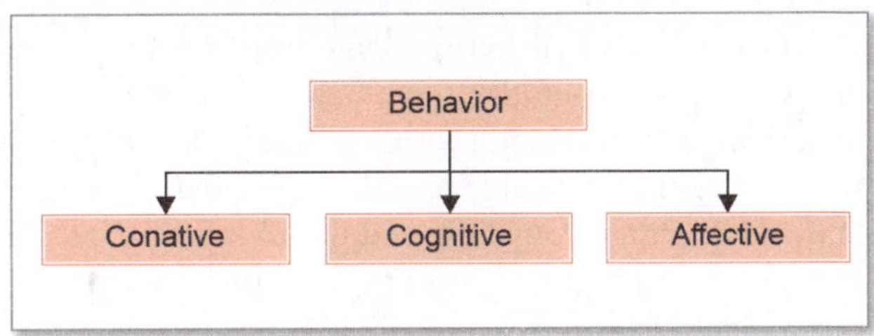

Fig. 1.4: Aspects of behaviorism

Psychoanalytic Psychology

The psychoanalytic branch of psychology was established by Sigmund Freud, emphasizing the profound influence of the unconscious mind on behavior. Alongside influential figures such as Anna Freud, Otto Rank, and other notable psychoanalytic thinkers, neo-Freudians like Erik Erikson, Alfred Adler, and Karen Horney also made significant contributions to the field. Freud's conceptualization of the human psyche delineated three distinct components: The id, ego, and superego, which he asserted interact to shape complex human behavior. Key tenets of psychoanalytic theory included the delineation between conscious and unconscious realms, Freud's psychosexual theory of personality development, and the concepts of life and death instincts. While Freud's ideas sparked substantial discourse and debate both in his era and in contemporary discussions, his contributions paved the way for the emergence of talk therapy as a viable treatment modality for mental illness. Despite the evolution away from many traditional Freudian therapeutic concepts, contemporary psychoanalytic approaches remain integral to psychology, with research highlighting the importance of self-reflection for emotional maturation and psychological well-being.[7]

Humanistic Psychology

This psychological approach underscores the paramount importance of individuals attaining their utmost potential and evolving into their most fulfilled selves. It posits that people's profound yearning for growth and fulfillment can only be realized through self-exploration and personal advancement. One notable humanistic psychologist, Abraham Maslow, places particular emphasis on fostering self-awareness and self-actualization, alongside exploring the subjective experiences of individuals.

The development of humanistic psychology was also influenced by the works of Clark Moustakas and Carl Rogers. Diverging from earlier psychological paradigms, humanistic psychology diverged by prioritizing the facilitation of individuals reaching their highest potential. Rather than focusing solely on addressing pathology, humanistic psychology delved into themes such as personal growth, the exercise of free will, and the attainment of ultimate achievements such as self-actualization, as delineated in Maslow's hierarchy of needs.

Cognitive Psychology

This field is dedicated to exploring human cognition and its impact on behavior. It operates on the premise that cognitive functions such as memory, problem-solving, and decision-making are subject to scientific inquiry, viewing the human mind as a sophisticated information-processing system. Cognitive psychologists, exemplified by figures like Jean Piaget, focus on understanding how individuals acquire, organize, and utilize information. The evolution of cognitive psychology in the 1950s was partly spurred by critiques of behaviorism, which were centered on its disregard for the role of internal processes in shaping behavior.

LEVELS OF EXPLANATION IN PSYCHOLOGY

The human mind and behavior are intricately woven tapestries. Understanding them requires a multifaceted approach, one that acknowledges the influence of various factors operating at different levels. In psychology, one explores these complexities through **levels of explanation**. Each level offers a distinct perspective on the "why?" behind our thoughts, feelings, and actions.[18]

Biological Level

This level delves into the biological foundations of behavior.[15] It examines the role of the brain, nervous system, genes, and hormones in shaping our experiences. Here are some key aspects:

- **Brain:** Psychologists explore how different brain structures contribute to specific functions like memory, emotion, and decision-making.[16] Techniques like neuroimaging allows to visualize brain activity and understand its role in behaviors.

- **Nervous system:** The intricate network of nerves throughout the body transmits information, allowing an individual to interact with the environment. Understanding how these systems function sheds light on reflexes, sensations, and responses.

- **Genetics:** Genetics plays a crucial role in predisposing an individual to certain traits and vulnerabilities. Studying the influence of genes will contemplate to understand an individual's difference in behaviors and mental health.

- **Hormones:** Often referred to as chemical messengers, hormones are produced by glands. They significantly impact one's emotions, level of motivation, and even basic needs like hunger and sleep cycle. Studying hormonal activity deepens our understanding of behavior across different stages of life.

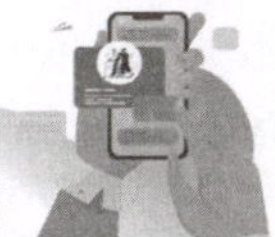
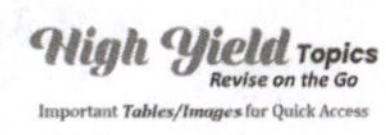

Psychological Level

This level focuses on internal mental processes like thoughts, emotions, motivations, learning, and personality. Here, psychologists explore:

- **Cognitive processes:** How an individual perceives, attends to, stores, retrieves, and uses information is crucial. This level examines memory, language, problem-solving, and decision-making.

- **Emotions:** An individual's feelings are powerful motivators and influence how we perceive and interact with the world. This level explores the nature of emotions, their physiological underpinnings, and their impact on behavior.

- **Learning:** How an individual acquires and modifies behavior is a fundamental aspect of psychology. This level examines different learning theories and how experiences shape our responses.

- **Personality:** The unique constellation of thoughts, feelings, and behaviors that defines an individual, falls under personality psychology.[14] This level explores individual differences and what makes a person who he is.

Social and Cultural Level

This level recognizes the profound influence of social and cultural contexts on an individual's behavior. It examines:

- **Social groups:** Our interactions with families, friends, communities, and social groups shape our values, beliefs, and behaviors. This level explores social pressure, conformity, and group dynamics.

- **Culture:** The customs, beliefs, values, and practices of the cultures we are raised in significantly impact our thoughts and actions.

Evolutionary Level

This level explores how our behavior is influenced by adaptations that benefited our ancestors. It examines how these adaptations might still be influencing our thoughts and actions today.

Interconnected Web

It is important to remember that these levels of explanation are not entirely separate entities. They interact and influence each other in a complex web. For instance, our biological makeup (level 1) can influence how we learn (level 2), which in turn can be shaped by our cultural background (level 3). Recognizing this interconnectedness provides a more holistic understanding of human behavior.

By exploring these levels of explanation, psychology equips us with a nuanced perspective on the human experience. It allows us to appreciate the intricate interplay between biology, mental processes, social context, and even our evolutionary history in shaping who we are and how we navigate the world.

UNDERLYING QUESTIONS ADDRESSED BY PSYCHOLOGY

Although psychology has changed dramatically over its history, the most important questions that psychologists address have remained constant, which are as follows:

- **Nature versus nurture:** This factor has a greater influence on a person's behavior and helps to explain individual variances in behavior—environment or genes? Although the majority of scientists today concur that genes and environment play significant roles in the majority of human behaviors, there is still much we do not know about the interaction between **Nature**—our biological make-up and **Nurture**—the experiences we have throughout our lives (Harris, 1998; Pinker, 2002). The phrase "heritability of the characteristic", which we use often, refers to the percentage of observed differences in traits across individuals (such as height, IQ or optimism) that are caused by genetics.[23] For illustration, that extraversion has a heredity of roughly 0.50, and intelligence has a very high heritability of about 0.85 out of 1.0. However, we will also see that there are intricate interactions between nature and nurture, making it challenging to determine whether something results from either (Fig. 1.5).[12]

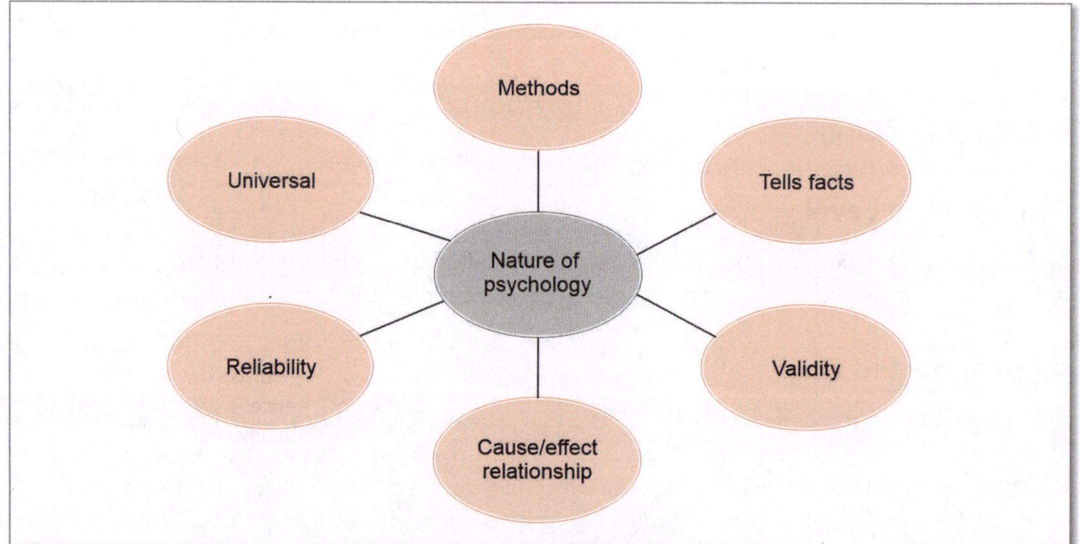

Fig. 1.5: Nature of psychology

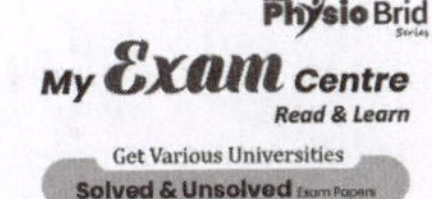

- **Free will versus determinism:** This inquiry focuses on how much control individuals actually have over their own behavior. Are we products of our surroundings, influenced by outside influences or do we have the ability to select the actions we take? The majority of us want to think that we have free will and can do anything we want, like get up and go fishing right now. Furthermore, the foundation of our legal system is the idea of free will;[11] we penalize offenders because we think individuals have the ability to control their actions and voluntarily choose to break the law. Recent research has suggested that we may have less control over our own behavior than we think we do.[16]

- **Accuracy versus inaccuracy:** How suitable are humans to process information? People are far from perfect, even when it seems like they are "good enough" to understand the world and make moral decisions. Errors in our cognitive processes, as well as biases and feelings, can impair human judgment.[1] For example, our emotional reactions to the things that happen to us and our ambitions to perceive ourselves favorably and accumulate financial prosperity may impact our judgment.

- **Conscious versus unconscious processing:** How much of our behaviors are influenced by forces we are unaware of, and how much are we aware of the causes of the acts we take? Numerous prominent psychological theories, from the psychodynamic theories of Freud to the latest research in cognitive psychology, contend that many of the factors influencing human behavior are hidden from our conscious awareness.[12]

- **Differences versus similarities:** How much do we all have in common, and how much do we all differ? For example, are men and women fundamentally different from one another in terms of psychology and mentality or are they similar overall? What about those who belong to other cultures and ethnic groups? Do people all throughout the world have similar backgrounds and settings or do they differ in certain ways? Cross-cultural, personality, and social psychologists try to address these timeless concerns.[33]

UNVEILING THE VAST LANDSCAPE: A DEEP DIVE INTO THE SCOPE OF PSYCHOLOGY

Psychology, the captivating exploration of the human experience, boasts a remarkably broad scope. It delves far beyond simply understanding why we think in a certain way or why we behave in particular situations. It encompasses the intricate interplay between our minds, our bodies, and the ever-evolving world around us. This section delves into the vastness of psychology, showcasing the diverse areas it explores and the profound impact it has on various aspects of our lives.[28, 29]

> **MUST KNOW**
>
> **Basic Tenets of Psychology**
> - **Debate on nature versus nurture:** The ongoing debate about the relative influence of genes (nature) and environment (nurture) on behavior and mental processes.
> - **Importance of critical thinking:** Psychology encourages critical evaluation of research findings and psychological theories.
> - **Evolving field:** Psychology is a constantly evolving field with new discoveries and advancements in understanding the mind and behavior.

A Spectrum of Human Experience

Psychology is not confined to a single domain; it investigates the entirety of the human experience across various subfields:

- **Biological psychology:** Explores the biological underpinnings of behavior, investigating the role of the brain, nervous system, hormones, and genes in shaping our thoughts, emotions, and actions. Techniques like neuroimaging allow psychologists to visualize brain activity and understand its influence on behavior.[35]

- **Cognitive psychology:** Delves into the fascinating realm of our thinking processes, including memory, learning, language, attention, problem-solving, and decision-making. This field explores how we take in information, process it, and use it to navigate the world.[34]

- **Developmental psychology:** Charts the course of human growth and development, examining how we change physically, cognitively, emotionally, and socially across the lifespan.[11] It explores how nature and nurture interact to shape who we become.

- **Social psychology:** Uncovers the power of social influence, group dynamics, conformity, prejudice, and social perception on our behaviors and attitudes.[8] This field sheds light on how we interact with others and how social contexts shape our experiences.[34, 35]

- **Personality psychology:** Seeks to understand individual differences in thoughts, feelings, and behaviors, exploring factors that shape our unique personalities. It investigates how personality traits emerge, develop, and influence our lives.

- **Abnormal psychology:** Studies mental disorders, their causes, symptoms, diagnosis, and treatment approaches. Psychologists in this field help individuals with mental health challenges to improve their well-being and functioning.[17]

- **Positive psychology:** Focuses on the strengths and positive aspects of human experience, such as happiness, well-being, resilience, and optimal functioning. This field explores how to cultivate these positive attributes and build a more fulfilling life.

This is just a glimpse into the diverse landscape of psychology. With its ever-expanding branches, psychology strives to comprehend the tapestry of human experience in all its richness and complexity.

A Window to a Richer Understanding

By understanding the vast scope of psychology, an individual gains a deeper appreciation for the human experience. It empowers us to not only comprehend ourselves better but also navigate the complexities of the world around us. Psychology equips us with tools and knowledge to:

- **Improve our mental health and well-being:** By understanding emotions, thoughts, and behaviors, we can learn to manage stress, build resilience, and cultivate positive mental health practices.[17]

- **Enhance our relationships:** Psychology provides insights into communication, conflict resolution, and social dynamics, fostering stronger and more fulfilling relationships.

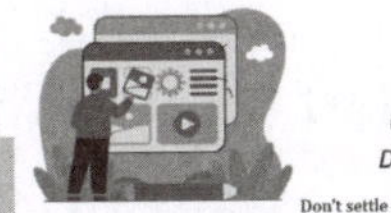

- **Make informed decisions:** Understanding how we think, learn, and make choices empowers us to be more conscious and deliberate in our decision-making processes.
- **Promote harmony:** The knowledge gained from psychology can be utilized to create true social change, fostering empathy, understanding, and building a better future for ourselves and others.

The scope of psychology is vast, ever-evolving, and constantly pushing the boundaries of our understanding of the human mind and behavior. As we delve deeper into this fascinating field, we unveil the richness and complexity that lies at the very core.[32, 33]

PSYCHOLOGY IN CLINICAL PRACTICE

Clinical practice is the cornerstone of applied psychology, where theoretical knowledge meets the real-world challenges faced by an individual. Here, the concept of psychology goes beyond simply understanding the human mind. It transforms into a powerful tool for assessment, diagnosis, intervention, and ultimately, promoting positive change and well-being.[31]

Understanding the Foundation

The core concept of psychology in clinical practice rests on several key pillars.

- **The scientific basis:** Clinical psychology is firmly rooted in scientific research. Evidence-based practices guide assessment tools, therapeutic interventions, and treatment approaches. Psychologists critically evaluate research findings to ensure the interventions they employ are effective and have a strong scientific grounding.
- **The power of the mind-body harmony:** Clinical practice acknowledges the intricate interplay between our thoughts, emotions, behavior, and biology. Psychologists consider the influence of factors like brain function, genetics, and the nervous system on mental health.[17]
- **Individuality at the forefront:** No two individuals are alike. Clinical practice emphasizes a personalized approach, recognizing the unique experiences, strengths, and challenges of each client.
- **Holistic assessment:** A comprehensive understanding of the client is crucial. Psychologists utilize various assessment tools, including interviews, psychological tests, and observations to evaluate a client's mental health, cognitive functioning,[9] personality traits, and social environment.

From Understanding to Intervention

The concept of psychology in clinical practice translates into a multifaceted approach:

- **Diagnosis:** By applying their knowledge of mental disorders and diagnostic criteria, psychologists can accurately diagnose mental health conditions. This diagnosis serves as a roadmap for treatment planning and intervention.[31]

- **Psychotherapy:** Psychologists utilize various therapeutic approaches, such as cognitive-behavioral therapy, psychodynamic therapy or humanistic therapy, to help clients manage their symptoms, improve their coping mechanisms, and develop healthier thought patterns and behaviors.

- **Intervention and treatment:** Treatment goes beyond psychotherapy. Psychologists might employ techniques like relaxation training, stress management strategies, and interpersonal skills training to equip clients with tools for managing their mental health challenges.[24]

- **Collaboration:** Clinical psychologists often collaborate with other mental health professionals, such as psychiatrists, social workers, and counselors, to provide clients with a comprehensive treatment plan.

Evolving Landscape

The concept of psychology in clinical practice is constantly evolving. Here are some key trends:

- **Culturally competent care:** Psychologists increasingly recognize the importance of cultural sensitivity in diagnosis and treatment. They strive to understand the influence of cultural background on mental health experiences and tailor interventions accordingly.[29]

- **Prevention and early intervention:** The focus is shifting toward preventative measures and early intervention to address mental health concerns before they escalate.[30]

- **Integration of technology:** Technology is playing a growing role in clinical practice. Tele-therapy and online interventions are making mental health services more accessible.[27]

- **The power of change:** The concept of psychology in clinical practice ultimately centers on empowering individuals to live fulfilling and meaningful lives. By providing a framework for understanding mental health, fostering positive change, and promoting well-being, psychology becomes a beacon of hope and a catalyst for positive transformation.

Practical Aspect

Psychology does not just about understand the mind; it is about applying that knowledge to real-world problems. Here's a glimpse into the practical side of psychology:

- **Improving mental health:** Psychologists diagnose and treat mental health disorders, helping individuals manage symptoms, develop coping mechanisms, and improve well-being.[28]

- **Enhancing relationships:** Understanding communication styles, conflict resolution, and social dynamics as explored by social psychology can lead to stronger, more fulfilling relationships.[13]

- **Boosting performance:** Sports psychologists help athletes manage anxiety, improve focus, and achieve peak performance.[24] Similarly, industrial-organizational psychologists create strategies for employee selection, training, and motivation in the workplace.

- **Informing education:** Educational psychologists help educators understand how students learn best, leading to improved teaching methods and fostering positive learning environments.

- **Guiding legal decisions:** Forensic psychology applies psychological knowledge to criminal investigations, jury selection, and offender rehabilitation, aiding the legal system.

- **Promoting positive change:** Understanding human behavior allows us to design interventions that address social issues, promote empathy, and create a better future.

Psychology's practical applications touch nearly every aspect of our lives, empowering us to improve ourselves, navigate our world more effectively, and contribute to a better society.

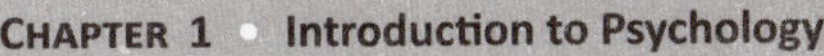

Physio CORNER

Psychological techniques used by physiotherapists during treatment:
- Encouraging positive self-talk
- Encouraging effective communication
- Enhancing self-confidence
- Reducing stress/anxiety
- Using relaxation techniques
- Mental visualization techniques
- Emotional control strategies

PHYSIOTHERAPY AND PSYCHOLOGY

Physiotherapy's Influence in Psychology: A Mind-Body Connection

Physiotherapy, traditionally focused on physical rehabilitation, plays a surprisingly significant role in psychology. Its integration into psychological treatment emphasizes the holistic approach to health and wellness. It goes beyond treating physical ailments and delves into the mind-body connection, influencing a person's mental well-being and overall recovery. Here is brief introduction to how physiotherapy intersects with psychology:

- **Pain management:** Chronic pain can significantly impact mental health, leading to anxiety, depression, and decreased motivation. Physiotherapy helps manage pain through exercise, manual therapy, and other techniques, thereby improving not just physical function but also psychological well-being.[36]

- **Bio-psychosocial approach:** Physiotherapy adds a physical dimension to psychological treatment, aligning with the bio-psychosocial model that acknowledges the interconnectedness of biological, psychological, and social factors in health and illness.[37]

- **Treatment of psychosomatic symptoms:** Physiotherapy techniques address physical manifestations of psychological distress, such as tension, pain, and muscle stiffness, offering relief and promoting relaxation.[24, 25]

- **Stress reduction:** Physiotherapy interventions, such as relaxation techniques, massage therapy, and exercise programs, help manage stress, anxiety, and mood disorders by promoting physical relaxation and enhancing overall well-being.[24]

- **Improved body image:** Physical limitations or impairments can negatively affect self-esteem and body image. Physiotherapy empowers individuals to regain control over their bodies, improving their confidence and overall sense of self.

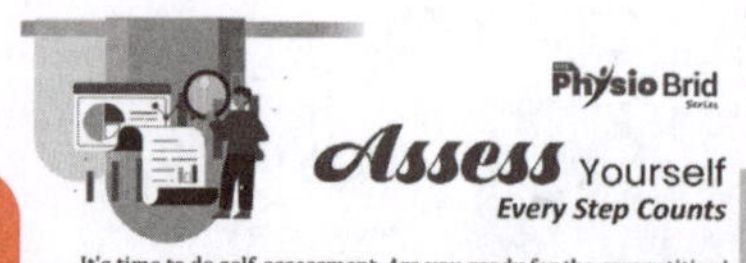

- **Movement and mental health:** Exercise has well-documented benefits for mental health. Physiotherapy programs often incorporate exercise routines, promoting the release of endorphins, which have mood-boosting effects, and reducing stress hormones.

- **Setting and achieving goals:** Physiotherapy often involves setting achievable goals for physical improvement. This goal-setting process can translate into other areas of life, fostering a sense of accomplishment and improving self-efficacy, a belief in one's ability to succeed.

- **Coping mechanisms for chronic conditions:** Physiotherapists help individuals to manage chronic conditions like arthritis or neurological disorders. This empowers patients to develop coping mechanisms, reducing stress and anxiety associated with their condition.

- **Improved sleep:** Pain and physical limitations can disrupt sleep patterns. Physiotherapy techniques aim at pain management and promoting physical well-being can indirectly improve sleep quality, which in turn has a positive impact on mental health.[26]

- **Patient-centered care:** Physiotherapists work collaboratively with clinical psychologists and other healthcare professionals to provide patient-centered care tailored to individual needs and preferences, ensuring a comprehensive approach to treatment.

- **Prevention of relapse:** Physiotherapy interventions aimed at improving physical health and fitness can contribute to the prevention of relapse in individuals with mental health conditions by promoting overall resilience and coping mechanisms.

- **Promotion of long-term wellness:** By addressing physical health concerns and promoting healthy lifestyle behaviors, physiotherapy in clinical psychology fosters long-term wellness and resilience, supporting individuals in achieving and maintaining optimal mental health.

In summary, the role of physiotherapy in clinical psychology extends beyond physical rehabilitation to encompass the holistic care of individuals, emphasizing the interconnectedness of physical and psychological well-being. Its integration into psychological treatment offers valuable benefits in promoting relaxation, managing stress and pain, improving functional ability, and enhancing overall treatment outcomes.

Psychology in Physiotherapy

Physiotherapists increasingly recognize the psychological aspects of their practice. They may:

- **Utilize cognitive behavioral therapy (CBT):** CBT techniques can be integrated into physiotherapy to help patients manage pain-related thoughts and anxieties, enhancing the effectiveness of treatment.

- **Promote relaxation techniques:** Techniques like deep breathing and meditation can be incorporated into physiotherapy sessions to manage stress and anxiety associated with physical limitations.

- **Provide support and motivation:** Physiotherapists can be a source of encouragement and support throughout the rehabilitation process, which can significantly impact a patient's mental state and adherence to treatment plans.

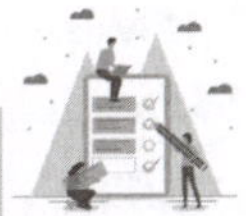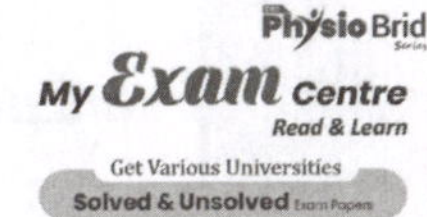

A GLIMPSE INTO THE FUTURE: RECENT ADVANCES IN PSYCHOLOGY

The ever-evolving field of psychology is constantly pushing the boundaries of our understanding of the human mind and behavior.[19] Some exciting recent advances in psychology are as follows:

- **The rise of neuroscience:** Techniques like neuroimaging are allowing us to map brain activity with greater detail, providing insights into the neural basis of emotions, memory, and decision-making.[27]

- **The power of big data:** Psychologists are leveraging vast datasets to identify patterns in human behavior and mental health, leading to more personalized treatment approaches and a deeper understanding of mental health trends.

- **The exploration of the microbiome:** The gut microbiome is increasingly recognized as influencing mental health. Research is exploring how gut bacteria might impact mood, anxiety, and even cognitive function.[11]

- **Virtual reality therapy:** Immersive technologies like virtual reality (VR) are being used to treat phobias, anxiety disorders, and post-traumatic stress disorder (PTSD), showing promising results in exposure therapy and skill development.[27]

- **Positive psychology flourishes:** The focus on strengths and positive aspects of human experience is gaining momentum. Research is exploring ways to cultivate happiness, well-being, and resilience.[11]

- **Artificial intelligence in psychology:** AI is being utilized to analyze data, personalize interventions, and even act as therapeutic chatbots, offering potential for increased accessibility of mental health services.[27]

SUMMARY

- Psychology, a discipline that delves into the intricacies of human thought and behavior, has evolved significantly over time, transitioning from philosophical musings to a robust scientific field. This chapter offers a comprehensive introduction to psychology, outlining its historical development, theoretical frameworks, and practical applications.

- **Historical development:** The journey of psychology is a fascinating one, beginning with early inquiries in ancient Greece and progressing through various stages of scientific evolution. Philosophers like Plato and Aristotle laid the groundwork by exploring the essence of the soul and perception. The shift toward a more scientific approach occurred in the 19th century, notably with Wilhelm Wundt's establishment of the first psychological laboratory in 1879. This marked a pivotal moment, where methodologies from the natural sciences were applied to the study of mental processes. The chapter highlights key milestones in the development of psychology, such as the rise of psychoanalysis with Sigmund Freud, the behaviorist movement led by John B. Watson, and the cognitive revolution that acknowledged the mind's active role in processing information.

Contd...

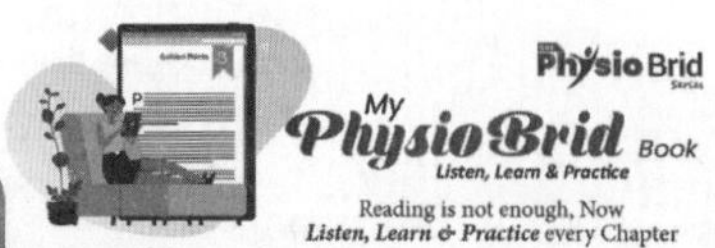

- **Branches of psychology:** Psychology is a vast field, and to make it more accessible, the chapter categorizes it into pure and applied branches. Pure psychology focuses on the fundamental principles and theories, while applied psychology deals with practical applications in various settings. Within these broad categories, the chapter discusses subfields such as educational psychology, clinical psychology, and industrial-organizational psychology, among others. Each branch contributes uniquely to our understanding and application of psychological principles.

- **Schools of psychology:** The chapter provides an in-depth exploration of the major schools of psychology, including structuralism, functionalism, Gestalt psychology, behaviorism, psychoanalysis, and humanistic psychology. Each school has its distinct approach and has significantly shaped the course of psychological research and practice. For instance, structuralism aimed to dissect mental processes into basic components, while functionalism focused on the adaptability of the mind. Behaviorism emphasized observable behavior and the role of the environment, whereas psychoanalysis delved into the unconscious mind. Humanistic psychology, on the other hand, highlighted the importance of self-actualization and personal growth.

- **Levels of explanation:** Understanding human behavior requires a multifaceted approach, and the chapter discusses four levels of explanation: Biological, psychological, social, and cultural. Each level provides a unique perspective on why individuals think and act the way they do. The biological level examines the role of the brain, nervous system, genes, and hormones. The psychological level focuses on internal mental processes like thoughts, emotions, and motivations. The social level explores the influence of social interactions and group dynamics, while the cultural level considers the impact of cultural norms and practices.

- **Practical applications:** Psychology has far-reaching practical applications, and the chapter highlights how it is used in various domains. In clinical practice, psychology plays a crucial role in diagnosing and treating mental health disorders. It also informs educational strategies, enhances workplace productivity, and guides legal decisions. Additionally, the chapter discusses the intersection of psychology with physiotherapy, emphasizing the mind-body connection and the role of physical rehabilitation in mental well-being.

- Psychology is a dynamic field that continues to evolve, offering profound insights into the human experience. By understanding its historical development, theoretical frameworks, and practical applications, readers can appreciate the complexity and diversity of human behavior. The chapter underscores the importance of integrating multiple perspectives to achieve a holistic understanding of psychology, making it an indispensable tool for addressing real-world issues and promoting individual and societal well-being.

REFERENCES

1. Cherniak, Christopher, Nisbett, Richard & Ross, Lee. Human Inference: Strategies and Shortcomings of Social Judgment. Philosophical Review. 1983; 92 (3):462

2. Cutler BL, Wells GL. Psychological science in the courtroom: Consensus and controversy. Expert testimony regarding eyewitness identification. 2009:100–23.

3. Seedat S, Scott KM, Angermeyer MC, Berglund P, Bromet EJ, Brugha TS, Demyttenaere K, De Girolamo G, Haro JM, Jin R, Karam EG. Cross-national associations between gender and mental disorders in the World Health Organization World Mental Health Surveys. Archives of general psychiatry. 2009 Jul 1;66(7):785–95.

Contd...

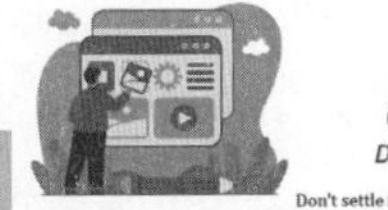
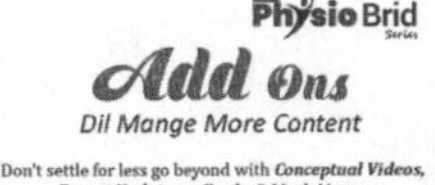

4. Benjamin Jr LT, Baker DB. From séance to science: A history of the profession of psychology in America. University of Akron Press; 2014.

5. Williams N, Simpson AN, Simpson K, Nahas Z. Relapse rates with long-term antidepressant drug therapy: A meta-analysis. Human Psychopharmacology: Clinical and Experimental. 2009 Jul;24(5):401–8.

6. Clark KE, Miller GA. The Behavioral and Social Science Survey. 1st ed. Psychology. 1970

7. Watson JB, Rayner R. Conditioned emotional reactions. Journal of experimental psychology. 1920 Feb;3(1):1.

8. Dijksterhuis A, Preston J, Wegner DM, Aarts H. Effects of subliminal priming of self and God on self-attribution of authorship for events. Journal of experimental social psychology. 2008 Jan 1;44(1):2–9

9. Ilardi SS, Feldman D. The cognitive neuroscience paradigm: A unifying metatheoretical framework for the science and practice of clinical psychology. Journal of Clinical Psychology. 2001 Sep;57(9):1067–88.

10. Chan DK. Tightness-looseness revisited: Some preliminary analyses in Japan and the United States. International Journal of Psychology. 1996 Mar 1;31(1):1–2.

11. Rosenthal R. Science and ethics in conducting, analyzing, and reporting psychological research. Psychological Science. 1994 May;5(3):127–34.

12. Kotowicz Z. The strange case of Phineas Gage. History of the Human Sciences. 2007 Feb;20(1): 115–31.

13. Karremans JC, Stroebe W, Claus J. Beyond Vicary's fantasies: The impact of subliminal priming and brand choice. Journal of experimental social psychology. 2006 Nov 1;42(6):792–8.

14. Darley JM, Gross PH. A hypothesis-confirming bias in labeling effects. Journal of personality and social psychology. 1983 Jan;44(1):20.

15. McCance-Katz EF, Kosten TR, Jatlow P. Concurrent use of cocaine and alcohol is more potent and potentially more toxic than use of either alone—a multiple-dose study. Biological psychiatry. 1998 Aug 15;44(4):250–9.

16. Ahn, W. Y., Vasilev, G., Lee, S. H., Busemeyer, J. R., Kruschke, J. K.,Bechara, A., andamp; Vassileva, J. (2014). Decision-making in stimulant and opiate addicts in protracted abstinence: Evidence from computational modeling with pure users. Frontiers in Psychology, 5, 849.

17. Alegría M, NeMoyer A, Falgàs Bagué I, Wang Y, Alvarez K. Social determinants of mental health: Where we are and where we need to go. Current psychiatry reports. 2018 Nov;20:1–3.

18. Briesch, A. M., Chafouleas, S. M., Nissen, K., andamp; Long, S. (2020). A Review of State- Level Procedural Guidance for Implementing Multitiered Systems of Support for Behavior (MTSS-B). Journal of Positive Behavior Interventions, 22(3), 131–144.

19. Braden JS, DiMarino-Linnen E, Good TL. Schools, society, and school psychologists: History and future directions. Journal of School Psychology. 2001 Mar 1;39(2):203–19.

20. Exner-Cortens D, Gaias L, Splett JW, Jones J, Walker W. Embedding equity into school mental health theory, research, and practice: An introduction to the special issue series. Psychology in the Schools. 2022 Oct;59(10):1941–7.

21. Runyan WM. A historical and conceptual background to psychohistory. Psychology and historical interpretation. 1988:3–60.

22. Friedman HS, Adler NE. The history and background of health psychology. Foundations of health psychology. 2007:3–18.

Contd...

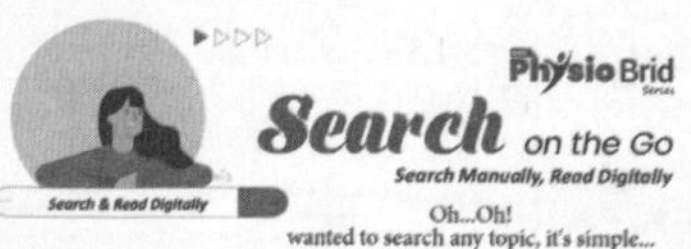

23. Danziger K. Universalism and indigenization in the history of modern psychology. Internationalizing the history of psychology. 2006 Oct 1:208–25.

24. Driver C, Kean B, Oprescu F, Lovell GP. Knowledge, behaviors, attitudes and beliefs of physiotherapists towards the use of psychological interventions in physiotherapy practice: A systematic review. Disability and rehabilitation. 2017 Oct 23;39(22):2237–49.

25. Moffett JA, Richardson PH. The influence of psychological variables on the development and perception of musculoskeletal pain. Physiotherapy Theory and Practice. 1995 Jan 1;11(1):3–11.

26. Saruhanjan K, Zarski AC, Bauer T, Baumeister H, Cuijpers P, Spiegelhalder K, Auerbach RP, Kessler RC, Bruffaerts R, Karyotaki E, Berking M. Psychological interventions to improve sleep in college students: A meta-analysis of randomized controlled trials. Journal of sleep research. 2021 Feb;30(1):13097.

27. Gado S, Kempen R, Lingelbach K, Bipp T. Artificial intelligence in psychology: How can we enable psychology students to accept and use artificial intelligence?. Psychology Learning andamp; Teaching. 2022 Mar;21(1):37–56.

28. Cameron RJ. Educational Psychology: The distinctive contribution. Educational Psychology in Practice. 2006 Dec 1;22(4):289–304.

29. Adair JG. Indigenisation of Psychology: The concept and its practical implementation. Applied Psychology. 1999 Oct;48(4):403–18.

30. Wood AM, Tarrier N. Positive clinical psychology: A new vision and strategy for integrated research and practice. Clinical psychology review. 2010 Nov 1;30(7):819–29.

31. Lilienfeld SO, Basterfield C. Reflective practice in clinical psychology: Reflections from basic psychological science. Clinical Psychology: Science and Practice. 2020 Dec;27(4):220.

32. Kallós D, Lundgren UP. Educational psychology: Its scope and limits. British Journal of Educational Psychology. 1975 Jun;45(2):111–21.

33. Staudinger UM, Glück J. Psychological wisdom research: Commonalities and differences in a growing field. Annual review of Psychology. 2011 Jan 10;62:215–41.

34. Ritchie PL, Grenier J. Branches of Psychology. PSYCHOLOGY–Volume I. 2009 Nov 29:62.

35. Lundh LG. Person, population, mechanism. Three main branches of psychological science. Journal for Person-Oriented Research. 2023;9(2):75.

36. Substance Abuse and Mental Health Services Administration. Managing Chronic Pain in Adults with or in Recovery From Substance Use Disorders. Treatment Improvement Protocol (TIP) Series 54. HHS Publication No. (SMA) 12–4671. Rockville, MD: Substance Abuse and Mental Health Services Administration, 2011.

37. Karime Mescouto, Rebecca E. Olson, Paul W. Hodges and Jenny Setchell. A critical review of the biopsychosocial model of low back pain care: Time for a new approach?, Disability and Rehabilitation, 2022, 44(13), 3270–84.

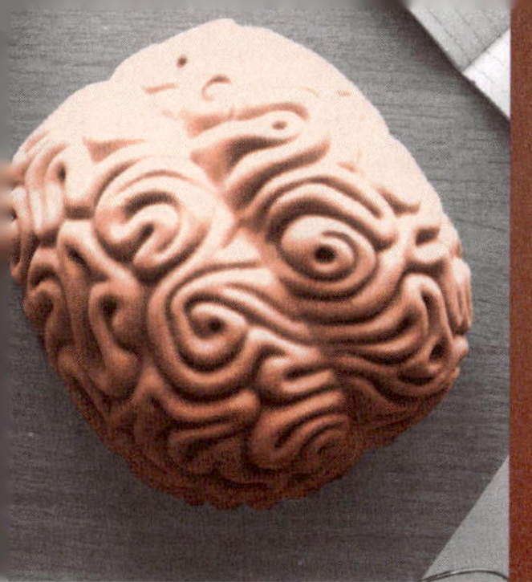

STUDENT ASSIGNMENT

LONG ANSWER QUESTIONS

1. What is psychology, and how does it contribute to our understanding of human behavior and mental processes? Explain various aspects of human cognition and behavior.
2. Write an overview of the historical development of psychology as a scientific discipline.
3. Different schools of psychology have shaped the evolution of psychological theory and research. Explain.
4. In what ways does pure psychology influence human behavior and mental processes? How do psychologists integrate pure psychology to form a comprehensive understanding of human psychology?
5. How does psychology contribute to addressing real-world issues and challenges, such as mental health disorders? What role do psychologists play in promoting individual and societal well-being?
6. Explain the scientific approach used in psychology to investigate questions about human behavior and mental processes.
7. How do psychologists and physiotherapists assess and diagnose mental health conditions, and what are the various approaches to treatment and therapy?
8. How do interdisciplinary collaborations enhance our understanding of complex psychological phenomena in diverse fields? Discuss.
9. What are some current trends and emerging areas of research in psychology? How do advancements in technology, such as artificial intelligence, virtual reality, and neuroimaging techniques, contribute to new discoveries and innovations in psychological science?

SHORT ANSWER QUESTIONS

1. What is psychology, and how does it contribute to our understanding of human behavior and mental processes?
2. What are the various aspects of human cognition and behavior that psychology explores?
3. Write about the historical development of psychology as a scientific discipline?
4. What are the core areas of practice, research, and application in psychology?
5. What are the ethical considerations and principles that guide psychological research and practice?
6. What are the levels of explanation in psychology?

MULTIPLE CHOICE QUESTIONS

1. **Which of the following is NOT a major goal of psychology?**
   a. Describing thoughts, feelings, and behaviors
   b. Predicting future actions and mental states
   c. Curing physical illnesses
   d. Explaining the causes of behavior

2. **The scientific study of both the mind and observable behaviors is the definition of:**
   a. Sociology
   b. Psychology
   c. Anthropology
   d. Neuroscience

3. **John B Watson, a prominent figure in psychology, is most associated with which school of thought?**
   a. Psychoanalysis
   b. Behaviorism
   c. Humanism
   d. Cognitive psychology

4. **Which of the following best describes the nature versus nurture debate in psychology?**
   a. The debate over free will versus determinism
   b. How much our genes and environment influence us
   c. The role of the conscious vs. unconscious mind
   d. Whether psychology should focus on thoughts or behaviors

5. **Who is credited with establishing the first psychology laboratory, marking a shift toward a more scientific approach?**
   a. Sigmund Freud
   b. William James
   c. BF Skinner
   d. Wilhelm Wundt

6. **The core tenet of Humanistic psychology emphasizes:**
   a. The role of the unconscious mind in behavior
   b. Learned behaviors through conditioning
   c. Breaking down the mind into basic elements
   d. Human potential and self-actualization

7. **Which school of thought views behavior and mental processes through the lens of natural selection and adaptation?**
   a. Functionalism
   b. Evolutionary psychology
   c. Structuralism
   d. Psychoanalysis

8. **The ethical principle of informed consent in psychological research ensures that participants:**
   a. Are aware of the study's purpose and potential risks
   b. Receive financial compensation for their participation
   c. Achieve a desired outcome from the research
   d. Will remain anonymous throughout the study

9. According to the cognitive perspective, what is the primary function of memory?
   a. To regulate emotions and motivations
   b. To store and retrieve information
   c. To drive us toward basic needs and desires
   d. To mediate conflict between the conscious and unconscious mind

10. The process of systematically collecting and analyzing data to answer psychological questions is known as:
   a. Introspection
   b. Self-actualization
   c. Hypothesis
   d. Psychological research

Note

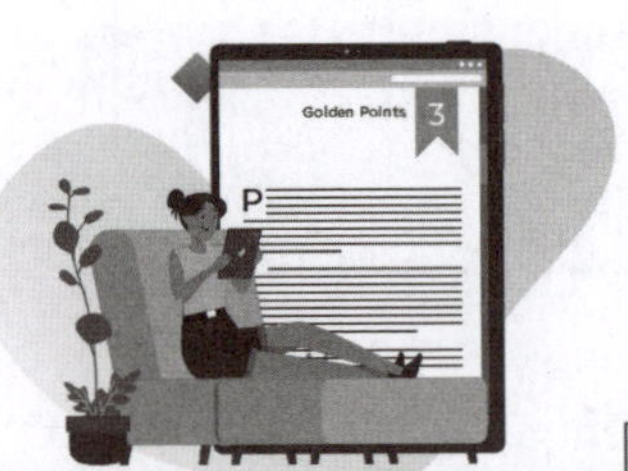

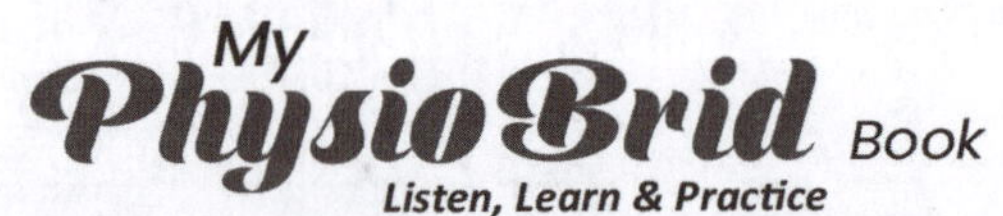

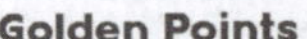

Golden Points	Solved Exercises	MCQs
Get Chapter-wise one liners in PODCAST form (audio) for quick revision of chapters	Subjective and objective exercises given in book with their solutions to evaluate and assess the complete chapter knowledge	Chapter-wise Multiple Choice Questions in Practice and Review mode to provide in-depth concept clarity

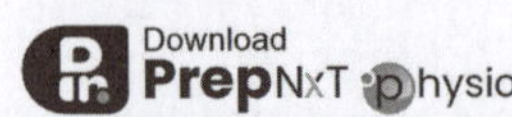

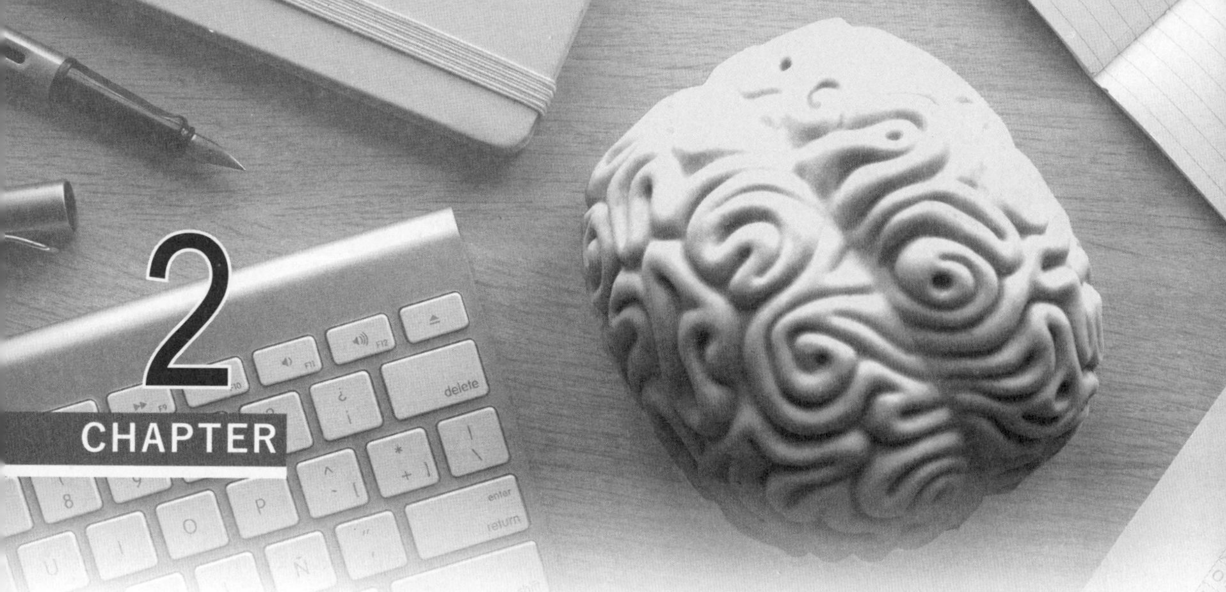

Growth and Development

Shweta Sharma, Ankita Sharma, Nishchint Banga, Parul Sharma

LEARNING OBJECTIVES

After the completion of the chapter, the readers will be able to:
- Differentiate between growth (increase in size) and development (functional maturation) across life stages.
- Explain key developmental theories, including those by Freud, Erikson, Piaget, and Vygotsky.
- Identify developmental milestones for cognitive, physical, and emotional growth.
- Assess the impact of genetic and environmental factors on growth and development.
- Discuss the role of social and cultural contexts in shaping individual development.
- Understand challenges and interventions in developmental psychology across different ages.

CHAPTER OUTLINE

- Introduction
- Definition and Importance
- Principles of Development
- Theoretical Perspectives
- Prenatal Development
- Infancy
- Early Childhood
- Middle Childhood
- Adolescence
- Adulthood
- Aging Process
- Cross-Cultural Variations in Developmental Milestones
- Applications of Developmental Psychology
- Current Research and Future Directions

KEY TERMS

Biological theories of aging: Theories that focus on the physiological processes that lead to aging, including the rate of living theory, free radical theory, and telomere shortening theory.

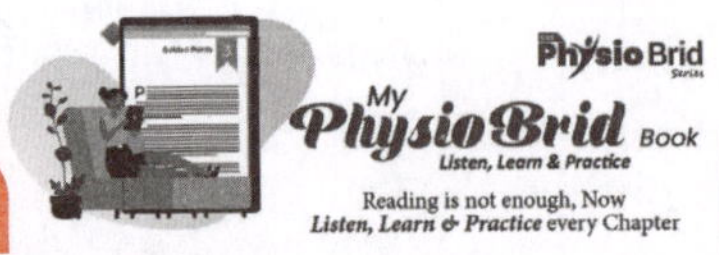

Bowlby's attachment theory: A theory developed by John Bowlby that emphasizes the importance of early interactions with caregivers for children's development and the lasting impact of attachment patterns on social life.

Empathy: The ability to understand and share the feelings of another.

Formal operational stage: A stage of cognitive development from about age 12 onward, characterized by the ability to think abstractly and engage in critical thinking.

Growth and development: Growth refers to the increase in size or mass, while development includes changes in shape, structure, and functions, leading to maturity.

Hypothesis: A proposed explanation or prediction made on the basis of limited evidence as a starting point for further investigation.

Neurolinguistics: The study of the neural mechanisms in the brain that control and underlie linguistic behaviors.

Protodeclarative pointing: Pointing by infants and young children to express interest or to communicate with others.

INTRODUCTION

This chapter provides a thorough exploration of the human developmental process from conception to late adulthood. It begins with a detailed introduction that delineates the distinctions between growth and development, emphasizing their interdependent nature. The initial sections are dedicated to defining these terms and explaining their significance across various stages of life, accompanied by an examination of the critical factors influencing developmental outcomes, such as genetic predispositions and environmental impacts.

Following the introduction, the chapter delves into the theoretical frameworks that have shaped our understanding of human development. This includes a discussion of major developmental theories proposed by Freud, Erikson, Piaget, and Vygotsky, each highlighting different aspects of psychological and physical maturation. Theories are contextualized within the stages of development they describe, from prenatal phases through childhood, adolescence, adulthood, and finally aging. Each section is structured to introduce the developmental milestones associated with each stage, supplemented by real-world applications and implications for education, parenting, and clinical practice.

The chapter concludes with a comprehensive look at the challenges and interventions related to developmental disorders. It outlines common developmental disruptions and their symptoms, explores the role of early diagnosis, and discusses intervention strategies. This segment underscores the importance of a nurturing environment and early intervention in mitigating developmental delays and enhancing the well-being of individuals across their lifespan. The chapter aims to provide readers with a foundational understanding of developmental psychology, equipping them with the knowledge to recognize normal and atypical development patterns.

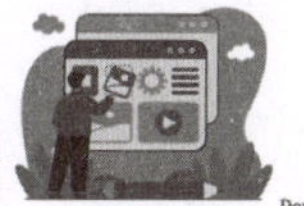

DEFINITION AND IMPORTANCE

The transition from childhood to adulthood is a period of growth and development, two separate but related processes. Quantitatively, growth represents the increase in size and mass of tissues over time but this is largely due to an accumulation of cells (cell proliferation) and intracellular substances rather than maturation of functions. Development as a process implies any quantitative change like growing bigger; including functionally regulatory processes led into maturation with advancement or differentiation especially well documented in the nervous system.[1]

The exponential increase in cell number during the early embryonic period reflects division and differentiation of fetal cells to populate tissues (and form organs). The rise in cell size is here associated mainly with the protein to deoxyribonucleic acid (DNA) ratio that presupposes a higher total cellular protein content after mid-pregnancy and stays elevated into early childhood. Cell size enlargement goes on until approximately 10 years of age.[1]

A delicate balance exists within the body with cells being renewed through aging and they cascade out as old, but new emerge. Different tissues have different rates of cell turnover (turnover time is the time to replace or repair all tissues that contain cells). Although growth and development are often considered in a separate light, they both remain interlinked as they are directly dependent on the root stakeholders influencing them.[1]

Growth and development are crucial natural changes that every individual goes through from the time of conception to maturity. Growth is the increase in size by number or mass while development includes change in shape, structure and functions like maturity (e.g., nervous system). There are continuous and reciprocal interactions between exposure processes, which change throughout an individual's life that lead to growth and development.[2]

There are principles for how things conveniently grow (or decay) which determine the path and texture of maturational change. These principles or properties of development portray typical growth as a more expected, systematic course. Children display unique personalities, activity levels, and developmental timing as part of their growth stages. However, there are universal principles and patterns-based on milestones and they guide their development.[3]

PRINCIPLES OF DEVELOPMENT

- **Development happens from the top down:** This is referred to as the **cephalocaudal** precept. This principle outlines the route of evolutionary growth. The child moves the head, then arms and finally legs as per this principle. By 2 months, infants begin to gain control of their head and face movements. They pull themselves up using their arms in the next several months. Infants are more likely to gain control of their legs between 6 and 12 months (use of the word "likely" because all babies develop at different rates) leading them closer toward crawling, standing or walking. Legs follow arms in acquiring coordination.[4]

- **Proximodistal trend in child development: From core to extremities:** This helps explain the onset of development or why one develops from 'the inside out,' as represented by what is known

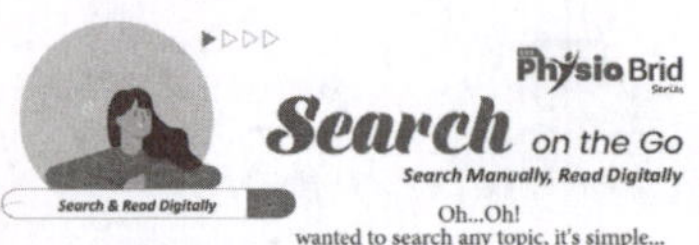

as the **proximodistal** principle of development. One of the examples is the way in which a spinal cord develops before the extremities. In contrast, the child will develop arms first then hands and feet before fingers over toes. Fine motor dexterity muscles—those of the fingers and toes, are among the last to develop in that area.[5]

- **Development requires maturity and learning:** Growth and development work sequentially leading to maturation. Biological events take place serially and confer new powers on a child. Brain and the nervous system-related changes explain growth to a great extent. These altercations in the brain, and nervous system make children learn faster or enhance other cognitive (thinking) as well as physical abilities. Additionally, children have to be developmentally ready for the next set of skills. For instance, a baby of 4 months does not possess the function to communicate through speech as the infant has not developed enough to speak and its brain is not prepared yet. By the age of 2 years, a child's brain has developed significantly, enabling them to speak a few words. The child has a vocabulary of around 50–100 words and can form simple sentences. A child who cannot hold a pencil/crayon will not be able to write or draw. Maturational patterns are hereditary which means that growth and development of every individual are determined genetically. Optimal development of the child is achieved through input from a healthy environment and learning that emerges out of experience. Good and different experiences provide an environment of excitement for the development of a child to reach its full potential.[4]

- **As with learning, development unfolds from the general (simple) to the specific:** This principle refers to the use of cognitive and language abilities for reasoning, thinking and sorting problems. A crucial ability used in cognitive development is learning the relationships between things. This is also known as classification. Learning how an apple and orange can be seen the same way is the process that begins by first thinking in even more simplest form or more concrete reasoning about the two items and what we know describes them. Devoid of any relationship, then the preschooler will name objects by some sort of property it possesses, for example, color. To prompt with, "an apple is red", (or green) and an orange is a certain shade of color, and a description or relationship between two objects, and objects can be considered to be alike when they possess the same attributes. Young children typically respond with "An apple and orange are round" or even, "an apple and orange are alike because we eat them!" For instance, when a child develops it cognitive ability, it can also formulate a concept at the higher level that says apple and orange belong to the category of fruit. The child could then categorize the information cognitively.[5]

- **Development is a never-ending process:** With the progress of a child from childhood to adulthood, additional skills are modified. Children grow abilities allowing for further improved masteries. The steps of development are mostly taken by the children. One period of growth sets the stage for another period of development. For example, with motor development, before a child walks there are predictable steps she will go through as eventual precursors to walking. The infants can raise and turn the head even before they can roll over. Before they can grasp an object, infants must be able to move their limbs (arms and legs).

Skills grow from hanging on to walking unaided even during ascending stairs. They usually walk up and down stairs using alternate feet at the age of 4-year-old. With development, it is necessary to first get the manual (hand) control of holding the pencil or crayon prior to writing any letters.[4]

- **Development and growth progress from the universal to individual:** In motor development, the infant might be able to grasp an object with the whole hand before using only the thumb and forefinger. The infant's first motor movements are very generalized, undirected, and reflexive; the infant waves arms or kicks before it can reach or creep toward an object. Growth is from large muscle movement to more refined or smaller muscle movement.[5]

- **Growth and development are personal:** Every single child is different and each individual grows at a totally unique rate. While the sequences and patterns for growth and development are typical, their rates vary greatly among individual children. This knowledge that children develop at different rates means to be careful about using typical age and stage descriptions or indeed ascribing to them regulatory settings for recognition by comparators. The accomplishment of any developmental need is spread over an age bracket. This is not the idea of the "typical kid". A few could possibly be walking at 10 months while others may not walk until 18 months of age. They may be a little more active than other kids. It does not mean the child who walks at 18 months will be an adult with less intelligence. Comparing one child and its path to that of another has no merit. Additionally, the rate of development is not even within a single child. An individual may, for instance have an intellectual development on the level of a much older enquiry rather than his emotional or social ways.[6]

THEORETICAL PERSPECTIVES

There have been perhaps thousands of proposed or planned theories about child development made by theorists and researchers over the years (Fig. 2.1). Most of the major child development theories are referred to as grand theories; they attempt to address all aspects of development, frequently in a staged approach. Some are called micro-theories and concentrate instead only on a rather small area of development, like cognitive or mental growth.

Freud's Theory of Psychosexual Development

Freud's theory of psychosexual development originated from the source of psychoanalysis, suggested to be the early work of Sigmund Freud. Freud himself was a clinician who had worked with mentally ill patients and he related the experiences of these people to early childhood events/ignored wishes.[7] One of the earliest and most influential grand theories is attributed to Freud, who described child growth as a series of psychosexual stages during which libido seeks gratification *via* different body zones.[8] The idea was that libido energy is concentrated on certain erogenous zones at different life stages—failing to move through one stage could result in unresolved conflict with lasting adult

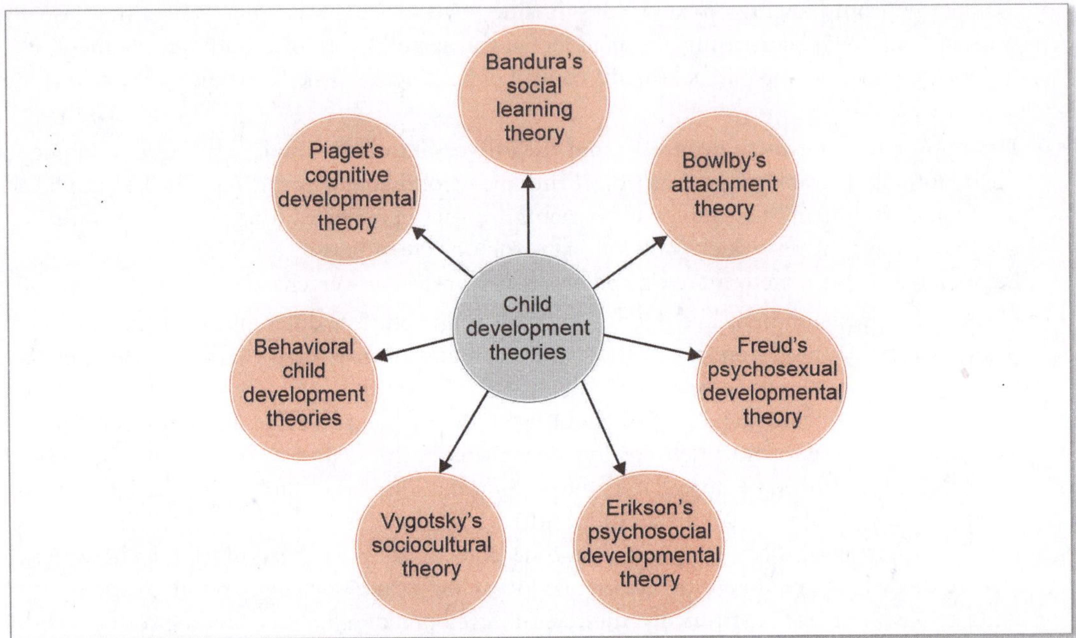

Fig. 2.1: Child development theories

personality traits.[9] If the conflicts of a stage are not successfully resolved, this can lead to fixations which may then be carried over into adult behavior.

Erikson's Psychosocial Developmental Theory

Psychoanalytic theory ruled the roost in mid-20th century. The work of Freud allowed his followers to modify and develop new theories. Erik Erikson's eight-stage theory of psychosocial development proved to be the most influential.[10] Erikson's theory differed from Freud's by emphasizing social interaction and experience over sexual interest as the essential motivating force in development.[11] This developmental biopsychosocial model covered development from birth to death, with each stage involving a crisis that significantly impacts the individual.[12] Navigating the difficulties of each stage results in a psychological virtue that is useful for life.

Behavioral Child Development Theories

Theories of learning that arose from 1913 through the mid-1940s constitute a new school of movement in psychology known as behaviorism. Behaviorists argued that psychology should only address behaviors that are observable and measurable.[13] John B Watson and B F Skinner proposed behaviorist theories that placed importance upon external environment as a determinate of behaviors.[14] This approach culminated in two essential types of learning—classical conditioning and

 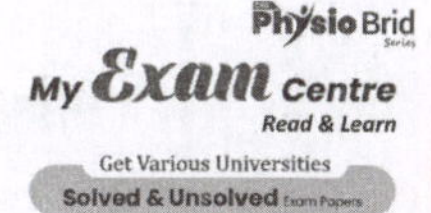

operant conditioning.[15] This theory is in stark contrast to many other child development theories as it does not consider any internal thoughts or feelings. Rather, it is entirely about what experience makes us.

Piaget's Cognitive Developmental Theory

Jean Piaget's theory of cognitive development suggests that children's cognitive development occurs in four stages mentioned below, each building on the previous one. Piaget's theory is based on the idea that children's thinking and behavior change as they progress through these stages. He also believed that children develop schemas or mental templates, to understand the world. These schemas are formed through experience and grow and adapt as children learn new things.

His schema includes sensorimotor, preoperational, concrete operational and abstract or formal operational stages.[16] Each stage is associated with distinct cognitive processes and ways of engaging in the world.

1. **Sensorimotor stage:** In Piaget's theory, the stage (from birth to about 2 years of age) during which infants know the world mostly in terms of object permanence is developed; first senses and motor activities, as its own reflexes.[17]

2. **Preoperational stage:** The second Piagetian stage lasts from 2 to 6 years during which a child learns language and continues to learn through prelogical thinking. Children at this stage have not developed concrete logic. This means they cannot yet mentally manipulate information and take on the point of view others.[17]

3. **Concrete operational stage:** A stage of cognitive development (about age 7–11) during which children gain a better understanding of mental operations. Children acquire the abilities to think logically, but their ability is limited comparing with what they are about to reach in a little later stage of cognitive faculty-ability to easily conceptualize hypotheticals or ideas.[17]

4. **Formal operational stage:** Age range from about 12 and the rest of the life where people develop critical thinking. This is the stage at which features like reasoning, deductive logic and methodical planning emerge.[17]

Bowlby's Attachment Theory

According to John Bowlby, one of the original authors of attachment theory, the earliest interactions with caregivers are of vital importance to children's development, and attachment patterns continue to affect one's social life later in life.[18] For example, "Children are biologically programmed to develop attachments. It is through attachment that human beings survive: Through attachment, infants ensure that they will be fed, cared for, and otherwise protected".[19] More studies into the attachment theory and its principles have been conducted since Bowlby. Nowadays, there are numerous attachment styles, secure, ambivalent, avoidant, disorganized, and so forth.[20] Thus, the behaviors designed to ensure proximity to caregivers are performed by both sides, and also providing proximity maintenance, the use of a caregiver as a secure base and safe haven for exploration by exploring children.[21]

Bandura's Social Learning Theory

According to Albert Bandura, we cannot explain human learning with just conditioning and reinforcement. According to the social learning theory, people learn from one another, *via* observation, imitation, modeling, attention, retention, reproduction, and motivation.[22] Modeling behaviors or information can lead to learning of new behavior and knowledge by children. For example, from a parent or otherwise peer.[23] Observational learning has long been mentioned as a way of acquiring new behaviors and knowledge.[24] The role of learning through observation is said to be pivotal in Bandura's child development theory.[25]

Vygotsky's Sociocultural Theory

According to the sociocultural theory of Lev Vygotsky, children learn dynamically and are rewarded for engaging in encounters that generate higher-order functions due to their organizational development.[26] In Vygotskian theory, the 'zone of proximal development' refers to the difference between what a person can achieve independently and what they can achieve with guidance and support. This concept highlights the potential for learning when assistance is provided, enabling individuals to function independently at a higher level.[27] Vygotsky-learning is a social process. Learning takes place as folktales interact with others on similar or higher skill levels through taking part in shared culturally valued activities and objects (Vygotsky, 1978).[28]

PRENATAL DEVELOPMENT

Stages of Prenatal Development

Prenatal period is also a critical stage in the development and to understand real-time brain changes, one has to consider child developmental stages starting with infancy. The stage of prenatal development, in turn is the period where most rapid changes occur and requires clean slate status to mimic future psychological developments.[29] The brain grows at an astonishing rate throughout the perinatal period and even more so during early childhood, as a substantial proportion of synapses would already be present by age 3.[30]

The first 2 weeks after fertilization are called the germinal stage, the third through eighth week is referred to as embryonic stage and from there until birth is called fetal stage.[31]

Germinal Stage

The initial stage starts from the day of fertilization when sperm gets penetrated through corona radiata and zona pellucida layers to reach the egg directly in (one of two) fallopian tubes.[32] The fertilized egg, now called a zygote, then begins to travel toward the uterus and it can take up to 7 days for this to complete.[33] Development of the new organism starts at around 24–36 hours after fertilization.[34] The single-celled zygote now sets off on its journey down the fallopian tube to reach maternal uterine cavity where it starts developing into a multicellular organism.[35] The zygote

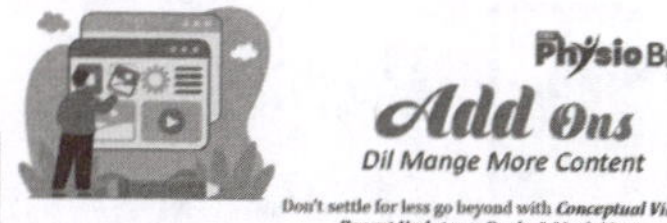

undergoes the process of cell division known as mitosis first to form two cells then four, eight and so on.[36] Many zygotes are lost at this stage of cell division; up to 50% of all zygotes may perish in the first few weeks.[37]

After this point, the cells start to differentiate into distinct types of cells which they eventually develop into.[38] When cells start to proliferate, they divide into two different populations; outer cell mass which will finally form the placenta and inner cell mass that gives rise to the embryo.[40] Cell division still happens at very fast rate and the cells are on their way to becoming what is called a blastocyst.[34] The blastocyst consists of three layers; the ectoderm (the future skin and nervous system); the endoderm (which will become digestive and respiratory systems) and the mesodermal layer.[32] The blastocyst is pushed out of the tube and into the uterus, where it sticks to its lining in a process called implantation.[35] The process of implantation is when these cells nestle themselves into the uterine lining, rupturing minuscule blood vessels. Thus, the connective web of blood vessels and intervening membranes will suffice to nourish the developing being for its subsequent nine months.[38] In short, implantation is not guaranteed.[34]

Embryonic Stage

This mass of cells is now called an embryo. The onset of the third week after conception introduces to embryonic period, a critical phase when this mass becomes recognizably human.[31] The embryonic phase of brain growth is crucial.[34] The blastocyst becomes the embryo creating three layers that later become main body systems.[37] The neural tube develops 22 days after the conception. This tube closely develops into nerves, including the spinal cord and brain.[35] Neural tube originates from an area known as the neural plate. In the human embryo, two ridges develop along each side of the neural plate as a first indication for neural development.[38] In the following days, more ridges form and then collapse inward to create a hollow tube. These cells start to migrate toward the center when this tube has been completely formed.[36] Closing of tube starts and brain vesicles form. Each of these vesicles grows into one part of the mature brain (different components in each case—the forebrain, midbrain, and hind brain) to which they correspond.[32] By week 4, the head begins to take shape starting with its eyes, nose, ears and mouth. The heart is the first organ to initiate function as a part of cardiovascular system. At 9th day, mesoblasts form blood vessel and primordium itself starts beating. During following week, buds develop into arms and legs sprout.[34] At the end of week 8, all basic parts and organs (other than the forming in baby's genitals) have been formed. It even has knees and elbows.[37] Now, the embryo is only 1 g in weight and approx. an inch long. At the end of this embryonic period, prime determinants for brain and central nervous system structure have been formed.[38] By this level of development, the general layout of both central and peripheral nervous system is also in place.[35]

Fetal Stage

When cell specialization is largely finished, the embryo enters into the next stage as a fetus.[31] Changes in the brain during fetal period of prenatal development are more significant.[29] This period

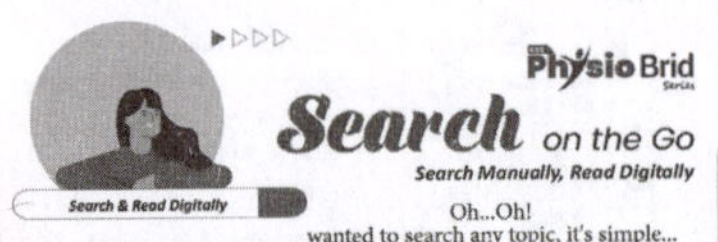

of development begins at week 9 and continues until birth.[30] It is at this time in prenatal development that the neural tube differentiates into the brain and spinal cord, with neurons continuing to be generated.[37] Once these neurons are born, they have to migrate into the correct locations.[38] However, other research suggests that synapses—the bridges between neurons—also start to grow.[36] Neonatal reflex programs begin at birth, leading to early repetitive limb movements that become more coordinated by 9–12 weeks.[36]

Factors Influencing Prenatal Development

Genetic Factors

Intelligence of parents and their education level has direct correlation with the final intelligence quotient (IQ) of the child. In addition, certain developmental patterns follow parental patterns, such as speech. There are countless causes of genetic developmental delay and subsequent Mental Retardation (MR). Prominent examples of such etiology are chromosomal abnormalities, X-linked MR, subtelomeric deletions, single-gene disorders causing disorders of brain formation, and other metabolic disorders.[41, 42]

Maternal Factors

A host of factors that impair growth in utero can also potentially affect brain growth, particularly if they are severe and/or sustained.

- **Maternal nutrition:** Malnutrition of maternal dietary intake (both macronutrients and micronutrients) is suggested to have long-term consequences on birth weight as well as postpartum child development. Research from resource-limited settings indicates potentially beneficial effects of nutritional supplementation for birth weight and possibly child development. Research throughout recent decades has indicated the ability of variations in global quality of maternal care to result in persistent stress-hyporesponsiveness, anxiety and abnormal memory formations in offspring.[43, 44]

- **Drugs and toxicants exposure:** Different types of drugs as well as toxins such as maternal drug abuse, alcohol, antiepileptic drugs, environmental factors can inhibit the development in child.[45]

- **Fetoplacental disorders:** In addition to acquired infections, like syphilis, toxoplasmosis, AIDS, malnutrition leading to starvation of the fetus, impairs both physical and brain growth. Oxidative stress in utero (e.g., chorioamnionitis) has been linked to cerebral palsy and developmental impairment.[46, 47]

INFANCY

Development proceeds from cephalocaudal end and also from the midline to lateral direction. The developmental milestone may be achieved within 3–4 months difference. An example of this is that social development, a cortical function rather than motor skill, develops before motor behavior.

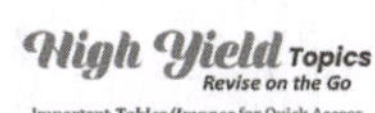

No social smile by 4 weeks is worrisome. Newborns are born with primitive reflexes. It is important to realize that some primitive reflexes serve a physiological role for the normal infant. When feeding is performed inefficiently, the sucking and rooting reflex aids it. The primitive reflex goes away in most cases to allow the normal aging process. For example, the grasp reflex dissipates at six months and mature grasp develops from 6 to 12 months.[2]

Physical Development

The physical development of a child includes growth in size and proportion, along with muscle coordination and control. This aspect of development is crucial as it lays the foundation for more complex motor skills. For example, around 5 months of age, a child typically begins to demonstrate significant physical milestones. During this period, infants start learning to roll over, an essential skill that indicates the strengthening of core muscles and coordination. Additionally, they gain better control over their head movements, being able to lift and hold their head steady while lying on their abdomen or sitting up with support. These early physical activities are crucial as they pave the way for subsequent developmental milestones such as sitting, crawling, and eventually walking. Proper nutrition, a stimulating environment, and opportunities for physical activity are essential factors that support this aspect of a child's growth and development.[48–52]

Cognitive Development

Cognitive development in children refers to their ability to learn and solve problems, a crucial aspect of their overall growth.[16] This process includes the acquisition and utilization of knowledge, problem-solving skills, and the capacity to think abstractly and logically. For example, a 2-month-old baby begins to explore the environment using its hands and eyes, a fundamental cognitive milestone.[53] This exploration allows the infant to start understanding the world around, developing sensory and motor coordination as it interacts with different objects and stimuli.[54] As children grow, their cognitive skills become more complex. By the age of 3 years, they are capable of more advanced tasks, such as memorizing and reciting poems. This ability to memorize not only highlights their improving memory capacity but also their understanding of language and rhythm.[27] These cognitive advancements are supported by various factors, including the child's interactions with caregivers, exposure to a stimulating environment, and opportunities for play and exploration. Proper cognitive development during early childhood lays the foundation for future learning and academic success.[55]

Social and Emotional Development

Social development in children involves learning and discovering the expectations and rules for interacting with others. This process starts early in life and continues throughout childhood. For instance, when a child smiles at the mother, it demonstrates an early form of social interaction, indicating the child's ability to recognize and respond to familiar faces.[19] This initial form of social communication is foundational, as it helps to build trust and attachment, which are crucial for later social relationships.

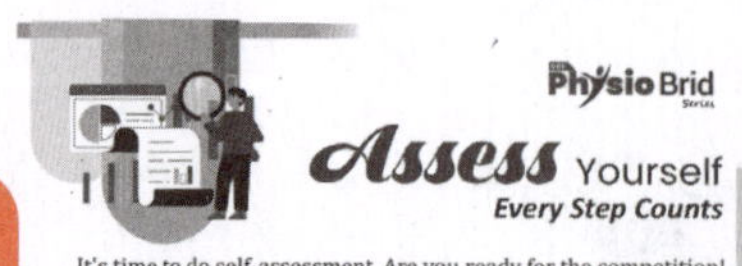

As children grow, their social skills become more sophisticated.[56] By engaging in cooperative play, children learn important social rules such as sharing, taking turns, and understanding others' perspectives. Cooperative play not only enhances their social skills but also their ability to work as part of a team, laying the groundwork for successful interactions in school and later in life.[57]

Emotional development is the ability to recognize and understand feelings and respond to them appropriately. This aspect of development is crucial for a child's overall well-being and mental health.[58] For example, a child may feel insecure at the arrival of a new baby in the family. This situation can trigger feelings of jealousy or fear of losing parental attention. Recognizing and addressing these emotions helps the child manage their feelings in a healthy way.[59] Emotional development also involves learning how to express emotions appropriately, such as using words to describe feelings rather than resorting to tantrums or aggression. Parents and caregivers play a vital role in modelling and teaching appropriate emotional responses, which helps children develop emotional intelligence and resilience (Fig. 2.2).[60]

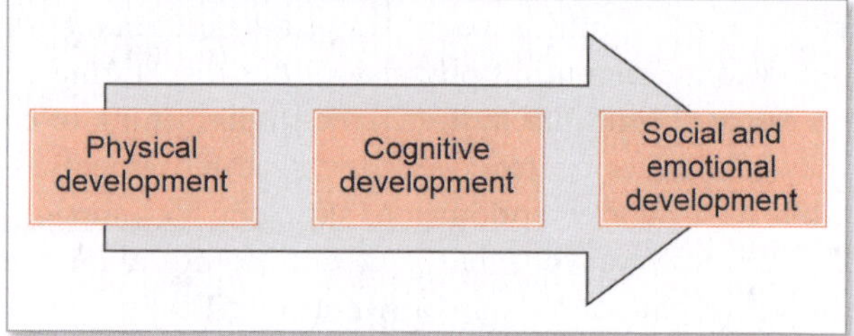

Fig. 2.2: Progression of developmental milestones

> **MUST KNOW**
>
> Key developmental milestones for physiotherapists to know and recognize:
> - **Gross motor skills:** Rolling over, sitting, crawling, standing, walking, running, jumping, and climbing.
> - **Fine motor skills:** Reaching, grasping, manipulating objects, hand-eye coordination.
> - **Social and emotional skills:** Interaction with caregivers and peers, expression of emotions.
> - **Cognitive skills:** Problem-solving, following instructions, attention span.

EARLY CHILDHOOD

Physical and Language Development

Developmental milestones have been established in gross and fine motor skills, self-help, problem-solving, social/emotional, and receptive and expressive language domains.

- **Neonatal:** The first 4 weeks after being born provide the groundwork for the baby's entire year. Parents, in turn, learn to meet the needs of their newborn by establishing feeding and sleeping schedules as well as times when infants are alert. Babies learn to follow faces, discriminate mothers' voices from others', cry, make sounds with their throats and lift the head when prone. Babies begin to form attachments with their parents through the voice that they hear when born and indeed prenatally. Babies learn that they can trust their caregivers to take care of them, so already at these early days the baby begins to feel safe.[61] All neonates should be risk-factor-screened; and babies beyond the newborn period, who do not startle to noise

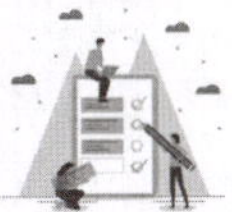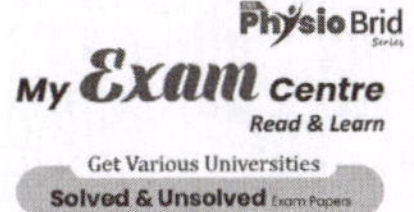

or follow objects within a few feet of their face, warrant referral for hearing (and vision) evaluations. Infants who are hypotonic and have difficulty feeding or moving should be referred for evaluation. When examining infants, neonatal protective reflexes are a good way for the clinician to gauge neurologic and motor function.[62]

- **2 months:** By around 6 weeks of age, infants typically begin to exhibit a 'social smile'. This smile, which is a response to interactions with caregivers rather than a reflex, marks the early development of social engagement, easily transitioning from a previously expressionless face to smiling when seeing their parents. By 2 months of age, infants begin to coo and gurgle in response to caregivers. With this ability, they begin to bring their hands together at midline.[63, 64]

- **4 months:** Head-lag with pull to sit is no longer present by 4 months of age. Baby is beginning to roll from front-to-back. Rolling from front to back might be delayed, but it is normal if the infant prefers sleeping on his abdomen and then tries sitting. Babies sometimes just roll one way first. Babies engage in both visually focused activities (like looking at photographs) and manual ones like reaching for objects effectively. Right around this time they can upright a stick or rattle it. Laughter erupts, blossoms unexpectedly from others; interaction blooms.[65, 66]

- **6 months:** Roll supine to prone; sit with hands propped in front. They can stand for a short time when held upright, push down on their legs in standing if supported and use both hands to transfer an object from one hand to the other whilst sitting. They can pick up things and hold them in the hand (two objects at once). Infants can feed themselves easy foods and may hold their own bottle. At this age, transition occurs from cooing (producing vowel sounds like aaah and oooo) to babbling (using consonants with replicating noises of sounds such as ba, ma, da), etc. They smile and coo in front of mirror. They experience separation anxiety with familiar faces and dislike being left with strangers; 6-month-old infants show more wariness toward strangers, but the presence of their caregivers comfort them.[67, 68]

- **9 months:** By 9 months, children pull to stand and creep or cruise around.

  - **Preseated play:** Infants can squat to the floor or a low seat and from this position they are able to start playing with toys (opening/closing objects, put in/take out of containers), bang toys/blocks together, hold food while taking bites.

  - **Eye gaze monitoring:** To watch for where an adult is looking (a precursor of joint attention) starts at this age. 9-month-old babies care about what is around and find them interesting and want to play along! These babies respond to commands, and they may start saying dada/papa or mama in babble.[69, 70]

- **12 months:** One year of age brings about a lot of changes in their little life. This is the age at which children begin to walk and talk.

  - As communication and mobility continue to increase, these changes have reverberations for learning across all disciplines.[71, 72] At 12 months, most but not all infants can stand well with legs wide set and arms out or overhead. They walk by themselves or with a caregiver's assistance. They have mastered the art of chucking objects and are able to experience gravity firsthand, deftly flinging items over the side of their high chair or stroller.

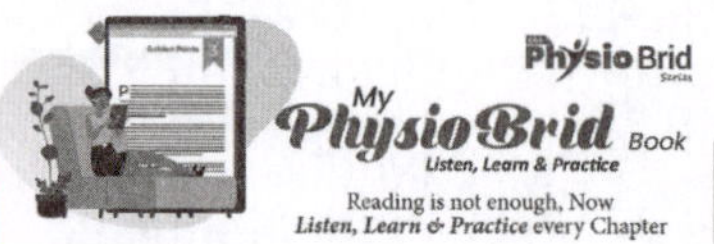

- **Dressing:** 1-year-old ones cooperate in dressing, remove own hat and socks. They finger feed themselves using a mature pincer grasp. They search for toys that they hide in places and complain to adults whenever they think they need help.

- **Protoimperative pointing** is the kind of pointing that children do to try and access something in which they are interested, a hugely significant behavior for newly mobile infants who must now learn about their own desires. It is an age where the children understand "no" and ask questions (albeit it doesn't mean they will obey) to using words.[71, 72]

- **15 months:** Past their first birthday, many new skills slowly emerge in children.

  - **Speaking:** Babbles or jargons (string of vowels and consonants that sounds like sentences, but with little or no meaningful words).

  - Children begin to identify body parts or point to real objects in books when asked and obey a command (e.g., go get your shoes so that we can go to the park). They can also hold and manipulate a book page (an essential step for early reading) and stack 10 cubes in a cup, pellets into small container, circle puzzle piece to targeted spot.

  - By this age, one key skill is **protodeclarative pointing** (pointing to show interest). They can draw with crayons on paper and can build a tower of 3 cubes. This is when empathy starts because children can now feel happy or sad with a friend or family member.[73, 74]

- **18 months:** Children at 18 months should run, sit down on a chair (with or without assistance), build four squares high tower with cubes and imitate vertical strokes using a crayon. They love to pretend they are talking on the phone, driving a car or having tea. At this stage, children become aware of the sense that some things belong to them and they start to talk like 'mine'. When they do something wrong, shame, guilt or sadness come at this age and also they can now decide what actions to take. Only 10–25% of children at 18 months use few words (kids with 'delayed' language). At this stage, they identify familiar faces (including recognize-self-in-mirror), point to pictures, occasionally snort toward reasoning-image/familiar object can be seen.[75, 76]

- **2 years:** Welcome to the 2-year-old world folks. A 24-month-old would be kicking a ball, throwing overhand and starting to practice jumping. They emulate black circles and horizontal lines. They start to undress themselves (a crucial marker in potty-training) and can even open certain doors by turning the knob. They play with peers doing the same activity together but rarely are they cooperatively doing it. They can also appear defiant or mask certain emotions when it is socially acceptable. At 2 years of age, children use 50–200 words and combine two or more words in sentences that have a noun and verb.[77, 78]

- **3 years:** At 3 years, imaginary play takes off into the stratosphere of interaction: Playing with others and being creative. From 3 years onward, most can label their own sex and that of same-sex friends. 3-year-old children can also begin to grasp their sense of right and left (from their perspective as the opposite side from mom) and they know where things are placed. Kids can learn to draw a circle, climb up on the jungle gym and run faster than before. Sentences become paragraphs, and children start to make contribution in two-way conversation. A gifted student

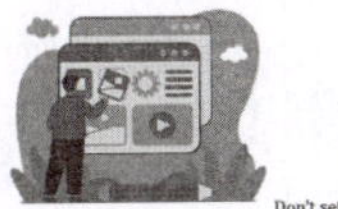

may be able to experience imaginative fears, just as a 3-year-old does, and talk about things that other might not understand.[79, 80]

- **4 years:** Children can achieve better balance and can hop on one foot a few times consecutively. They can stand on one foot for 4–8 seconds, hop a few inches forward, and gallop. 4-year-old children can make a cross and square with crayon, draw by copying, tie a knot or cut paper. In all probability, they can draw a person with 4–6 parts. They can tell 5–6 colors and random letters, may count out loud from one-to-four but often not beyond that by rote memorization and some may even be able to point or recognize other signs (like STOP) of things they are interested in areas/stores/brands. They can go to the bathroom by themselves, brush and wash their face/hands mannerly, and start using fork. They may have certain friends they prefer over others, recognize different feelings and begin to play with other children.[81, 82]

- **5 years:** Once the children turn 5, they are entering the "school age" years.

    - Their balance increases to over 8 seconds per side, they can hop on one foot for 15 repetitions on each leg and are able to skip. They can imitate a triangle, cut scrapes with scissors, string their names and build stairs using block. They get themselves ready in the morning, can take a bath on their own. Some examples of children without disability include generate person figure with 8–10 parts, identify coins.

    - Language—recite alphabet, count out loud, etc. Children at this age may even skip letters or give a set of numbers out of sequence[85] and they may still reverse write letters or numerals. Rhyming is a skill of potentially greater importance than others in the same category. Some studies suggest that it may be a more effective predictor of early success in phonemic awareness and literacy development. Kindergarteners recognize the sounds of most consonants and short vowels, can read 25 words (or more) relevant to them by year's end. Kindergarten: Making friends and feeling happy for their friends when good things happen. Children at this age should know 2,000 or more words and be able to define a simple word; use sentences appropriately; memorize his phone number or address. They can answer why questions. Most children are fond of reading and they can even remember stories.[83, 84]

Psychosocial Development

Erikson endorses eight stages of psychosocial development (Fig. 2.3):

1. **Trust and mistrust:** Infant develops trust only if a warm caretaker who attends to his needs responds. The opposite is true, and children develop mistrust under the same conditions.

2. **Autonomy and doubt:** Infants are encouraged to be autonomous and not doubt their abilities.

3. **Initiative and guilt:** Preschool children explore to realize their potentiality by playing imagination. However, children will be guilty of their origin if the parent fails to develop a sense of initiative.

4. **Industry and inferiority:** Early school children begin to cooperate with others, and if peers are mean, children believe they are inferior.

5. **Identity and role diffusion:** Self-identity is a multidimensional aspect during adolescence.

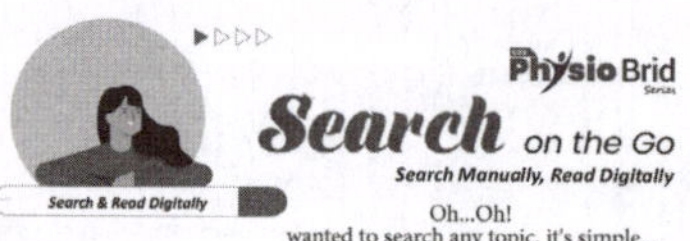

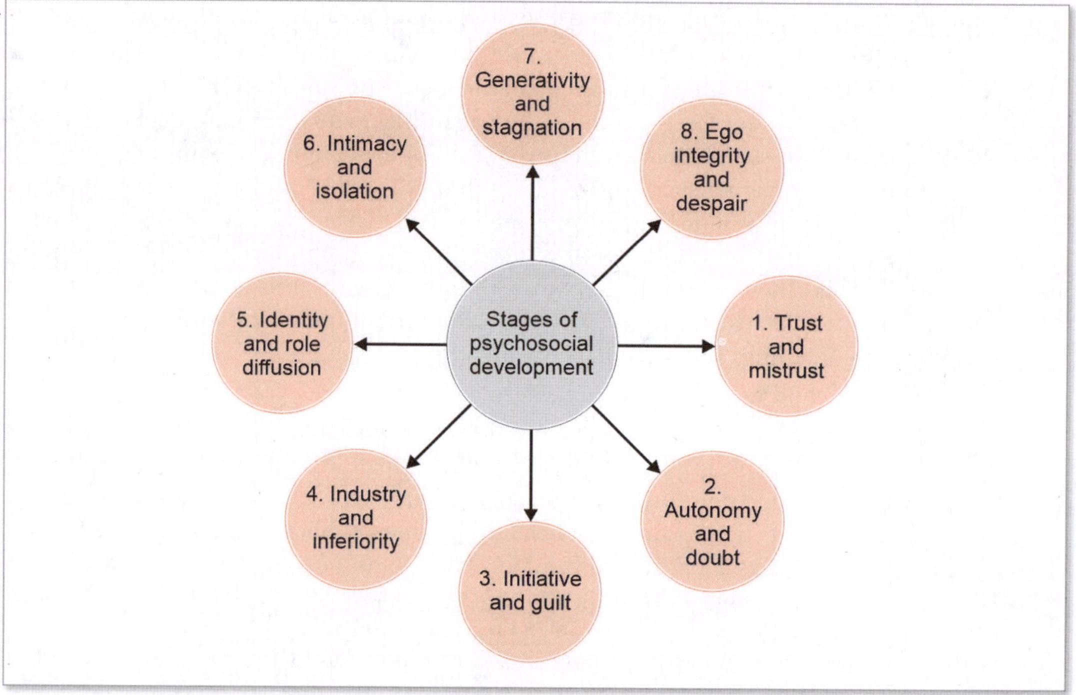

Fig. 2.3: Stages of psychosocial development

6. **Intimacy and isolation:** In early adulthood, failure to form an association leads to solitariness.
7. **Generativity and stagnation:** In middle adulthood, children learn how to properly guide others, and parenting is the best model.
8. **Ego integrity and despair:** In late adulthood, teaching the youth helps people to feel contempt or despair.[5]

MIDDLE CHILDHOOD

Cognitive Development

Piaget called the period of time between 6- and 11-years, concrete operational thought. While later research has shown that certain forms of logical thought take root much earlier in middle childhood, Piaget established that by the school years, children have mastered flexible use of mental categories and can apply them simultaneously and inductively. In middle childhood, the child can classify objects into categories-based on some common property and in conformity to the development of their own schema, forming complex cognitive sets or connections. Today, however, researchers believe that transitive inference is more complex and simpler than Piaget had imagined. Inferential reasoning is connected to another logical concept termed seriation by Piaget.[86–88]

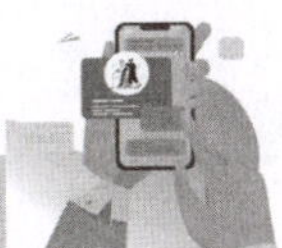

Like Piaget, Vygotsky was primarily interested in the concrete thinking of children; however, unlike Piaget, Vygotsky considered that access to participation scaffolded or mediated by peers and teachers who assisted a child with more advanced knowledge activated crucial cognitive processes.[89] Similarly, to Piaget, Vygotsky leaned heavily on the importance of social and cultural context for learning (Vadeboncoeur & Stanners, 2005); however, this view contrasts markedly with Piaget's more maturational take.[90, 91]

Culture has been found to influence the processes of learning—not just material.[92] Incoming stimuli are held just long enough to be processed into a bin or forgotten almost immediately following, according to information-processing theory. Working memory (a school term for short-term memories designed to do some type of mental task at any moment) is only able to work on material which has been deposited into it from long-term store. There are two parts to working memory that has been shown to increase: the phonological loop, which is essentially sound storage and the visual-spatially sketch pad or sight stores. Information is stored in the long-term memory for days, but also months and years.[93, 94] The ability to store and retrieve information from long-term memory is important for development. Some memories are easier to retrieve than others.[95] Children become better learners in middle childhood for a new reason: "They have more extensive knowledge".[96] The processes that assemble memory, processing speed, and content are executive control systems (processes), encompassing selective attention/meta-cognition/emotion regulation. Explicit instruction or discovery learning drives control processes.[97] School children also outperform preschoolers in metacognition, which is the ability to evaluate a cognitive task in order to determine how best (speed and accuracy) it can be accomplished, then monitor and adjust performance.[98]

Social Development

The social development of children during middle childhood is roughly between the ages of 6–11 years. This stage is particularly important as children start school and begin to significantly interact outside the family circle.

During middle childhood, children deepen their social interactions and develop more complex social skills. They learn to understand and follow social rules, and their peer relationships become increasingly important. This is the age when children start to form friendships based on shared interests and mutual respect, rather than just convenience or proximity. Social development in this stage also includes the ability to cooperate with others, understand different perspectives, and manage conflicts and competition in healthy ways.

The development of these social skills is crucial for children's overall emotional and psychological health. It lays the foundation for later social interactions in adolescence and adulthood, influencing their future relationships, academic performance, and ability to work collaboratively in team settings. Additionally, the text discusses how this social development is supported by the child's cognitive advances that allow them to better process and understand social information, rules, and norms.

ADOLESCENCE

Physical Changes

Volumetric and functional imaging studies reveal subtle changes in the structure of the developing adolescent human brain, which manifests as differential growth. The precise meaning of these changes is mostly unclear, but likely represents a reorganizational or compensatory change in parallel with the manifold increase in its functions and capabilities.[99, 100]

- **Initial stage:** In early childhood, this is the 'concrete thinking model' where children still process concepts in a more 'literal' sense than metaphors. Teens are generally reflexive and have precarious mental capacities to consider the long-term outcomes of their conduct. They prefer same-sex peers. Most are too sensitive on what other people may think about their looks as well as the things they do. This stage also typically leads to curiosity about sexual anatomy and comparison with same-sex peers.[101, 102]

- **Intermediate phase:** This is where the challenge in emotional independence becomes visible. The young mind transcends selfhood, and the capacity for abstract thought emerges. They can now question and validate. This is the period when they become more detached from family. The peer group acceptance becomes of great importance. Sexual experimentation (e.g., masturbation) typically begins before this age.[103, 104]

- **Late phase:** All the pubertal changes have already taken place. Moral principles and strong self-identity are clearly outlined. Now, they can shut down impulsive responses and are more resistant to peer pressure. The family dynamics become more of a thing than the peer group. The youth turns serious and starts doing both short term and long-term planning to achieve his targets in life. Many start sexual activity.[105, 106]

Cognitive Changes

The critical cognitive and communication developments occur during adolescence. It is a dynamic period characterized by significant growth in brain functions and language abilities. Adolescence marks a phase of rapid changes in processing speed, which increases notably at the ages of 5 and 11 years, followed by more gradual improvements by age 18. This period also sees a profound evolution in executive functions, defined as the supervisory cognitive processes that orchestrate the planning and regulation of behavior.[107] These functions are essential for developing metacognitive skills, such as the ability to self-monitor one's performance on complex and demanding tasks, which become increasingly sophisticated during adolescence.

Furthermore, there are nuances of social cognition and language development during this pivotal stage. Social cognition, which involves the processing of information essential for successful social interaction, matures significantly as adolescents enhance their capabilities in understanding and navigating social environments.[108] This development is closely tied to improvements in language skills, where adolescents achieve greater syntactic complexity and pragmatic nuances in communication. Language development during adolescence is not only about acquiring a larger

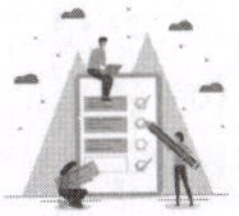
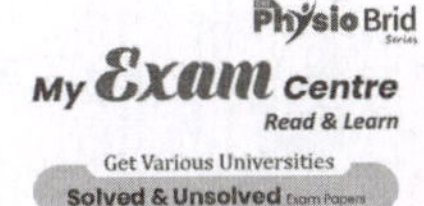

vocabulary but also about mastering the use of language in diverse social and academic settings, supported by the simultaneous advances in cognitive abilities such as working memory and abstract reasoning.[109] These cognitive and linguistic milestones are crucial for adolescents as they prepare for more complex social interactions and academic challenges in later life.

Identity Formation

This adolescent identity construction is a major part of psychological development, as illustrated by Erikson's stages of psychosocial expansion. This period in a person's life is marked by the exploration of personal identity, where they experiment with various roles and lifestyles. This exploration is often embraced as a way to establish a coherent sense of self. The concept he labeled as "Identity versus role confusion", in which the successful consolidations of this stage were to a strong identity and failure at lack of stability among adolescents.[110]

During adolescence, individuals experiment with different social roles, behaviors, and activities. This exploration is influenced by their peers, family, culture, and the larger societal context. As adolescents try out various roles, from academic and social to vocational, they begin to integrate these experiences into their personal identity that feels most true to themselves. This process is also affected by their emerging cognitive abilities to think abstractly and consider future possibilities, which allows them to conceptualize different "selves" they might become.[111]

Social interactions play a pivotal role in this developmental phase. As adolescents engage with peers and observe reactions to their behaviors, they receive feedback that helps them refine their self-concept. This social feedback, whether positive or negative, serves as a mirror reflecting the adequacy of their role explorations and helps them make decisions about personal values and beliefs.

Moreover, identity formation is not just about choosing between different paths but also about negotiating identity issues within various contexts such as gender, sexuality, ethnicity, and religion. These factors can complicate the identity formation process, as adolescents may face challenges related to acceptance and discrimination. How they resolve conflicts related to these aspects of their identity significantly affects their overall psychological well-being and self-esteem.

ADULTHOOD

Adulthood is a significant period in the lifespan characterized by multiple developmental stages, each marked by distinct psychological and physiological changes. This chapter explores the transitions and challenges individuals face during early, middle, and late adulthood, focusing on Erikson's psychosocial stages, career development, and the physical and cognitive transformations that occur.

Early Adulthood

- **Career development:** Early adulthood is a phase where individuals are deeply engaged in building their careers. This period involves the exploration of different job opportunities and the establishment of a professional identity.[10] Career development during this stage is influenced by one's education, personal goals, and the socioeconomic context. Success in this area is often seen as a foundation for future stability and satisfaction.

- **Intimacy versus isolation:** Erikson's psychosocial stage for early adulthood, intimacy versus isolation, revolves around the development of intimate relationships with others. Achieving intimacy means establishing relationships that are consensual, close, and committed. If successful, it leads to strong friendships and romantic partnerships. Failure to achieve intimacy can result in social isolation, loneliness, and depression.[112] This stage is crucial for emotional and psychological well-being as individuals balance their needs and desires with those of others.

Middle Adulthood

- **Physical changes:** Middle adulthood is typically marked by noticeable physical changes that include a decline in muscle mass, metabolic rate, and often an increase in body fat. Vision, hearing, and overall physical strength tend to diminish during this stage. These changes are a natural part of aging and can affect an individual's lifestyle and psychological state, influencing their self-concept and behaviors.

- **Generativity versus stagnation:** This stage of Erikson's theory focuses on generativity, which involves contributing to the next generation through parenting, productive work, and community involvement. It reflects a broadening concern for future generations and a commitment to improving the world.[113] Stagnation occurs when individuals become self-absorbed or unable to contribute effectively to society, leading to feelings of unproductiveness and disconnect.

Late Adulthood

- **Physical and cognitive changes:** Late adulthood is characterized by more pronounced physical declines, including increased fragility, decreased mobility, and higher susceptibility to chronic diseases such as arthritis, cardiovascular diseases, and dementia. Cognitively, this period may see a decline in speed of clarifying, memory, and problem-solving skills, although significant variation exists among individuals.[114]

- **Integrity versus despair:** In Erikson's final stage, the focus is on reflecting back on life. Individuals strive to achieve ego integrity, a sense of fulfilment and completeness, accepting their lives as they have lived them and achieving a sense of wisdom.[115] Despair may arise if individuals look back with regret, feeling that their lives have been wasted. Successfully resolving the conflict of integrity versus despair leads to wisdom and the ability to face the end of life with a sense of peace and fulfilment.

These stages in adulthood highlight the continuous development and adaptation required in the face of physiological changes and evolving social roles. Each stage presents unique challenges and opportunities for personal growth and redefinition of one's roles in society.

AGING PROCESS

Aging is an inevitable, complex process that involves various biological, psychological, and social changes. This section of the chapter delves into the theories that explain the aging process and the psychosocial adjustments that accompany it, providing a comprehensive overview of how aging impacts individuals across different domains of life.[116]

Aging Theories

Theories of aging[117] explore the dimensions of aging given as follows (Fig. 2.4).

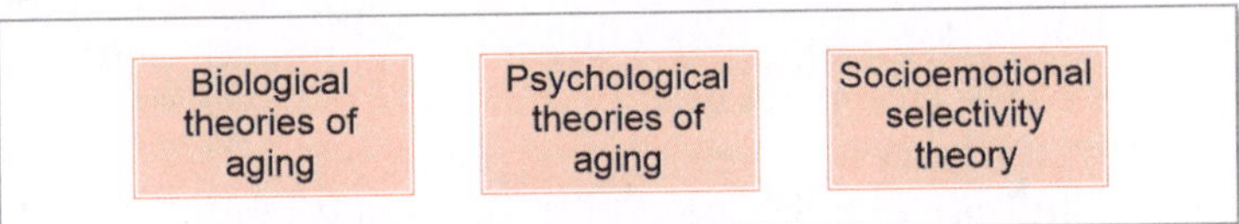

Fig. 2.4: Theories of aging for different dimensions

- **Biological theories of aging:** These ideas revolve around the physiological processes that have triggered in one's body to bring about those old, usual changes and subsequent decline. The **Rate of Living Theory** is the idea that metabolism controls lifespan, so if a living thing's metabolic rate is high then its biological clock clicks more quickly. **Free Radical Theory**, which holds free radicals, unstable molecules capable of damaging cellular components, induce biological damage and contribute to aging. In their place, the **Telomere Shortening Theory** tells us that with each cell division, telomeres which are the protective segments at the end of chromosomes become shorter and eventually cause cellular aging, then organismal decline.

- **Psychological theories of aging:** These include the **Disengagement Theory**, which suggests that aging naturally involves withdrawal from social and professional roles, which can be mutually beneficial for the individual and society by freeing up roles for younger people. Conversely, the **Activity Theory** argues for the benefits of maintaining active social engagements, suggesting that those who remain active and socially involved tend to be more satisfied and better adjusted.

- **Socioemotional selectivity theory:** It offers another perspective, proposing that older adults narrow their social networks because they prioritize emotional over informational goals, focusing on relationships that are most emotionally satisfying in the time they perceive as remaining.

Psychosocial Adjustment

- **Adjustment to aging:** Adjusting to the aging process is multifaceted, involving acceptance of physical limitations and changes, adapting to different social roles, and finding new sources of satisfaction and purpose.[118] Successful adjustment often depends on the individual's ability to maintain a sense of control and independence despite physical declines.

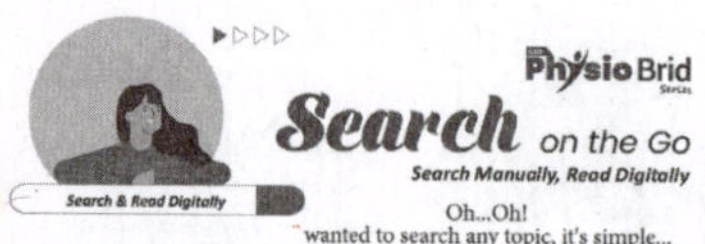

- **Coping with loss:** Aging is frequently associated with various losses, including the loss of loved ones, health, and independence. Effective coping mechanisms, such as seeking social support and engaging in meaningful activities, are critical for maintaining mental health and well-being.[119] Resilience plays a crucial role here, as it helps individuals recover from setbacks and maintain or regain their psychological well-being.

- **Mental health in late life:** Maintaining mental health in later years can be challenging due to the various changes and losses experienced.[118] Depression and anxiety are common but often underdiagnosed in this population. Promoting mental health involves regular social interaction, physical activity, and cognitive stimulation, along with professional interventions when necessary.

- **Identity and self-perception:** As individuals age, their self-perception can change significantly. It is vital for aging adults to integrate their past experiences with their current capabilities, forming a coherent identity that includes the acceptance of aging. This self-perception impacts their overall happiness and psychosocial adjustment.

Understanding these aspects of aging helps frame the later stages of life not merely as a time of decline but as a period rich with opportunities for growth, reflection, and fulfilment. This comprehensive approach offers insights into not only the challenges but also the potential for positive aging experiences (Fig. 2.5).

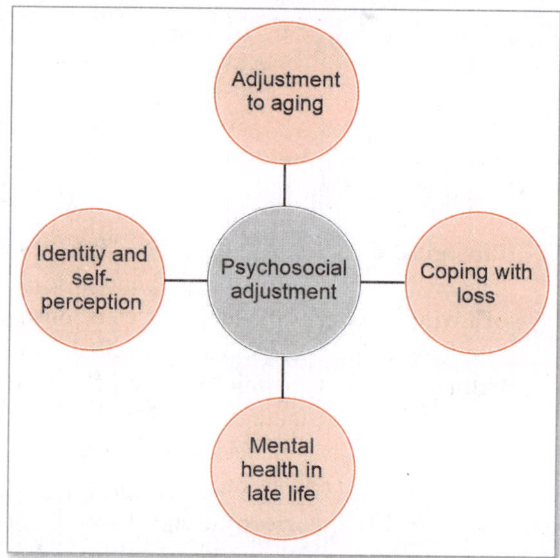

Fig. 2.5: Components of psychosocial adjustment

CROSS-CULTURAL VARIATIONS IN DEVELOPMENTAL MILESTONES

The study of cross-cultural variations in developmental milestones illuminates how different cultural contexts shape developmental trajectories. This section explores the cultural differences in developmental milestones and the profound impact of cultural factors on the paths of individual growth and development.

Cultural Variations in Developmental Milestones

Developmental milestones, such as walking, talking, and social interaction, can occur at different ages and in various contexts across cultures. For instance, children in some cultures may achieve certain motor skills earlier due to specific practices that encourage early movement, such as the use of floor beds instead of cribs. Similarly, language development milestones can vary significantly; in communities where multilingualism is the norm, children might begin speaking later but develop a more complex linguistic repertoire over time. These variations highlight the role of cultural practices and expectations in shaping developmental processes.[120] Research also indicates that parenting styles, which are deeply influenced by cultural beliefs and values, significantly impact the speed and manner in which developmental milestones are reached.[121] For example, cultures that value independence tend to encourage self-reliant behaviors earlier, whereas those valuing communal living might foster interdependence among family members from a young age.

Impact of Culture on Developmental Trajectories

Culture profoundly influences the entire developmental trajectory, from infancy through adulthood. Cultural norms dictate not only the milestones that are considered important but also the methods by which development is fostered and measured. For instance, educational attainment, a significant developmental milestone in many societies, is highly influenced by cultural attitudes toward education, gender roles, and economic factors.

Cultural context also affects the psychosocial development stages proposed by Erik Erikson.[10] The importance of achieving specific outcomes like autonomy in adolescence or generativity in middle adulthood can vary with cultural expectations and values. For example, the Western emphasis on individualism may lead to different challenges and resolutions in Erikson's stages compared to Eastern cultures, which might emphasize community and family integration.

Furthermore, cultural differences in the perception and treatment of the elderly can influence the developmental stage of late adulthood, impacting how individuals view their roles and effectiveness in society as they age. Cultures that revere the elderly and integrate them into daily family life often provide more positive roles for aging individuals, affecting their sense of integrity and despair.

Developmental Challenges

Development throughout life stages is not always smooth and linear; various challenges can influence growth and progress. This section examines the common developmental disorders, and the risk and protective factors that can impact developmental trajectories.

Developmental Disorders

Developmental disorders encompass a broad range of neurological issues that affect children, often from birth, influencing their development across multiple domains including physical, learning, language, and behavior.[122] Common disorders include Autism Spectrum Disorders (ASD), Attention-Deficit/Hyperactivity Disorder (ADHD), and learning disabilities such as dyslexia. These disorders can significantly impact a child's ability to achieve developmental milestones at typical ages. For instance, children with ASD may show delayed language and social skills, while those with ADHD might exhibit difficulties with attention, executive function, and impulse control, affecting their academic and social development.

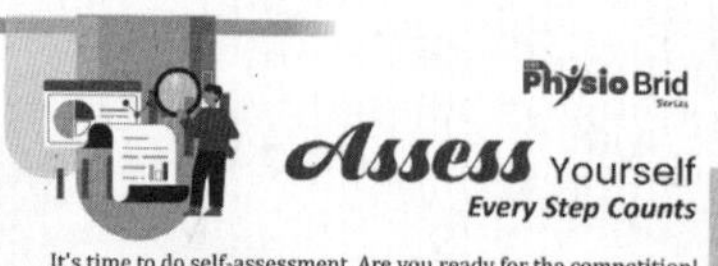

Physio CORNER

Developmental delays in autism spectrum disorder (ASD) can vary widely, as ASD is a complex neurodevelopmental condition characterized by challenges in social interaction, communication, and repetitive behaviors. Understanding these developmental delays is crucial for early identification, intervention, and support. Here are the key areas where developmental delays are often observed in children with autism:

Social and Emotional Development

- **Social interaction:**
  - **Limited eye contact:** Difficulty making or maintaining eye contact.
  - **Difficulty with social cues:** Challenges in understanding and responding to social cues, such as facial expressions and body language.
  - **Lack of interest in peers:** Limited interest in playing or interacting with other children, preferring solitary activities.
- **Emotional regulation:**
  - **Difficulty expressing emotions:** Trouble expressing emotions appropriately, leading to tantrums or outbursts.
  - **Empathy challenges:** Difficulty understanding or responding to the emotions of others.

Communication Development

- **Language delays:**
  - **Delayed speech:** Late onset of speaking; some children may not speak at all (nonverbal).
  - **Limited vocabulary:** Reduced number of words used compared to typically developing peers.
- **Communication skills:**
  - **Echolalia:** Repetition of words or phrases without understanding their meaning.
  - **Difficulty with pragmatics:** Problems with the social use of language, such as taking turns in conversation, understanding jokes or using appropriate greetings.
- **Nonverbal communication:**
  - **Limited gestures:** Few or no use of gestures like pointing or waving.
  - **Atypical body language:** Unusual body movements or lack of expressive gestures.

Behavioral Development

- **Repetitive behaviors:**
  - **Stereotyped movements:** Repetitive movements such as hand-flapping, rocking or spinning.
  - **Insistence on sameness:** Strong preference for routines and resistance to changes in routine.
- **Restricted interests:**
  - **Intense focus:** Intense interest in specific topics or objects, often to the exclusion of other activities.
  - **Unusual interests:** Interest in atypical objects or parts of objects (e.g., spinning wheels, fans).

Sensory Processing

- **Sensory sensitivities:**
  - **Hypersensitivity:** Overreaction to sensory stimuli, such as loud noises, bright lights or certain textures.
  - **Hyposensitivity:** Underreaction to sensory input, seeking out intense sensory experiences.

Contd...

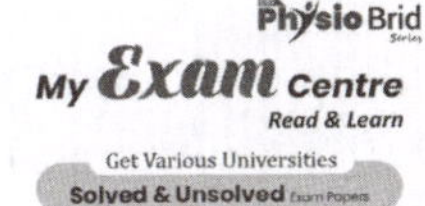

- **Sensory-seeking behaviors:**
  - **Seeking stimulation:** Engaging in activities that provide strong sensory input, such as spinning, jumping or chewing on objects.

Cognitive Development
- **Variable intellectual functioning:**
  - **Range of abilities:** Cognitive abilities can range from intellectual disability to average or above-average intelligence.
  - **Uneven skill development:** Some children may have strengths in certain areas (e.g., memory, visual-spatial skills) and weaknesses in others (e.g., abstract thinking, problem-solving).

Motor Development
- **Gross motor skills:**
  - **Coordination issues:** Delays or difficulties with coordination and balance, affecting activities like running or jumping.
- **Fine motor skills:**
  - **Handwriting and manipulation:** Difficulty with tasks requiring fine motor control, such as handwriting, using utensils or buttoning clothes.

Risk Factors and Protective Factors

The trajectory of an individual's development can be influenced by various risk and protective factors. Risk factors are conditions or attributes that increase the likelihood of developing a disorder or negative outcomes. These can include genetic predispositions, prenatal exposure to toxins, poor nutrition, and socioeconomic challenges such as poverty.[123] Conversely, protective factors mitigate risks and enhance resilience, potentially leading to positive developmental outcomes despite the presence of risk factors. These include supportive family environments, strong social connections, positive school experiences, and access to quality healthcare and educational opportunities. The interplay between these factors can significantly influence the extent to which developmental challenges affect an individual.

APPLICATIONS OF DEVELOPMENTAL PSYCHOLOGY

Developmental psychology provides valuable insights that can be applied in various practical contexts, notably in parenting and education. This section explores how understanding developmental principles can enhance parenting styles and educational practices.

Parenting Styles and Child Development

The influence of parenting styles on child development is profound and far-reaching. Developmental psychologists have identified several key styles, including authoritative, authoritarian, permissive, and neglectful parenting. Each style impacts children differently. For example, authoritative parenting which combines warmth and structure is often linked to the best developmental outcomes, fostering

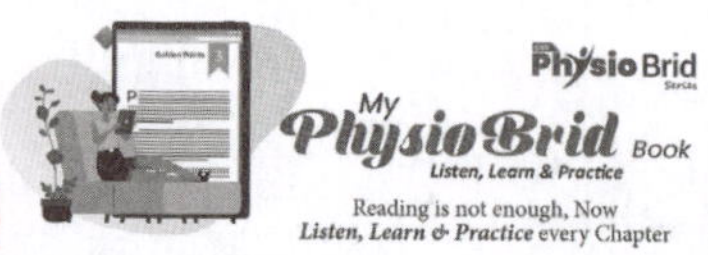

independence, high self-esteem, and social competence.[124] In contrast, authoritarian parenting, which is strict and less emotionally warm, may lead to lower self-esteem and higher levels of aggression in children. Understanding these styles and their impact can help parents make informed choices that foster healthier psychological and social development in their children.

Case Study

Patient Profile
Name: Michael Smith
Age: 2 years
Gender: Male
Medical history: Premature birth at 32 weeks, neonatal jaundice, and mild respiratory distress syndrome
Family history: No known neurological disorders

Presenting Symptoms
- Delayed motor milestones (not sitting independently, not crawling, not walking)
- Muscle stiffness (spasticity) in the legs
- Poor trunk control and balance
- Difficulty using hands for fine motor tasks (grasping toys, self-feeding)
- Limited speech and communication skills

Initial Assessment
- **Neurological exam:** Hypertonia in the lower limbs, brisk reflexes, and clonus in both ankles. Upper limbs show mild spasticity with delayed fine motor skills.
- **Developmental assessment:** Significant delay in gross and fine motor skills. Social and cognitive skills are mildly delayed.
- **Imaging:** MRI of the brain shows periventricular leukomalacia (PVL), which is often associated with spastic diplegia, a form of cerebral palsy.

Clinical Diagnosis
Spastic diplegic cerebral palsy (SDCP)

Treatment Plan
- **Medical management:**
  - **Medications:** Baclofen to manage spasticity, with the possibility of botulinum toxin injections in the future.
  - **Nutritional support:** Ensure adequate nutrition to support growth and development, considering potential feeding difficulties.
- **Physiotherapy:**
  - **Goals:** Improve muscle strength, flexibility, and functional mobility. Enhance trunk control and balance.
  - **Techniques:**
    - *Stretching exercises:* Regular stretching to reduce muscle tightness and prevent contractures.

Contd...

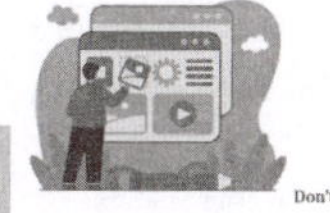
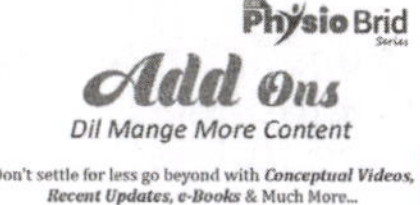

- *Strengthening exercises:* Activities to build muscle strength, particularly in the core and lower extremities.
  - *Balance and coordination:* Exercises like sitting on a therapy ball, supported standing, and playing with balance toys.
  - *Mobility training:* Encourage crawling, using walkers or other assistive devices to promote independent movement.
- **Occupational therapy:**
  - **Goals:** Improve fine motor skills, self-care abilities, and sensory processing.
  - **Techniques:**
    - *Fine motor skills:* Activities to improve hand-eye coordination and manual dexterity (e.g., stacking blocks, manipulating small objects).
    - *Adaptive techniques:* Use of adaptive utensils and tools to facilitate self-feeding and other daily activities.
    - *Sensory integration:* Exercises to help Michael process sensory information more effectively.
- **Speech and language therapy:**
  - **Goals:** Enhance communication skills and address any feeding difficulties.
  - **Techniques:**
    - *Speech development:* Encouraging babbling, single words, and simple phrases through play and interaction.
    - *Alternative communication:* Introduction of basic sign language or picture boards if verbal communication remains limited.
    - *Oral motor skills:* Exercises to improve muscle control for speech and eating.
- **Family support and education:**
  - **Parental training:** Educate parents on how to perform stretches and exercises at home, use adaptive equipment, and encourage developmentally appropriate play.
  - **Support groups:** Connect the family with local support groups for parents of children with cerebral palsy.
- **Early intervention program:**
  - **Comprehensive services:** Enroll Michael in an early intervention program that provides a multidisciplinary approach, including therapy, education, and socialization opportunities.

Progress Monitoring
- **Regular assessments:** Monthly evaluations to monitor Michael's progress in therapy, adjusting the treatment plan as needed.
- **Developmental milestones:** Track progress in achieving specific motor, communication, and cognitive milestones.
- **Parental feedback:** Regular meetings with parents to discuss Michael's progress and address any concerns.

Outcome
After 6 months of consistent therapy, Michael showed improvement in muscle tone and strength, with better trunk control and balance. He began to sit independently and crawl with some assistance. His fine motor skills improved, allowing him to grasp and manipulate small toys more effectively. Communication skills also showed progress, with increased babbling and the use of a few simple words and signs.

Contd...

Follow-Up
- Continued physiotherapy and occupational therapy as outpatient services.
- Ongoing speech and language therapy sessions.
- Regular follow-up with a pediatric neurologist to monitor medical management and overall development.

Conclusion
Early diagnosis and a comprehensive, multidisciplinary intervention plan have significantly improved Michael's functional abilities and quality of life. Continued therapy and support will be essential to maximizing his developmental potential and promoting independence.

Educational Implications

Developmental psychology has crucial implications for education, offering insights that can shape curricular designs, teaching methods, and educational policies. For instance, knowledge about cognitive development stages can help educators design age-appropriate learning experiences that align with students' cognitive capabilities at each developmental stage. Moreover, understanding the specific needs of children with developmental disorders such as dyslexia or ADHD can lead educators to adopt more inclusive and supportive teaching practices that accommodate diverse learning needs and help all students achieve their potential.[124]

Overall, the application of developmental psychology in parenting and education not only enhances individual outcomes but also promotes healthier, more supportive environments where all children can thrive.

CURRENT RESEARCH AND FUTURE DIRECTIONS

The field of developmental psychology is continually evolving, with new research shedding light on how humans grow and change throughout their lives. This section discusses the latest trends in the field and the ethical considerations that guide research.

Emerging Trends in Developmental Psychology

Recent trends in developmental psychology emphasize the integration of technology and neuroscience, enhancing our understanding of developmental processes. Neurodevelopmental research is exploring how brain structures and functions change from infancy through adulthood, providing insights into the neurological underpinnings of developmental milestones and disorders. Technological advancements, such as eye-tracking and wearable technology, are being used to study developmental stages in real-time, offering more precise and continuous data collection.

Another significant trend is the growing focus on lifespan development, recognizing that significant growth and change continue into and throughout old age. Researchers are also increasingly addressing cultural diversity in developmental studies, which helps to understand how context, environment, and culture impact the developmental trajectory across global populations.

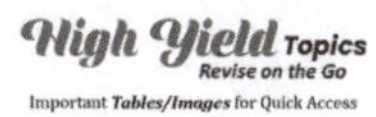

Ethical Considerations in Developmental Research

Ethical considerations are paramount in developmental research, particularly because it often involves vulnerable populations such as children and the elderly. Key ethical concerns include obtaining informed consent, ensuring the right to privacy, and maintaining the welfare of participants. For children and individuals with cognitive impairments, obtaining consent involves not only communicating with the individual at a level appropriate to their understanding but also involving parents or legal guardians in the consent process.

Researchers must also consider the potential psychological impact of developmental assessments and interventions. Studies are designed to minimize distress and disruption to the participants' daily lives, and any long-term follow-up must be handled with sensitivity to changes in the participant's developmental stage and personal circumstances.

SUMMARY

- This chapter has explored the comprehensive journey of human development from infancy through late adulthood, highlighting the complexities of growth and the impact of various factors on developmental trajectories. It has examined the influence of genetics, environment, and culture on development and discussed the challenges and disorders that can affect individuals at different life stages.
- Future directions in developmental psychology promise to deepen our understanding of the developmental processes through innovative research methods and technologies. By continuing to explore and integrate new findings, developmental psychology can offer more effective interventions and support systems tailored to the needs of diverse populations at different stages of life. This ongoing research not only enhances academic knowledge but also has practical implications for improving educational, clinical, and social outcomes, ensuring that individuals across the lifespan have the support they need to achieve their potential.

REFERENCES

1. Cherniack NS. The basis of human development. New York: Harper & Row; 1973.
2. Balasundaram P, Avulakunta ID. Human growth and development. In: StatPearls [Internet]. Treasure Island (FL): StatPearls Publishing; 2023 Jan-. Available from: https://www.ncbi.nlm.nih.gov/books/NBK536962/
3. Scharf RJ, Scharf GJ, Stroustrup A. Developmental milestones. Pediatrics in Review. 2016 Jan;37(1):25. Available from: http://publications.aap.org/pediatricsinreview/article-pdf/37/1/25/824665/pedsinreview_20140103.pdf
4. Freud S. Three Essays on the Theory of Sexuality. New York: Basic Books; 1905.
5. Freud S. Beyond the Pleasure Principle. London: The Hogarth Press; 1920.
6. Freud S. The Interpretation of Dreams. New York: Macmillan; 1900.
7. Erikson EH. Childhood and Society. New York: Norton; 1950.
8. Erikson EH. Identity and the Life Cycle. New York: International Universities Press; 1959.
9. Erikson EH. The Life Cycle Completed. New York: Norton; 1982.

Contd...

10. Watson JB. Psychology as the Behaviorist Views It. Psychological Review. 1913;20(2):158–177.

11. Skinner BF. The Behavior of Organisms: An Experimental Analysis. New York: Appleton-Century; 1938.

12. Skinner BF. Beyond Freedom and Dignity. New York: Knopf; 1971.

13. Piaget J. The Origins of Intelligence in Children. New York: International Universities Press; 1952.

14. Bellman M, Byrne O, Sege R. Developmental assessment of children. BMJ. 2013;346. doi:10.1136/bmj.e8687

15. Piaget J. The Construction of Reality in the Child. New York: Basic Books; 1954.

16. Bowlby J. Attachment and Loss. Volume I: Attachment. New York: Basic Books; 1969.

17. Ainsworth MD, Blehar MC, Waters E, Wall S. Patterns of Attachment: A Psychological Study of the Strange Situation. Hillsdale, NJ: Erlbaum; 1978.

18. Marwaha S, Goswami M, Vashist B. Prevalence of Principles of Piaget's Theory Among 4-7-year-old Children and their Correlation with IQ. J Clin Diagn Res. 2017;11(8). doi:10.7860/JCDR/2017/28435.10513

19. Bandura A. Social Learning Theory. Englewood Cliffs, NJ: Prentice-Hall; 1977.

20. Bandura A. Self-Efficacy: The Exercise of Control. New York: Freeman; 1997.

21. Bandura A, Walters RH. Social Learning and Personality Development. New York: Holt, Rinehart & Winston; 1963.

22. Barnes GL, Woolgar M, Beckwith H, Duschinsky R. John Bowlby and contemporary issues of clinical diagnosis. Attachment (Lond). 2018;12(1):35–47.

23. Vygotsky LS. Mind in Society: The Development of Higher Psychological Processes. Cambridge, MA: Harvard University Press; 1978.

24. Vygotsky LS. Thought and Language. Cambridge, MA: MIT Press; 1986.

25. Vygotsky LS. The Collected Works of L.S. Vygotsky. Volume 1: Problems of General Psychology. New York: Plenum Press; 1987.

26. Gazzaniga MS, Ivry RB, Mangun GR. Cognitive Neuroscience: The Biology of the Mind. 4th ed. New York: W.W. Norton; 2013.

27. Kandel ER, Schwartz JH, Jessell TM, Siegelbaum SA, Hudspeth AJ. Principles of Neural Science. 5th ed. New York: McGraw-Hill; 2013.

28. Carlson NR. Physiology of Behavior. 11th ed. Boston: Pearson; 2012.

29. Sadler TW. Langman's Medical Embryology. 13th ed. Philadelphia: Lippincott Williams & Wilkins; 2014.

30. Larsen WJ. Human Embryology. 4th ed. Philadelphia: Churchill Livingstone; 2001.

31. Moore KL, Persaud TVN, Torchia MG. The Developing Human: Clinically Oriented Embryology. 10th ed. Philadelphia: Elsevier; 2015.

32. Gilbert SF. Developmental Biology. 11th ed. Sunderland: Sinauer Associates; 2013.

33. O'Rahilly R, Müller F. Human Embryology and Teratology. 3rd ed. New York: Wiley-Liss; 2001.

34. Sadler TW. Langman's Medical Embryology. 13th ed. Philadelphia: Lippincott Williams & Wilkins; 2014.

35. Schoenwolf GC, Bleyl SB, Brauer PR, Francis-West PH. Larsen's Human Embryology. 5th ed. Philadelphia: Churchill Livingstone; 2014.

36. Carlson BM. Human Embryology and Developmental Biology. 5th ed. Philadelphia: Elsevier; 2014.

37. Plomin R, DeFries JC, Knopik VS, Neiderhiser JM. Behavioral Genetics. 6th ed. New York: Worth Publishers; 2013.

38. Rutter M. Gene-environment interplay and developmental psychopathology. J Child Psychol Psychiatry. 2007;48(3-4):359–61.

Contd...

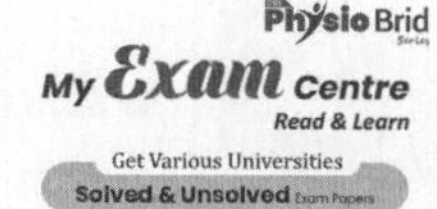

39. Black RE, Victora CG, Walker SP, et al. Maternal and child undernutrition and overweight in low-income and middle-income countries. Lancet. 2013;382(9890):427–51.

40. Bhutta ZA, Das JK, Rizvi A, et al. Evidence-based interventions for improvement of maternal and child nutrition: What can be done and at what cost? Lancet. 2013;382(9890):452–77.

41. Abbott LC, Winzer-Serhan UH. Smoking during pregnancy: Lessons learned from epidemiological studies and experimental studies using animal models. Crit Rev Toxicol. 2012;42(4):279–303.

42. Goldenberg RL, Culhane JF. Infection as a cause of preterm birth. Clin Perinatol. 2003;30(4):677–700.

43. Romero R, Espinoza J, Kusanovic JP, et al. The preterm parturition syndrome. BJOG. 2006;113 (Suppl 3):17–42.

44. Berk LE. Child Development. 9th ed. Boston: Pearson; 2013.

45. Kail RV, Cavanaugh JC. Human Development: A Life-Span View. 7th ed. Boston: Cengage Learning; 2019.

46. Johnson MH, de Haan M. Developmental Cognitive Neuroscience: An Introduction. 4th ed. Hoboken: Wiley-Blackwell; 2015.

47. Volpe JJ. Neurology of the Newborn. 6th ed. Philadelphia: Elsevier; 2017.

48. Thelen E, Smith LB. A Dynamic Systems Approach to the Development of Cognition and Action. Cambridge: MIT Press; 1994.

49. Gopnik A, Meltzoff AN, Kuhl PK. The Scientist in the Crib: What Early Learning Tells Us About the Mind. New York: William Morrow & Co; 1999.

50. Siegler RS, Alibali MW. Children's Thinking. 4th ed. Upper Saddle River: Prentice Hall; 2005.

51. Diamond A. Executive Functions. Annu Rev Psychol. 2013;64:135–68.

52. Piaget J. The Moral Judgment of the Child. London: Routledge & Kegan Paul; 1932.

53. Parten MB. Social Participation among Preschool Children. J Abnorm Soc Psychol. 1932;27(3):243–69.

54. Ainsworth MD, Bell SM. Attachment, Exploration, and Separation: Illustrated by the Behavior of One-Year-Olds in a Strange Situation. Child Dev. 1970;41(1):49–67.

55. Eisenberg N, Fabes RA. Emotion, Regulation, and the Development of Social Competence. In: Clark MS, ed. Emotion and Social Behavior. New York: Springer; 1992. p. 119–50.

56. Saarni C. The Development of Emotional Competence. New York: Guilford Press; 1999.

57. Klaus MH, Fanaroff AA. Care of the High-Risk Neonate. 6th ed. Philadelphia: Elsevier Health Sciences; 2012.

58. American Academy of Pediatrics. Pediatric Clinical Practice Guidelines & Policies. 20th ed. Elk Grove Village, IL: American Academy of Pediatrics; 2020.

59. Feldman R. Parent-infant synchrony and the construction of shared timing; physiological precursors, developmental outcomes, and risk conditions. J Child Psychol Psychiatry. 2007;48(3-4):329–54.

60. Papousek M, Bornstein MH, Nageishi N. Early Development: Parent-infant Interaction and Developmental Disabilities. Hillsdale, NJ: Lawrence Erlbaum Associates; 1992.

61. Gerber RJ, Wilks T, Erdie-Lalena C. Developmental milestones: motor development. Pediatr Rev. 2010;31(7):267–77.

62. Diamond A. Close interrelation of motor development and cognitive development and of the cerebellum and prefrontal cortex. Child Dev. 2000;71(1):44–56.

63. Emde RN, Robinson J. The first relationship: Infant and mother. Cambridge, MA: Harvard University Press; 1979.

Contd...

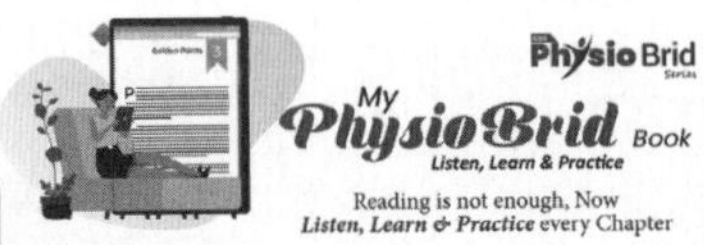

64. Fogel A, Garvey A. Alive communication. Infant Behav Dev. 2007;30(2):251–57.

65. Campos JJ, Anderson DI, Barbu-Roth MA, Hubbard EM, Hertenstein MJ, Witherington D. Travel broadens the mind. Infancy. 2000;1(2):149–219.

66. Mundy P, Newell L. Attention, joint attention, and social cognition. Curr Dir Psychol Sci. 2007; 16(5): 269–74.

67. Kuhl PK. Early language acquisition: Cracking the speech code. Nat Rev Neurosci. 2004;5(11):831–43.

68. Nelson CA. The development and neural bases of face recognition. Infant Child Dev. 2000;9(1):69–79.

69. Shonkoff JP, Phillips DA. From Neurons to Neighborhoods: The Science of Early Childhood Development. Washington, DC: National Academies Press; 2000.

70. Brooks-Gunn J, Markman LB. The contribution of parenting to ethnic and racial gaps in school readiness. Future Child. 2005;15(1):139–68.

71. Meltzoff AN. 'Like me': A foundation for social cognition. Dev Sci. 2007;10(1):126–34.

72. Raver CC. Placing emotional self-regulation in sociocultural and socioeconomic contexts. Child Dev. 2004;75(2):346–53.

73. Gopnik A, Wellman HM. The theory theory. In: Hirschfeld L, Gelman S, editors. Mapping the mind: Domain specificity in cognition and culture. Cambridge: Cambridge University Press; 1994. p. 257–93.

74. Wellman HM, Liu D. Scaling of theory-of-mind tasks. Child Dev. 2004;75(2):523–41.

75. Vygotsky LS. Mind in Society: The Development of Higher Psychological Processes. Cambridge, MA: Harvard University Press; 1978.

76. Berk LE. Child Development. 8th ed. Boston: Pearson; 2006.

77. Elkind D. The Power of Play: Learning What Comes Naturally. Cambridge, MA: Da Capo Press; 2007.

78. Piaget J. Play, Dreams, and Imitation in Childhood. New York: Norton; 1962.

79. Bruner J. Child's Talk: Learning to Use Language. New York: Norton; 1983.

80. Hart B, Risley TR. Meaningful Differences in the Everyday Experience of Young American Children. Baltimore: Paul H. Brookes Publishing Co.; 1995.

81. Scharf RJ, Scharf GJ, Stroustrup A. Developmental milestones. Pediatr Rev. 2016;37(1):25–38.

82. Piaget J. The Origins of Intelligence in Children. New York: International Universities Press; 1952.

83. Siegler RS. Emerging Minds: The Process of Change in Children's Thinking. New York: Oxford University Press; 1996.

84. Case R. The Mind's Staircase: Exploring the Conceptual Underpinnings of Children's Thought and Knowledge. Hillsdale, NJ: Lawrence Erlbaum Associates; 1992.

85. Halford GS, Andrews G. The Development of Logical Thinking: A Neo-Piagetian Perspective. Mahwah, NJ: Lawrence Erlbaum Associates; 2006.

86. Vygotsky LS. Mind in Society: The Development of Higher Psychological Processes. Cambridge, MA: Harvard University Press; 1978.

87. Rogoff B. Apprenticeship in Thinking: Cognitive Development in Social Context. New York: Oxford University Press; 1990.

88. Greenfield PM. The cultural evolution of IQ. In: Sternberg RJ, Grigorenko EL, editors. Intelligence, Heredity, and Environment. Cambridge: Cambridge University Press; 1997. p. 127–70.

89. Baddeley A. Working Memory, Thought, and Action. New York: Oxford University Press; 2007.

90. Cowan N. Working Memory Capacity. New York: Psychology Press; 2005.

91. Tulving E. Elements of Episodic Memory. New York: Oxford University Press; 1983.

Contd...

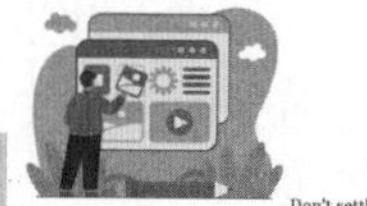 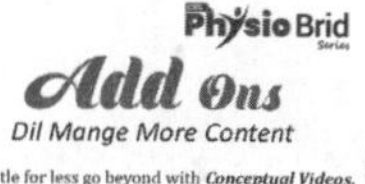

92. Chi MTH. Knowledge structures and memory development. In: Chi MTH, Glaser R, Farr MJ, editors. The Nature of Expertise. Hillsdale, NJ: Lawrence Erlbaum Associates; 1988. p. 75–105.

93. Flavell JH. Cognitive Development. Englewood Cliffs, NJ: Prentice-Hall; 1985.

94. Kuhn D. Metacognitive development. Curr Dir Psychol Sci. 2000;9(5):178–81.

95. Blakemore SJ, Choudhury S. Development of the adolescent brain: Implications for executive function and social cognition. J Child Psychol Psychiatry. 2006 Mar;47(3-4):296–312.

96. Giedd JN. The teen brain: insights from neuroimaging. J Adolesc Health. 2008 Apr;42(4):335–43.

97. Keating DP. Cognitive and brain development. In: Lerner RM, Steinberg L, editors. Handbook of Adolescent Psychology. 2nd ed. Hoboken, NJ: Wiley; 2004. p. 45–84.

98. Casey BJ, Jones RM, Hare TA. The adolescent brain. Ann N Y Acad Sci. 2008 Mar;1124(1):111–26.

99. Steinberg L. Cognitive and affective development in adolescence. Trends Cogn Sci. 2005 Feb;9(2):69–74.

100. Smetana JG, Campione-Barr N, Metzger A. Adolescent development in interpersonal and societal contexts. Annu Rev Psychol. 2006;57:255–84.

101. Arnett JJ. Emerging adulthood: A theory of development from the late teens through the twenties. Am Psychol. 2000 May;55(5):469–80.

102. Erikson EH. Identity: Youth and Crisis. New York: Norton; 1968.

103. Ciccia AH, Meulenbroek P, Turkstra LS. Adolescent brain and cognitive developments: Implications for clinical assessment in traumatic brain injury. Top Lang Disord. 2009 Jul 1;29(3):249–65.

104. Barch DM, Albaugh MD, Avenevoli S, Chang L, Clark DB, Glantz MD, Hudziak JJ, Jernigan TL, Tapert SF, Yurgelun-Todd D, Alia-Klein N. Demographic, physical and mental health assessments in the adolescent brain and cognitive development study: Rationale and description. Dev Cogn Neurosci. 2018 Aug 1;32:55–66.

105. Keating DP. Cognitive and brain development in adolescence. Enfance. 2012;3(3):267–79.

106. Crocetti E. Identity formation in adolescence: The dynamic of forming and consolidating identity commitments. Child Dev Perspect. 2017 Jun;11(2):145–50.

107. Marcia JE, Waterman AS, Matteson DR, Archer SL, Orlofsky JL, Waterman AS. Developmental perspectives on identity formation: From adolescence to adulthood. Ego identity: A handbook for psychosocial research. 1993:42–68.

108. Heckhausen J, Dixon RA, Baltes PB. Gains and losses in development throughout adulthood as perceived by different adult age groups. Dev Psychol. 1989 Jan;25(1):109.

109. Slater CL. Generativity versus stagnation: An elaboration of Erikson's adult stage of human development. J Adult Dev. 2003 Jan;10:53–65.

110. Arenaza-Urquijo EM, de Flores R, Gonneaud J, Wirth M, Ourry V, Callewaert W, Landeau B, Egret S, Mézenge F, Desgranges B, Chételat G. Distinct effects of late adulthood cognitive and physical activities on gray matter volume. Brain Imaging Behav. 2017 Apr;11(2):346–56.

111. Hearn S, Saulnier G, Strayer J, Glenham M, Koopman R, Marcia JE. Between integrity and despair: Toward construct validation of Erikson's eighth stage. J Adult Dev. 2012 Mar;19:1–20.

112. Harman D. Aging: overview. Ann N Y Acad Sci. 2001 Apr;928(1):1–21.

113. Cefalu CA. Theories and mechanisms of aging. Clin Geriatr Med. 2011 Nov 1;27(4):491–506.

114. Coleman PG, O'Hanlon A. Ageing and adaptation. Handbook of the clinical psychology of ageing. 2008 Jan 11:15–32.

115. Parkes CM. Coping with loss: Bereavement in adult life. BMJ. 1998 Mar 14;316(7134):856–9.

Contd...

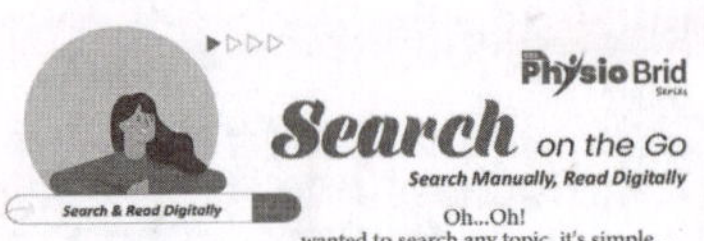

116. Kagan J, Klein RE. Cross-cultural perspectives on early development. Am Psychol. 1973 Nov;28(11):947.

117. Zervides S, Knowles A. Generational changes in parenting styles and the effect of culture. E-J Appl Psychol. 2007 Apr 5;3(1):65.

118. Thomas MS, Annaz D, Ansari D, Scerif G, Jarrold C, Karmiloff-Smith A. Using developmental trajectories to understand developmental disorders.

119. Werner EE. Protective factors and individual resilience. Handbook of early childhood intervention. 2000 May 22;2:115–32.

120. Joseph MV, John J. Impact of parenting styles on child development. Glob Acad Soc J Soc Sci Insight. 2008;1(5):16–25.

121. Pellegrini DS. Psychosocial risk and protective factors in childhood. J Dev Behav Pediatr. 1990 Aug 1;11(4):201–9.

122. Kuppens S, Ceulemans E. Parenting Styles: A Closer Look at a Well-Known Concept. J Child Fam Stud. 2019;28(1):168-181. doi: 10.1007/s10826-018-1242-x.

123. Darling-Hammond L, Flook L, Cook-Harvey C, Barron B, Osher D. Implications for educational practice of the science of learning and development. Appl Dev Sci. 2019;24(2):97–140. doi: 10.1080/10888691.2018.1537791

124. Berk, LE. Child Development. 8th ed. USA: Pearson Education, Inc; 2009.

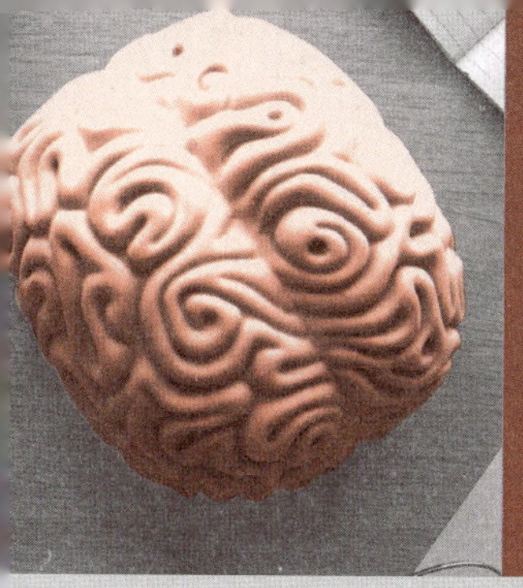

STUDENT ASSIGNMENT

LONG ANSWER QUESTIONS

1. Discuss the role of neurodevelopmental research in understanding the biological underpinnings of developmental milestones. Provide examples of how this research can inform interventions.
2. Analyze the impact of culture on developmental trajectories, providing examples of how different cultural expectations can influence developmental stages from childhood through adulthood.
3. Evaluate the ethical considerations in developmental psychology research, particularly when involving vulnerable populations such as children or the elderly.
4. Describe how developmental psychology can inform educational practices, specifically through the application of cognitive developmental theories in curriculum design.
5. Explore the relationship between aging theories such as the 'Free Radical Theory' and practical health interventions aimed at prolonging health during late adulthood.
6. Discuss the interplay between genetic predispositions and environmental influences in the development of developmental disorders.
7. Examine the effects of different parenting styles on children's emotional and social development. Include a discussion of cross-cultural variations in parenting norms.
8. Write in detail how developmental psychology research can be applied to improve outcomes for individuals with developmental disorders, focusing on educational and social interventions.
9. Analyze the contributions of Erikson's psychosocial stages to understand the challenges faced during different life stages.
10. Describe how advancements in technology, like wearable devices, are changing the landscape of developmental psychology research.

SHORT ANSWER QUESTIONS

1. What is the primary distinction between the 'Free Radical Theory' and the 'Telomere Shortening Theory' of aging?
2. How the 'Socioemotional Selectivity Theory' explains changes in social networks during late adulthood?
3. What are the implications of authoritarian parenting on child development?
4. What is the concept of 'Generativity vs. Stagnation' during middle adulthood according to Erikson?
5. What role does culture play in the developmental milestones during childhood?
6. How does the use of eye-tracking technology enhance our understanding of developmental stages?

7. Why is resilience considered important in the context of aging?
8. Identify two risk factors and two protective factors in child development.
9. What is the significance of puberty in developmental psychology?
10. What is the difference between active and passive aging theories?

MULTIPLE CHOICE QUESTIONS

1. **Which theory of aging suggests that aging results from the damage caused by unstable molecules known as free radicals?**
   - a. Rate of living theory
   - b. Telomere shortening theory
   - c. Free radical theory
   - d. Neuroendocrine theory

2. **Erikson's stage of 'Intimacy versus Isolation' occurs during which life stage?**
   - a. Adolescence
   - b. Early adulthood
   - c. Middle adulthood
   - d. Late adulthood

3. **Which parenting style is characterized by high responsiveness and high demands?**
   - a. Authoritative
   - b. Authoritarian
   - c. Permissive
   - d. Neglectful

4. **In developmental psychology, what is the term used to describe a period of rapid physical growth and sexual maturation that occurs mainly in early adolescence?**
   - a. Puberty
   - b. Infancy
   - c. Senescence
   - d. Adulthood

5. **Which developmental theory focuses on the impact of culture on development?**
   - a. Psychoanalytic theory
   - b. Cognitive development theory
   - c. Sociocultural theory
   - d. Behavioral theory

6. **What is the primary focus of the 'Activity Theory' regarding aging?**
   - a. Increased metabolic processes
   - b. Maintenance of social engagement
   - c. Biological deterioration
   - d. Cognitive decline

7. **Which type of developmental research tool involves tracking and where and how long a person gazes when looking at a stimulus?**
   - a. MRI
   - b. CT scan
   - c. Eye-tracking
   - d. EEG

8. **'Generativity versus Stagnation' is a stage described by Erikson that typically occurs during which period of life?**
   - a. Adolescence
   - b. Early adulthood
   - c. Middle adulthood
   - d. Late adulthood

9. Which of the following is NOT typically considered a risk factor for developmental disorders?
   a. Genetic predisposition
   b. High socioeconomic status
   c. Prenatal exposure to toxins
   d. Poor nutrition

10. At what stage does Erikson's theory suggest individuals deal with the conflict between integrity and despair?
    a. Early adulthood
    b. Adolescence
    c. Middle adulthood
    d. Late adulthood

Note

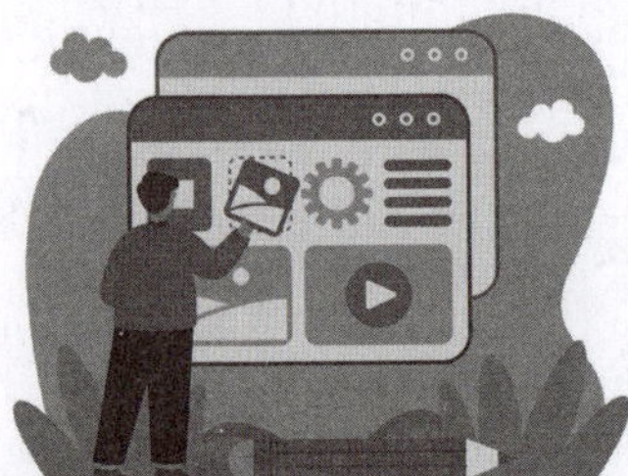

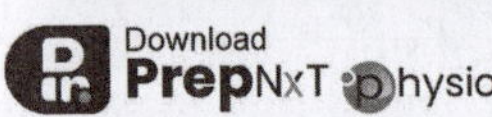

Physio Brid Series

Add Ons
Dil Mange More Content

Recent Update	e-Book
Regular updates related to Recent advancements & Book Errata	Get PDFs of important chapter/section (Annexures /Appendices) of book *(optional and exclusive for Pro-users and Institutions)*

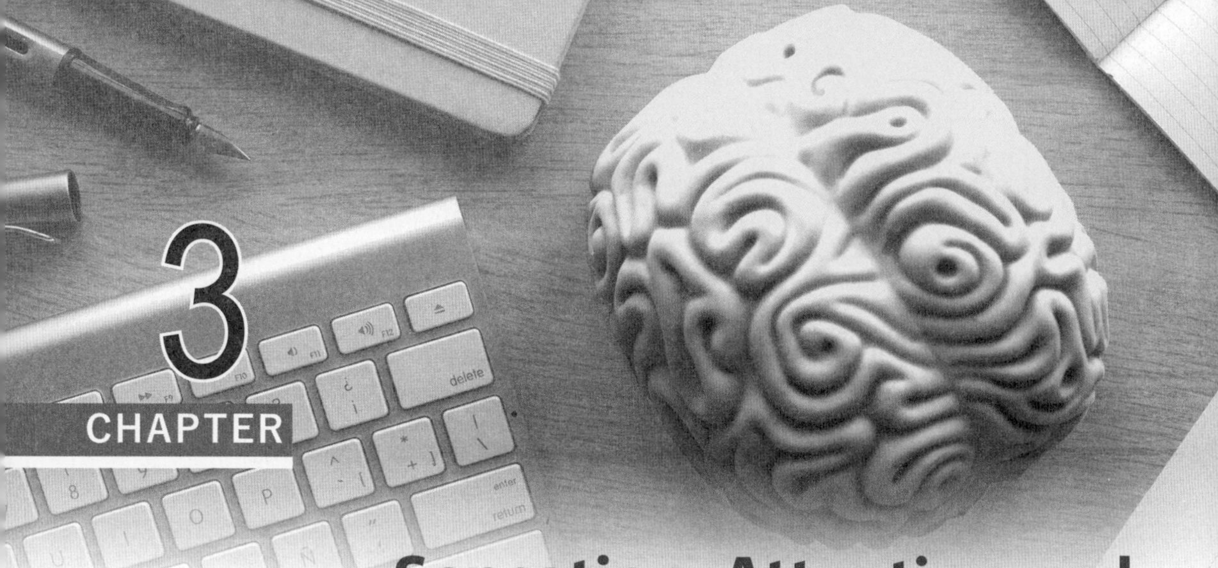

Sensation, Attention and Perception

Hina Vaish

LEARNING OBJECTIVES

After the completion of the chapter, the readers will be able to:
- Understand the meanings of sensation, attention and perception.
- Define the characteristics and types of attention.
- Understand the importance of attention.
- Enumerate the factors influencing attention, nature and characteristics of perception.
- Explain the differences between sensation and perception.
- Analyze the factors influencing perception.
- Learn about errors of perception.

CHAPTER OUTLINE

- Introduction
- Sensation
- Attention
- Perception
- Interconnection of Sensation, Attention and Perception
- Concept to Clinic

KEY TERMS

Attention: It is the perception process of selecting certain inputs to be included in our conscious awareness at any given time.

Bottom-up processing: The process of recognizing the process from discrete components to the whole.

Depth perception: The ability to measure the distance an object is with an observer or from the front of a solid object to the back.

Divided attention: Dividing attention between two or more sets of stimuli.

Gestalt principles: The concept that our brains typically perceive objects as part of a larger whole and are components of more complex systems (e.g., similarity, closure, continuity, etc.).

Perception: It can be defined as the sensory information and the way of processing the information.

Perceptual constancy: The perceptual ability to extrapolate from perceptual activity patterns comparable information about the external world.

Phi phenomenon: The appearance of motion in rapid succession between visual stimuli.

Selective attention: Focusing consciousness on a specific stimulus.

Sensation: It is a psychological process resulting from an immediate external stimulus to a sensory organ.

Top-down processing: A methodological approach that goes from the whole to the individual parts.

Visual illusions: Illusions created visually.

INTRODUCTION

Cognitive psychology is based on a complex of human emotions, feelings, and attention that explains how people interact with their environment. The term "perception" describes how sensory processes that convert physical energy into brain impulses first perceive stimuli. This initial phase is important because it provides unprocessed information that enables higher level cognitive functions. In other words, perception involves organizing and interpreting these sensory impulses to create a mentally coherent representation of the external world. People use it as a dynamic process, influenced by context, expectations and prior knowledge, making sense of complex and often confusing input.

Cognitive processing of attention contributes to the accuracy and efficiency of cognition by allowing specific information to be selected for further processing. It acts as a filter, consuming certain inputs before others, avoiding cognitive overload. Goals and objectives can guide the process of voluntary attention, whereas primary stimuli can inadvertently attract attention. The dynamic interaction of different kinds of attention illustrates the dynamic nature of cognitive control and change in an ever-changing environment.

Understanding how these processes work together is essential to interpret and interact with the environment in better way.

This chapter goes into further detail on the definition, meaning and details of sensation, attention and perception.

SENSATION

Color, light, tone and taste of a particular food are examples of sensations. Sensation can be defined as a psychological process resulting from an immediate external stimulus to a sensory organ.[1] Sense organs are the gateways by which we acquire knowledge of the world around us. In fact, stimulation stimulates or activates the receptors of the sensory organs involved.[2] These receptors release nerve impulses, which are transmitted to an associated area of the brain where they are interpreted. These are called effectors.

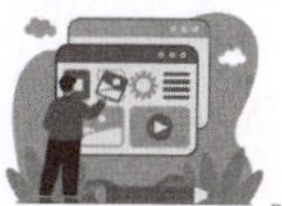

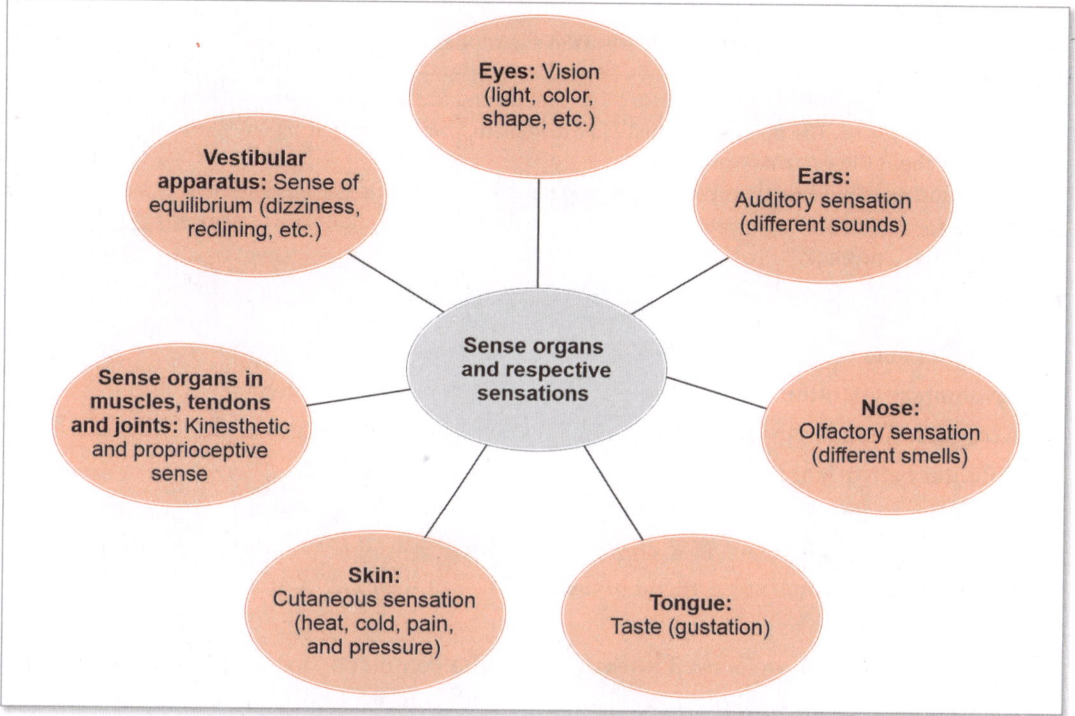

Fig. 3.1: Sense organs and respective sensations

This gives the information of object stimulating. These sensations differ in amount, intensity or quality.[3] The basic sensations concerning various forms of experiences are shown in Figure 3.1.[4, 5]

Threshold is essential for stimulus to be detected. Absolute threshold is the lowermost intensity at which a stimulus can be detected and difference threshold is the minimum perceived difference between the two stimuli.

Sensory Process to Perception

Whatever is experienced by a person can be defined as perception.

Simple perception or sensation are related to the activity in the sensory channels themselves.[3]

Perception = Sensory input + Way of processing of the sensory information

ATTENTION

Attention is a principal process and perception is impossible without attentional processes. Attention leads to perception. Attentional processes aid several functions in the organization of perceptions and additional cognitive functions.[6, 7]

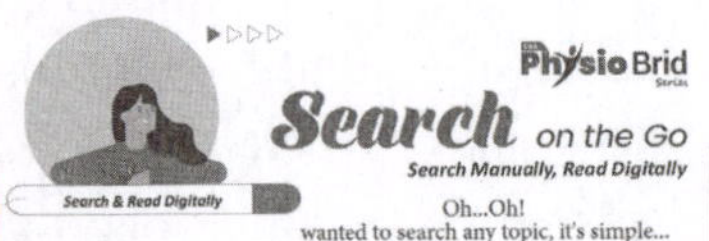

Attention is the perception process of selecting certain inputs to be included in our conscious awareness at any given time. It is possible for us to attempt to only one object or experience at a time.[8] But we can attend to two objects at a time when one is mechanical and other needs our attention.[9]

"Attention is the concentration of consciousness upon one object rather than upon another."

—Dumville

"Attention is being keenly alive to some specific factor in our environment. It is a preparatory adjustment for response."

—Morgan and Gilliland

Types

Attention is of following types:[10–13]

1. **Involuntary attention:** It does not require any conscious effort to attend to an object.

   Examples: Attention to lurid noises, bright colored lights and pungent odors.

2. **Voluntary attention:** Effort is must.

   Examples: Uninteresting lectures, difficult assignments.

3. **Habitual attention:** There is a conscious effort or sensation so prominent to attract the involuntary attention. People attend to them because of their habits or interests.

   Example: Attention to patients.

4. **Sustained, directed or focused attention:** It is the continuous focus on a specific stimulus or task over a long period of time. This type of attention involves sustained mental effort and distractions are resisted.

5. **Divided attention:** It is also known as multitasking, involves simultaneous attention to multiple stimuli or multiple tasks. When cognitive resources are allocated to two or more tasks simultaneously, individuals experience divided attention.

   Examples: Driving while listening to music or texting while attending a congregation meeting.

6. **Selective attention:** It is the ability to focus attention on specific stimuli while excluding irrelevant or distracting information. Such a view allows individuals to prioritize certain stimuli for processing while inhibiting others.

   Examples: Paying attention to a conversation in a noisy environment or focusing on a specific task despite environmental distractions.

Span of Attention

The maximum information processed in a single attention duration. For adults, the typical attention span on a particular task ranges from approximately 10 to 20 minutes before the onset of mental fatigue or distraction. In contrast, the attention span for children differs considerably with their age. For instance, a 5-year-old may be able to maintain focus for 5–10 minutes, whereas an adolescent is capable of sustaining concentration for 20–30 minutes.

Factors Determining Attention

There are objective and subjective factors that determine attention as discussed here:[10–13]

Objective Factors

- **Intensity:** Our attention is attracted more by intense stimuli such as loud sounds, bright colors, intense odors and sharp pain. Here, the selection of stimuli depends upon nature of sense receptor and the amount of energy stimulated.

- **Size:** Large size of an object or bigger patch of color draws our attention more easily than small object or small patch of color.

- **Repetitions:** Though the stimulus is weak in intensity, it draws our attention if repeated several times.

  Examples: A repeated cry, repeated ringing of a call bell, persistent tapping.

MUST KNOW	
Factors affecting attention	

Objective factors	Subjective factors
Intensity	Interest
Size	Habits
Repetitions	Motives
Movement	Emotions
Change	Attitudes and prejudices
Systemic form	
Novelty	
Location	
Nature of stimulus	

- **Movement:** Anything that moves if that is small can attract our attention more than one, which is stationary.

  Example: Moving toys attract children.

- **Change:** A sudden change in intensity or in size or sudden cessation (disappearing) of the continuous stimulus catches our attention.

  Examples: Loud noise, bright color, continuous sound when they stop.

- **Systemic form:** A systemic form or rhythm attracts our attention more than the stimulus which is not systemic and nonrhythmic.

  Examples: A melodious music, a beautiful picture, a symmetrical building.

- **Novelty:** Anything that is unusual or new or strange will draw our attention.

  Example: A new fashion dress.

- **Location:** The object or the picture, which is directly in front of our eyes or picture at the center, attracts our attention more than the one in the corner.

- **Nature of stimulus:** In an advertisement the picture attracts more than the words.

Subjective Factors

- **Interest:** If a person is interested in a particular object, it attracts attention much earlier than others. For example, a scholar who is attracted to a specific book is fascinated by it earlier than the other books.

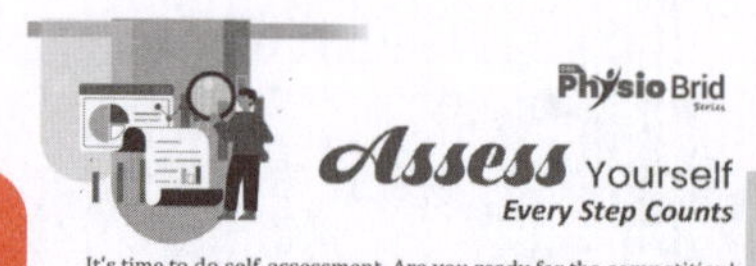

- **Habits:** Habits help in sensation of stimulus. All individuals are habituated to react to the sound of a coin. In a busy street also, this sound catches the attention.
- **Motives:** A sleeping mother may not be disturbed even by a loud noise outside but a faint cry of her child may attract her attention. A hungry person will be attracted more by an eatable.
- **Emotions:** If a person is angry with another person, in a group that person will catch their attention. Under stressful conditions individuals fail to perceive the surroundings fully.
- **Attitudes and prejudices:** Whenever attitude is unfavorable toward a group or a person, even a small mistake committed by that person will attract others, attention. In the same way, prejudices also influence attention.

PERCEPTION

Perception is the course by which we discriminate among stimuli and interpret their meanings and appreciate their significance.[14]

Example: When we touch an object, we can identify its shape, texture and what it is?

Perception gives meaning to sensation.

"All the processes involved in creating meaningful patterns out of a jumble of sensory impressions fall under the general category of perception." *—Charles G Morris*

"Perception is the experience of objects, events or relationships obtained by extracting information from and interpreting sensations." *—J H Jackson, O Desiderato and D B Howieson*

Principles of Perception (Perceptual Organization)

- **Bottom-up processing:** The process of recognizing the process from discrete components to the whole.
- **Top-down processing:** A methodological approach that goes from the whole to the individual parts.
- **Depth perception:** The ability to measure the distance an object is with an observer or from the front of a solid object to the back.

Gestalt Principles

The concept that our brains typically perceive objects as part of a larger whole and are components of more complex systems.[14, 15]

- **Principle of proximity:** Objects/things or items which are nearby to each other tend to be clustered together (Fig. 3.2).

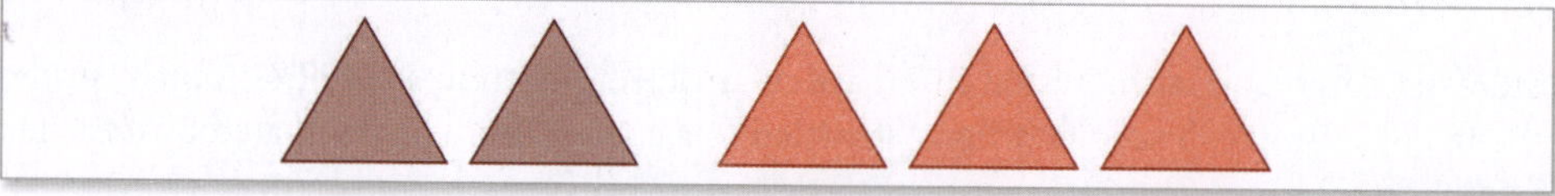

Fig. 3.2: One set of two triangles and one set of three triangles and not five separate triangles

- **Principle of similarity:** Items or figures which are alike in form or figure, however, mixed up with additional things have the propensity of perceiving them collected in form of a unit or pattern (Fig. 3.3).

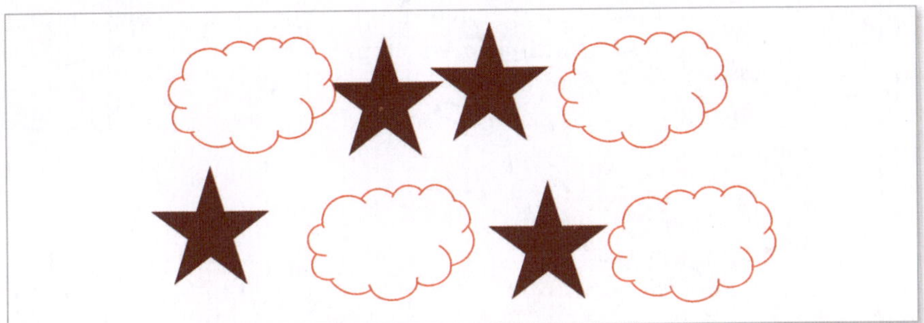

Fig. 3.3: Four white clouds and four blue stars

- **Principle of continuity:** States that individuals perceive continuous, flowing lines instead of rough or fragmented lines (Fig. 3.4).

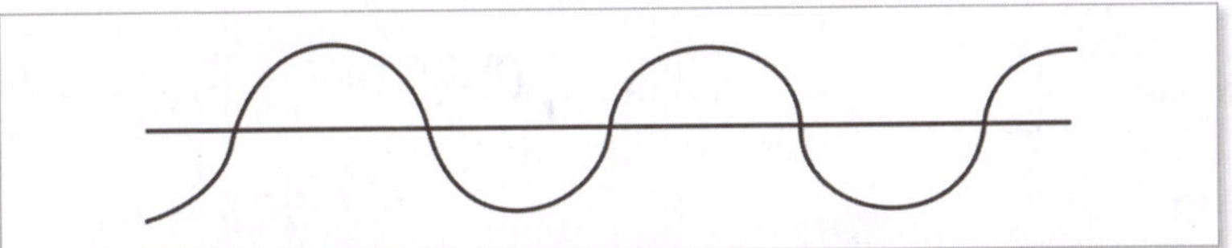

Fig. 3.4: A straight line and a curved line; not seen as straight line with semicircles above and below the line

- **Principle of closure:** States that we organize our perceptions into whole things rather than a series of fragments (Fig. 3.5).
- **Principle of simplicity:** Individuals tend to perceive the simplest likely arrangement or pattern as they aid the individual to perceive the full from some of its parts.
- **Principle of context:** An assessor may grant more grades to the equal solution book in a neat context than in untidy one.
- **Principle of contour:** The contour is the boundary between the figure and its ground. It is the shape of the contour that separates figure from landscape that enables individuals to organize certain objects or objects into meaningful patterns.

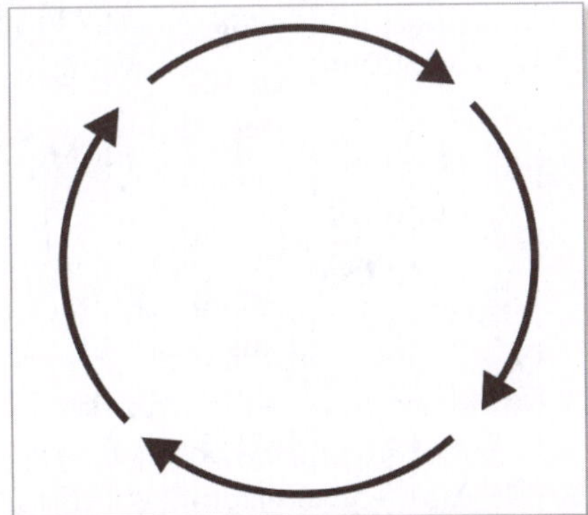

Fig. 3.5: A whole circle is perceived instead of sequence of segments

- **Principle of adaptability:** Perceptual organization for certain stimuli is based on the perceiver's adaptive ability to recognize similar stimuli. A person who adjusts to working in brightness will find normal sunlight to be relatively dim.

- **Principle of contrast:** Perceptual organization is strongly influenced by contrast effects because stimuli that are highly contrasting with adjacent stimuli can capture our attention more and carry perceptual effects (Figs 3.6A and B).

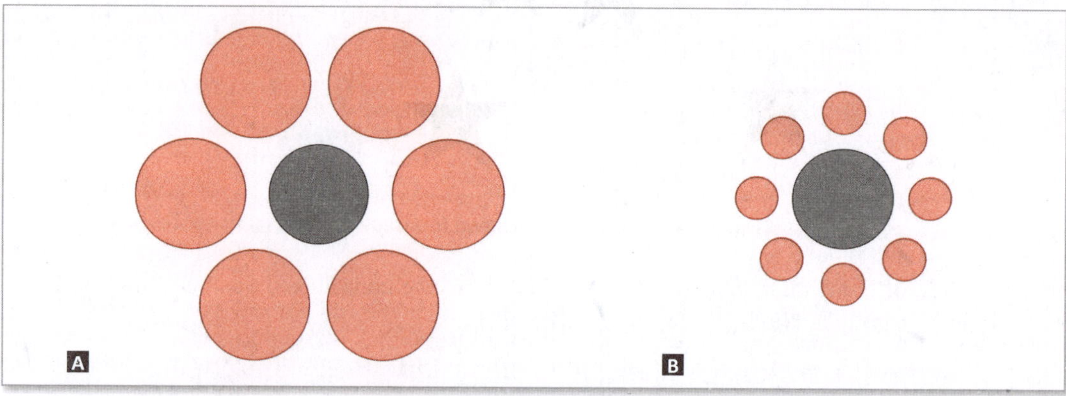

Figs 3.6A and B: The center circle looks smaller due to the surrounding circles in **(A)** than the center circle in **(B)**, though the two circles are of the same size

- **Principle of figure-ground relationship:**
  - The principle of figure-ground relation states that an image is perceived in context to the background of the figure. The perception of a thing or image for color, shape and intensity, etc. depends on the image-ground relationship. An individual perceives an image against the background or background of an image based on the characteristics of the person perceiving it as well as the strength of the image or ground.

  - A proper figure-ground relationship is vital from the angle of perception of the figure or the ground. In case, where such relationship does not exist, there exists ambiguity in terms of clear perception.

  - Sensory experiences other than visual experiences may also be perceived as figure and ground. Sometimes, when there are different parts within the general field of awareness, with equally balanced qualities, a conflict may occur and two or more figures may form. In such a case, there will be a shifting of the ground and the figure.

  - A part can be the ground one moment and the image of the ground the next (Fig. 3.7).

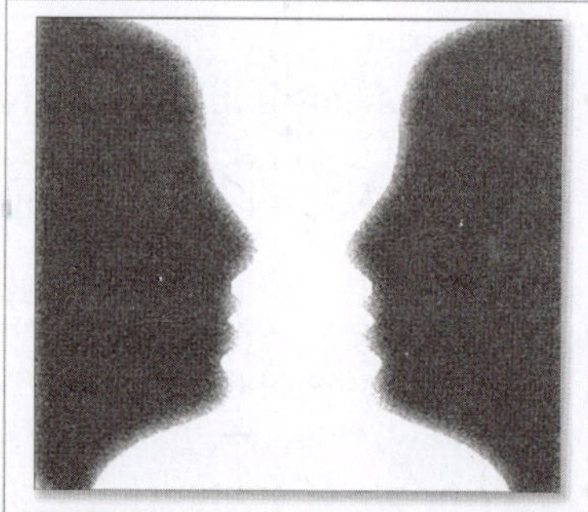

Fig. 3.7: An image is perceived against the background or background of an image based on the characteristics of the perceiver as well as the relative strength of the image or ground

Physio CORNER

Neurological perceptual disorders, such as agnosia and apraxia, involve impairments in perception and the ability to perform purposeful movements, respectively. These disorders can significantly affect an individual's daily functioning and quality of life. Here is a brief overview:

- **Agnosia:**
  - **Definition:** Agnosia is a disorder characterized by the inability to recognize or identify objects, people, sounds, shapes or smells, despite having intact sensory function. It results from damage to specific areas of the brain, particularly in the occipital or temporal lobes.
  - **Types:**
    - **Visual agnosia:** Inability to recognize objects or faces visually.
    - **Auditory agnosia:** Difficulty recognizing sounds, including speech.
    - **Tactile agnosia:** Inability to recognize objects by touch.
  - **Causes:** Common causes include stroke, traumatic brain injury, brain tumors, and neurodegenerative diseases.
  - **Symptoms:** Symptoms vary based on the type of agnosia but typically involve difficulties in recognizing familiar objects, sounds or people.
  - **Treatment:** Focuses on rehabilitation strategies, including compensatory techniques, cognitive therapies, and sometimes occupational therapy to help patients adapt to their impairments.

- **Apraxia:**
  - **Definition:** Apraxia is a motor disorder caused by damage to the brain, particularly the parietal and frontal lobes, leading to difficulties in planning and executing voluntary movements despite having normal muscle function.
  - **Types:**
    - **Ideomotor apraxia (IMA):** Difficulty in executing movements in response to verbal commands, despite understanding the task.
    - **Ideational apraxia:** Inability to plan and sequence complex motor actions involving multiple steps.
    - **Constructional apraxia:** Difficulty in drawing or constructing objects, often seen in tasks like assembling puzzles.
  - **Causes:** Often results from stroke, traumatic brain injury, Alzheimer's disease or other conditions affecting the brain.
  - **Symptoms:** Patients may struggle with simple tasks like waving goodbye, using tools or dressing themselves.
  - **Treatment:** Involves occupational and physical therapy, focusing on repetitive practice, using visual or verbal cues, and developing alternative strategies to perform daily activities.

Factors Affecting Perception

There are several factors affecting perception as listed here:[15, 16]

- **Sense organs:** Perception depends on the sense organs or receptors, on which the stimuli act and sensory neurons, which transmit the nerve current from the receptors to the sensory area of the brain. For example, colors cannot be perceived if cones are not well developed.

- **Brain:** Perception depends upon the sensory area and the association areas of the brain. For example, if the olfactory area is destroyed, olfactory perception will be absent.
- **Memory images of the past experience:** Memory images help individuals in the understanding of the thing or stimulus before them. Generally, perception involves the integration of sensory experience and existing psychological situations. Experiments have shown that whenever we encountered new stimuli, we are inclined to interpret them in terms of our experiences with similar stimuli in the past. For example, a child who encountered a dog for the first time and has already seen a goat. When asked what it (dog) is, they may say it is a goat.
- **Personal interests and mindset:** Individuals perceive those things rapidly, which are concerned with their interests and mindset. Acquired interests also determine the objects, which individuals perceive. For example, a person, who is interested, in cars will rapidly notice any new car in the market.
- **Needs and desires:** Needs and desires also modify perceptions. In addition to these, opinions, views and social norms also modify perception of things, circumstances and substances. Furthermore, the structural factors, which affect perception, are nature of physical stimuli and their arrangements and the neural effects they arouse in the systema nervosum of the individual.
- **Emotions:** These factors may influence the perceptual ability of an individual.

Errors or Abnormalities in Perception

As stated by Fish, perceptual anomalies may be explained as sensory distortions (Example: Hyperacusis) and sensory deceptions (Example: Illusions and hallucinations).[17, 18]

Sensory Distortions

These are the changes in perception due to changes in intensity, quality of stimulus, spatial form of perception, splitting of perception or distortion of experience of time.

Sensory Deceptions

Illusion

Illusion is a misinterpretation of actual perception. When the interpretation of a specific stimulus goes inappropriate, it leads to incorrect perception or illusion. For instance, a rope in the dim light may be perceived as a snake. Illusions are caused by insufficiencies of sense organs, distance of the object from the sense organ which perceives it, disingenuous stimuli in the setting, perceived notions and expectancy.

- **Horizontal-vertical illusion:** The vertical line drawn from mid-point to the horizontal line. Nonetheless, the two lines are equivalent in length, the erect line appears lengthier than the horizontal line. This is because of the movement of the eyes along the vertical line (Fig. 3.8).

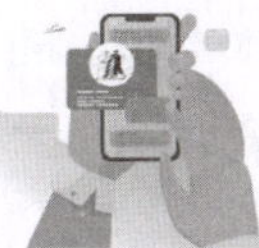
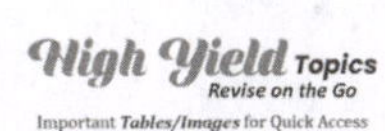

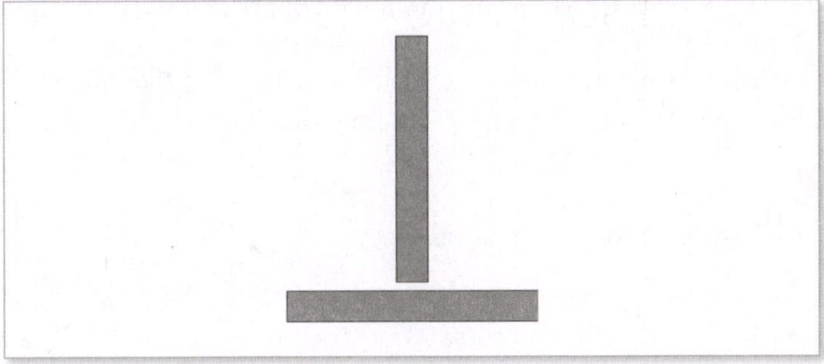

Fig. 3.8: Horizontal and vertical illusion

- **Muller-Lyre illusion:** This illusion emphasizes that open figure looks longer or larger than the enclosed area. For example, in Figure 3.9, the line B looks longer than line A. This is because of the line A has arrowhead which is enclosed whereas B is with featherhead which looks more open.

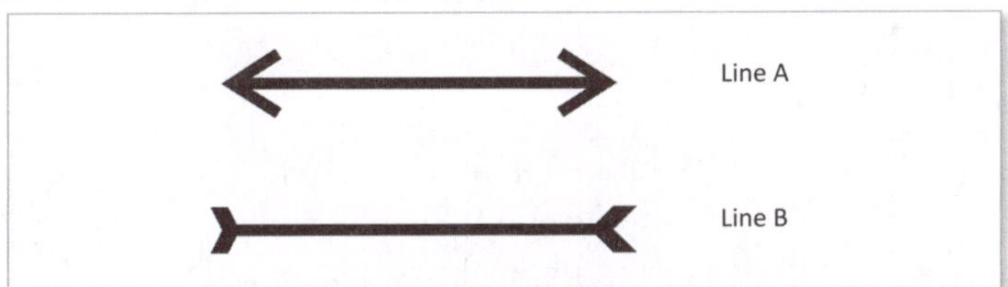

Fig.3.9: Muller-Lyre illusion

- **Illusion of movement or Phiphenomenon:** The perception of apparent movement is due to primitive organization of perception.

  Example: In cinema, there are no real movements but a series of still pictures projected on the screen at a particular speed.

> **MUST KNOW**
>
> **Errors or perception**
> - **Illusion:** Misinterpretation of actual perception.
> - **Hallucination:** Sensory perception without corresponding external sensory stimuli.

Hallucination

Hallucination is identified as a most important error of perception. Hallucinations are sensory perceptions without corresponding external sensory stimuli. They are imaginary perceptions, seeing or hearing something that others around do not see or hear. An alcoholic may see "a wall moving", a schizophrenic may hear voices in absence of any voices.

Hallucinations are more common in mentally ill people. Accurate perception is necessary to record an accurate observation. It is possible to make errors in perception due to several reasons. Depending on the specific sensory channel, people experience various hallucinations, such as visual, auditory, olfactory, etc.

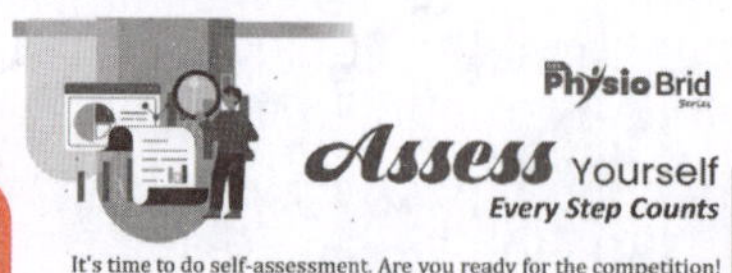

INTERCONNECTION OF SENSATION, ATTENTION AND PERCEPTION

Sensation occurs when outside stimuli are detected and encoded while attentional mechanism allows individual to focus on related information for further processing.

MUST KNOW

Different kinds of sensation and their experiences

Sensation	Sense organ involved	Sensory experience
Vision	Eye and retina	Light, color, shape, etc.
Auditory	Ear	Sounds
Taste	Tongue and taste buds	Sweet, sour, bitter, salty, etc.
Olfaction	Nose	Odor
Cutaneous touch	Skin receptors	Temperature, pressure, pain
Kinesthetic	Muscle and joint receptors	Movement in space

CONCEPT TO CLINIC

The study of sensation, perception, and attention facilitates learning about basic psychological processes and how they interact with each other. These findings not only enhance theoretical understanding but also provide guidance for real-world applications in areas such as clinical psychology, education, and human-computer interaction, and ultimately all improve human performance and well-being.

The knowledge of sensation, perception and attention will also aid in identifying psychological disorders such as sensory processing disorders (condition where the brain has problem receiving and responding to records that is available in *via* the senses), attention deficit hyperactivity disorder (ADHD) (a neurodevelopmental ailment characterized *via* troubles with recognition, hyperactivity, and impulsiveness) and perceptual disorders (conditions affecting the manner sensory facts is interpreted like agnosia, wherein patients can't recognize items regardless of having everyday vision).[19]

Physio CORNER

- Attention aids in bringing attentiveness and readiness. Consequently, the physiotherapist becomes mentally alert and efforts to exercise mental powers as efficiently as likely for providing care.
- Attention helps the physical therapist by focusing consciousness on one thing at a time instead of two.
- Attention helps the physiotherapist have better perceptual field for understanding of the patient's situation.
- Focus provides the ability to continue the cognitive functional task, despite the obstacles created by the distractions.

Contd...

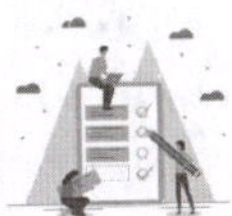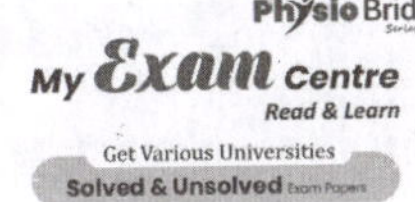

- The physical therapist can use the psychology of attention to call upon not only their voluntary work, but also involuntary attention.
- Accurate perception and observation are very important for a physiotherapist to provide quality care to a patient.
- All assessment and management activities require accurate observation and perception. For example, checking vital signs, assessing patient, administering correct dosage of, etc. If physiotherapist is not a keen observer, physiotherapist will not be able to note some very critical or important symptoms with the result that sometimes the patient may die premature.
- Accurate perception, and observation will help the physiotherapist to gather accurate information and knowledge, which will help the physiotherapist to learn more easily, adjust more quickly to new situations.
- It also prevents accidents and incidents harmful to the patient.
- With accurate perception, physiotherapists memory improves, recording and reporting is more accurate and is helpful for the patient and other health, team members.
- All types of false perceptions, illusions should be scrupulously avoided by physiotherapist.

CASE STUDY

A 65-year-old male patient with a history of hypertension, type 2 diabetes, smoking suffered from ischemic stroke.

The following are the findings:

Presenting Symptoms
- Loss of sensation on the right side of the body
- Difficulty in recognizing objects by touch (tactile agnosia)
- Difficulty performing purposeful movements with the right hand (ideomotor apraxia)

Initial Assessment
- **Neurological exam:** Confirmed sensory deficits in the right arm and leg, right-sided weakness (hemiparesis), and difficulty in performing tasks on verbal command.
- **Imaging:** Magnetic Resonance Imaging (MRI) revealed an infarct in the left parietal and frontal lobes, areas commonly associated with sensory processing and motor planning.

Clinical Diagnosis
- Ischemic stroke resulting in loss of sensation on the right side (contralateral to the lesion).
- Tactile agnosia and ideomotor apraxia due to damage in the left parietal and frontal lobes.

Treatment Plan
- **Medical management:**
  - Antiplatelet therapy (Aspirin)
  - Blood pressure control (ACE inhibitors)
  - Blood sugar management (Insulin therapy)
  - Smoking cessation program

Physiotherapy
- **Goal:** Improve sensory perception, motor function, and daily living activities.

Contd...

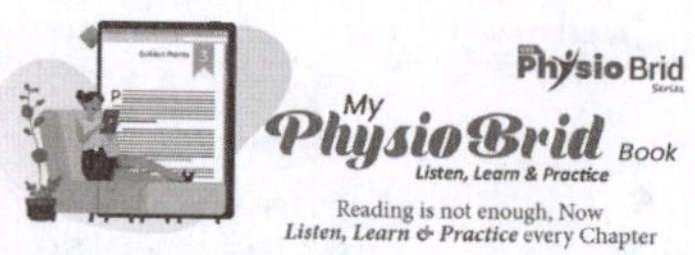

- **Techniques:**
  - **Sensory re-education:** Exercises to improve sensory awareness and discrimination (e.g., identifying objects with closed eyes).
  - **Proprioceptive training:** Activities to enhance the sense of body position and movement.
  - **Strengthening exercises:** Targeted exercises to strengthen the right-sided muscles.
  - **Task-oriented training:** Practicing specific tasks like buttoning a shirt, using utensils, and other daily activities to improve motor planning and execution.
  - **Mirror therapy:** Using the reflection of the unaffected limb to stimulate the affected side and improve motor function.
  - **ADL training:** Activities of daily living (ADL) (e.g., dressing, grooming) with adaptive equipment, if necessary.
  - **Cognitive strategies:** Techniques to improve planning and execution of tasks.
  - **Environmental modifications:** Adjustments at home to ensure safety and ease of movement.
  - **Speech therapy (if needed):** Assessment and treatment of any speech or swallowing difficulties.

Psychological Support

- Counseling to address emotional and psychological impacts of stroke.
- Support groups for stroke survivors.

The interdisciplinary approach, combining medical management, physiotherapy, occupational therapy, and psychological support, all are essential in addressing the patient's sensory and perceptual deficits and improving his overall quality of life after the stroke.

Recent Advances

Attention spans the fields of psychology, neuroscience, and artificial intelligence (AI).[20] Attention has been studied with many topics in neuroscience and psychology including consciousness, distinctiveness, executive management, and learning. It has also lately been extensively used in machine learning.

The AI development, with precise conclusions about the best ways to focus attention on cognitive processes or on specific projects seems promising.

The use of attention in artificial neural networks emerged like the necessity for attention in the brain to make neural systems more convenient.[20] Attention in machine learning enables trained single-processing neural networks to perform well on several tasks or tasks with inputs of varying dimensions or order.

These attention processes are, therefore, a form of repeated rebalancing. This makes it context-dependent, like a biological perspective. While sequence modeling already has a time element implied, this can also be applied to static inputs and outputs and consequently acquaint with dynamics into the model.

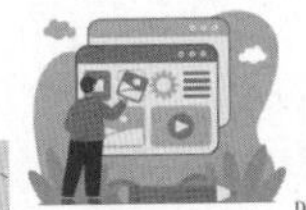
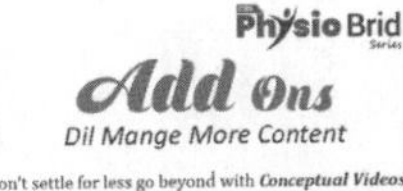

SUMMARY

- Sensation, attention and perception are interrelated subjects that have helped to understand human mind in a more profound way.
- By combining sensory inputs, selective attention mechanisms and perceptual processes, people can shape their own views about the world they live in.
- Sensation occurs when outside stimuli are detected and encoded while attentional mechanism allows individual to focus on related information for further processing.
- Attention is an ability of the brain to allocate mental resources to pick out certain stimuli or activities.
- Perception then organizes these sensations into coherent representations that guide our actions as well as shape our consciousness.
- In other words, sensation, attention and perception is a crucial part of cognitive science which provides insights into the remarkable abilities of a human brain.

REFERENCES

1. Bigley GK. Sensation. In: Walker HK, Hall WD, Hurst JW, editors. Clinical Methods: The History, Physical, and Laboratory Examinations. 3rd ed. Boston: Butterworths; 1990. Chapter 67. Available from: https://www.ncbi.nlm.nih.gov/books/NBK390/.

2. Wolfe JM, Kluender KR, Levi DM, Bartoshuk LM, Herz RS, Klatzky RL, Lederman SJ, Merfeld DM. Sensation & perception. Sunderland, MA: Sinauer; 2006.

3. Feinstein JS, Stein MB, Castillo GN, Paulus MP. From sensory processes to conscious perception. Consciousness and cognition. 2004 Jun 1;13(2):323–35.

4. Goldstein E. B. Sensation and perception. In: Goldstein E. B., Brockmole J. R., editors. Sensation and Perception. 11th ed. Boston: Cengage Learning; 2022.

5. Stevens S. S. Psychophysics. In: Goldstein E. B., Brockmole J. R., editors. Sensation and Perception. 10th ed. Boston: Cengage Learning; 2017: 75–112.

6. Pitts MA, Lutsyshyna LA, Hillyard SA. The relationship between attention and consciousness: An expanded taxonomy and implications for 'no-report' paradigms. Philos Trans R Soc Lond B Biol Sci. 2018;373(1755):20170348. doi:10.1098/rstb.2017.0348.

7. Bowins B. Sliding Scale Theory of Attention and Consciousness/Unconsciousness. Behav Sci (Basel). 2022 Feb 10;12(2):43. doi: 10.3390/bs12020043.

8. Posner M. I., Petersen S. E. The attention system of the human brain. In: Posner M. I., editor. Foundations of Cognitive Science. Cambridge, MA: The MIT Press; 1989: 243–257.

9. Carrasco M. Visual attention: The past 25 years. In: Nobre A. C., Kastner S., editors. Oxford Handbook of Attention. Oxford, UK: Oxford University Press; 2014: 25–46.

10. Ballard JC. Computerized assessment of sustained attention: A review of factors affecting vigilance performance. Journal of clinical and experimental neuropsychology. 1996 Dec 1;18(6):843–63.

11. Wang W. Factors Affecting Learners' Attention to Teacher Talk in Nine ESL Classrooms. Tesl-Ej. 2015 May;19(1):n1.

Contd...

12. Zeef EJ, Sonke CJ, Kok A, Buiten MM, Kenemans JL. Perceptual factors affecting age-related differences in focused attention: Performance and psychophysiological analyses. Psychophysiology. 1996 Sep;33(5):555–65.

13. Palmer J, Ames CT, Lindsey DT. Measuring the effect of attention on simple visual search. Journal of Experimental Psychology: Human Perception and Performance. 1993 Feb;19(1):108.

14. Koffka K. Principles of Gestalt psychology. Mimesis International; 2014.

15. Foley HJ. Sensation and perception. Routledge; 2019 Aug 14.

16. Foley HJ, Matlin MW. Sensation and perception. 5th ed. Boston: Allyn and Bacon; 2010.

17. Coren S, Ward LM, Enns JT. Sensation and perception. 6th ed. New York, NY: John Wiley and Sons; 2004.

18. Nour MM, Nour JM. Perceptual distortions and deceptions: What computers can teach us. BJPsych Bull. 2017 Feb;41(1):37-40. doi: 10.1192/pb.bp.115.052142. PMID: 28184316; PMCID: PMC5288092.

19. Passarello N, Tarantino V, Chirico A, Menghini D, Costanzo F, Sorrentino P, et al. Sensory Processing Disorders in Children and Adolescents: Taking Stock of Assessment and Novel Therapeutic Tools. Brain Sci. 2022 Oct 31;12(11):1478. doi: 10.3390/brainsci12111478.

20. Lindsay GW. Attention in Psychology, Neuroscience, and Machine Learning. Front Comput Neurosci. 2020 Apr 16;14:29. doi: 10.3389/fncom.2020.00029. Erratum in: Front Comput Neurosci. 2021 May 26;15:698574.

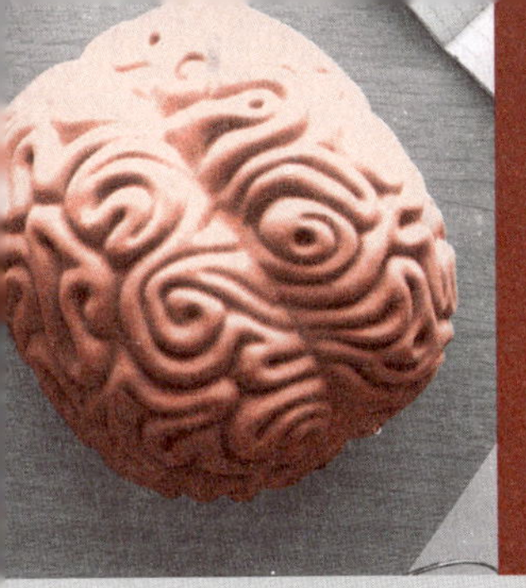

LONG ANSWER QUESTIONS

1. Define perception and discuss the organization of perception.
2. Explain the factors influencing perception. What is the relation between sensation and perception?
3. What is attention? Explain the factors affecting attention.
4. What are errors in perception? Write the differences.
5. Discuss the salient features of sensation and perception.
6. Enumerate different types of attention. Explain whether attention can be divided.
7. Define perception. What are the factors affecting perception?
8. Describe the principles of perceptual organization.

SHORT ANSWER QUESTIONS

1. Write a few features of attention.
2. List the determinants of attention.
3. Define sensation.
4. What do you mean by perception?
5. Define illusion.
6. Define hallucination.
7. Write any two principles of perception.

MULTIPLE CHOICE QUESTIONS

1. **An example of sensory distortions is:**
   a. Illusion
   b. Hallucination
   c. Hyperacusis
   d. Phi Phenomenon
2. **Illusion of movement is:**
   a. Divided attention
   b. Delusion
   c. Phi Phenomenon
   d. None of these
3. **When certain stimuli are selected from a bunch of others is cited as:**
   a. Amplitude
   b. Attention
   c. Pitch
   d. Path

4. **Which of the following is an internal factor affecting the process selective attention?**
   a. Internal stimuli
   b. Size of stimuli
   c. Interest
   d. Repetition of stimuli

5. **Completing your assignments while listening to music is an instance of:**
   a. Selective attention
   b. Sustained attention
   c. Concentration
   d. Divided attention

6. **Perception is associated to:**
   a. Olfaction
   b. Unconscious
   c. Interpretation
   d. Vision

7. **Which of the following personal variable influence our perception?**
   a. Need
   b. Emotion
   c. Values
   d. All of these

8. **Misperception resultant from interpretation of information received by sensory organs is called:**
   a. Delusion
   b. Illusion
   c. Hallucinations
   d. None of these

9. **An example of external factor of attention is:**
   a. Memory
   b. Forgetting
   c. Competitive Spirit
   d. Interest

10. **Perception that happens in the absence of external stimuli is:**
    a. Delusion
    b. Hallucinations
    c. Illusion
    d. None of these

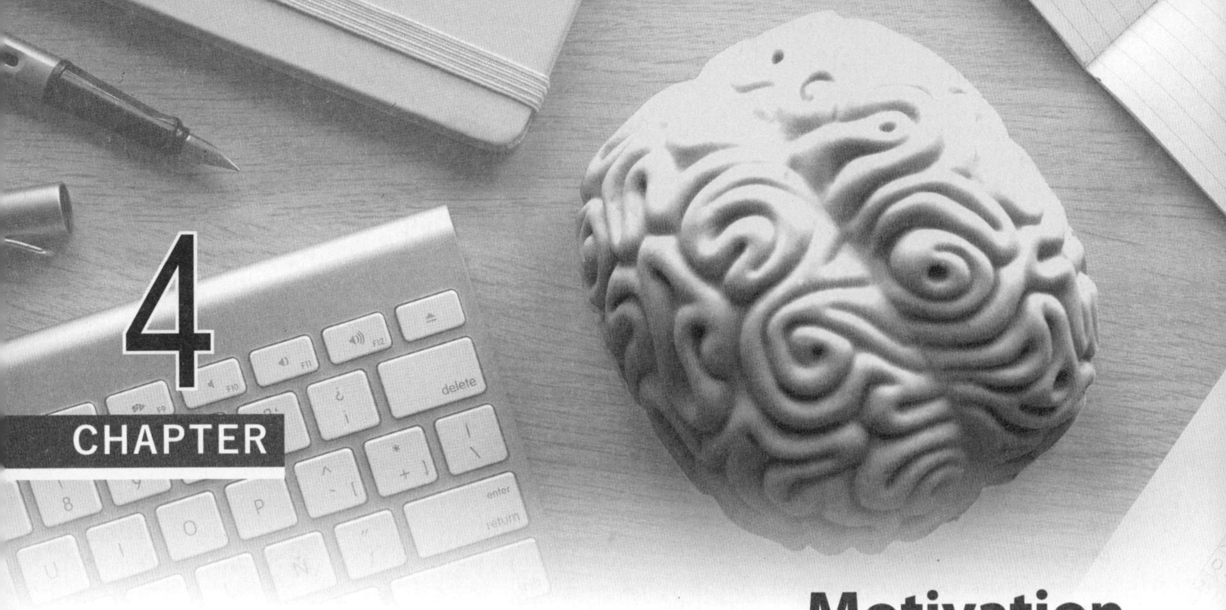

Motivation

Aditi Popli, Hem Jivani, Lakshay Panchal

LEARNING OBJECTIVES

After the completion of the chapter, the readers will be able to:
- Define motivation, its role in human behavior, and its importance for physiotherapist.
- Differentiate between intrinsic and extrinsic motivation.
- Identify common factors affecting motivation and describe stages involved in motivational cycle.
- Understand how Maslow's hierarchy classifies human needs and how it relates to motivation.
- Explain how a physiotherapist can use the knowledge of motivation to improve patient adherence to treatment.

CHAPTER OUTLINE

- Introduction
- Definitions
- Concept
- Importance
- Classification of Motives
- Motivation Cycle
- Types
- Theories of Motivation
- Applications of Motivation: Moving from Theory to Practice

KEY TERMS

Action: The actual behavior or response that a person takes to satisfy a need or desire.

Arousal: The first phase of the motivation cycle, where a person becomes conscious of a need or want.

Drive: The phase in which a person feels tension or arousal, prompting them to seek ways to fulfill or lessen their need or want.

Extrinsic motivation: Activities pursued with the specific aim of attaining a particular goal, contrasting with intrinsic motivation.

Fear motivation: This is the desire to avoid unpleasant or dangerous situations. This type of motivation is driven by the fear of negative outcomes, prompting individuals to take action to avoid harm or danger.

Incentive motivation: The drive to perform actions in order to achieve favorable results or avoid unfavorable ones.

Intrinsic motivation: The inclination to engage in activities for the inherent satisfaction they provide, rather than for external rewards or incentives.

Maslow's hierarchy of needs: A theory proposed by Abraham Maslow that categorizes human needs into five levels: Physiological, safety, love and belonging, esteem, and self-actualization.

McClelland's theory of motivation: A theory proposed by David McClelland that identifies three core human needs: Power, achievement, and affiliation.

Motivation: The process that influences an individual's actions to achieve their goals. It can be intrinsic (internal) or extrinsic (external).

Motivation cycle: The process by which people are motivated to start, maintain, and focus their behavior toward particular objectives or results. It typically includes stages, like arousal, drive, action, and reinforcement.

Reinforcement: It is results of a person's actions that can either increase or decrease their desire to repeat the same actions in the future.

Self-actualization: This is the highest level of Maslow's hierarchy of needs, where individuals are motivated by a strong sense of inner fulfillment and purpose.

INTRODUCTION

Motivation is a process that influences an individual's action in order to achieve their goals. Motivation can be intrinsic (internal) or extrinsic (external). It is used to stimulate and propel an individual toward desirable needs. After studying this chapter, learners will understand different theories of motivation and how to apply the concept of motivation in real life.

DEFINITIONS

Motivation can be described as a series of events where-in a requirement or longing is stimulated, and an internal psychological impetus propels us toward satisfying those needs and desires. Being moved to an action is a motivation to do something.[1] The Latin word 'movére', which meanings "to move", is derived from the word motivation.[2] There are many definitions of motivation, and some of them are as follows:

- "The elements that direct and energize the action of humans and other organisms" is how Feldman (2015) described motivation.[3]

- Motivation is described as "the urge to move toward one's goals, to accomplish tasks" by Feist and Rosenberg (2015).[4]

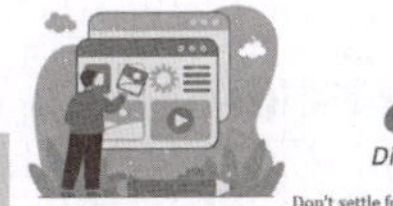
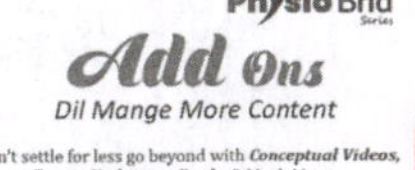

- Motivation is described as "an internal state, dynamical rather than static in nature, that propels action, directs behavior, and seeks toward satisfying both instincts and cultural needs and goals" by Chamorro-Premuzic (2015).[5]
- Motivation is defined as "a condition that stimulates behavior and gives it direction" by Nolen Hoeksema, Fredrickson, Loftus, & Lutz (2009, p. 419).[6]

CONCEPT

Motivation, as conceptualized in psychology, is an internal force that fuels and directs an individual's actions toward a specific goal.[7, 8] It serves as a driving mechanism, igniting the desire to achieve and sustain efforts toward a desired outcome. This multifaceted phenomenon involves intricate interactions between behavior, environment, cognition, and individual characteristics.[9]

Drawing from cognitive perspectives, Brown delineates three distinct categories to define motivation (Table 4.1). Firstly, the drive theory posits that motivation originates from inherent, innate drives, implying its presence since birth. Secondly, the hierarchy of needs theory suggests that motivation arises from fulfilling individual needs. Lastly, the self-control theory suggests that motivation emerges when individuals have the autonomy to make choices, exercising self-control over their pursuits. Collectively, these definitions underscore motivation's pivotal role as a catalyst in teaching-learning dynamics, compelling learners to strive toward their objectives.[1]

The essence of motivation extends beyond mere activation and direction of behavior; it serves three fundamental purposes: Providing energy, guiding actions, and aiding in decision-making processes.[9] Furthermore, motivation encompasses the intricate interplay between desires, needs, and the intensity and direction of behavior toward goal attainment.[8]

Table 4.1: Different theories of motivation

Aspect	Drive theory	Hierarchy of needs theory	Self-control theory
Basic concepts	Motivation arises from biological needs	Motivation stems from fulfilling needs	Motivation depends on self-regulation
Primary focus	Biological drives (e.g., hunger thirst)	Hierarchical progression of needs	Management of impulses and behaviors
Origin	Freudian psychology	Psychological theory by Maslow	Social cognitive theory by Baumeister
Key proponents	Clark Hull, Sigmund Freud	Abraham Maslow	Roy Baumeister
Key concepts	Drive reduction, homeostasis	Five levels of needs hierarchy	Limited resource model, ego depletion
Example	Eating when hungry	Seeking self-actualization	Resisting temptation to procrastinate

IMPORTANCE

Motivation, as its name suggests, is the driving force behind one's actions. It intricately influences human psychology and behavior, dictating how individuals allocate their time, exert effort in tasks, perceive their work, and persist in their endeavors.[10] At its core, motivation involves a complex interplay of biological and psychological processes, spanning from molecular mechanisms to species-specific social dynamics (Fig. 4.1).

While inherent motivational processes are fundamental to physical well-being, humans may encounter two distinct types of motivation disorders. The first category encompasses conditions such as apathy and pathological motivation deficiencies, commonly observed in individuals grappling with affective disorders and schizophrenia. On the other hand, the second group comprises disorders characterized by pathological motivational misdirection and detrimental behavioral excesses, including addiction. These manifestations underscore the profound impact of motivation on human behavior and well-being.[11]

CLASSIFICATION OF MOTIVES

Motivation serves as a fundamental element in one's interactions both externally and interpersonally, acting as the driving force that steers behavior toward a desired objective. Across all creatures, the

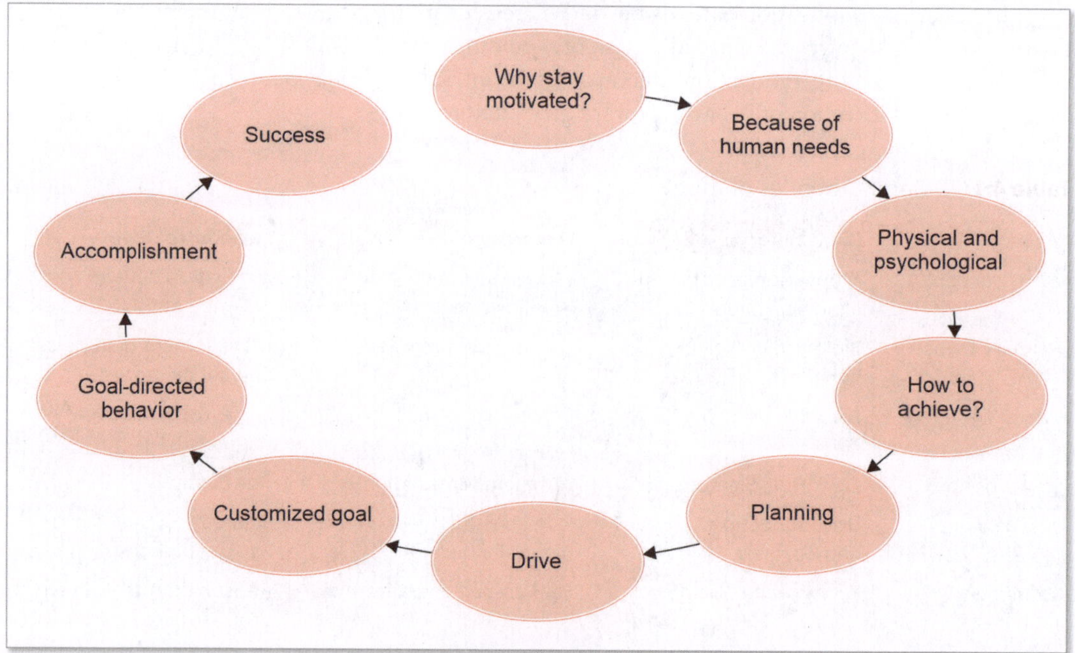

Fig. 4.1. Importance of motivation

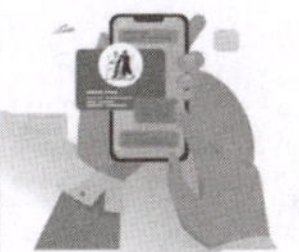
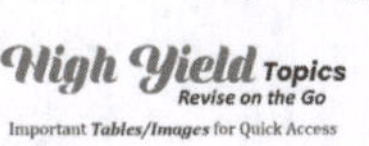

pursuits of fundamental needs such as sustenance, hydration, reproduction, and social engagement serve as the impetus for action.[11]

Motives underpin human behavior, channeling energy toward fulfilling both essential and aspirational objectives. They are broadly divided into primary motives, driven by innate biological necessities, and secondary motives, shaped by social contexts and psychological aspirations.

Table 4.2 differentiates primary motives from secondary motives.

Table 4.2: Differences between primary and secondary motives

Primary motives	Secondary motives
Connected to basic biological needs	Associated with sociopsychological needs
Examples include hunger, thirst, sex	Examples include achievement, affiliation, power
Essential for survival and physical well-being	Influence social interactions, self-esteem and personal growth
Innate and universal	Influenced by culture, upbringing and individual experiences

MOTIVATION CYCLE

The method by which people are motivated to start, maintain, and focus their behavior toward particular objectives or results is known as the motivation cycle (Fig. 4.2). Arousal, drive, action, and reinforcement are some of the stages that this cycle usually entails. It is impacted by a number of internal and external factors. Let's examine each step with an illustration:

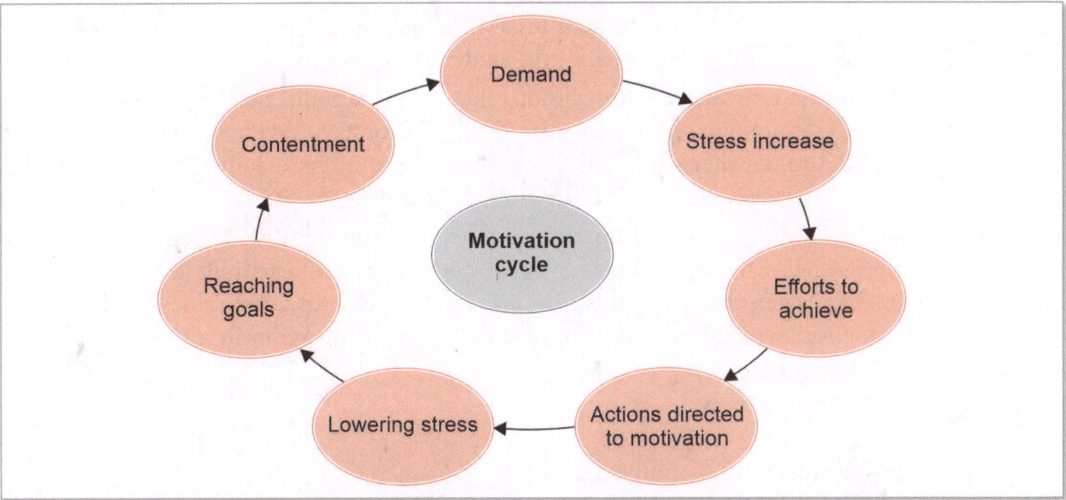

Fig. 4.2: Motivation cycle

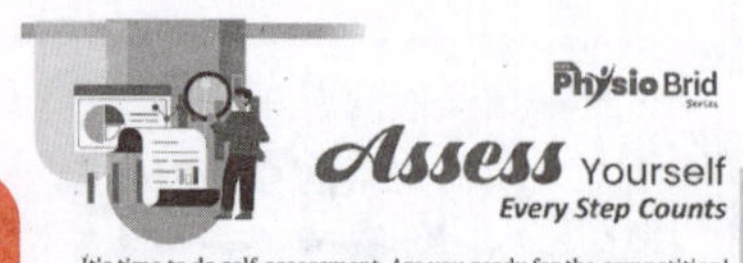

- **Arousal:** It is the first phase of motivation, during which a person becomes conscious of a need or want. This could be brought on by external stimuli, like reading an advertisement for a new product or internal physiological situations, like hunger or thirst. Consider a student who believes, they must study in order to do well on an impending exam.

- **Drive:** It refers to the phase in which a person feels tensed or aroused, prompting them to seek methods to fulfill or lessen their need or want. This puts the person in a motivated state and compels them to act. In our scenario, the student feels motivated to study so as to ace the test and release the stress brought on by failure-related anxiety.

- **Action:** The actual behavior or response that a person takes to satisfy a need or desire and lessen their drive is referred to as action. This could entail a range of mental, emotional or physical actions meant to accomplish the intended outcome. Using the example above once more, the student begins studying by going over their notes, reviewing textbooks, and doing practice questions.

- **Reinforcement:** The results of a person's actions or consequences, can either increase or decrease their desire to repeat those actions in the future. Presenting a rewarding stimulus is known as positive reinforcement, while removing an unpleasant stimulus is known as negative reinforcement. Positive reinforcement for the student could come from getting a good score as a reward for doing well in exam. They might become more motivated to learn in the future, as a result. However, in the event that the student obtains a low grade despite the efforts, they might feel disappointed or guilty, which could make them less motivated to study for future exams.

After the reinforcement stage, the person feels satisfied if their activities were successful in meeting their needs or desires or frustrated if they were not successful in reaching their objectives. An individual's future motivational tendencies and behaviors are influenced by this assessment of the result. In our scenario, a student who does well in the test can feel pleased with their performance and stay inspired to study hard for upcoming tests. If in spite of their best efforts, they perform poorly, they could become irritated and change the study methods or look for more help.

The dynamic interactions between the various phases of the motivation cycle might vary in terms of strength and duration based on environmental conditions, individual characteristics, and the type of goal or desire. Furthermore, people may experience numerous motivations at once or move to and fro between stages, so the cycle may not necessarily be linear.

This heightened state propels individuals to take action that aligns with their objectives. For instance, when experiencing thirst, the need for water motivates one to search for it. Upon satisfying this need by obtaining water, the motivation diminishes. Consequently, after achieving the desired outcome, motivation recedes, and the individual returns to a state of equilibrium.[2]

TYPES

Figure 4.3 exhibits various types of motivation.

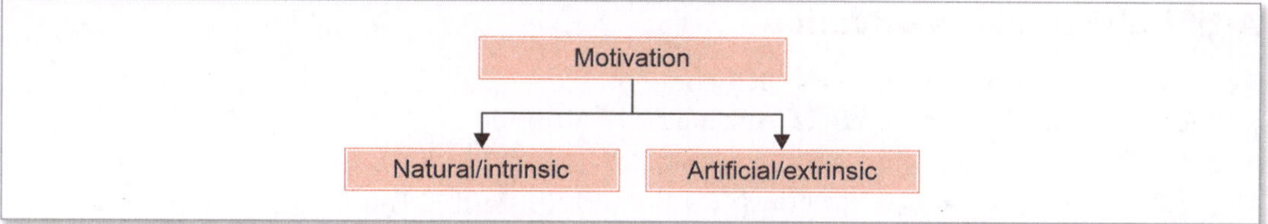

Fig. 4.3: Types of motivation

Natural/Intrinsic Motivation

Natural or intrinsic motivation refers to the inclination to engage in activities for the inherent satisfaction they provide, rather than for external rewards or incentives. When driven by intrinsic motivation, individuals are motivated by the enjoyment or challenge inherent in the task itself, rather than by external pressures or inducements.[1] The primary objectives of intrinsic motivation are pleasure and satisfaction derived directly from the activity.

Intrinsic motivation arises from internal drives and a sense of fulfillment (Fig. 4.4). It is:

- **Organic:** Rooted in personal growth and self-determination.
- **Psychological:** Fueled by a desire for competence, autonomy, and mastery.
- **Incorporeal:** Driven by intangible rewards like joy, curiosity, and purpose.
- **Social:** Enhanced by meaningful relationships and a sense of belonging.

Activities driven by intrinsic motivation evoke feelings of pleasure, contentment, and happiness, as they inherently bring about a sense of ease and joy. It is essential to note that activities cannot be considered fully intrinsically motivated if they serve purposes beyond the enjoyment of the activity itself.[12] The concept of intrinsic motivation was initially recognized through experimental studies of animal behavior, where creatures engaged in exploratory and playful behaviors even in the absence of external feedback or incentives.[8]

These instinctive actions, while advantageous for the organism's adaptability, are not driven by utilitarian goals but rather by the gratifying experience of utilizing one's abilities. Focusing on the characteristics of tasks and their intrinsic appeal holds practical significance as it enhances task design or selection, thereby enhancing motivation.[8]

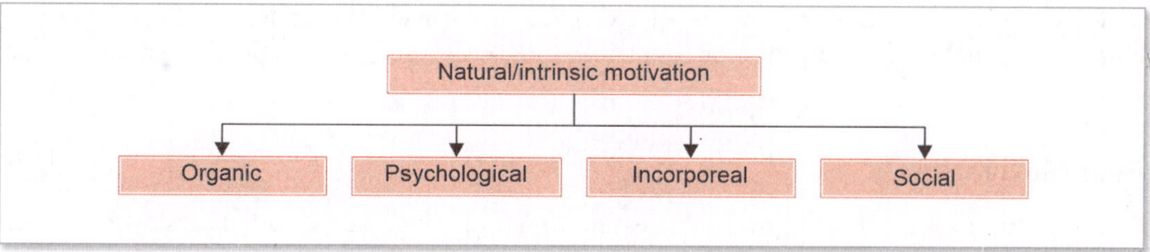

Fig. 4.4: Types of natural/intrinsic motivation

Artificial/Extrinsic Motivation

Extrinsic motivation encompasses activities pursued with the specific aim of attaining a particular goal, contrasting with intrinsic motivation, which involves engaging in an activity solely for the pleasure it brings.[8]

Extrinsic motivation is driven by external rewards or pressures (Fig. 4.5).

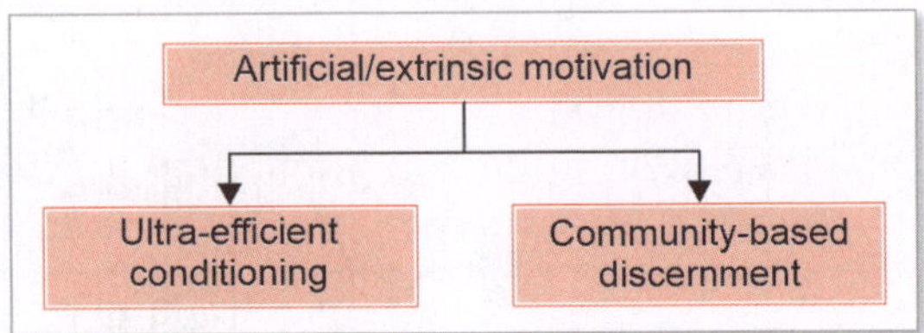

Fig. 4.5: Types of artificial/extrinsic motivation

- **Ultra-efficient conditioning:** Achieved through structured reinforcements like incentives, deadlines or recognition to maximize performance.
- **Community-based discernment:** Shaped by societal expectations, peer influence, and collective goals that guide behavior toward external validation.

Early psychological frameworks of extrinsic motivation focused on the influence of goal expectation on behavior and control, asserting that the attainment of goals is facilitated by willpower and intention. According to this framework, an individual's actions in pursuit of a goal—particularly their mental representation of the goal—are influenced by both environmental factors and internal states or memories. This necessitates the establishment, maintenance, and updating of various cognitive representations, with a particular emphasis on learning and external stimuli.[13]

The self-determination theory further categorizes extrinsic motivation into three distinct types: (1) Identification, (2) External regulation, and (3) Introjections. External tools such as rewards and constraints are employed to regulate behavior from the outside. Through interjected regulation, individuals begin to internalize the motivations behind their actions. Moreover, the incorporation of extrinsic reasons is guided by identification, particularly to the extent that the behavior is valued and perceived as essential by the individual, especially if it is viewed as a personal choice.[14]

Incentive Motivation

Anticipating benefits or penalties is what drives incentive motivation. It is a basic feature of human behavior that drives people to do actions in order to achieve favorable results or stay away from unfavorable ones. Rewards might be material, like cash or gifts or they can be immaterial, like recognition or admiration. People use this kind of incentive to balance the costs and advantages of a decision before acting, which has a big impact on behavior. An understanding of incentive motivation aids in the justification of people's actions, decisions, and reactions to environmental cues.

Fear Motivation

Fear motivation is the desire to avoid unpleasant things or dangerous situations. It's a strong force that drives people to take precautions to keep themselves safe from injury, danger or unfavorable outcomes. Fear can take on diverse manifestations, including fear of bodily damage, rejection or failure.

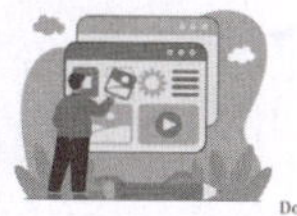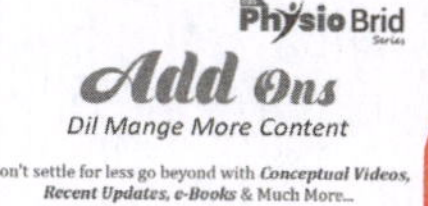

This kind of drive sets off the fight-or-flight reaction, which compels people to either face their fears or flee from them. Recognizing the motivations behind fear helps us better understand how fear affects people's behavior, risk assessment, and decision-making as they work to reduce danger and protect themselves.

THEORIES OF MOTIVATION

Maslow's Hierarchy of Needs

The 20th-century psychologist Abraham Maslow formulated the novel theory of the hierarchy of needs, which offers a systemic structure for comprehending human motivation and behavior. The basic idea of Maslow's theory is that individuals are motivated by a hierarchy of needs, which moves from the most primary physiological demands to more complex psychological needs. The idea of self-actualization, which represents the apex of human fulfilment and personal growth, is fundamental to this hierarchy. Physiological requirements which include primary needs for human sustenance and well-being, represent the basic level of Maslow's hierarchy.

The Maslow's five stage framework (Fig. 4.6) includes:

1. **Physiological needs:** Physiological needs or the bare minimum needed to survive, are at the beginning of Maslow's pyramid. Air, water, nourishment, shelter, and sleep are among these

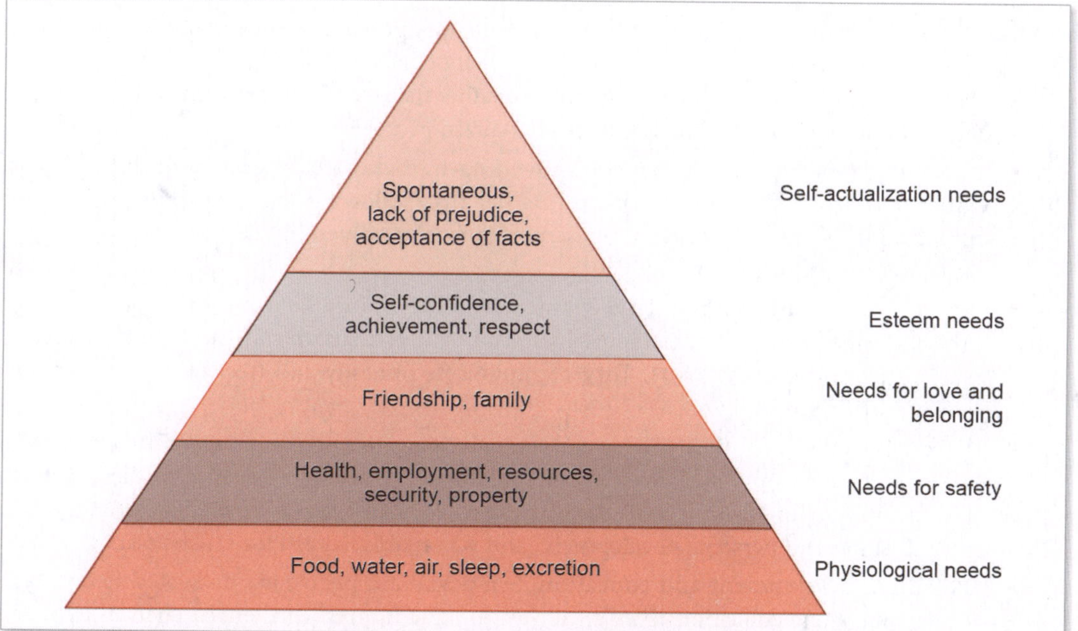

Fig. 4.6: Maslow's Hierarchy of needs

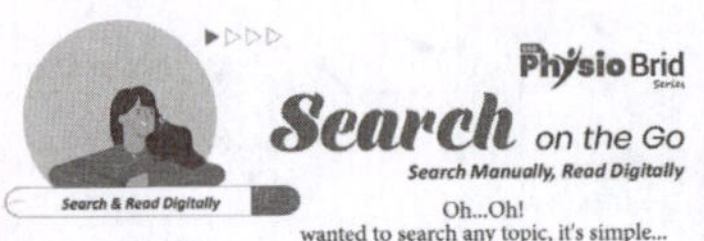

necessities. People cannot advance to the next level of the hierarchy if these physiological demands are not met. Therefore, it is critical to provide access to these necessities for human functioning and well-being.

2. **Needs for safety:** People shift their focus to safety needs after their physiological needs are satisfied. Seeking safety from emotional and physical harm as well as creating security and steadiness in one's surroundings are all part of one's desires for safety. This comprises monetary security, stability in work, well-being, and personal safety. When people's safety needs are met, they feel confident and at ease, which frees them up to concentrate on other needs.

3. **Needs for love and belonging:** Maslow's hierarchy of requirements places a strong emphasis on the value of social ties and interpersonal interactions at level three, which deals with wants for love and belonging. Since humans are social creatures by nature, having a sense of love, affection, and belonging is essential to psychological health. Meaningful interactions with family, friends, love partners, and social groups fulfill these requirements.

4. **Esteem needs:** Esteem needs include both internal esteem—which comes from a sense of value and respect for oneself—and external esteem, which comes from acknowledgment and appreciation from others. Acquiring respect, standing, and gratitude from others by accomplishments is the foundation of external esteem. Internal esteem, on the other hand, is associated with growing a sense of competence, confidence, and a good self-image. The development of self-actualization and self-confidence depends on the satisfaction of esteem requirements.

5. **Self-actualization needs:** The pinnacle of psychological growth and fulfilment that people can attain is self-actualization. Realizing one's full potential, pursuing personal development, and putting one's special skills and abilities to use are what define it. Self-actualized people are driven by a strong sense of inner fulfilment and purpose rather than by incentives from external factors, as stated by Maslow.[21-23] The features of self-actualized people include:

    -   **Autonomy and independence:** People who have reached self-actualization have a great sense of independence and autonomy. Rather than following social standards or outside expectations, they make decisions based on their own values, beliefs, and wants. They are self-directed and self-regulated.

    -   **Self-expression and authenticity:** Self-actualized people are known for their authenticity. They are sincere and loyal to themselves, leading lives that are consistent with their own goals, values, and convictions. They communicate honestly and freely without worrying about criticism or rejection.

    -   **Creativity and innovation:** Highly creative and innovative people are self-actualized. They are able to come up with fresh concepts and answers to issues because of their distinct viewpoint on the world. Creativity encompasses many facets of life, including work, relationships, and personal development, and is not just reserved for artistic pursuits.

    -   **Persistent development and education:** Self-actualized people are dedicated to constant development and education. They are always looking for fresh challenges, chances to better themselves, and methods to learn more about the world and themselves.

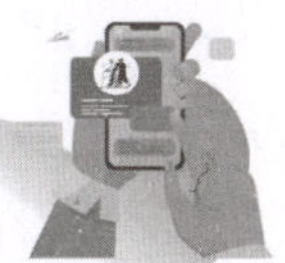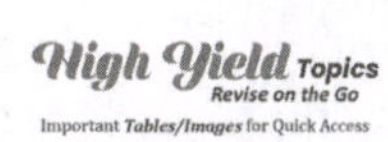

- **Acceptance and realism:** People who are self-actualized are realistic in their acceptance of others, themselves, and their surroundings. They accept and don't feel defensive or judgmental about their flaws. In addition, they have a profound understanding of the complexity of society and human nature, seeing that life isn't always ideal but nevertheless finding value and beauty in its flaws.

Limitations of Maslow's Theory

Refer to Table 4.3 to understand the limitations of Maslow's hierarchy of needs.

Table 4.3: Limitations of Maslow's hierarchy of needs

Limitation	Description
Cultural variability	Maslow's theory may not apply universally across cultures. The prioritization and interpretation of needs can vary significantly based on cultural norms and values.
Individual differences	People have different needs and motivations, and these can change over time. Maslow's theory oversimplifies human behavior by assuming a universal hierarchy of needs.
Lack of empirical evidence	Maslow's theory lacks strong empirical support. It is primarily based on anecdotal evidence and case studies rather than rigorous scientific research.
Overemphasis on self-actualization	Maslow's hierarchy places a strong emphasis on self-actualization as the pinnacle of human motivation, potentially neglecting the importance of other needs and goals.
Rigidity of the hierarchy	Maslow's hierarchy implies a strict hierarchical structure, suggesting that lower-level needs must be completely satisfied before higher-level needs become relevant.
Dynamic nature of needs	Human needs are dynamic and can change in response to various factors such as life events, experiences, and socioeconomic conditions. Maslow's theory does not account for this dynamic nature adequately.
Incomplete and simplistic model	Maslow's hierarchy presents a simplified model of human motivation, overlooking the complexity and interplay of various factors that influence behavior and decision-making.

McClelland's Theory of Motivation

David McClelland introduced the theory of needs, delineating three core human needs: Power, affiliation, and achievement (Table 4.4). This theory, established in 1961 and further elaborated upon in 1987, has garnered significant attention across various academic fields such as social psychology, education, political science, economics, and management sciences.[15]

Drawing from Maslow's research, McClelland pinpointed three primary human motivators in the early 1960s. He emphasized the needs for power, achievement, and affiliation, incorporating

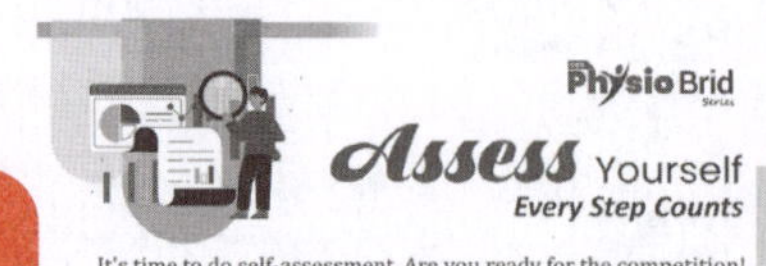

them into his classifications of needs. Unlike the theories of Maslow and Alderfer, which prioritize satisfying existing needs over creating new ones, McClelland's framework diverges. Our upbringing and life experiences significantly shape our predominant motivators, which encompass power, affiliation, and achievement.[16]

Table 4.4: McClelland's theory of motivation

Aspect	Description
Theory name	McClelland's theory of motivation, also known as the three needs theory.
Basic premise	Individuals have three primary needs: Achievement, affiliation and power.
Need for achievement	• Desire for challenging tasks and opportunities to excel. • Preference for tasks with a moderate level of difficulty where success depends on personal effort and skill.
Need for affiliation	• Desire for positive relationships, social approval and acceptance. • Preference for cooperative and supportive environments.
Need for power	• Desire to influence, lead or control others and situations. • **May manifest in different forms:** Personalized (focused on individual goals) or socialized (focused on group goals).
Application in work settings	• Job design: Matching tasks to individuals' dominant needs. • Leadership: Understanding leader' and followers' motivational needs to enhance effectiveness. • Team dynamics: Recognizing and leveraging diverse motivational profiles for improved collaboration and performance.
Assessment	McClelland developed Thematic Apperception Test (TAT) and self-report measures to assess individuals needs.
Criticisms and limitations	• Cultural bias in assessment tools. • Lack of empirical support for the universality of needs across cultures. • Oversimplification of complex human motivation.

Needs for Achievement (Fig. 4.7)

McClelland (1961, 1985) characterized the need for achievement as the drive to excel based on established standards. When individuals can achieve their goals autonomously, irrespective of external circumstances, their need for achievement is satisfied. High achievers do not rely on luck to determine their success; instead, they seek discernible reasons for their achievements or failures. Additionally, individuals with high achievement needs, experience happiness or dissatisfaction based on the observable outcomes of their efforts.[19]

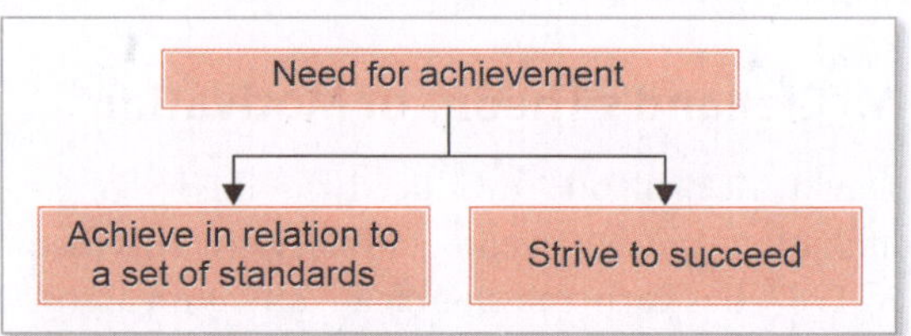

Fig. 4.7: Need for achievement

According to McClelland, individuals with a strong drive for achievement actively seek out opportunities to tackle challenges in innovative ways, often driven by a desire to alleviate concerns about their future within the organization. They demonstrate persistence and determination when solving problems. Research indicates that those with high achievement needs often exhibit effective leadership qualities. However, there is evidence suggesting a tendency to act opportunistically in pursuit of fulfilling this need.[19]

Need for Affiliation (Fig. 4.8)

The need for affiliation in individuals is prompted by both positive emotions like happiness and negative experiences such as feelings of vulnerability or powerlessness. Those with a strong inclination toward affiliation are motivated to establish friendships and actively seek the company of others. Most individuals desire some level of social interaction or companionship, as few find solace in prolonged solitude. Human tendency leans toward forming groups upon discovering common interests or developing emotional bonds. The capacity to forge connections and build collectives is a fundamental aspect of human nature. People consistently endeavor to connect with others, seek their support, and become part of their social circles. Affiliation encompasses the pursuit of interpersonal relationships, both physical and emotional, reflecting the intrinsic motivation for social engagement.[20]

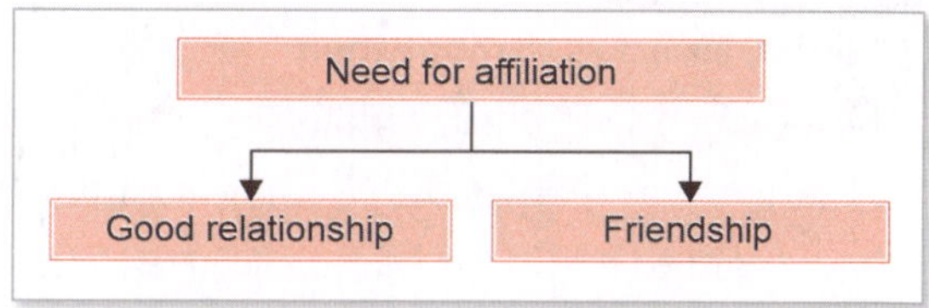

Fig. 4.8: Need for affiliation

Need for Power

The urge of people to exert influence or control over others is referred to as their "need for power" (Fig. 4.9). The study suggests that this desire stems from an unconscious drive to impact others. Salespeople with a strong need for power often employ various strategies to assert themselves in interpersonal interactions. They actively seek out leadership positions within sales teams, professional organizations, and social circles. The study indicates that salespeople can satisfy this urge through facing challenges, pursuing self-improvement, attaining status, and receiving acknowledgment.

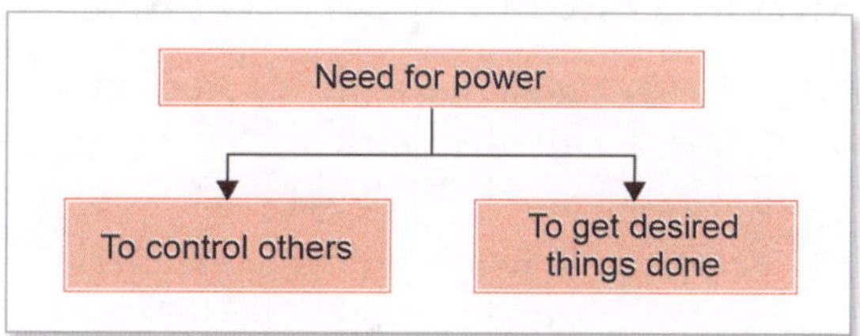

Fig. 4.9: Need for power

Considering the insights from Maslow's Hierarchy of Needs and the findings of this study, it is recommended that sales managers recognize and validate the achievements of salespeople as a means to enhance sales performance. This recognition can be offered privately or publicly through adjustments, expressions of appreciation, promotions, advanced training opportunities, involvement in special projects, and increased authority and responsibility.[17]

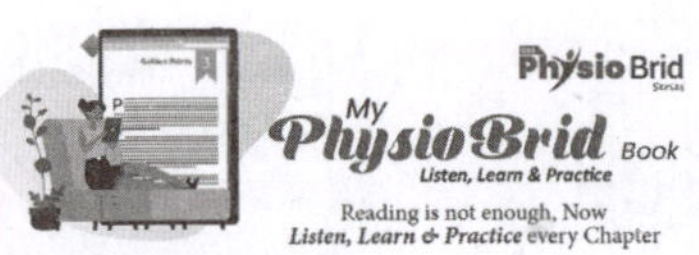

According to David McClelland's 1975 delineation, the power motive can manifest in four primary ways. Initially, individuals may seek to derive a sense of strength and authority from external sources by reading about sports stars or identifying with popular figures. Secondly, power can also emanate from within, expressed through efforts to strengthen one's physicality and exert control over impulses. Thirdly, individuals may take independent action to influence others, such as engaging in conflict or rivalry to exert influence over another person. Lastly, individuals may act within organizational frameworks to exert influence over others.[18]

MUST KNOW

Major approaches to motivation

Theory	Main points
Instinct	Innate biological instincts guide behavior.
Drive reduction	Behavior is guided by biological needs and learned wants of reducing drives arising from those needs.
Arousal	People seek to maintain an optimal level of physiological arousal, which differs from person to person. Maximum performance occurs at optimal arousal level.
Incentive	External stimuli direct and energize behavior.
Hierarchy of needs	Needs form a hierarchy; lower order needs must be fulfilled before higher order needs are met.

APPLICATIONS OF MOTIVATION: MOVING FROM THEORY TO PRACTICE

Managers are keenly interested in effective employee motivation and seek practical advice for implementation. The theories of motivation offer valuable insights, leading to the following recommendations:

- **Recognize individual differences:** Every motivation theory acknowledges the uniqueness of employees, each with distinct personalities and needs.

- **Set clear objectives and provide feedback:** Supervisors should ensure that staff members have well-defined goals and offer regular feedback on their progress toward achieving them.

- **Match personnel to roles thoughtfully:** Aligning individuals with suitable roles is essential for maximizing motivational benefits.

- **Tie rewards to performance:** Managers should link rewards, such as salary increases and promotions, to specific performance targets, incentivizing employees to excel.

- **Enhance visibility of rewards:** Making rewards more visible can increase employees' effectiveness as motivators.

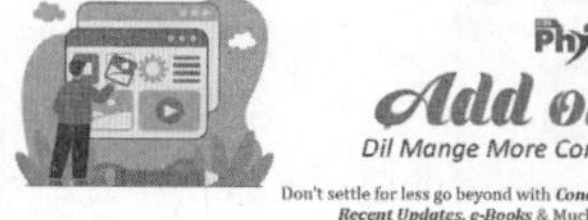

- **Establish equity:** Employees should perceive a fair balance between their contributions (inputs) and the rewards they receive (outputs).

- **Demonstrate care and support:** When managers show genuine concern for their employees, it fosters a positive work environment and enhances employee performance.[24]

Improving motivation in physiotherapy is essential for enhancing patient's adherence and achieving better outcomes. Here are some physiotherapy techniques and strategies to boost motivation:

Physio CORNER

Methods to Implement Motivational Strategies for Rehabilitation

- **Goal setting:**
  - **SMART goals:** Set Specific, Measurable, Achievable, Relevant, and Time-bound goals. Breaking down long-term goals into smaller, manageable milestones helps patients see progress and stay motivated.
  - **Patient involvement:** Involve patients in the goal-setting process to ensure goals are meaningful and personalized.

- **Progress tracking:**
  - **Visual feedback:** Use charts, graphs or apps to visually track progress. Seeing tangible improvements can boost motivation.
  - **Regular assessments:** Conduct regular assessments and provide feedback on progress. Celebrating small victories can enhance motivation.

- **Positive reinforcement:**
  - **Praise and encouragement:** Offer verbal praise and encouragement during sessions to reinforce positive behavior and effort.
  - **Rewards:** Implement a reward system for achieving milestones. Rewards can be as simple as certificates or small incentives.

- **Patient education:**
  - **Understanding the process:** Educate patients about their condition, the benefits of physiotherapy, and the expected outcomes. Knowledge empowers patients and can increase their commitment.
  - **Realistic expectations:** Set realistic expectations to prevent frustration and maintain motivation.

- **Variety and fun:**
  - **Diverse exercises:** Incorporate a variety of exercises to prevent monotony and keep sessions engaging.
  - **Gamification:** Use games and playful activities to make exercises more enjoyable and competitive.

- **Patient-centered approach:**
  - **Personalized programs:** Tailor exercise programs to match patients' interests, preferences, and lifestyle.
  - **Empathy and rapport:** Build a strong therapeutic relationship based on empathy, trust, and open communication.

- **Social support and group therapy:**
  - **Group exercises:** Group sessions can foster a sense of community, provide peer support, and create a motivating environment.
  - **Support networks:** Encourage involvement of family and friends to provide additional support and encouragement.

Contd...

- **Use of technology:**
  - **Telehealth:** Offer virtual sessions to increase accessibility and convenience for patients.
  - **Fitness apps:** Use fitness and health apps to monitor progress, set reminders, and provide motivational content.
- **Biofeedback and wearable devices:**
  - **Biofeedback:** Use biofeedback to help patients visualize their progress and understand the impact of exercises.
  - **Wearables:** Utilize wearable devices to track physical activity, monitor vital signs, and provide feedback.
- **Motivational interviewing:**
  - **Active listening:** Engage in active listening to understand patients' motivations, barriers, and concerns.
  - **Reflective statements:** Use reflective statements to validate patients' feelings and encourage self-motivation.
  - **Action planning:** Collaboratively develop action plans to overcome barriers and achieve goals.
- **Mindfulness and relaxation techniques:**
  - **Mindfulness exercises:** Incorporate mindfulness exercises to help patients focus, reduce stress, and stay present during sessions.
  - **Relaxation techniques:** Teach relaxation techniques such as deep breathing, progressive muscle relaxation, and guided imagery.
- **Professional development for physiotherapists:**
  - **Continuing education:** Stay updated with the latest research and techniques in motivational strategies and patient engagement.
  - **Interpersonal skills:** Develop strong interpersonal and communication skills to effectively motivate and support patients.

Case Study

Rehabilitation and Motivation: The Case of John Doe's Journey to Overcoming Chronic Lower Back Pain

Patient Profile
Name: John Doe
Age: 45 years
Condition: Chronic Lower Back Pain

Motivational Strategies Implemented
- **Goal setting:** Set a long-term goal of returning to recreational basketball and short-term goals like improving flexibility and reducing pain.
- **Progress tracking:** Used a digital app to track daily exercises and pain levels, providing visual feedback on progress.
- **Positive reinforcement:** Praised John for his efforts during each session and rewarded him with a milestone certificate for completing 4 weeks of consistent therapy.
- **Patient education:** Educated John about the causes of his back pain and the importance of exercises in managing his condition.

Contd...

- **Variety and fun:** Included basketball drills in his therapy sessions to keep him engaged and motivated.
- **Social support:** Involved John's family in his rehabilitation process, encouraging them to participate in some exercises at home.
- **Technology:** Used telehealth for follow-up sessions to ensure consistency and convenience.
- **Motivational interviewing:** Regularly discussed John's progress, addressing any concerns and collaboratively setting new goals.

Outcome

John's motivation and adherence to the therapy program improved significantly. He experienced a reduction in pain, improved flexibility, and eventually returned to playing recreational basketball, achieving his long-term goal.

By incorporating these techniques, physiotherapists can enhance patient's motivation, leading to better adherence to therapy programs and improve overall outcomes.

SUMMARY

- The chapter begins by defining motivation, a concept that propels individuals toward his goals. It distinguishes between intrinsic motivation, driven by internal satisfaction, and extrinsic motivation, which is fueled by external rewards. This foundational understanding sets the stage for a deeper exploration of the motivational cycle, which includes stages such as arousal, drive, action, and reinforcement. Each stage is meticulously explained, with real-life examples illustrating how these phases unfold in the context of human behavior.
- **Maslow's hierarchy of needs:** The chapter delves into Abraham Maslow's ground-breaking theory, which categorizes human needs into five levels: (1) Physiological, (2) Safety, (3) Love and belonging, (4) Esteem, and (5) Self-actualization. This hierarchy provides a framework for understanding how individuals are motivated to fulfill their needs, progressively moving from basic physiological requirements to the pinnacle of self-actualization.
- **McClelland's theory of motivation:** David McClelland's theory is introduced, focusing on three core human needs: Power, achievement, and affiliation. The chapter discusses how these needs shape behavior and can be leveraged to enhance motivation in various settings, including physiotherapy.
- **Practical applications in physiotherapy:** The critical role of motivation in physiotherapy has been described, where patient adherence to treatment is paramount. They provide practical strategies for physiotherapists to employ, grounded in the theories of motivation. These include recognizing individual differences, setting clear goals, providing feedback, and aligning rewards with performance. By understanding and applying these principles, physiotherapists can create a more motivating environment, leading to better patient outcomes.
- In conclusion, there is importance of motivation in driving human behavior and its specific application in the field of physiotherapy. By exploring various theories and practical applications, the chapter equips readers with a robust understanding of motivation, enabling them to apply these insights effectively in their professional practice.

REFERENCES

1. Ryan RM, Deci EL. Intrinsic and extrinsic motivations: Classic definitions and new directions. Contemporary educational psychology. 2000;25(1):54–67.
2. Brandstätter V, Schüler J, Puca RM, Lozo L. Motivation und emotion. Berlin: Springer; 2013.
3. Feldman RS. Understanding psychology. McGraw-Hill; 2015.
4. Feist G, Rosenberg E. Psychology: Perspectives and Connections, 5th Edition" Faculty Research, Scholarly, and Creative Activity. 2022.
5. Warne RT, Astle MC, Hill JC. What do undergraduates learn about human intelligence? An analysis of introductory psychology textbooks. Archives of Scientific Psychology. 2018;6(1):32.
6. Nolen-Hoeksema, S., Fredrickson, B., Loftus, G., & Lutz, C. Atkinson & Hilgard's Psychology. In: An Introduction to Psychology. United Kingdom: Cengage Learning. 2009.
7. Kong Y. A brief discussion on motivation and ways to motivate students in English language learning. International Education Studies. 2009;2(2):145–9.
8. Huitt W. Motivation to learn: An overview. Educational psychology interactive. 2001;12(3):29–36.
9. Filgona J, Sakiyo J, Gwany DM, Okoronka AU. Motivation in learning. Asian Journal of Education and social studies. 2020;10(4):16–37.
10. Simpson EH, Balsam PD. The behavioral neuroscience of motivation: An overview of concepts, measures, and translational applications. In: Simpson, E., Balsam, P. (eds) Behavioral Neuroscience of Motivation. Current Topics in Behavioral Neurosciences, vol 27. Springer, Cham.; 2016; 27,1–12.
11. Locke EA, Schattke K. Intrinsic and extrinsic motivation: Time for expansion and clarification. Motivation Science. 2019;5(4):277.
12. Morris LS, Grehl MM, Rutter SB, Mehta M, Westwater ML. On what motivates us: A detailed review of intrinsic v. extrinsic motivation. Psychological medicine. 2022;52(10):1801–16.
13. Ayub N. Effect of intrinsic and extrinsic motivation on academic performance. Pakistan business review. 2010;8(1):363–72.
14. Osemeke M, Adegboyega S. Critical review and comparism between Maslow, Herzberg and McClelland's theory of needs. Funai journal of accounting, business and finance. 2017;1(1):161–73.
15. Acquah A, Nsiah TK, Antie EN, Otoo B. Literature review on theories of motivation. EPRA International Journal of Economic and Business Review. 2021;9(5):25–9.
16. Uduji, J. I., & Ankeli, M. O. Needs for Achievement, Affiliation, and Power: The Possible Sales Manager's Actions for Exceptional Salesforce Performance. In Research Journal of Finance and Accounting. 2013;4(9).
17. Acquah A, Nsiah TK, Antie EN, Otoo B. Literature review on theories of motivation. EPRA International Journal of Economic and Business Review. 2021;9(5):25–9.
18. Royle MT, Hall AT. The relationship between McClelland's theory of needs, feeling individually accountable, and informal accountability for others. International Journal of management and marketing research. 2012;5(1):21–42.
19. Trivedi AJ, Mehta A. Maslow's hierarchy of needs-theory of human motivation. International Journal of Research in all Subjects in Multi Languages. 2019;7(6):38–41.
20. McLeod S. HCC Certificate in Counselling Skills Maslow's Hierarchy of Needs. Simple Psychology Psychology. Org. 2007;2(5).

Contd...

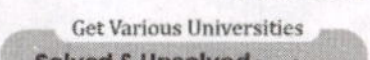

21. Mustofa AZ. Hierarchy of human needs: A humanistic psychology approach of Abraham Maslow. Kawanua International Journal of Multicultural Studies. 2022;3(2):30–5.

22. Zalenski RJ, Raspa R. Maslow's hierarchy of needs: A framework for achieving human potential in hospice. Journal of palliative medicine. 2006;9(5):1120–7.

23. Gawel JE. Herzberg's theory of motivation and Maslow's hierarchy of needs. Practical Assessment, Research, and Evaluation. 2019;5(1):11.

24. Badubi RM. Theories of motivation and their application in organizations: A risk analysis. International Journal of Innovation and Economic Development. 2017;3(3):44–51.

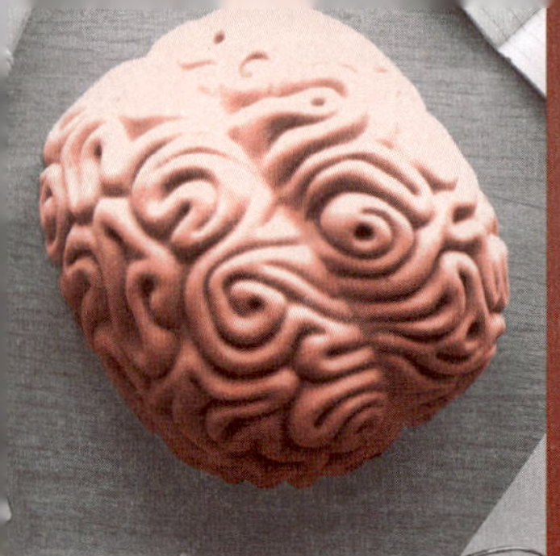

LONG ANSWER QUESTIONS

1. What is motivation? Explain its significance in various aspects of life.
2. Elaborate how human behavior is influenced by motivation.
3. Discuss the relationship between motivation and setting up a goal.
4. Explain intrinsic motivation with suitable examples. How does intrinsic motivation influence behavior?
5. Explain extrinsic motivation in detail with its suitable examples to human subject.
6. Discuss the concept of self-determination theory and its relevance in daily life.
7. Summarize the role and importance of biological factors in framing motivational behavior.
8. Explain Maslow's hierarchy of needs in detail.
9. Discuss the key role of leadership and its implication in motivating humans at workplace.
10. How social factors, such as family, relatives, peers, and cultural difference determine individual's motivation toward goal directed behavior?

SHORT ANSWER QUESTIONS

1. Define motivation.
2. What are the two main types of motivation?
3. What are the stages of the motivation cycle?
4. How does Maslow's hierarchy of needs classify human needs?
5. What are the three core human needs according to McClelland's theory of motivation?
6. What is the difference between intrinsic and extrinsic motivation?
7. How can physiotherapists use the concept of motivation to improve patient adherence to treatment?
8. What is the role of reinforcement in the motivation cycle?
9. What is the primary objective of intrinsic motivation?
10. How does fear motivation influence behavior?

MULTIPLE CHOICE QUESTIONS

1. **Which of the following is NOT a core function of motivation?**
   a. Energizing behavior
   b. Directing behavior
   c. Facilitating critical thinking
   d. Aiding decision-making

2. **In the motivation cycle, the stage where an unmet need or desire creates tension is called:**
   a. Arousal
   b. Drive
   c. Action
   d. Reinforcement

3. **A patient is highly motivated to regain mobility after a stroke because it will allow them to return to their independent lifestyle. This type of motivation is most likely:**
   a. Incentive motivation
   b. Fear motivation
   c. Intrinsic motivation
   d. External regulation

4. **Which of the following statements about McClelland's needs theory is FALSE?**
   a. People with a high need for power are driven to influence others.
   b. Individuals with a strong need for affiliation seek close social connections.
   c. A high need for achievement is associated with a desire for external validation.
   d. These needs can influence a patient's adherence to a physiotherapy program.

5. **Maslow's hierarchy of needs proposes that individuals prioritize fulfilling:**
   a. Esteem needs before safety needs
   b. Physiological needs before social needs
   c. Self-actualization needs before love and belonging
   d. All needs are equally important

6. **A physiotherapist notices a patient is less motivated to complete exercises after initially making good progress. This could be due to:**
   a. Deficient intrinsic motivation
   b. Lack of clear goals
   c. Absence of external rewards
   d. All of the above

7. **Which strategy would MOST likely enhance intrinsic motivation in a physiotherapy patient?**
   a. Offering praise and encouragement after each session
   b. Providing tangible rewards for completing exercises
   c. Helping them identify the personal benefits of physiotherapy
   d. Setting short-term, easily achievable goals

8. **A physiotherapist uses graphic charts to track a patient's progress visually. This approach is most closely aligned with the concept of:**
   a. Incentive motivation
   b. Fear motivation
   c. External regulation
   d. Self-determination theory

9. **Ethical considerations are important when using fear motivation in physiotherapy because it can lead to:**
   a. Increased pain perception
   b. Feelings of inadequacy
   c. Reduced trust in the therapist
   d. All of these

10. **A patient with a high need for affiliation may benefit from physiotherapy exercises that:**
    a. Focus on individual goals and independence
    b. Encourage group participation and social interaction
    c. Offer opportunities for competition with other patients
    d. Emphasize the potential for pain relief

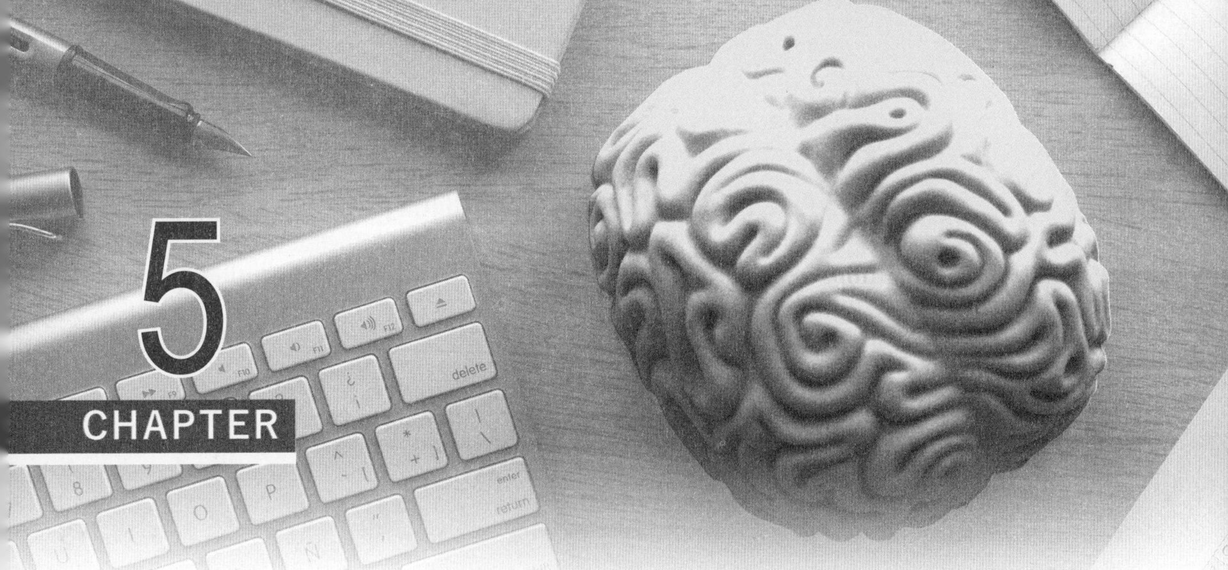

Frustration and Conflict

Ankita Sharma, Moattar Raza Rizvi

LEARNING OBJECTIVES

After the completion of the chapter, the readers will be able to:
- Describe and explain key psychological theories related to frustration and conflict, including the frustration-aggression hypothesis and conflict theory.
- Recognize emotional, cognitive, physiological, and behavioral signs of frustration in various settings, particularly in clinical and therapeutic environments.
- Apply various conflict management styles—such as accommodation, avoidance, compromise, competition, and collaboration—and determine the most appropriate style based on context, goals, relationships, and dynamics.
- Develop and implement effective strategies for managing and coping with frustration, including educational interventions, enhanced communication techniques, and psychological strategies such as positive self-talk and mindfulness.
- Assess different types of conflicts including, intrapersonal, interpersonal, intragroup, and organizational conflicts, and apply appropriate interventions to manage or resolve these conflicts effectively.
- Understand how internal and external factors, such as cognitive limitations, physical barriers, economic factors, and social dynamics, contribute to frustration and conflict.
- Promote emotional and psychological well-being in themselves and others, particularly in settings that involve interpersonal interactions.
- Identify and understand various defense mechanisms such as denial, projection, and displacement, and their impact on patient behavior and therapy outcomes, and strategies to address these mechanisms constructively in clinical settings.

CHAPTER OUTLINE

- Introduction
- Frustration
- Sources of Frustration
- Frustration in Clinical Practice
- Conflict

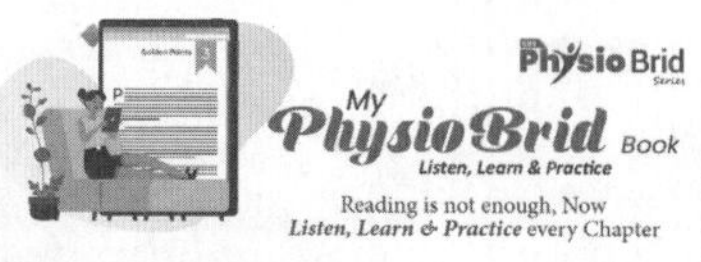

KEY TERMS

Active listening: Fully concentrating on what is being said, understanding the message, and responding thoughtfully.

Aggressive tendencies: Behavior characterized by overt or covert aggression as a discharge of emotional tension.

Cognitive distortions: Negative thinking patterns like exaggerating problems or catastrophizing outcomes.

Conflict management techniques: Strategies used to manage and resolve conflicts effectively.

Emotional arousal: Intense emotions such as anger, irritation, and agitation that cloud perception and make challenges seem larger.

Empathy: Understanding and sharing the feelings of others, going beyond mere sympathy.

Flexibility: Being open to compromise and adapting to different perspectives.

Frustration: An emotional response to opposition or the blocking of goal-directed behavior, characterized by feelings of anger, annoyance, and disappointment.

Humor: The intentional use of light-hearted or witty remarks to create a positive atmosphere, reduce stress, and foster connection. When used appropriately, it can de-escalate tensions by diffusing conflict, easing emotional strain, and encouraging open, cooperative communication.

Impaired decision-making: Difficulty making balanced decisions due to high emotional arousal and skewed perceptions.

Informal mediation: Resolving disputes through casual conversation and guidance by a neutral party.

Intragroup conflict: Disagreements within a group over task priorities, relationships or processes, affecting cohesion, decision-making, and performance.

Intrapersonal conflict: Internal struggles due to opposing desires, needs or emotions, impacting decision-making, emotional well-being, and mental health.

Interpersonal conflict: Disputes between individuals caused by differences, miscommunication or disagreements over values, methods or goals, affecting personal and professional relationships.

Learned helplessness: A state of resignation from repeated frustrations where one believes that their actions cannot bring about change.

Maladaptive coping strategies: Unhealthy coping mechanisms like avoidance or substance abuse that complicate situations further.

Negative affect: Accompanying negative emotions like sadness, anxiety or hopelessness that contribute to a cycle of negativity. These emotions can significantly diminish a person's capacity to cope effectively with challenges, reducing motivation and adherence to treatment.

Organizational conflict: Conflicts within an organization arising from role distinctions, hierarchical structures or functional discrepancies.

Persistence and perseverance: Stubborn adherence to familiar, yet ineffective, methods due to frustration.

Physiological arousal: Physical responses such as increased heart rate, higher blood pressure, and muscle tension.

Societal conflict: Conflicts stemming from broader societal issues like politics, race, class or gender, influencing workplace dynamics.

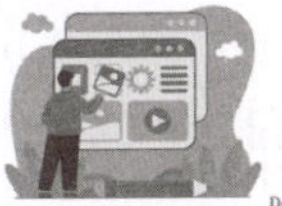
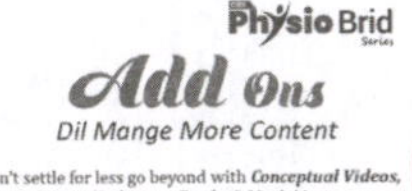

INTRODUCTION

The word frustration has been derived from a Latin word 'Frustra' meaning 'obstruct'. Frustration refers to the blocking of behavior directed toward the goal. In psychology, frustration is defined as a common emotional response to opposition, encompassing feelings of anger, annoyance, and disappointment arising from perceived resistance to achieving an individual's will or goal.[1] This emotional response can be internal, stemming from personal challenges in fulfilling goals or desires or external, caused by factors beyond one's control like physical obstacles or difficult tasks.

Frustrated behavior manifests as a range of responses when individuals are blocked from achieving their goals. Common signs include irritability, anger outbursts, and social withdrawal. It can also lead to aggression, increased anxiety, and a decline in motivation and productivity.[2] Understanding and addressing these behaviors are crucial for effective management and resolution.

FRUSTRATION

Definition

According to Dollard et al., (1939) in their seminal work, "Frustration and Aggression", frustration is defined as "an interference with the occurrence of an instigated goal-response at its proper time in the behavior sequence".[3] This definition was further described for frustration as "a condition that results from blocking of a tendency to respond when the block itself is perceived as unpleasant or unjustified".[4]

> **MUST KNOW**
>
> Frustration is a natural emotional response to obstacles or unmet expectations, and it serves as a signal that something in your environment or approach may need adjustment. Interestingly, frustration can either lead to positive problem-solving and motivation when managed constructively or escalate into stress and aggression if left unchecked. Understanding and addressing the root cause of frustration is key to maintaining emotional well-being and fostering personal growth.

Characteristics

Various characteristics of frustration encountered by physiotherapists are described in Table 5.1.

Table 5.1: Characteristics of frustration

Characteristics	Description	Examples in physiotherapy settings
Emotional arousal	Intense emotions such as anger, irritation, and agitation that cloud perception and make challenges seem larger. Emotional arousal often makes it difficult to focus on solutions or positive aspects.	Physiotherapy and sports rehabilitation patients feeling irritable when progress is slow.
Cognitive distortions	Negative thinking patterns like exaggerating problems or catastrophizing outcomes. These distorted thoughts can often prevent individuals from recognizing realistic solutions.	Clients catastrophizing minor setbacks as total failures in recovery processes.

Contd...

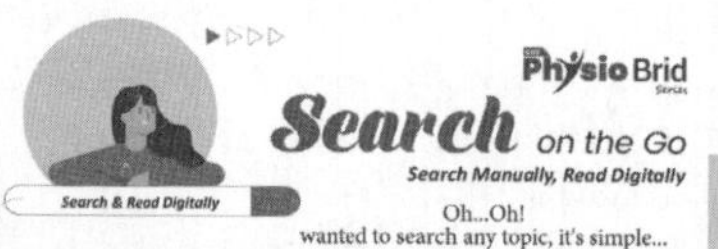

Characteristics	Description	Examples in physiotherapy settings
Impaired decision-making	Difficulty making balanced decisions due to high emotional arousal and skewed perceptions. This often leads to choices that are more emotional than logical, increasing the likelihood of poor outcomes.	Physiotherapy patients insisting on painful exercises under the belief that they are necessary for gain, risking further injury.
Aggressive tendencies	Frustration can lead to overt or covert aggressive behaviors as a discharge of emotional tension. This aggression can disrupt interactions and exacerbate existing conflicts.	Verbal outbursts or passive-aggressive behavior toward healthcare providers in rehab settings.
Persistence and perseveration	Stubborn adherence to familiar, yet ineffective, methods due to frustration. This behavior is often counterproductive, as it prevents adaptation and innovation in approach.	Patients in sports rehabilitation sticking to specific exercises that do not aid in recovery, hoping to accelerate progress.
Physiological arousal	Physical responses such as increased heart rate, higher blood pressure, and muscle tension. These responses can often exacerbate the perception of stress and hinder relaxation needed for recovery.	Increased muscle tension interfering with effective therapeutic exercises and increasing injury risk in physiotherapy.
Maladaptive coping strategies	Unhealthy coping mechanisms like avoidance or substance abuse that complicate situations further. These strategies often provide temporary relief but lead to more significant issues in the long-term.	Skipping therapy sessions or using substances to cope with pain and emotional distress in long rehabilitation processes.
Negative affect	Accompanying negative emotions like sadness, anxiety or hopelessness that contribute to a cycle of negativity. These emotions can significantly diminish a person's capacity to cope effectively with challenges.	Sadness or anxiety in sports rehabilitation reducing a client's motivation and adherence to treatment protocols.
Interpersonal conflicts	Strained relationships due to projecting feelings onto others or lashing out, leading to conflicts and misunderstandings. These reactions can damage trust and communication, adding social turmoil to stress.	Misunderstandings and tension between clients and therapists in therapy settings, potentially harming the therapeutic alliance.
Learned helplessness	A state of resignation from repeated frustrations where one believes that their actions cannot bring about change. This mindset can lead to a significant drop in effort and engagement in therapeutic activities.	Clients feeling helpless about the pace or direction of therapy, leading to decreased motivation and engagement.

MUST KNOW

- Emotional arousal often makes it difficult to focus on solutions or positive aspects.
- Negative thinking patterns can often prevent individuals from recognizing realistic solutions.

Signs

Understanding the psychological dynamics within physiotherapy is essential for achieving successful patient outcomes. Recognizing signs of psychological frustration is particularly crucial, as these can severely hinder the rehabilitation process.[5] Here's a closer examination of the emotional manifestations of frustration[6] that physiotherapists frequently encounter:

Emotional

- **Irritability or short temper:** Patients may exhibit a lower tolerance for minor irritations, which they might have previously ignored. This change in demeanor can affect their interaction with the therapy and the therapist.

- **Anger outbursts:** These are often sudden and severe, appearing out of proportion to the precipitating event. Such episodes can interrupt therapy sessions and strain the patient-therapist relationship.

- **Feelings of hopelessness:** Slow progress can lead patients to believe their condition is unchanging, resulting in despair and a reduced motivation to engage in their treatment plan.

- **General sadness:** Patients may consistently feel low or sad, which is often a reaction to the continuous challenges and restrictions their ailment brings.

Cognitive

The mental load of dealing with chronic pain or slow recovery can lead to several cognitive signs of frustration:[7]

- **Difficulty concentrating:** Pain and emotional distress can scatter mental focus, making it hard for patients to follow through with therapy instructions or maintain regular therapy schedules.

- **Persistent negative thoughts:** These often revolve around the efficacy of treatment, fears of nonrecovery or a preoccupation with pain, which can spiral into a negative feedback loop that hampers recovery.

- **Impaired decision-making:** The stress from ongoing pain or disability might cloud judgment, leading to poor decision-making regarding treatment options or compliance.

Special Considerations

- **Neurological patients:** These individuals may face additional challenges due to the direct impact of their conditions on cognitive functions. Cognitive impairments can exacerbate frustrations, as these patients might struggle more with memory, problem-solving, and adapting to new therapy routines.[8] Physiotherapists should employ clear, repetitive, and simplified instructions to aid understanding and retention.

- **Geriatric patients:** Older adults often deal with multiple health issues that can slow down their recovery and increase their frustration levels. Cognitive decline associated with aging can further complicate their therapy adherence. It's crucial for physiotherapists to use patience, frequent reinforcement, and adapt therapeutic approaches to match the cognitive capacities of older patients, ensuring they feel supported and understood throughout their treatment journey.

Behavioral

Frustration can also manifest through various behaviors[9] that physiotherapists should be alert to:

- **Changes in eating and sleeping habits:** These might include insomnia or hypersomnia and overeating or loss of appetite, which can affect physical health and therapy outcomes.

- **Avoidance of rehabilitation sessions:** This might be due to discouragement from perceived lack of progress or due to the pain associated with exercise.

- **Decreased communication:** Patients might become less communicative about their pain or progress, which can hinder the therapist's ability to adjust treatment effectively.

- **Dependency on substances:** In an attempt to manage their frustration or pain, some patients might increase their use of substances like alcohol, nicotine or even pain medication beyond prescribed limits.

Physiological

The physical manifestations of psychological stress include:[10]

- **Muscle tension and headaches:** Chronic stress after underlying frustration can lead to increased muscle tension, particularly around the neck and shoulders, which can exacerbate pain and discomfort.

- **Changes in heart rate and breathing:** Stress brought by frustration can trigger the body's fight or flight response, leading to elevated heart rates and rapid, shallow breathing, which are not conducive to healing.

- **Gastrointestinal issues:** Stress can significantly impact digestive functions, leading to symptoms like nausea, diarrhea or constipation.

> **MUST KNOW**
>
> - Frustration can lead to overt or covert aggressive behaviors as a discharge of emotional tension.
> - Persistence and perseverance in familiar, yet ineffective, methods are often counterproductive.
> - Physical responses such as increased heart rate and muscle tension can exacerbate the perception of stress.

SOURCES OF FRUSTRATION

The concept of frustration in psychology is multifaceted, involving an emotional response triggered when an individual's progress toward a goal is blocked or when expectations are not met. This can arise from various sources, such as influencing behavior and emotional well-being.

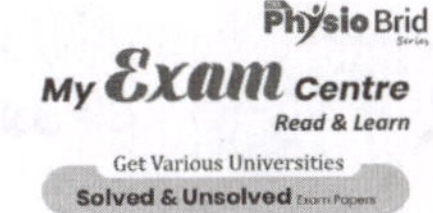

Frustration in physiotherapy can be defined as an emotional state that occurs when a patient or therapist encounters barriers to achieving therapeutic goals. This emotional response can stem from internal factors (like pain or fear) or external factors (such as treatment limitations or healthcare policies) (Fig. 5.1). It is characterized by feelings of anger, irritation, and a sense of helplessness or defeat.[11] These emotions can significantly impact the motivation and compliance of patients, as well as the professional satisfaction and effectiveness of therapists.

Depending on Conditions

External Sources of Frustration

External sources of frustration involve conditions and barriers that are outside an individual's control, such as environmental obstacles, social conflicts, and economic limitations.[12] These sources can hinder progress toward goals, leading to feelings of helplessness and dissatisfaction.

Physical Factors

In physiotherapy, environmental stressors and faulty ergonomics significantly impact frustration and recovery. Urban challenges such as noise, traffic, and high costs can perpetually block personal and professional achievements, as explained by Lazarus and Folkman's (1984) stress and coping theory. Additionally, improper workstation setups, nonergonomic home environments, and poorly designed rehabilitation spaces further hinder physical rehabilitation, exacerbating pain and limiting effective treatment. This continual frustration can affect individuals' quality of life, leading to chronic stress and decreased well-being. In a physiotherapy context, these physical barriers can delay recovery processes, leading to frustration among patients who are unable to progress as expected.[13, 14] Addressing these ergonomic issues is crucial for creating optimal conditions that support patient recovery and reduce frustration.

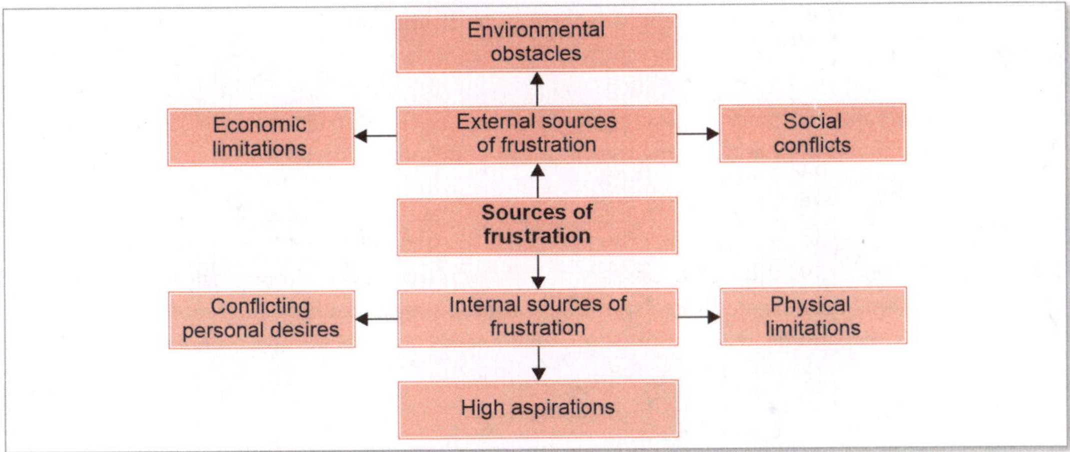

Fig. 5.1: Sources of frustration

Social Factors

Interpersonal conflicts and societal expectations can be significant sources of frustration. Disputes with colleagues, misunderstandings with patients or restrictive cultural norms can all lead to tensions that complicate professional interactions and therapy processes.[15] Moreover, societal laws or healthcare policies that limit treatment options or access to necessary resources can heighten feelings of injustice and frustration among patients and therapists alike.

Interpersonal conflicts can catalyze frustration, particularly when such conflicts block personal objectives. In professional settings, ongoing disputes with colleagues or supervisors can substantially frustrate individuals, negatively impacting their job satisfaction and productivity.[16] These conflicts often stem from miscommunications, mismatched expectations or competition for resources, requiring effective resolution strategies to restore harmony and reduce frustration.

For neurological patients, who may require more nuanced communication and tailored treatment approaches due to cognitive or behavioral challenges, the impact of such conflicts can be even more pronounced. For instance, a physiotherapist might need to navigate additional barriers when societal norms and healthcare policies do not accommodate the specific needs of neurological patients, such as requiring longer session times or specialized equipment.[17] Moreover, the behavior of physiotherapists in managing these interactions is crucial; demonstrating patience, empathy, and clear communication can mitigate the potential for misunderstandings and enhance the therapeutic relationship, ultimately reducing frustration and facilitating more effective treatment outcomes.

Economic Factors

Financial constraints often lead to frustration in settings where resources are limited or expensive. According to Lazarus and Folkman, insufficient resources or support can be a major source of frustration, impeding goal attainment.[18] In educational settings, students may become frustrated if they lack access to necessary learning materials or academic support, which can limit their educational achievements and future opportunities. This form of frustration often calls for systemic changes to ensure equitable access to educational resources. In physiotherapy and sports rehabilitation, patients may become frustrated if they cannot afford the necessary treatments or if their insurance does not cover certain therapeutic interventions.[19] Economic factors can restrict access to the required care, directly impacting recovery and leading to significant emotional distress.

Internal Sources of Frustration

Internal sources of frustration stem from within the individual, including physical limitations, conflicting personal desires, and high aspirations. These internal conflicts and constraints can lead to emotional distress and decreased motivation when personal expectations are not met.[12]

Personal Limitations

Berkowitz identified that personal limitations, whether cognitive, physical or skill-based, can lead to frustration when they prevent individuals from achieving their desired outcomes.

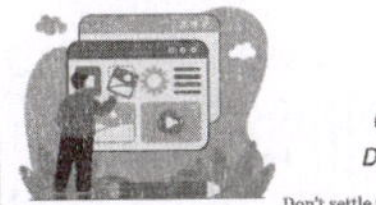

In sports, for example, athletes recovering from injuries often face significant frustration if physical limitations hinder their performance or delay their return to preinjury levels.[20] For instance, an amputee athlete undergoing physiotherapy may experience heightened frustration when faced with the challenges of relearning movements or adapting to a prosthetic limb. The frustration can be profound when comparing their current capabilities to their preamputation performance. Managing this frustration involves setting realistic goals, gradual rehabilitation, and psychological support to adjust expectations and cope with the recovery process.[21]

Conflicting Desires or Goals

Kurt Lewin's field theory (1935) provides a framework for understanding how conflicting internal forces can lead to psychological tension and frustration.[22] This occurs when individuals hold incompatible desires or goals that compete for their mental and emotional resources. For example, someone may wish to save money for future security while simultaneously desiring to travel extensively. The inability to fully pursue either goal without compromising the other can lead to significant internal conflict and resultant frustration.

Blocked Goals or Unmet Expectations

The frustration-aggression hypothesis suggests that frustration arises when there is an obstruction to achieving a desired goal, potentially leading to aggressive responses. This theory is particularly relevant in contexts like physiotherapy, where patients often have specific expectations about their recovery timelines and outcomes.[23] When these expectations are not met, whether due to slow progress, unexpected complications or persistent pain, patients may experience high levels of frustration. This emotional state can impede further progress by reducing motivation and adherence to prescribed therapy routines, thereby creating a cycle of frustration and insufficient recovery.

Perceived Unfairness or Injustice

It is also explored how perceptions of unfairness or injustice trigger emotional responses like frustration and anger. This response is prevalent in societal contexts where individuals or groups feel marginalized or subjected to discriminatory practices.[24] Such perceptions of injustice can lead to significant frustration, motivating individuals and communities to seek fairness and rectification through social justice movements or legal avenues.

Lack of Control or Autonomy

Wortman and Brehm's reactance theory (1975) highlights the psychological reaction to diminished personal autonomy or control, which can trigger frustration and efforts to regain lost freedoms.[25] In workplace settings, this type of frustration is commonly observed among employees who are subject to micromanagement. Such environments restrict employees' autonomy, leading to decreased job satisfaction and productivity. When individuals cannot make decisions that influence their roles or outcomes, the resultant frustration can diminish their overall engagement and effectiveness at work.

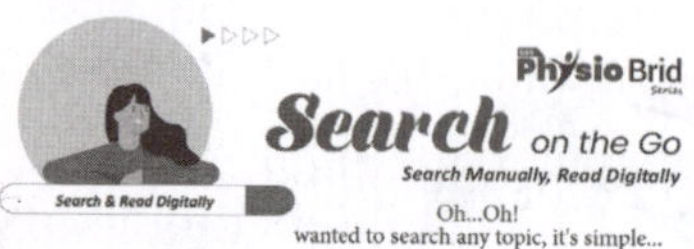

Depending on Causes

- **Patient-related causes:**

    ▪ **Chronic pain management:** Physiotherapists may feel frustrated when treating patients with persistent pain that is resistant to standard interventions, complicating therapy effectiveness and patient progress.[26]

    ▪ **Limited progress in patients:** Frustration can arise for physiotherapists when patients do not show expected levels of recovery, despite adhering to treatment plans. This can challenge the therapist's sense of professional efficacy and satisfaction.[27]

    ▪ **Repeated setbacks:** Handling cases where patients experience recurring injuries or deteriorating symptoms can be disheartening for physiotherapists, increasing their stress levels and potentially leading to feelings of helplessness or failure in their role.[28]

- **Therapist-related causes:**

    ▪ **Skill and resource limitations:** Physiotherapists may experience frustration when their current skill set or available resources fall short of adequately addressing complex patient conditions, impacting the effectiveness of treatment.[29]

    ▪ **Caseload pressure:** The stress of handling a large number of patients can overwhelm physiotherapists, leading to frustration due to the challenges of delivering individualized care and maintaining treatment quality.

- **System-related causes:**

    ▪ **Time limitations:** The pressure to adhere to strict session times often frustrates therapists, especially when they feel more time is needed to address complex patient issues adequately.

    ▪ **Administrative burdens:** Excessive paperwork and bureaucratic procedures can detract from clinical work, leading to frustration among physiotherapists.

    ▪ **Insurance limitations:** Constraints imposed by insurance providers regarding approved treatments or session limits can cause significant frustration, as they may prevent therapists from delivering optimal care.

Physio CORNER

Exercise can significantly improve feelings of frustration through various physiological, psychological, emotional, social and behavioral mechanisms. Here are the key ways in which exercise helps alleviate frustration:

Physiological Mechanisms:

- **Endorphin release:**

    ▪ **Endorphins:** Exercise stimulates the release of endorphins, which are natural mood lifters. These chemicals interact with receptors in the brain to reduce the perception of pain and trigger positive feelings.

Contd...

- **Stress hormone reduction:**
  - **Cortisol:** Regular physical activity helps reduce levels of cortisol, a hormone associated with stress. Lower cortisol levels can lead to decreased feelings of stress and frustration.
- **Improved sleep:**
  - **Sleep quality:** Exercise can improve the quality and duration of sleep. Better sleep is associated with improved mood and reduced irritability and frustration.

Psychological Mechanisms:
- **Distraction:**
  - **Mental break:** Engaging in physical activity provides a distraction from the sources of frustration, offering a mental break and allowing the mind to reset.
- **Sense of accomplishment:**
  - **Achievement:** Completing a workout or achieving fitness goals can provide a sense of accomplishment and boost self-esteem, counteracting feelings of frustration.
- **Cognitive function:**
  - **Brain health:** Exercise enhances cognitive function, including improved focus, memory, and decision-making abilities, which can help in managing frustrating situations more effectively.

Emotional Mechanisms:
- **Mood enhancement:**
  - **Serotonin and dopamine:** Exercise increases the production of neurotransmitters like serotonin and dopamine, which are associated with improved mood and reduced feelings of frustration.
- **Anxiety reduction:**
  - **Calmness:** Regular physical activity is known to reduce anxiety levels, promoting a sense of calm and well-being that can mitigate feelings of frustration.

Social Mechanisms:
- **Social interaction:**
  - **Community:** Participating in group exercises or team sports provides social interaction and support, which can improve mood and reduce feelings of isolation and frustration.
- **Support networks**
  - **Peer support:** Engaging with others in a fitness setting can create a support network, offering encouragement and shared experiences that help in managing frustration.

Behavioral Mechanisms:
- **Healthy habits:**
  - **Routine:** Establishing a regular exercise routine can lead to the development of other healthy habits, such as better nutrition and time management, which contribute to overall well-being and reduced frustration.
- **Improved coping skills:**
  - **Resilience:** Regular physical activity can enhance resilience and improve coping skills, making it easier to handle and recover from frustrating situations.

CASE STUDY 1

Chronic Pain Management

- **Background:** Jane, a 45-year-old with chronic lower back pain, experiences significant frustration due to her persistent discomfort and limited mobility. Her frustration grows as she struggles to see improvements despite regular physiotherapy sessions.
- **Intervention:** Her physiotherapist introduces a multidisciplinary approach, incorporating psychological support and pain management education. Techniques such as cognitive-behavioral therapy (CBT) and mindfulness are used to help Jane manage her pain perceptions and enhance her coping strategies.
- **Outcome:** Jane learns to set realistic expectations and develop better coping mechanisms for her pain, which alleviates her frustration and gradually improves her engagement with the physiotherapy process.

CASE STUDY 2

Overcoming Setbacks in Sports Injury

- **Background:** Alex, a young athlete recovering from a knee surgery, faces repeated setbacks that delay his return to sport, leading to significant frustration and decreased motivation.
- **Intervention:** The physiotherapist sets up a clear, phased recovery plan with short-term achievable goals to help maintain Alex's motivation. Regular feedback sessions are implemented to discuss his concerns and adjust the plan as needed.
- **Outcome:** With clear milestones and constant communication, Alex feels more in control and less frustrated, seeing each small achievement as progress toward his ultimate goal of returning to sports.

MUST KNOW

- Learned helplessness is a state of resignation from repeated frustrations where one believes that their actions cannot bring about change.
- Understanding and addressing frustrated behavior is crucial for effective management and resolution in physiotherapy.

FRUSTRATION IN CLINICAL PRACTICE

Frustration tolerance is essentially the ability to withstand stressors and setbacks during the therapeutic and recovery processes.[28] It's not only about enduring difficulties but also managing emotional responses constructively.[30]

Coping Strategies

Factors contributing to low frustration tolerance include neurological conditions like Attention-deficit/hyperactivity disorder (ADHD) and autism, which directly impact cognitive processing and

emotional regulation.[31] Chronic physical conditions such as persistent pain can also diminish an individual's tolerance, as continuous discomfort skews perception and reduces resilience.

To bolster frustration tolerance, physiotherapists can adopt specific psychological strategies. For instance, positive self-talk encourages a more optimistic outlook, transforming thoughts like "I can't do this" into "I can manage this challenge." Mindfulness practices are also crucial, as they anchor the individual in the present moment, reducing the impact of stressors and improving emotional regulation.[32] For younger patients, tailored approaches such as guiding through example (demonstration), distraction techniques, and cognitive reframing are beneficial. These interventions help children develop adaptive responses to frustration, which are critical in both therapeutic settings and daily life.

Building and maintaining high levels of frustration tolerance is key to effective physiotherapy. It requires a nuanced approach that integrates psychological resilience-building techniques to enhance patient care and outcomes. By understanding and addressing the roots of low frustration tolerance, therapists can significantly improve their practice's effectiveness.

Reactions to Frustrations

Frustration is a complex emotional response that arises when obstacles impede one's goals, triggering a range of reactions that can profoundly impact behavior and mental health. These reactions are not uniform and vary greatly among individuals, shaped by personality, context, and coping mechanisms.[33] Understanding these reactions is crucial as they determine how effectively we can manage challenges and navigate stressful situations.

Aggression

Frustration often triggers aggression, which can be directed in two primary ways: (1) Directly and (2) Indirectly. Direct aggression involves overt behaviors aimed at harming another person or object, which might include verbal outbursts or physical altercations.[34] For example, in physiotherapy settings, a patient experiencing high levels of frustration may lash out at healthcare professionals with angry words or, in severe cases, physical actions. Indirect aggression, on the other hand, involves behaviors that are aimed at hurting someone without direct confrontation. This can include passive-aggressive actions, such as noncompliance with therapy regimens or spreading negative comments about the healthcare staff.[35]

The frustration-aggression hypothesis suggests that when individuals are blocked from achieving a desired goal, their frustration can convert into aggressive impulses. This might manifest in the workplace as conflicts with colleagues or at home as arguments or physical confrontations. Internally directed aggression, which is another aspect of indirect aggression, involves self-criticism or self-destructive behaviors such as negative self-talk and self-harm. These behaviors are often more subtle and can be equally damaging, affecting both psychological well-being and physical recovery.

In physiotherapy, recognizing both direct and indirect aggression is crucial. This understanding helps therapists tailor their approaches to effectively manage and mitigate these behaviors, ensuring a safer and more constructive environment for both patients and healthcare providers.

Depression

Chronic frustration can be a significant precursor to depression, particularly when individuals face persistent obstacles that prevent them from achieving their goals. When progress is consistently impeded without any perceived relief or success, it can lead to feelings of hopelessness and helplessness.[2] Depression can reduce motivation, making patients less likely to adhere to their treatment plans. It can also worsen the perception of pain, making physical therapy sessions more challenging and less effective.[36] Additionally, depression can lead to decreased energy levels and altered sleep patterns, further hindering physical recovery. Recognizing and addressing depression early in physiotherapy is crucial to ensure that patients can continue to progress and achieve their rehabilitation goals effectively.

Low Self-Esteem

Low self-esteem often develops from repeated failures or the perceived inability to meet personal or external expectations, which is common in situations of prolonged frustration. For instance, patients who repeatedly struggle to reach recovery milestones in physiotherapy may start to doubt their abilities and intrinsic worth. This self-doubt can significantly affect their motivation and commitment to the therapeutic process, potentially leading to poorer outcomes.[37] Physiotherapists need to be aware of these risks and strive to reinforce positive achievements, no matter how small, to bolster their patients' self-esteem and encourage continued effort toward recovery.

Unhealthy Coping Behaviors

To cope with the pain of frustration, some people may turn to unhealthy behaviors such as substance abuse, overeating or engaging in compulsive behaviors like excessive gambling or shopping. These activities might provide temporary relief from frustration but typically lead to additional problems, perpetuating a cycle of frustration and poor coping.[38]

Some patients may turn to unhealthy behaviors like substance abuse, overeating or other addictive activities to manage frustration associated with physiotherapy or their physical limitations. These coping mechanisms can further impede progress and negatively affect overall health and well-being.

Increased Effort

When confronted with frustrating situations, one common response is to increase effort. This response is rooted in the determination to overcome the barriers hindering one's goals.

 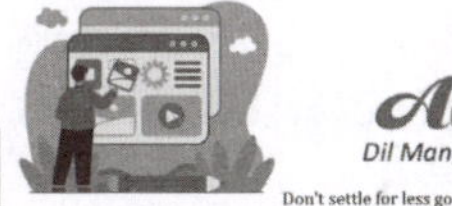

For instance, a student who is frustrated with poor academic performance might study harder or an athlete might intensify his training to surpass a performance plateau.[39] This increase in effort can be constructive but may also lead to burnout if the goals continue to be unmet despite heightened efforts.

When faced with frustration during physiotherapy sessions or rehabilitation programs, patients may respond by intensifying their efforts to overcome the obstacles and achieve their recovery goals. This could involve pushing themselves harder during exercises, adhering more strictly to treatment plans or persisting through challenging or painful interventions.

Withdrawal/Avoidance

Some individuals respond to frustration by withdrawing from the source of their frustration or avoiding it altogether. This might involve physically removing oneself from a frustrating environment or emotionally disengaging from a situation. For example, an employee overwhelmed by job demands might start calling in sick frequently or a person in a challenging relationship might become emotionally distant. While sometimes protective in the short-term, this strategy can prevent resolution of the underlying issues.[40]

Some patients may cope with frustration by withdrawing from physiotherapy sessions or avoiding specific exercises or interventions that are perceived as the source of frustration. This avoidance behavior can hinder progress and impede the rehabilitation process.

Submissiveness

In response to frustration, some individuals may adopt a submissive attitude, passively accepting the situation without attempting to alter it. This response can stem from feelings of helplessness or defeat, believing that no action can change the outcome. Submissiveness can lead to missed opportunities for growth and resolution, maintaining the status quo even when it is detrimental.[41]

In certain cases, patients may respond to frustration by becoming passive and submitting to the obstacles or sources of frustration, such as accepting limitations or setbacks without actively trying to overcome them. This submissive reaction can lead to decreased motivation and engagement in physiotherapy.

Anger and Hostility

Frustration is closely linked to feelings of anger and hostility. These emotions often arise when individuals perceive that they are being prevented from achieving something unjustly.[4] The expression of anger and hostility can vary from verbal outbursts to resentful silence, affecting personal and professional relationships, and if not managed properly, can escalate into more intense conflicts.

Frustration in physiotherapy is often accompanied by feelings of anger, irritability, and hostility toward healthcare professionals, the treatment plan or the patient's own physical limitations.[42]

These emotions can strain therapeutic relationships and impede progress if not addressed appropriately.

Impulsivity

The distress associated with frustration can lead individuals to act impulsively. Impulsive behaviors—such as making hasty decisions, engaging in risky activities or reacting without full consideration of consequences—are attempts to quickly relieve the discomfort of frustration.[43] However, these actions may complicate situations or create new problems.

Frustration can lead to impulsive and reckless behaviors in physiotherapy settings, such as disregarding safety precautions, ignoring instructions or engaging in activities that may exacerbate injuries or conditions. Prolonged or unresolved frustration during the rehabilitation process can contribute to feelings of sadness, hopelessness, and a diminished sense of self-worth in patients. This can negatively influence motivation, adherence to treatment, and overall recovery.

Physiological Reactions

Frustration can trigger various physiological reactions in patients, such as increased heart rate, elevated blood pressure, muscle tension, and hormonal changes (e.g., increased cortisol levels). These physiological responses can affect pain perception, recovery rates, and overall treatment outcomes.

Interventions to Manage Frustration

- **Educating patients and setting realistic goals:**

  It is crucial for physiotherapists to help patients set realistic expectations right from the beginning of the treatment. Education about the recovery process and potential challenges can prepare patients mentally and emotionally, reducing frustration from unexpected setbacks. In addition to stretching or yoga, physiotherapists should incorporate other gentle exercises such as Pilates or tai chi, which not only enhance physical flexibility but also promote mental relaxation.[44] This broad approach helps in setting comprehensive and realistic goals by physically preparing patients for the recovery journey and mentally equipping them to handle setbacks. Such education fosters a deeper understanding of the body's healing process, enabling patients to adjust their expectations and actively participate in managing their recovery.[45]

- **Enhanced communication techniques:**
  - Physiotherapists can utilize motivational interviewing to deepen understanding and address patients' specific concerns, fostering a collaborative relationship that reduces misunderstandings.[29]
  - Regular, structured feedback sessions further enhance patient engagement by keeping them informed of their progress, mitigating feelings of helplessness.

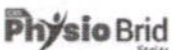
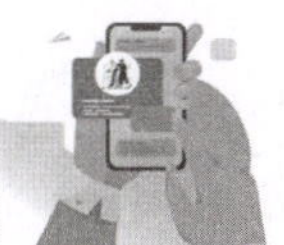
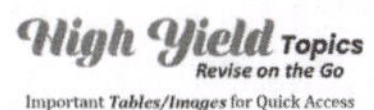

- Additionally, incorporating anger management techniques such as deep breathing and guided imagery, alongside cognitive-behavioral strategies like challenging negative thoughts and journaling, can significantly improve emotional regulation and reduce frustration during the rehabilitation process.[46]

- **Addressing therapist burnout:**
  - Implementing regular peer support meetings and supervision can help therapists manage their own frustrations and stress, promoting a healthier work environment and better patient care.[47]
  - Time management training and administrative support can alleviate the burden of overwhelming caseloads and administrative tasks, allowing therapists to focus more on patient care.
  - Additionally, physiotherapists should engage in physical self-care exercises such as yoga, Pilates or aerobic activities to manage stress, enhance physical health, and prevent burnout, ensuring they remain effective and motivated in their roles.

- **Systemic changes in healthcare:**
  - Advocating for policy changes within healthcare institutions to increase session durations or flexibility can significantly reduce system-related frustrations for both patients and therapists.
  - Training on dealing with insurance and administrative issues can equip therapists with better tools to handle external pressures and focus on delivering optimal care.

> **MUST KNOW**
>
> - Physiotherapists should employ clear, repetitive, and simplified instructions to aid understanding and retention, especially for neurological and geriatric patients.
> - Building and maintaining high levels of frustration tolerance is key to effective physiotherapy.

CONFLICT

Conflict is often described by psychologists as a state marked by opposition, disagreement or the inability of two or more parties or groups to find common ground, sometimes even leading to physical confrontations.[48] In the realm of psychology, conflict also refers to the emergence of two or more compelling desires or motives within an individual, which are irreconcilable at the same time.[49] For example, a teenager might experience internal conflict when deciding whether to attend a dance to align with his peer group, despite personal reservations.

Frustration often escalates into conflict, especially when persistent barriers prevent individuals or groups from achieving their goals.[50] This sense of being thwarted can lead to heightened emotional responses such as anger, which if not managed properly, can strain interpersonal relationships and create adversarial situations. In both personal and professional contexts, unaddressed frustration can result in confrontations, deteriorating communication, and the breakdown of teamwork, as parties increasingly see each other as obstacles rather than collaborators. Managing these feelings constructively is crucial to preventing conflict escalation.

Definition

Echoing a similar sentiment, Thomas defined conflict as "the process which begins when one party perceives that the other has negatively affected or is about to negatively affect something that the first party cares about." This definition reiterates the role of perception in the initiation of conflict.[51]

- **Organizational behavior:** This definition focuses on the perception that initiates the conflict. According to Robbins and Judge, conflict arises when one party perceives that another party has affected or will affect, something important to them negatively. This viewpoint highlights the subjective nature of conflict, emphasizing that it is not necessarily about actual interference or harm, but the perception of potential harm. This perception is crucial in organizational settings where different stakeholders may have diverse interests and priorities.[52]

- **Group dynamics:** Forsyth simplifies the concept by describing conflict as a perceived incompatibility of actions, goals or ideas. This definition is significant because it underscores the idea that conflict is not just about tangible clashes but can also arise from differences in ideologies or plans. This perspective is particularly relevant in team dynamics where the alignment of goals is critical for coherence and efficiency.[53]

- **Interpersonal conflict:** This definition adds layers to our understanding by introducing the elements of expressed struggle and interdependence. Conflict, in this context, is not just about internal perceptions but involves an outward expression of discord between parties who rely on each other in some way. The notion of interdependence suggests that the parties in conflict are in a relationship where each one's actions affect the other, highlighting the complexity of managing interpersonal conflicts where shared goals or resources are at stake.[54]

- **World religions in practice:** Thompson broadens the definition by incorporating differences in beliefs, values or practices that are significant to the parties involved. This definition is particularly insightful as it extends the idea of conflict beyond immediate personal or organizational goals to encompass broader cultural and ideological disparities. This perspective is crucial in global and multicultural contexts where differing worldviews can lead to conflict.[55]

MUST KNOW

- Conflict is often a perception that begins when one party perceives another and has negatively affected something they care about.
- Intrapersonal conflict involves opposing desires within an individual, significantly impacting decision-making and emotional well-being.

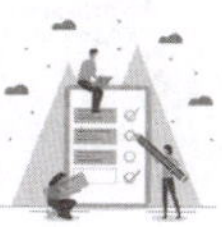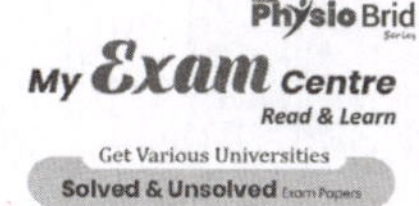

Types

Various types of conflicts[56, 57] are described in Table 5.2.

Table 5.2: Types of conflicts

Types	Definition
Intrapersonal	Conflicts within an individual due to opposing desires or emotions, impacting decision-making and emotional well-being.
Interpersonal	Conflicts between individuals due to personal differences or disagreements over data, values or methods.
Intragroup	Conflicts within a group, involving disagreements over task priorities, relationships or processes.
Organizational	Conflicts within an organization arising from role distinctions, hierarchical structures or functional discrepancies.
Societal	Conflicts stemming from broader societal issues like politics, race, class or gender, influencing workplace dynamics.

Intrapersonal Conflict

- **Approach-approach conflict:** This type of conflict occurs when an individual is faced with two equally tempting options, but choosing one necessitates forgoing the other. For example, a patient may need to decide between two equally beneficial treatment modalities that suit different aspects of their recovery. Each option offers desirable benefits, yet choosing one means missing out on the advantages of the other. Understanding such conflicts can help physiotherapists in guiding patients to make choices that align best with their long-term health goals.[58]

- **Avoidance-avoidance conflict:** In this scenario, an individual must choose between two unappealing outcomes, making it a case of choosing the lesser of two evils. A common example in physiotherapy might involve a patient deciding whether to undergo a painful rehabilitation procedure or continue living with debilitating pain. Both options are undesirable, which can lead to significant stress and hesitation. Physiotherapists can assist by providing clear, compassionate guidance and support, helping the patient weigh the long-term benefits against the immediate discomfort.[59]

- **Approach-avoidance conflict:** This conflict arises when a single goal has both appealing and unappealing aspects. For instance, a patient might desire the benefits of a particular treatment but dread the associated pain or discomfort. This type of conflict is common in physiotherapy settings, where the anticipation of pain can deter patients from pursuing beneficial treatments. Effective communication about the pros and cons, as well as reassurance and motivational interviewing, can be crucial in these scenarios.[60]

- **Multiple approach-avoidance conflict:** More complex than the other types, this conflict involves several options, each with its own set of pros and cons. A physiotherapy patient, for example, may need to choose a treatment plan that balances various factors such as recovery time, potential risks, cost, and personal or professional commitments. Physiotherapists need to facilitate a thorough decision-making process, guiding the patient through each option's potential outcomes to find the most suitable course of action.[61]

- **Internal conflict:** As a broader category, internal conflict encompasses any psychological struggle stemming from opposing desires, thoughts, values or emotions within an individual. For physiotherapy students, it is important to recognize that these conflicts can profoundly affect a patient's emotional and physical well-being. By understanding the nature of these internal struggles, future physiotherapists can better support their patients through empathetic engagement and tailored intervention strategies, aiming to resolve conflicts in ways that enhance treatment adherence and effectiveness.[62]

Interpersonal Conflict

- **Relationship conflict:** These conflicts stem from personal incompatibilities or emotional disputes.[63] In physiotherapy settings, such conflicts might occur between colleagues due to personality clashes or between therapists and patients due to misaligned expectations about treatment goals or methodologies. Such misalignment can lead to tension, reduced cooperation from the patient, and a potential decline in therapeutic outcomes if not resolved through understanding and compromise.

- **Data conflict:** This type involves disagreements over factual data and information interpretation.[64] For physiotherapy professionals, this could arise during discussions on treatment effectiveness, differing patient assessments or when evaluating the latest research impacting clinical decisions. This might manifest when physiotherapists from different training backgrounds interpret the efficacy of a new treatment differently based on their understanding and experience. Such disputes could affect team cohesion and the overall treatment plan, requiring clear communication and perhaps third-party mediation to align on the best approach.

- **Value conflict:** These conflicts are rooted in differing belief systems, ethics or values, which can significantly influence professional interactions and treatment decisions.[65] If a clinic introduces a new protocol that prioritizes efficiency over individual patient needs, a physiotherapist who values patient-centered care might object to the change. This conflict between personal ethics and organizational policy can lead to moral distress and dissatisfaction, impacting professional performance.

- **Structural conflict:** Caused by external pressures such as organizational roles, resource limitations or environmental factors, structural conflicts can influence interpersonal dynamics. These often manifest in disagreements over job responsibilities, workspace arrangements or schedule management within a physiotherapy clinic.[66]

Intragroup Conflict

- **Task conflict:** This conflict often arises in settings where team members have different views on the priorities or methodologies of a project. It can be constructive if managed properly, leading

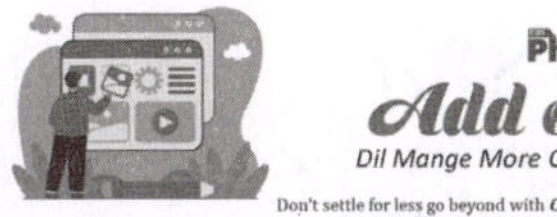
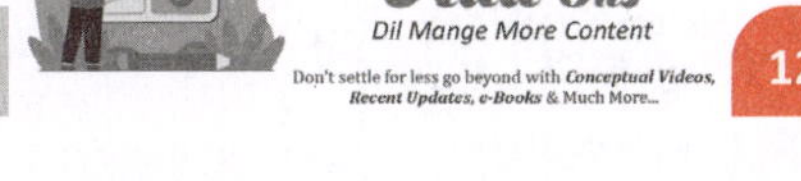

to innovative solutions and enhanced decision-making as different perspectives are considered. In physiotherapy teams, this might include conflicting views on the priority of treatment goals for a patient or differing opinions on which rehabilitation techniques to employ.[67]

- **Relationship conflict:** Deep-seated interpersonal disputes can severely disrupt team dynamics. These conflicts often stem from personality clashes or unresolved grievances and can lead to a toxic work environment if not addressed. Such conflicts might stem from personal grievances or competitive tensions among team members.[67]

- **Process conflict:** This type of conflict focuses on the logistics of task execution within a team, such as the division of responsibilities and the methods used to complete tasks. Mismanagement of process conflict can lead to inefficiency and dissatisfaction among team members, but when resolved effectively, it can improve organizational procedures and workflow efficiency. For example, disagreements over the allocation of tasks in a patient's treatment plan or conflicts about the delegation of administrative responsibilities.[67]

Realistic and Nonrealistic Conflict

- **Realistic conflict:** Often revolves around tangible resources like space, equipment or budget allocations. In a healthcare setting, this could involve disputes between different departments over the allocation of clinic resources or space utilization.[68]

- **Nonrealistic conflict:** Encompasses conflicts based on identities, beliefs or values. These conflicts can emerge in diverse workplace settings where varied cultural backgrounds and personal values are present, potentially leading to misunderstandings or biases affecting group interactions.[68]

Organizational Conflict

- **Line-staff conflict:** Emerges between line employees, who are directly involved in patient care, and staff employees, who provide support and administrative services. Disputes might revolve around the perceived value of each role or misunderstandings about the contributions of different roles to patient outcomes.[69]

- **Hierarchical conflict:** Arises from power differentials and communication barriers between different levels of an organization's hierarchy. This type of conflict can affect decision-making processes and the implementation of organizational policies.[70]

- **Functional conflict:** Occurs between different departments or functional areas with competing priorities or goals. For example, the physiotherapy department might have conflicts with the administration over budget priorities or with the nursing staff over patient care coordination.[71]

Societal Conflict

Political, racial/ethnic, class, and gender conflicts: These conflicts reflect broader societal issues that can infiltrate the workplace and affect professional interactions and policies. Such conflicts might influence patient interactions, hiring practices, and workplace culture within a physiotherapy setting.[72]

> **MUST KNOW**
>
> - Interpersonal conflict arises from disagreements between individuals, often due to personal differences or misunderstandings.
> - Intragroup conflict within teams can stem from differing views on task priorities or methods.

Defense Mechanisms in Clinical Practice

In the realm of physiotherapy, understanding the psychological dimensions of patient care is crucial. Defense mechanisms, common psychological strategies employed by individuals to manage stress and conflicts, can significantly influence patient behavior and therapy outcomes.[77]

- **Denial:** This mechanism involves a refusal to accept reality or facts, acting as if a distressing event or situation did not happen or does not exist. People using denial can block external events from their consciousness. In a clinical setting, this might manifest as a patient ignoring medical advice or denying the severity of their condition.

- **Repression:** Repression serves as a way to keep disturbing or threatening thoughts from becoming conscious. This process involves pushing away thoughts, feelings or memories that are too difficult to handle. For example, a patient may repress the emotional implications of a chronic illness, affecting their ability to fully participate in treatment.

- **Projection:** Projection involves attributing one's own unacceptable or unwanted thoughts, feelings or motives to another person. By projecting these attributes onto others, the individual can avoid acknowledging them in themselves. This can lead to misunderstandings and conflicts in therapeutic relationships, as patients might accuse healthcare providers of negative behaviors or attitudes that are actually their own.

- **Rationalization:** Rationalization allows individuals to justify or explain their behavior or feelings in a seemingly rational or logical manner, avoiding the true explanation which is typically unacceptable or threatening. Patients might rationalize skipping therapy sessions by claiming they are not necessary despite medical advice to the contrary.

- **Displacement:** This mechanism involves shifting feelings from their original object to a safer, substitute target. Displacement can reduce anxiety by allowing the expression of the feelings but in a way that will not disrupt primary relationships. For example, a patient frustrated with their progress might displace their anger onto the clinic staff instead of their condition.

- **Reaction formation:** Reaction formation reduces anxiety by taking up the opposite feeling, impulse or behavior. An individual who feels a strong dislike toward someone may instead express excessive affection. Within a therapy context, a patient who actually feels very vulnerable might act overly confident or dismissive of their rehabilitation needs.

- **Sublimation:** Sublimation is a way of dealing with unacceptable impulses by unconsciously transforming them into more acceptable forms of behavior. This might be seen in a patient who channels frustration with their physical limitations into a relentless dedication to their therapeutic exercises, thus using the energy from their frustrations constructively.

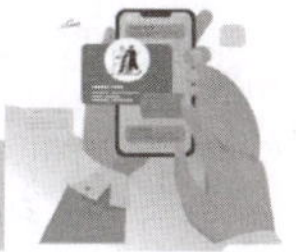
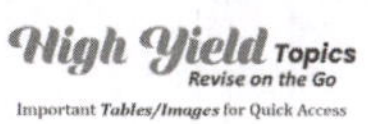

- **Intellectualization:** This mechanism involves avoiding uncomfortable emotions by focusing on facts and logic. Individuals may create a distance from their anxieties by discussing their situation in complex terms. For instance, a patient might focus minutely on the details of their surgical procedure or diagnosis instead of addressing their fears about the surgery.

- **Regression:** Regression involves moving back to a previous developmental stage in order to feel safe or to have certain psychological needs met. Adults might regress when under a great deal of stress, displaying childlike behaviors. In a clinical setting, a patient might regress to dependency, seeking comfort from caregivers beyond what is typical for their age or situation.

- **Compensation:** Compensation is a strategy whereby people counterbalance perceived weaknesses by emphasizing strengths in other areas. This can often be seen in the physical therapy setting where patients, unable to perform certain tasks due to their condition, might focus intensively on excelling in other areas of their health or life to maintain self-esteem.

> **MUST KNOW**
>
> - Societal conflicts reflect broader issues like politics, race, class or gender that influence workplace dynamics.
> - Effective conflict resolution strategies include active listening, empathy, flexibility, and open communication.
> - Maintaining professional relationships is crucial in managing conflicts and ensuring successful outcomes.

Conflict Management

Conflict Management Styles (Fig. 5.2)

Competition (Assertive and Uncooperative)

This style is characterized by a high concern for one's own interests and a low concern for the interests of others. It involves using whatever power or resources one has to win the conflict and achieve one's goals at the expense of the other party's goals. Competition can be an effective approach when the issue is extremely important, there is an emergency situation requiring quick decisive action or when one party holds a position of legitimate authority or greater expertise on the matter.[78, 79]

However, competition often leads to resentment, damaged relationships, and potential retaliation or escalation of the conflict. It should be used judiciously and sparingly. For physiotherapists, using competition judiciously is important, as it can lead to resentment and strained relationships with colleagues and patients, potentially compromising collaborative care.

Accommodation (Unassertive and Cooperative)

With accommodation, one party neglects their own interests entirely to satisfy the interests or concerns of the other party. This approach is focused on preserving harmony and avoiding confrontation in the relationship, even if it means subjugating one's own needs or goals.[79]

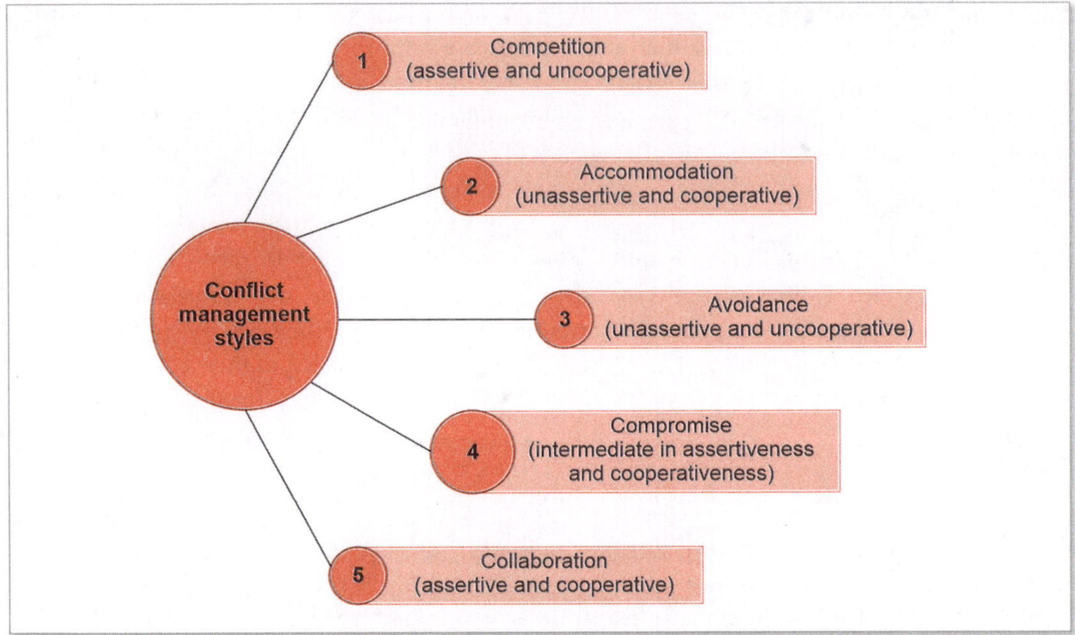

Fig. 5.2: Conflict management styles

Accommodation can be appropriate when the issue is more important to the other party or when continued competition would lead to severe disruption or damage. It can also foster goodwill. However, it may breed resentment if used too frequently, and the accommodating party's interests are consistently neglected. In physiotherapy, this might manifest when a therapist defers to a patient's resistance to a particular treatment plan to maintain rapport or when navigating priorities within a multidisciplinary team. While fostering goodwill, overuse can lead to burnout and dissatisfaction if the therapist's professional judgments are consistently set aside.

Avoidance (Unassertive and Uncooperative)

Avoidance involves sidestepping or postponing the conflict entirely by withdrawing, changing the subject or choosing not to address the disagreement. It allows parties to temporarily circumvent confrontation.[79]

Avoidance can be useful when the issue is trivial, there is little chance of resolving the conflict constructively or when one needs time to gather more information or regain perspective. However, it is an ineffective long-term approach, as important issues may remain unresolved and fester. In clinical settings, avoidance may serve as a short-term solution in high-tension scenarios to prevent escalation, such as when deferring a discussion with an emotionally charged patient. However, it is generally ineffective as a long-term strategy. Unresolved issues can lead to incomplete patient care and ongoing conflicts within the healthcare team.

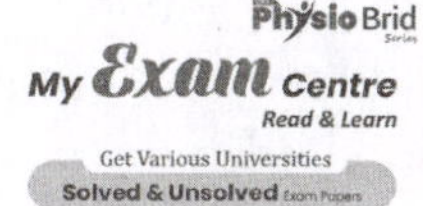

Compromise (Intermediate in Assertiveness and Cooperativeness)

With compromise, both parties give up elements of their original interests through negotiation and bargaining to reach a mutually acceptable solution. Both sides make concessions, and no one is fully satisfied, but the conflict is partially resolved on a temporary basis.[79]

Compromise is useful when parties have equal power/motivation or when they have failed to negotiate a more satisfactory solution. It allows tangible issues to be settled promptly. However, compromise may be unsatisfying if core values or concerns are compromised excessively. For physiotherapists, compromise might be necessary when coordinating care with other healthcare providers, each with different treatment approaches. While it can resolve issues quickly, the risk is that the best possible patient outcome may not be fully achieved if compromises are made on essential aspects of care.

Collaboration (Assertive and Cooperative)

Collaboration involves cooperating to fully understand each party's interests and working together to find a mutually beneficial solution that satisfies both sets of concerns. It integrates multiple perspectives through open dialogue and creative problem solving.[79]

Collaboration leads to superior outcomes, builds commitment, and strengthens relationships, but it requires significant time, effort, trust, and effective communication skills. It is ideal for complex issues where a higher-quality solution is needed and where the long-term relationship is important. In clinical settings, collaboration is ideal for complex scenarios where a comprehensive understanding of a patient's condition necessitates input from various specialties. This approach promotes a holistic view of patient care, resulting in high-quality outcomes and enhanced professional relationships.

Ultimately, the appropriate conflict style depends on the specific situation, goals, power dynamics, relationships, and the willingness of parties to be assertive about their interests or cooperative in addressing others' concerns. An effective conflict manager will be able to assess situations and employ multiple styles flexibly as needed.

> **MUST KNOW**
>
> Conflict can be constructive if managed properly, leading to innovative solutions and enhanced decision-making.

Collaboration in conflict resolution can lead to superior outcomes and strengthen relationships between frustration and conflict in physiotherapy settings. They gain insights into the psychological underpinnings of frustration, how it manifests in various behaviors, and its impact on therapy outcomes. The chapter also equips students with strategies for identifying and managing both personal and professional conflicts effectively, emphasizing the importance of communication, empathy, and problem-solving skills. This knowledge is crucial for fostering a supportive therapeutic environment and enhancing both patient care and professional relationships.

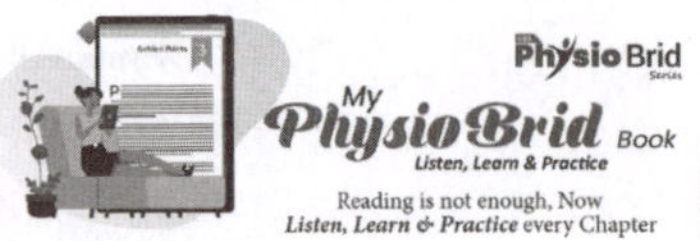

Techniques

In physiotherapy, where collaboration and interaction with patients and colleagues are integral to everyday operations, understanding and applying informal conflict-management techniques is essential. These practical strategies, often highlighted in psychology resources for physiotherapy students, help manage and resolve conflicts within clinical settings without resorting to formal interventions.[73, 74]

- **Active listening** is particularly valuable in physiotherapy. It involves fully concentrating on what is being said, understanding the message, and responding thoughtfully. This approach is crucial when resolving disputes over treatment approaches, ensuring all parties involved—be it colleagues or patients—feel heard and understood, which can significantly de-escalate potential conflicts.[75]

- **Open communication** plays a critical role in a physiotherapy setting. Maintaining transparency in sharing thoughts, feelings, and rationales can prevent misunderstandings and misinterpretations that often lead to conflicts, whether in discussing patient care plans or in team management decisions.[76]

- **Empathy** is another essential skill for physiotherapists. It involves understanding and sharing the feelings of others, which goes beyond mere sympathy. Demonstrating genuine emotional outreach can build trust and understanding, crucial for resolving personal and emotional conflicts, particularly in interactions with patients who may be experiencing stress and discomfort due to their conditions.[75]

- **Flexibility** in decision-making is particularly useful in physiotherapy, where treatment plans may need to be adapted based on patient progress or feedback. Being flexible and open to compromise can help manage structural and process conflicts within the team, especially concerning scheduling, treatment planning, and role assignments.[75]

- **Informal mediation** by a neutral or more experienced colleague can effectively mediate disputes in a nonconfrontational manner. This informal approach, involving casual conversation and guidance, can be particularly effective in a physiotherapy context, helping to resolve disagreements over clinical decisions or interpersonal issues without escalating to formal disciplinary channels.[75]

- **Humor**, used appropriately, can serve as a stress reliever and a way to lighten the atmosphere in stressful clinical environments. When used sensitively and appropriately, humor can de-escalate tensions during team meetings or in daily interactions, contributing to a more relaxed and cooperative work environment.[75]

- Lastly, **building relationships** is vital in physiotherapy. Engaging in team-building activities and fostering strong, positive relationships among staff can prevent many conflicts. In physiotherapy, where teamwork and cooperation can significantly affect treatment outcomes, having strong interpersonal relationships can simplify the resolution of minor disagreements and enhance overall workplace harmony.

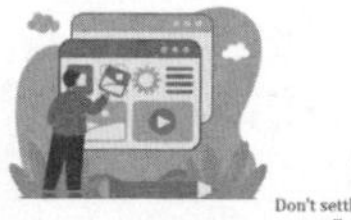
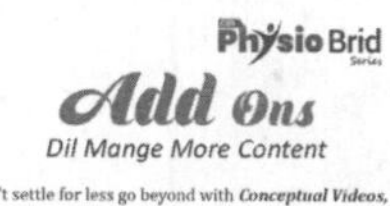

SUMMARY

- In the realm of physiotherapy and rehabilitation, the dynamics of frustration and conflict are both significant and multifaceted. These emotional and interpersonal challenges can profoundly impact the therapeutic process, patient outcomes, and the overall well-being of both patients and healthcare providers. This unit delves into the intricacies of frustration and conflict, examining their psychological underpinnings, manifestations, and the strategies necessary to navigate and mitigate their effects.

- Frustration, an emotional response to opposition or the blocking of goal-directed behavior, is a common experience in physiotherapy. It can arise from both internal sources, such as cognitive limitations or physical barriers, and external sources, including environmental obstacles and societal factors. The chapter elaborates on the various characteristics of frustration, such as emotional arousal, cognitive distortions, and physiological arousal, and how they manifest in clinical settings. For instance, patients may exhibit irritability, anger outbursts or feelings of hopelessness when faced with slow progress or setbacks in their recovery.

- The chapter categorizes the sources of frustration into internal and external factors, providing a detailed examination of each. External sources include physical factors like environmental stressors and social factors such as interpersonal conflicts and societal expectations. Internal sources encompass cognitive limitations, conflicting desires, and perceived unfairness or lack of control. These factors can significantly hinder the therapeutic process and lead to emotional distress and decreased motivation among patients.

- The impact of frustration on physiotherapy is multifaceted. It can lead to impaired decision-making, aggressive tendencies, and maladaptive coping strategies among patients, thereby complicating the recovery process. For instance, patients may become noncompliant with treatment plans, exhibit passive-aggressive behavior or resort to substance abuse to cope with the emotional distress caused by frustration.

- Conflict, often a byproduct of frustration, can arise in various forms within physiotherapy settings. The chapter explores different types of conflicts, including intrapersonal conflicts (internal struggles), interpersonal conflicts (disagreements between individuals), intragroup conflicts (within a team), and organizational conflicts (within an institution). These conflicts can stem from personal incompatibilities, disagreements over data or values, and structural issues like resource limitations.

- Effective management of frustration and conflict is crucial for the success of physiotherapy interventions. The chapter discusses several strategies for managing these challenges, including educating patients about the recovery process, enhancing communication techniques, and addressing therapist burnout. It emphasizes the importance of empathy, active listening, and open communication in resolving conflicts and fostering a supportive therapeutic environment. Additionally, it explores the role of defense mechanisms in clinical practice and provides insights into the various conflict management styles, such as competition, accommodation, avoidance, compromise, and collaboration.

- Understanding and effectively managing frustration and conflict are essential components of successful physiotherapy practice. By recognizing the signs of frustration, employing appropriate conflict resolution strategies, and fostering a supportive therapeutic relationship, physiotherapists can enhance patient engagement, improve recovery outcomes, and maintain professional satisfaction. This chapter provides a comprehensive framework for navigating these complex emotional and interpersonal challenges, equipping physiotherapists with the tools needed to create a positive and productive therapeutic environment.

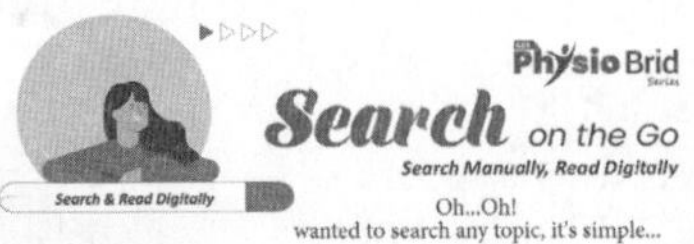

REFERENCE

1. Roeckelein JE. Elsevier's dictionary of psychological theories: Elsevier; 2006.

2. Novaco RW. Anger dysregulation. Anger, aggression, and interventions for interpersonal violence: Routledge; 2023. p. 3–54.

3. Dollard J, Coob L, Miller N, Mowrer O, Sears R. Frustration and Aggression. Yale University. Press, New Haven. 1939.

4. Mallick SK. Frustration-reinterpretation and Catharsis of Hostility: Indiana University; 1964.

5. Linton SJ. Understanding pain for better clinical practice: A psychological perspective. 2005.

6. Gard G, Gyllensten AL. The importance of emotions in physiotherapeutic practice. Physical Therapy Reviews. 2000;5(3):155–60.

7. Gullacksen A-C, Lidbeck J. The life adjustment process in chronic pain: Psychosocial assessment and clinical implications. Pain Research and Management. 2004;9(3):145–53.

8. Rolland JS. Neurocognitive impairment: Addressing couple and family challenges. Family Process. 2017;56(4):799–818.

9. Sherman M, Jost H. Frustration reactions of normal and neurotic persons. The Journal of Psychology. 1942;13(1):3–19.

10. Jost H. Some physiological changes during frustration. Child Development. 1941:9–15.

11. De Castella K, Goldin P, Jazaieri H, Ziv M, Dweck CS, Gross JJ. Beliefs about emotion: Links to emotion regulation, well-being, and psychological distress. Basic and applied social psychology. 2013;35(6):497–505.

12. Brisset M, Nowicki S. Internal versus external control of reinforcement and reaction to frustration. Journal of personality and social psychology. 1973;25(1):35.

13. Krohne HW. Stress and coping theories. Int Encyclopedia of the Social Behavioral Sciences [cited 2021]. 2002.

14. Cohen S, Evans GW, Stokols D, Krantz DS. Behavior, health, and environmental stress: Springer Science & Business Media; 2013.

15. Fykaris I, Rantzou M, Matiaki V, Karolidou S. Frustration of Expectations and Aspirations in Pre-adolescents as a Cause of Emotional and Social Conflict. Journal of Education, Society and Behavioural Science. 2020;33(5):26–35.

16. Gilbert MA, Bushman BJ. Frustration-aggression hypothesis. Encyclopedia of personality and individual differences: Springer; 2020. p. 1683–5.

17. Finkelstein SA, Adams C, Tuttle M, Saxena A, Perez DL, editors. Neuropsychiatric treatment approaches for functional neurological disorder: A how to guide. Seminars in Neurology; 2022: Thieme Medical Publishers, Inc.

18. Folkman S, Lazarus RS, Gruen RJ, DeLongis A. Appraisal, coping, health status, and psychological symptoms. Journal of personality and social psychology. 1986;50(3):571.

19. Folkman S, Chesney M, McKusick L, Ironson G, Johnson DS, Coates TJ. Translating coping theory into an intervention. The social context of coping. 1991:239–60.

20. Chen Y. Relationships of frustrators with affective, behavioral, and physical reactions: The effects of potential moderators: University of South Florida; 1989.

21. Chen PY, Spector PE. Relationships of work stressors with aggression, withdrawal, theft and substance use: An exploratory study. Journal of occupational and organizational psychology. 1992;65(3):177–84.

Contd...

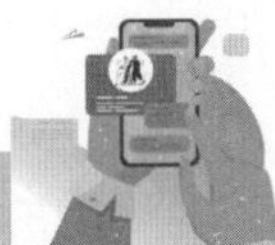

22. Burnes B, Cooke B. K urt L ewin's Field Theory: A Review and Re-evaluation. International journal of management reviews. 2013;15(4):408–25.

23. Lange F. Frustration? aggression. A reconsideration. European Journal of Social Psychology. 1971;1(1):59–84.

24. Barclay LJ, Skarlicki DP, Pugh SD. Exploring the role of emotions in injustice perceptions and retaliation. Journal of applied psychology. 2005;90(4):629.

25. Wortman CB, Brehm JW. Responses to uncontrollable outcomes: An integration of reactance theory and the learned helplessness model. Advances in experimental social psychology. 8: Elsevier; 1975. p. 277–336.

26. Szczegielniak A, Skowronek A, Krysta K, Krupka-Matuszczyk I. Aggression in the work environment of physiotherapists. Psychiatria Danubina. 2012;24(suppl 1):147–52.

27. Wiles R, Ashburn A, Payne S, Murphy C. Discharge from physiotherapy following stroke: The management of disappointment. Social science & medicine. 2004;59(6):1263–73.

28. Topley DT. The Repeated Re-referral of Chronic Pain Patients into Musculoskeletal Physiotherapy Outpatient: Ulster University; 2019.

29. Driver C, Kean B, Oprescu F, Lovell GP. Knowledge, behaviors, attitudes and beliefs of physiotherapists towards the use of psychological interventions in physiotherapy practice: A systematic review. Disability and rehabilitation. 2017;39(22):2237–49.

30. Leyro TM, Zvolensky MJ, Bernstein A. Distress tolerance and psychopathological symptoms and disorders: A review of the empirical literature among adults. Psychological bulletin. 2010;136(4):576.

31. Seymour KE, Macatee R, Chronis-Tuscano A. Frustration tolerance in youth with ADHD. Journal of attention disorders. 2019;23(11):1229–39.

32. Hülsheger UR, Alberts HJ, Feinholdt A, Lang JW. Benefits of mindfulness at work: The role of mindfulness in emotion regulation, emotional exhaustion, and job satisfaction. Journal of applied psychology. 2013;98(2):310.

33. Berkowitz L. Frustrations, appraisals, and aversively stimulated aggression. Aggressive behavior. 1988;14(1):3–11.

34. Onyike C, Lyketsos C. Aggression and violence. Textbook of Psychosomatic Medicine: Psychiatric Care of the Medically Ill. 2011;101:153–74.

35. Beck S, Tong L. Psychiatry in the Primary Care Setting: Managing Chronic Illness: Psychiatric Issues. Biopsychosocial Approaches in Primary Care: State of the Art and Challenges for the 21st Century: Springer; 1997. p. 45–63.

36. Jensen MP. Enhancing motivation to change in pain treatment. Psychological approaches to pain management: A practitioner's handbook. 1996:78–111.

37. Resnick B, Avers D. Motivation and Patient Education: Implications for Physical Therapist. Geriatric Physical Therapy, 3rd ed. (Guccione AA, Avers D, Wong R, Eds), Elsevier Mosby, USA. 2011:183–206.

38. Zorrilla EP, Koob GF. The dark side of compulsive eating and food addiction: Affective dysregulation, negative reinforcement, and negative urgency. Compulsive eating behavior and food addiction: Elsevier; 2019. p. 115–92.

39. Clarke DC, Skiba PF. Rationale and resources for teaching the mathematical modeling of athletic training and performance. Advances in physiology education. 2013.

40. Yu C. The display of frustration in arguments: A multimodal analysis. Journal of Pragmatics. 2011;43(12):2964–81.

Contd...

41. Tiedens LZ, Fragale AR. Power moves: Complementarity in dominant and submissive nonverbal behavior. Journal of personality and social psychology. 2003;84(3):558.

42. Burns JW, Higdon LJ, Mullen JT, Lansky D, Wei JM. Relationships among patient hostility, anger expression, depression, and the working alliance in a work hardening program. Annals of Behavioral Medicine. 1999;21(1):77–82.

43. Ramirez JM, Andreu JM. Aggression, and some related psychological constructs (anger, hostility, and impulsivity) Some comments from a research project. Neuroscience & biobehavioral reviews. 2006;30(3):276–91.

44. Burckhardt CS. Educating patients: Self-management approaches. Disability and rehabilitation. 2005;27(12):703–9.

45. Jacobson N, Greenley D. What is recovery? A conceptual model and explication. Psychiatric services. 2001;52(4):482–5.

46. Mateer CA, Sira CS. Cognitive and emotional consequences of TBI: Intervention strategies for vocational rehabilitation. NeuroRehabilitation. 2006;21(4):315–26.

47. Burri SD, Smyrk KM, Melegy MS, Kessler MM, Hussein NI, Tuttle BD, et al. Risk factors associated with physical therapist burnout: A systematic review. Physiotherapy. 2022;116:9–24.

48. Golovey L, Danilova MV, Rykman L, Gruzdeva I, Danilova M. Conflict Between Self-Esteem and Aspirations Related to Psychological Well-being of Adolescents. European Proceedings of Social and Behavioural Sciences. 2020;94.

49. Golovey LA, Danilova MV, Gruzdeva IA, Rykman LV. Psychological Well-Being and Intra-personal Conflicts in Adolescence. Psychology in Russia. 2021;14(3):132.

50. Keashly L, Nowell BL. Conflict, conflict resolution and bullying. Bullying and emotional abuse in the workplace: CRC Press; 2002. p. 357–76.

51. Thomas KW. Conflict and conflict management: Reflections and update. Journal of organizational behavior. 1992:265–74.

52. Robbins SP, Judge TA. Organizational behavior 15th edition: Prentice Hall; 2012.

53. Forsyth DR. Group dynamics. 2011.

54. Hocker JL, Wilmot WW. Interpersonal conflict: McGraw-Hill Education New York, NY; 2018.

55. Thompson L. Religion and Diplomacy. The Hague Journal of Diplomacy. 2015;10(2):197–214.

56. Fisher R. Sources of conflict and methods of conflict resolution. International Peace and Conflict Resolution, School of International Service, The American University. 2000;1965:1–6.

57. Cox KB. The effects of intrapersonal, intragroup, and intergroup conflict on team performance effectiveness and work satisfaction. Nursing administration quarterly. 2003;27(2):153–63.

58. Bell AO. Examination of the ease or difficulty of resolving an approach-approach conflict 2013.

59. Campbell BA, Smith NF, Misanin JR. Effects of punishment on extinction of avoidance behavior: Avoidance-avoidance conflict or vicious circle behavior? Journal of Comparative and Physiological Psychology. 1966;62(3):495.

60. Garcia-Guerrero S, O'Hora D, Zgonnikov A, Scherbaum S. The action dynamics of approach-avoidance conflict during decision-making. Quarterly Journal of Experimental Psychology. 2023;76(1):160–79.

61. Corr PJ. Approach and avoidance behaviour: Multiple systems and their interactions. Emotion Review. 2013;5(3):285–90.

62. Brown ME. The international dimensions of internal conflict: Mit Press; 1996.

Contd...

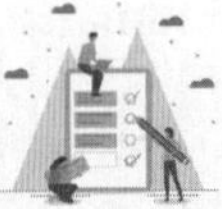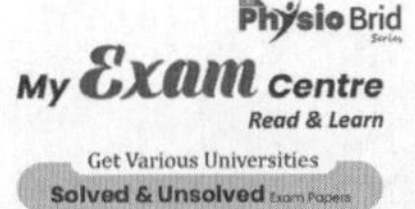

63. Canary DJ, Cupach WR, Messman S. Relationship conflict: Conflict in parent-child, friendship, and romantic relationships: Sage Publications; 1995.

64. Zhong Z, Zhang C. Technologies for detecting data conflicts in distributed situation. Control Engineering and Information Systems: CRC Press; 2015. p. 821–6.

65. Donohue WA. Managing interpersonal conflict: Sage Publications; 1992.

66. Kim S, Bochatay N, Relyea-Chew A, Buttrick E, Amdahl C, Kim L, et al. Individual, interpersonal, and organisational factors of healthcare conflict: A scoping review. Journal of interprofessional care. 2017;31(3):282–90.

67. Medina FJ, Munduate L, Dorado MA, Martínez I, Guerra JM. Types of intragroup conflict and affective reactions. Journal of managerial psychology. 2005;20(3/4):219–30.

68. Jehn KA. Types of conflict: The history and future of conflict definitions and typologies. Handbook of conflict management research: Edward Elgar Publishing; 2014. p. 3–18.

69. Agarwal A, Vrat P. Line and staff functions in organizations revisited: A bionic system analogy using ISM. Vision. 2015;19(2):89–103.

70. Thompson VA. Hierarchy, specialization, and organizational conflict. Administrative science quarterly. 1961:485–521.

71. Medina FJ, Dorado MA, Munduate L, Martínez I, Cisneros IF, editors. Types of conflict and personal and organizational consequences. Comunicación presentada a la Internacional Association for Conflict Management Conference, Park City USA; 2002.

72. Oberschall A. Theories of social conflict. Annual review of sociology. 1978;4:291–315.

73. Bochatay N, Bajwa NM, Cullati S, Muller-Juge V, Blondon KS, Perron NJ, et al. A multilevel analysis of professional conflicts in healthcare teams: Insight for future training. Academic Medicine. 2017;92(11S):S84–S92.

74. Ayandiran E, Ola O. Experiences of Conflicts and Conflict Management Styles among Healthcare Professionals: Do Conflict's Perception and Attitude Matter? Life Social Sciences Review. 2015;24(2):1–15.

75. Ronquillo Y, Ellis VL, Toney-Butler TJ. Conflict management. StatPearls [Internet]: StatPearls Publishing; 2023.

76. Overton AR, Lowry AC. Conflict management: difficult conversations with difficult people. Clinics in colon and rectal surgery. 2013;26(04):259–64.

77. Wolf M, Gerlach A, Merkle W. Conflict, trauma, defence mechanisms, and symptom formation. Psychoanalytic Psychotherapy: Routledge; 2018. p. 61–78.

78. 78. Slabbert A. Conflict management styles in traditional organisations. The Social Science Journal. 2004;41(1):83–92.

79. Thomas KW, Thomas GF. Introduction to conflict. California Management Review. 1978;21:56–9.

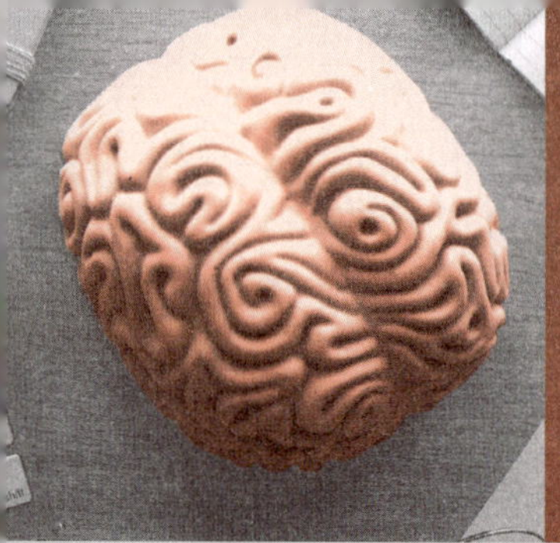

LONG ANSWER QUESTIONS

1. Explain the concept of 'Learned Helplessness' and how it relates to frustration in physiotherapy. Discuss its effect on patient involvement.
2. Discuss the differences between intrapersonal and interpersonal conflicts with examples.
3. Describe the various reactions to frustration.
4. Describe the various characteristics of frustration seen in physiotherapy settings with relevant examples.
5. Discuss conflict management in detail.

SHORT ANSWER QUESTIONS

1. Define frustration and conflict using relevant examples.
2. Describe the causes of frustrations for physiotherapists.
3. Explain organizational conflict.
4. What role does empathy play in managing conflicts within physiotherapy?
5. How does effective communication prevent conflicts?

MULTIPLE CHOICE QUESTIONS

1. **What does frustration primarily stem from in psychology?**
   a. Achieving goals too easily
   b. Facing unexpected successes
   c. Encountering obstacles that block goals
   d. Experiencing relief from stress

2. **Which theory connects frustration directly to aggression?**
   a. Behaviorism
   b. Frustration-aggression hypothesis
   c. Humanism
   d. Cognitive dissonance theory

3. **According to Dollard et al. (1939), frustration occurs when there is an interference with:**
   a. An expected reward
   b. The occurrence of an instigated goal-response
   c. General emotional stability
   d. Cognitive processing

4. **What type of factors are primarily responsible for causing external frustration?**
   a. Motivational conflicts
   b. Physical barriers and social constraints
   c. Psychological disorders
   d. Personal achievements

5. **In the context of physiotherapy, which is a common internal source of frustration?**
   a. Noise in the therapy environment
   b. High treatment costs
   c. Physical limitations of the patient
   d. Lack of public healthcare policies

6. **What does 'learned helplessness' in response to frustration involve?**
   a. Enhanced motivation to try harder
   b. Belief that one's actions have no effect on outcomes
   c. Immediate resolution of the stressful situation
   d. Increased cognitive abilities

7. **What does empathy in a physiotherapy setting help to resolve?**
   a. Financial disputes
   b. Personal and emotional conflicts
   c. Organizational goals
   d. Scheduling issues

8. **Which conflict type arises from differences in belief systems, ethics or values?**
   a. Data conflict
   b. Value conflict
   c. Task conflict
   d. Structural conflict

9. **In physiotherapy, humor can be used to:**
   a. De-escalate tensions
   b. Increase productivity
   c. Worsen conflicts
   d. Complicate communication

10. **Building strong relationships in a physiotherapy team helps to:**
    a. Increase resource allocation issues
    b. Prevent many conflicts
    c. Reduce treatment effectiveness
    d. Create task conflicts

11. **Informal mediation in a physiotherapy context is used to:**
    a. Formally discipline team members
    b. Resolve disagreements through casual conversation
    c. Implement strict administrative policies
    d. Increase the budget for the physiotherapy department

12. **Which defense mechanism involves refusing to acknowledge reality?**
    a. Projection
    b. Denial
    c. Rationalization
    d. Repression

13. **Regression as a defense mechanism can manifest as:**
    a. Taking a logical approach to emotional stress
    b. Exhibiting behaviors typical of a younger age
    c. Assigning personal unacceptable qualities to others
    d. Justifying actions with acceptable reasons

14. **Sublimation is best described as:**
    a. Avoiding emotional stress through logic and facts
    b. Transforming unacceptable impulses into acceptable behaviors
    c. Denying the reality of a stressful situation
    d. Regressing to behaviors of an earlier developmental stage

15. **Displacement might occur in a clinical setting when a patient:**
    a. Ignores the severity of their condition
    b. Redirects anger from their condition to the clinic staff
    c. Justifies missing treatment sessions
    d. Exhibits the opposite of their actual feelings

ANSWER KEY

1. c	2. b	3. b	4. b	5. c	6. b	7. b	8. b
9. a	10. b	11. b	12. b	13. b	14. b	15. b	

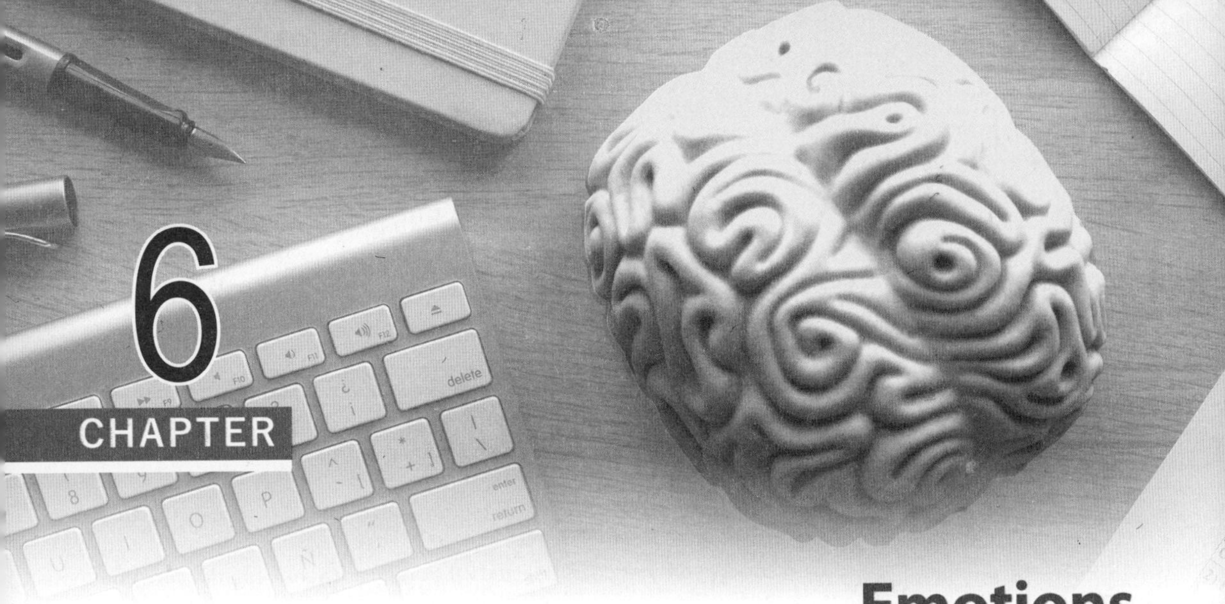

Emotions

Manu Goyal, Kanu Goyal, Prateek Sharda

LEARNING OBJECTIVES

After the completion of the chapter, the readers will be able to:
- Understand emotions and its anatomy.
- Identify the types and models of basic emotions.
- Explain the different theories of emotions.
- Understand the physiological mechanisms of emotions.
- Know emotional regulation strategies.
- Describe role of emotions in physiotherapy practice and its Implications.

CHAPTER OUTLINE

- Introduction
- Neuroanatomy and Physiology
- Theories of Emotion
- Psychophysiological Measures of Emotions
- Emotional Regulation
- Role of Emotions in Physiotherapy Practice

KEY TERMS

Amygdala: An almond-shaped set of neurons located deep in the brain's medial temporal lobe, critical for processing fear, aggression, and emotional memories.

Anterior cingulate cortex (ACC): A region of the brain involved in emotional regulation, decision-making in an ethical manner, and avoiding negative outcomes.

Cognitive reappraisal: A strategy for emotion regulation that involves reframing the meaning of a situation to alter its emotional impact.

Distraction: A strategy for emotion regulation that involves redirecting attention away from emotionally arousing stimuli toward neutral or positive distractions.

Emotion: A complex psychological state that involves subjective feelings, physiological responses, and expressive behaviors. Emotions can be intense and short-lived, and they influence human behavior and cognitive processes.

Emotion regulation: The process through which individuals monitor, evaluate, and modify their emotional experiences, expressions, and responses to better align with their goals, values, and situational demands.

Emotional intelligence: The ability to recognize, understand, and manage one's own emotions and the emotions of others.

Hippocampus: A region of the brain involved in forming and retrieving memories, especially those associated with emotional experiences.

Hormones: Chemical messengers produced by endocrine glands that regulate various bodily functions. Examples: Cortisol, adrenaline, noradrenaline.

Hypothalamus: A small region of the brain that regulates the autonomic nervous system and the endocrine system, affecting physiological responses to emotional stimuli.

Insula: A region of the cerebral cortex that integrates somatosensory, autonomic, and cognitive-affective components to form subjective emotional experiences.

Limbic system: A complex set of interconnected brain regions that play a crucial role in emotion processing, memory, and behavior.

Neurobiology of emotions: The study of the biological mechanisms in the brain and nervous system that underlie emotional experiences. This includes the role of specific brain regions and neurochemical processes.

Neurotransmitters: Chemical messengers in the brain that transmit signals between neurons. Examples: Serotonin, dopamine, norepinephrine.

Orbitofrontal cortex (OFC): A region of the prefrontal cortex involved in evaluating the reward/ punishment outcomes of an action and in emotion regulation.

Parasympathetic nervous system (PNS): The part of the autonomic nervous system that promotes relaxation and conserves energy by decreasing heart rate, blood pressure, and respiration.

Suppression: A strategy for emotion regulation that involves inhibiting the outward expression of emotions while still experiencing them internally.

Sympathetic nervous system (SNS): The part of the autonomic nervous system that prepares the body for action by increasing heart rate, blood pressure, and respiration.

Ventromedial prefrontal cortex (vmPFC): A region of the prefrontal cortex involved in risk and decision-making, helping to regulate emotional responses by dampening the activity of the amygdala.

INTRODUCTION

Emotion is a multifaceted process with a component of subjective feelings characterized by change in physical and mental state that may influence human behavior.[1,2] Subjective experience, physiological reaction, and expressive response are its three separate components. Though they can be used interchangeably, emotions, feelings, and mood have slightly different meanings. Emotions produce feelings, which are then impacted by the circumstances. Emotions are the result of stimuli and remain short-lived normally but intense in nature. Mood is a temporary emotional state and it could be happy or gloomy.

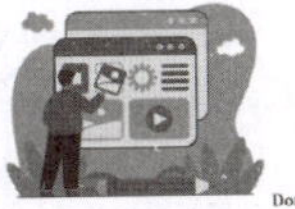

Emotions are not only psychological phenomena but also intricate physiological processes that engage various brain regions, neurotransmitters, hormones, and bodily systems. Bodies perceive, process, and respond to emotional stimuli in complex manner.

NEUROANATOMY AND PHYSIOLOGY

Anatomy

In the emotion processing, the limbic system plays a pivotal role. Its putative role is described by an American neuroscientist, James Papez in his anatomical model referred to as Papez circuit[3, 4] as shown in Figure 6.1. The major structures that form the limbic system are the amygdala, hippocampus, hypothalamus, ventromedial prefrontal cortex (vmPFC), orbitofrontal cortex (OFC), insula, anterior cingulate gyrus are discussed here:[5]

- **Amygdala:** An almond-shaped group of neurons that are essential for processing fear, aggression, and emotional memories is situated in the medial temporal lobe of the brain. It triggers the body's fight-or-flight response by interacting with the hypothalamus, leading to immediate physiological reactions.[6, 7] Amygdala hyperactivity has been linked to anxiety disorders and heightened emotional reactivity.[8]

- **Hippocampus:** Located adjacent to the amygdala, the hippocampus is integral for forming new memories about experienced events. Emotionally charged memories stored here can be stronger and last longer, influencing how emotions are experienced in similar future scenarios. It is one of the diagnostic markers of poor cognition as in senile dementia.[9, 10]

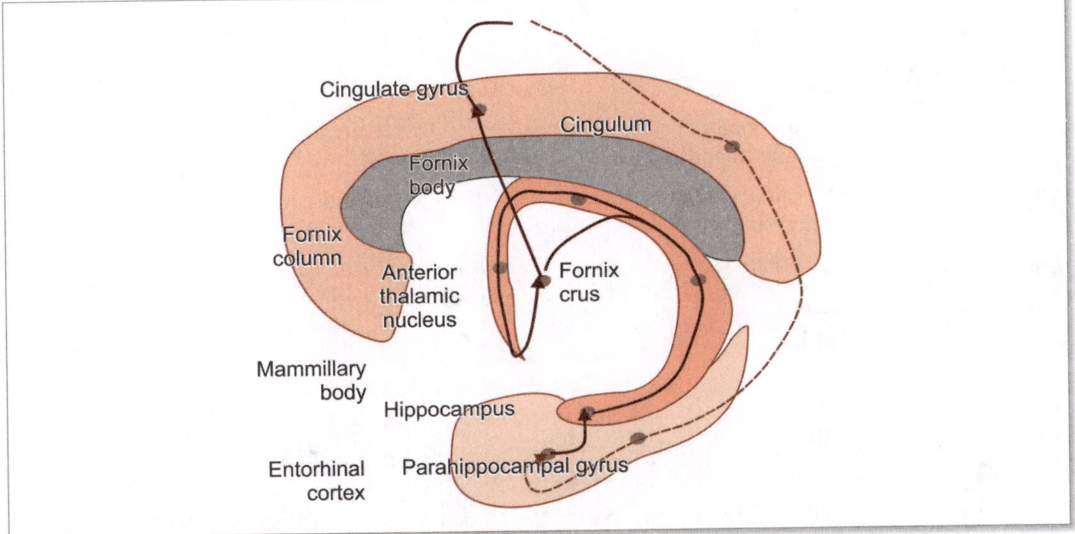

Fig. 6.1: Papez circuit

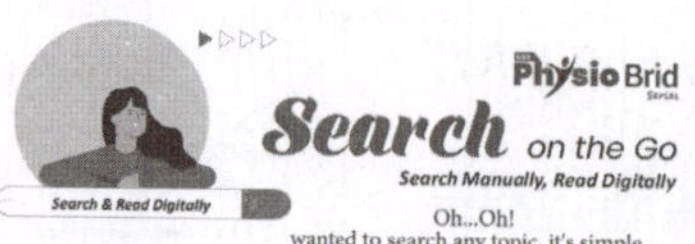

- **Hypothalamus:** It regulates the autonomic nervous system and the endocrine system, affecting physiological responses to emotional stimuli by controlling the release of hormones such as cortisol.[11, 12]

- **Ventromedial prefrontal cortex (vmPFC):** Involved in risk and decision making, the vmPFC helps regulate emotional responses by dampening the activity of the amygdala, providing a balance between emotional and rational behaviors.[13]

- **Orbitofrontal cortex (OFC):** This region is key for evaluating the reward/punishment outcomes of an action and is critical in emotion regulation and impulse control.[14]

- **Insula:** The insula is a small region of the cerebral cortex that has widespread connections to the limbic system, associative cortex, and sensory areas. It integrates somatosensory, autonomic, and cognitive-affective components to form subjective emotional experiences.[15]

- **Anterior cingulate cortex (ACC):** It is vital for emotional control, ethical decision-making, and avoiding and predicting unpleasant outcomes. It mediates both autonomic and social cognitive functions.[16]

Neurotransmitters and Hormones

Neurotransmitters and hormones play a critical role in regulating emotions by influencing brain activity and physiological responses. Key neurotransmitters like serotonin, dopamine, and norepinephrine affect mood and arousal, while hormones such as cortisol and oxytocin regulate stress and social bonding.

Tables 6.1A and B below highlights the important neurotransmitters and hormones impacting emotion and their function.

Table 6.1A: Neurotransmitters

Neurotransmitter	Function
Serotonin[17]	Influences mood, anxiety, and happiness. Low levels are associated with depression and other mood disorders.
Dopamine[18]	Associated with the brain's reward system and pleasure center, playing a major role in motivation and pleasure-seeking behaviors.
Norepinephrine[19]	Acts primarily in the brainstem, increasing arousal and alertness, promoting vigilance, improving memory formation and retrieval, and focusing attention.

Table 6.1B: Hormones

Hormone	Function
Cortisol[11]	Known as the "stress hormone", it regulates changes in the body in response to physical or psychological stress.
Adrenaline and noradrenaline[11]	These hormones increase heart rate, blood pressure, and blood glucose levels, part of the rapid response mechanism to stress.

Physiology

The autonomic nervous system (ANS) and neuroendocrine pathways mediate the physiological changes in the various body systems associated with emotions. These changes can have profound effects on physical function, pain perception, and recovery processes relevant to physiotherapy practice.

Emotions trigger sympathetic and parasympathetic nervous system, affecting various bodily functions. Sympathetic activation leads to increase heart rate, blood pressure, respiration, pupil dilation, and inhibition of digestive processes.[20] Parasympathetic activation leads to decrease heart rate, blood pressure, and respiration, and increased digestive activity.[21] These autonomic responses may potentially contribute to exacerbate musculoskeletal disorders by influencing muscle tension, sensitivity to pain and function.

Musculoskeletal System

Heightened stiffness and reduced elasticity have found to be the characteristics of myofascial tissue in depressive patients. It may be resulted due to stress-related dysregulations of ANS, resulted in dysfunction of immune system elevated levels of transforming growth factor-$\beta 1$ (TGF-$\beta 1$) leads to increase in contractility of fascia.[22] Reduced positive affect and increased accessibility of negative memories appear to be associated with stiff and inflexible myofascial tissue. This could lead to increased stress, which could further impair elasticity and increase stiffness in the tissue.[23]

Pain Perception

Emotions can modulate the experience of pain through descending pathways from the brain to the spinal cord, influencing the transmission and perception of nociceptive signals. Negative emotions, such as anxiety and depression, can amplify pain perception, while positive emotions can reduce pain sensitivity.[24] Emotional pictures induced emotions activate the pain modulation descending pathways distressing the amplitude of the spinal nociceptive reflex mechanism.[25]

Models

Models of basic emotions categorize and describe fundamental emotions, such as happiness, sadness, anger, fear, surprise, and disgust, which are considered universal and evolutionarily significant. These models focus on identifying specific emotions and their expression across cultures.

Russell's Two-Dimensional Circular Model

It is divided into couple of quadrants with two crossed axes. Emotional variables, valence and arousal represent each axis and emotions are displayed upon this two-dimensional plane (Fig. 6.2).[26] Arousal is the extent of association between emotion and energy consciousness of an individual. Valence is the extent to which an emotion reflects the state of mind either positive or negative.[27]

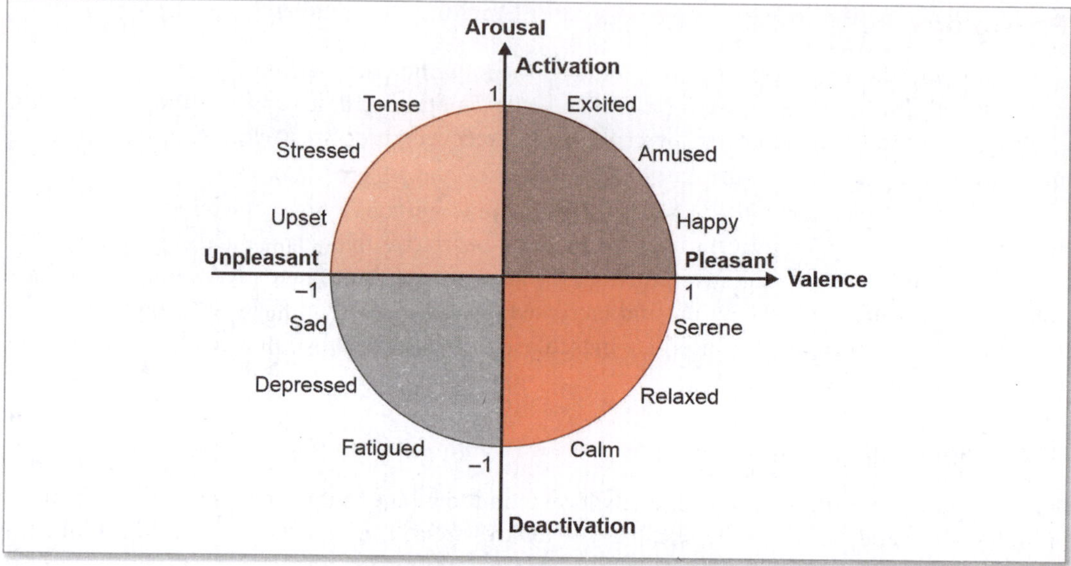

Fig. 6.2: Two-dimension emotion system[28, 29]

Circumplex Model of Affect

This model suggests that affective states arise from cognitive interpretations of core sensations of subjective feelings, mediated by two neurophysiological mechanisms: Valence and arousal, within a given situational context.[30, 31] The cognitive function as determined by the nature of a task is of paramount importance to observe a correlation between stimulus properties of an affective state and the region of activity in a brain.[32] This model is valid and utilized to dissociate the functions of amygdala, cerebellum, thalamus, brainstem and vmPFC, OFC in modulation and representation of the affective assessment of

MUST KNOW

Dennis Coon, a prominent psychologist, identified several components of emotions to help in understanding how emotions are experienced and expressed. According to Coon, the primary components of emotions are:

- **Physiological arousal:** This refers to the physical changes in the body that accompany emotions, such as increased heart rate, sweating, and hormonal changes. These physiological responses are regulated by the autonomic nervous system and are often a key indicator of emotional states.
- **Cognitive processes:** These mental activities influence emotions, including perceptions, thoughts, and interpretations of events. Cognitive appraisal of a situation plays a crucial role in determining the type and intensity of the emotion experienced.
- **Behavioral expressions:** Emotions are often expressed through observable behaviors, including facial expressions, body language, and vocal tone. These expressions communicate emotional states to others and are frequently recognized universally.
- **Subjective feelings:** This refers to the personal and internal experience of emotions, which can vary widely from person to person. Subjective feelings are the conscious experience of emotions, such as feeling happy, sad, angry or scared.

human expressions. This model accompanies data from the various studies such as developmental, neuroimaging and behavioral genetics of disorders of the affective state.

THEORIES OF EMOTION

In contrast, theories of emotions aim to explain how and why emotions occur by exploring their underlying mechanisms. They examine the interplay between physiological responses, cognition, and behavior in generating emotional experiences. Key theories include the James-Lange theory, which links emotions to physiological changes, the Cannon-Bard theory, which proposes simultaneous emotional and physiological responses, and appraisal theories, which highlight the role of individual evaluations in shaping emotions. While models focus on categorization, theories provide insights into emotional processes.

James-Lange Theory

In the late 19th century, William James and Carl Lange proposed the James-Lange Theory. It offers a distinctive perspective on the relationship between physiological responses and emotional experiences. According to this theory, emotions are not directly triggered by external stimuli but instead emerge as a result of physiological reactions within the body. When an individual encounters a stimulus, the body initiates a specific physiological response. Subsequently, the individual perceives these bodily changes and interprets them as specific emotions. In other words, emotions are considered to be the perception of one's physiological state in response to a stimulus. The sequence of the events is shown in Figure 6.3.

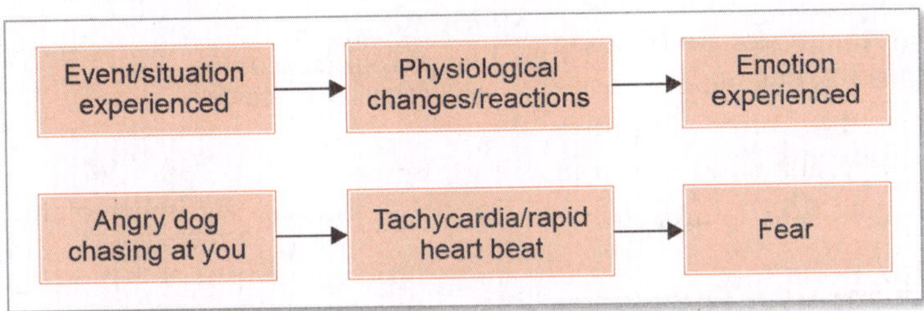

Fig. 6.3: Emergence of emotions according to James-Lange theory

The theory was criticized as sometimes, an emotion experience may arise prior to physiological changes. Also, the physiological change every time is not the result of an emotion. For example, an elevated heart rate may be attributed to exercise rather fear.

Cannon-Bard Theory

In the 1920s, Walter Cannon and Philip Bard presented an alternative perspective on the relationship between emotions and physiological responses. This theory challenges the idea that emotions are solely the result of bodily reactions to stimuli. Instead, it suggests that emotions and physiological responses occur simultaneously and independently in response to a stimulus. According to this theory, the thalamus plays a central role in both initiating emotional experiences and coordinating physiological responses. Figure 6.4 reflects the key features of this theory.

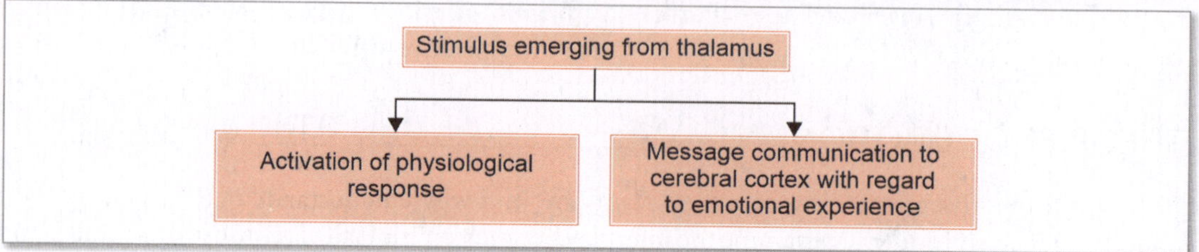

Fig. 6.4: Key features of Cannon-Bard theory

This theory rejected the view of James-Lange Theory. However, the limbic system and hypothalamus rather than thalamus plays a role in emotional experience.

Schachter-Singer Theory

The theory proposed by Stanley Schachter and Jerome Singer in the 1960s, introduces the concept of cognitive appraisal as a crucial determinant of emotional experiences. This theory suggests that emotions result from a combination of physiological arousal and cognitive interpretation within a particular context. According to Schachter and Singer, physiological arousal is a nonspecific state that can be interpreted in various ways depending on the situational context and the individual's cognitive appraisal of the situation. Emotions are thus seen as the result of labelling the physiological arousal-based on cognitive interpretation as shown in Figure 6.5.

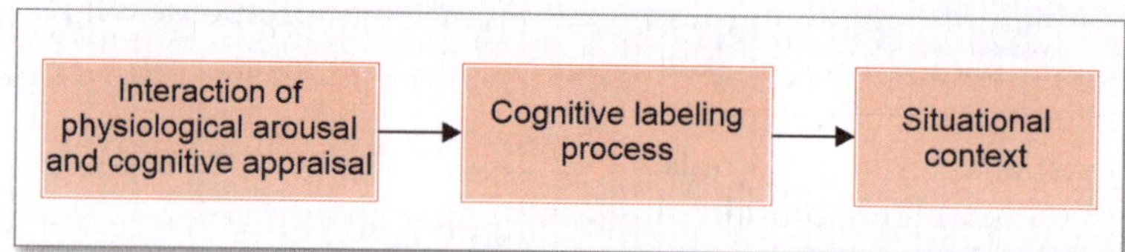

Fig. 6.5: Key aspects of the Schachter-Singer theory

Appraisal Theory[33]

Appraisal theory emphasizes the role of cognitive appraisal processes in generating emotions. According to these theories, individuals evaluate the significance of a situation or event-based on personal goals, beliefs, and expectations. The appraisal process involves assessing the relevance, meaning, and implications of the stimulus, which in turn elicits emotional responses. Appraisal theories highlight the subjective and context-dependent nature of emotions, emphasizing the importance of cognitive appraisal in shaping emotional experiences.

PSYCHOPHYSIOLOGICAL MEASURES OF EMOTIONS

Electrodermal Activity

Electrodermal activity (EDA), also known as galvanic skin response, reflects changes in the electrical conductivity of the skin in response to emotional arousal. EDA is commonly used as a psychophysiological measure of sympathetic nervous system activity and emotional arousal. Increased EDA is observed during states of emotional arousal, such as fear, excitement or stress.[34]

Skin conductance, a component of EDA, includes two main types: (1) Tonic and (2) Phasic. Tonic skin conductance or skin conductance level (SCL), reflects the baseline level of arousal influenced by general mood, stress or environmental factors. Phasic skin conductance or skin conductance response (SCR), represents short-term changes triggered by specific stimuli, such as emotional or sensory events. Key features include amplitude (response intensity), latency (time from stimulus to response), and frequency (number of responses over time). These components provide insights into baseline physiological states and reactions to external triggers, making skin conductance a valuable measure of emotional arousal. Figure 6.6 describes the components of skin conductance.

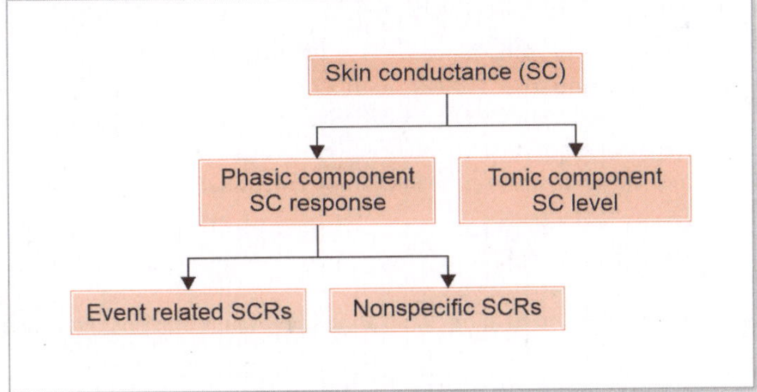

Fig. 6.6: Components of skin conductance[35]

Heart Rate Variability

It refers to the variation in the time interval between successive heartbeats. Heart rate variability (HRV) is influenced by autonomic nervous system activity and reflects the dynamic interplay between sympathetic and parasympathetic branches of the autonomic nervous system. Reduced HRV is associated with increased emotional arousal and impaired emotion regulation, while higher HRV is indicative of greater emotional flexibility and resilience.[36] The amygdala and the vmPFC are involved for both HRV and regulation of emotion.[37] Research has indicated that increased HRV is associated with structural thickness in regions of prefrontal cortex in both younger and older adults respectively.[38] It has been concluded that emotion can be enhanced by HRV by attuning brain rhythms in a manner that augment brain regulatory network.[39]

Neuroimaging Techniques

Advances in neuroimaging technologies, such as functional Magnetic Resonance Imaging (fMRI) and positron emission tomography (PET), have revolutionized understanding of the neural basis of emotions. These techniques allow researchers to investigate brain activity patterns associated with specific emotional experiences and identify the neural circuits involved in emotion processing and regulation.[40]

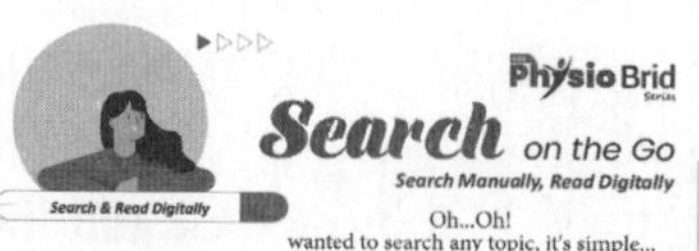

Physio CORNER

Emotions play a significant role in physiotherapy, influencing both the patient's experience and the outcome of treatment. Here's how emotions can affect physiotherapy:

- **Pain perception:**
  - **Anxiety and stress:** High levels of anxiety and stress can increase the perception of pain. Patients who are anxious about their condition or treatment may report higher pain levels.
  - **Depression:** Depressive symptoms can amplify pain perception and reduce the effectiveness of physiotherapy.
- **Motivation and compliance:**
  - **Positive emotions:** Patients with a positive outlook and emotions are often more motivated to follow through with physiotherapy exercises and recommendations, leading to better outcomes.
  - **Negative emotions:** Negative emotions like frustration, anger or hopelessness can decrease a patient's motivation to participate in therapy and adhere to prescribed exercises.
- **Recovery and healing:**
  - **Stress response:** Chronic stress can hinder the body's healing process by affecting the immune system and inflammation levels.
  - **Relaxation and healing:** Relaxation techniques and positive emotional states can promote healing and enhance the effectiveness of physiotherapy.
- **Therapist-patient relationship:**
  - **Trust and rapport:** A good therapeutic relationship, where the patient feels understood and supported, can positively influence treatment outcomes. Emotions play a critical role in building this relationship.
  - **Communication:** Effective communication, which is influenced by emotional intelligence on both sides, is crucial for understanding the patient's needs and tailoring the treatment accordingly.
- **Psychosomatic factors:**
  - **Mind-body connection:** Emotions can manifest physically, such as muscle tension in response to stress. Addressing these emotional factors can be crucial for comprehensive physiotherapy.
- **Behavioral aspects:**
  - **Coping strategies:** Patients' emotional responses can influence their coping strategies. Positive coping mechanisms can enhance physiotherapy outcomes, while negative coping strategies can impede progress.

EMOTIONAL REGULATION

Emotional regulation (ER) refers to the process through which individuals monitor, evaluate, and modify their emotional experiences, expressions, and responses to better align with their goals, values, and situational demands. Effective emotional regulation is essential for psychological well-being, interpersonal relationships, and overall adaptive functioning. This process involves various strategies, individual differences, and implications for mental health and well-being.

Developmental Perspectives

Understanding the development of emotions across the lifespan involves examining how emotional experiences, expression, and regulation evolve from infancy through childhood, adolescence, and into adulthood. This developmental journey is influenced by various factors, including biological maturation, cognitive development, social interactions, and cultural contexts.

Infancy

An essential aspect of growth and development of children is the ER in a socially adaptive manner.[41] Lack of ER is predictive of cognitive and social development problems through preschool and initial school years.[42] Infants ER abilities are based upon temperament characteristics and influences of environment.[41] Children may be more sensitive to their environment if they are temperamentally reactive, with greater likelihood of dependent, frustrated to situations and greater risk for maladjustment.[43, 44] During infancy, emotion regulation is primarily facilitated through caregiver interactions and the establishment of attachment relationships. Infants express a range of basic emotions, such as joy, sadness, fear, and anger, through facial expressions, vocalizations, and body movements. Caregivers play a critical role in supporting infants' emotional development by responding sensitively to their cues, providing comfort and reassurance, and helping them regulate physiological arousal.[45] Table 6.2 displayed the key aspects of ER in infancy.

Table 6.2: Key aspects of emotional regulation in infancy

Aspect	Description
Social referencing	Use of social cues from caregivers by infants for ER and protection from nonfamiliar situations. To interpret and respond to environmental stimuli, caregivers' emotional expressions were served as guide for infants.[46]
Co-regulation	Caregivers regulate infants' emotions to promote safety and security by means of lullaby and amicable behavior. It fosters the development of auto regulation of skills and emotional resilience.[47, 48]
Attachment and secure base	Caregivers' availability, responsiveness, and sensitivity contribute to the development of trust and emotional security in infancy.[49]

Childhood and Adolescence

During growth and development, children and adolescents acquire increasingly sophisticated emotion regulation skills, emotional understanding, and socialization processes. Greater fluctuations and increased intensity of emotions, maturation of brain prefrontal cortex are the characteristics of adolescent emotional regulation.[48–51] In the studies, it has been found that girls exhibit minimal use of emotional regulation strategies in an efficient way and greater difficulties in regulating emotions than boys.[52, 53] They learn to identify, label, and express a wider range of emotions, understand the causes and consequences of emotions, and regulate their emotional responses in social contexts. The key aspects are displayed in Table 6.3.

Table 6.3: Key aspects of emotional regulation in childhood and adolescence

Aspect	Description
Emotion regulation skills (ERS)	ERS such as cognitive reappraisal, distraction, problem-solving, and seeking social support enable children and adolescents to manage stress, cope with challenges, and navigate social relationships effectively.[54, 55]
Emotional understanding	With age and cognitive development, children and adolescents become increasingly proficient in recognizing and understanding emotions in themselves and others. They learn to differentiate between different emotional states, identify the causes and consequences of emotions, and recognize the role of social and cultural factors in shaping emotional experiences.[56]
Socialization processes (SP)	In shaping the emotional development of children and adolescents', social interactions and agents play a pivot role. Through SP, they learn social norms, values, and expectations related to emotional expression, regulation, and communication.[57]

Continuity and Change in Emotional Functioning Across the Lifespan

Emotional functioning continues to evolve across the lifespan, with both continuity and change observed in emotional experiences, regulation strategies, and socioemotional functioning. Aging and life transitions bring new challenges and opportunities for emotional development, while socioemotional selectivity theory suggests that older adults prioritize emotionally meaningful goals and relationships as they age. Table 6.4 describes the important aspects of continuity and change in emotional functioning across the lifespan.

Table 6.4: Key aspects of continuity and change in emotional functioning across lifespan

Aspect	Description
Aging and emotional well-being	Emotional well-being changes with an ageing process across the life span. Geriatric population develops greater emotional resilience and may prioritize emotional goals and relationships.[58]
Life transitions	Life transitions, such as retirement, bereavement, and health changes, can impact emotional functioning and well-being. Older adults may experience both positive and negative emotions in response to life changes, with resilience and coping strategies playing a crucial role in adaptation.[59]
Socioemotional selectivity theory	With an increasing age, an individual becomes more selective in their social and emotional goals, focusing on relationships and activities that are personally meaningful and emotionally rewarding. This shift in priorities may contribute to greater emotional satisfaction and well-being in later life.[60]

Strategies

Strategies for emotional regulation are essential to manage intense emotions, reduce stress, and improve decision-making. They help individuals maintain emotional balance, enhance interpersonal relationships, and adapt effectively to challenging situations. The various strategies are mentioned in Table 6.5 as under.

Table 6.5: Different strategies

Strategy	Description
Cognitive reappraisal	It involves reframing the meaning of a situation to alter its emotional impact. Individuals reinterpret events in less threatening or distressing ways, leading to changes in emotional experiences. For example, someone might reinterpret a challenging situation as an opportunity for growth or learning, thereby reducing feelings of anxiety or stress.[61, 62]
Suppression	It entails inhibiting the outward expression of emotions while still experiencing them internally. This strategy involves exerting conscious control over emotional displays to avoid social consequences or regulate interpersonal interactions. However, it may lead to increase physiological arousal and negative effect over time, making it less effective as a long-term emotion regulation strategy.[63]
Distraction	It involves redirecting attention away from emotionally arousing stimuli toward neutral or positive distractions. Engaging in activities such as hobbies, exercise or socializing can help individuals temporarily shift their focus away from distressing emotions and reduce their intensity. However, distraction may not address the underlying causes of emotional distress and may be less effective for regulating intense or persistent emotions.[64]

Individual Differences

Emotion regulation varies across individuals due to factors like personality traits, life experiences, cultural background, and biological predispositions. Some people naturally use adaptive strategies like cognitive reappraisal, while others rely on less effective methods like suppression. Factors such as resilience, emotional intelligence, and social support also influence one's ability to regulate emotions. These differences affect how individuals respond to stress, manage relationships, and maintain mental well-being. It can be influenced by various factors as mentioned in Table 6.6.

Table 6.6: Factors influencing individual differences in emotion regulation

Factor	Description
Personality traits	Neuroticism, extraversion, and conscientiousness have been associated with differences in emotion regulation strategies. For example, individuals high in neuroticism may be more likely to use maladaptive strategies such as rumination or emotional suppression, whereas those high in conscientiousness may prefer adaptive strategies such as cognitive reappraisal or problem-solving.[65]
Self-esteem	It can influence how individuals regulate their emotions. High self-esteem has been linked to greater emotional resilience and the use of adaptive emotion regulation strategies, such as positive reappraisal and seeking social support. In contrast, low self-esteem may be associated with greater reliance on maladaptive strategies, such as avoidance or self-blame.[66]

Contd...

Factor	Description
Coping styles	It refers to stable patterns of responding to stress and adversity. Individuals may adopt problem-focused coping strategies, which involve actively addressing and resolving stressors or emotion-focused coping strategies, which involve managing emotional responses to stressors. They can influence the effectiveness of emotion regulation efforts and contribute to individual differences in emotional well-being.[67]

Implications for Mental Health and Well-Being

Emotion regulation plays a critical role in mental health and well-being, with adaptive regulation strategies associated with positive outcomes and maladaptive strategies linked to psychological distress and psychopathology (Table 6.7).

Table 6.7: Emotion regulation strategies for mental health and well-being

Strategy	Description
Adaptive emotion regulation	Cognitive reappraisal, problem-solving, and seeking social support, have been associated with better psychological adjustment, reduced symptoms of anxiety and depression, and enhanced overall well-being. These strategies promote emotional flexibility, resilience, and effective coping with stressors.[68]
Maladaptive emotion regulation	Emotional suppression, rumination, and avoidance, are associated with increased psychological distress, heightened symptoms of anxiety and depression, and reduced overall well-being. These strategies may exacerbate emotional difficulties, maintain negative mood states, and interfere with adaptive coping responses.[68]

ROLE OF EMOTIONS IN PHYSIOTHERAPY PRACTICE

In the literature, the influence of emotions on several aspects of physiotherapy including, patients' perspectives and experiences, therapeutic liaisoning, adherence, and decision-making in clinical practice have been examined.

Patients' Perspectives and Experiences

Pain (chronic), functional limitations, and uncertain conditions due to disease or injury can evoke variety of emotional states including fear–avoidance, false beliefs, frustrations and sadness in patients.[69] Several studies have explored the emotional experiences of patients undergoing physiotherapy in outpatient and inpatient settings. A study was conducted in outpatient setting for the musculoskeletal conditions often experience the feelings of vulnerability, frustration, neglect and lack of control.[70] In another study, related to experience of stroke patients in inpatient settings have noticed emotional experiences as anxiety, depression and fear of burden on caregivers.[71, 72]

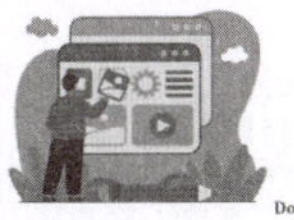
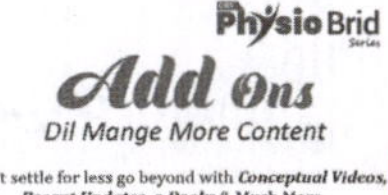

Therapeutic Liaisoning

Therapeutic liaisoning between the physiotherapists and patients is a critical component for an effective rehabilitation. This liaisoning is based upon both competent skills and emotional factors such as empathy, trust, and communication.[73–75] Healthy therapeutic liaisoning helps in building rapport of the therapist among patients and also compliance of the patients toward rehabilitation plan.

Research has shown that physiotherapists who exhibit high levels of emotional intelligence and engage in effective emotional labor can better connect with their patients, build trust, and create a supportive environment conducive to positive treatment outcomes.[76–78]

Adherence

For successful physiotherapy outcomes, adherence toward prescribed physiotherapy treatment is integral. However; the adherence has been found to be suboptimal, with a significant role of factors associated with emotions.[79–81] Emotions such as fear, anxiety, and frustration can negatively impact adherence by influencing patients' motivation, self-efficacy, and perceived barriers to treatment.[79] Conversely, positive emotions, such as hope, encouragement, and a sense of empowerment, can enhance adherence by fostering a more optimistic outlook and a stronger commitment to the rehabilitation process.[81]

Clinical Decision-Making

The clinical decision-making of the physiotherapists is not only based upon subjective and objective assessments, but emotional factors also play a vital role. The emotions experienced by physiotherapists themselves, as well as their ability to recognize and respond to patients' emotions, can shape clinical reasoning and treatment decisions.[82–84] A study conducted found that physiotherapists' emotional responses to patients' pain behaviors could influence their clinical decisions, with some therapists adopting more cautious or more aggressive treatment approaches based on their emotional reactions.[84]

Implications for Physiotherapy Practice

There are several implications of role of emotions in various aspects of physiotherapy practice. Table 6.8 describes various implications.

Recent Advancements

A holistic approach that addresses both physical and emotional aspects of rehabilitation is becoming increasingly crucial for providing patient-centered, comprehensive care. Recent advancements as highlighted from the research have shown the recognition of emotional aspect of care and competencies in physiotherapy practice and clinical education. Table 6.9 highlights various recent advancements related to emotional competencies in the physiotherapy practice.

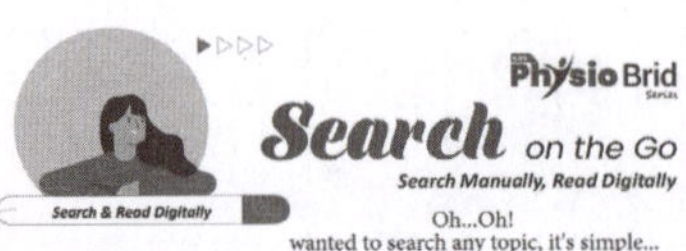

Table 6.8: Implications for physiotherapy practice

Implication	Description
Emotional awareness and regulation	Physiotherapists should develop emotional intelligence skills to better recognize and manage their own emotions, as well as those of their patients. This can facilitate more effective therapeutic relationships, enhance patient adherence, and inform clinical decision-making.
Empathetic communication	Effective communication that conveys empathy and emotional understanding is crucial in physiotherapy practice. Physiotherapists should strive to create a supportive and emotionally safe environment for patients to express their concerns, fears, and frustrations.
Holistic approach	In addition to addressing physical impairments and functional limitations, physiotherapists should consider the emotional well-being of their patients. Incorporating strategies to address emotional barriers, foster hope and motivation, and provide emotional support can enhance overall treatment outcomes.
Interprofessional collaboration (IPC)	Physiotherapists should collaborate with other healthcare professionals, such as psychologists, counselors, and social workers, to provide comprehensive care that addresses both the physical and emotional needs of patients.
Education and training	Emotional intelligence, emotional labor, and the role of emotions in physiotherapy should be integrated into physiotherapy education programs and continuing professional development opportunities. This will equip physiotherapists with the necessary skills and knowledge to navigate the emotional complexities of their profession effectively.

Table 6.9: Emotional competencies in physiotherapy practice

Competency	Description
Emotional intelligence training (EIT)	Emotional competencies such as self-awareness, self-regulation, empathy, and interpersonal skills can be enhanced through EIT programs. A recent study implemented 12 weeks EIT program on physiotherapy students by means of group discussions, lectures, and practical training has showed significant improvement in their emotional intelligence scores, self-reported empathy and communication skills. It further improved their understanding toward the emotional role in physiotherapy practice.[85]
Emotional labor strategies (ELS)	It involves the conscious regulation of emotions to create a desired emotional state in patients.[77] Several ELS such as surface acting (portraying emotions not genuinely felt), deep acting (modifying inner feelings to align with desired emotions), and genuine emotional expression were explored in a study[86] and findings obtained highlighted the importance of authentic emotional connections and the potential risks of emotional dissonance (a mismatch between felt and expressed emotions) on physiotherapists' well-being and job satisfaction.
Emotional disclosure and patient-centered care	It has been found in the research that patients who were engaged in emotional disclosure reported greater therapeutic alliances and satisfaction toward physiotherapy treatment.[87] Better compliance levels to physiotherapy and positive outcomes can be encouraged by patient's self-efficacy.[88]

Contd...

Competency	Description
Emotion-focused interventions	These interventions aim to address emotional barriers, foster emotional regulation, and enhance overall well-being alongside physical rehabilitation. A pilot study investigated the feasibility and acceptability of an emotion focused intervention for patients undergoing physiotherapy for chronic musculoskeletal conditions. The intervention included components such as emotional awareness exercises, cognitive-behavioral techniques, and mindfulness practices. The results showed promising improvements in emotional well-being, pain management, and adherence to physiotherapy recommendations among participants who received the emotion-focused intervention.[89]
Technology-assisted emotional support	A recent study developed and evaluated a mobile application designed to offer emotional support and encourage self-reflection for patients undergoing physiotherapy rehabilitation. The app featured interactive modules for emotional expression, goal-setting, and mindfulness exercises. The results indicated that patients who used the app reported higher levels of emotional well-being, increased motivation, and better adherence to their physiotherapy programs compared to a control group receiving standard care.[90]

SUMMARY

- Emotions are at the core of human experience, shaping thoughts, behaviors, and interactions with the world. From the earliest stages of development to later stages in life, emotions play a fundamental role in every aspect of life, influencing perceptions and responses to the various situations and challenges encountered.

- Throughout this exploration, the multifaceted nature of emotions has been examined, including their definition, components, and various theoretical perspectives from psychology. Differences between emotions and related constructs such as moods and affective states have been explored, along with the intricate interplay between emotions, cognition, and physiology.

- The role of emotions in various contexts, including social interactions, decision-making, and work and organizational settings, has been explored. Emotions influence individual well-being, shape interpersonal relationships, impact organizational culture, and affect leadership effectiveness.

- Acknowledging and addressing the emotional dimensions of physiotherapy enhance patient-centered care, improve treatment outcomes, and contribute to the overall well-being of both patients and physiotherapists. Developing emotional intelligence skills, fostering empathetic communication, adopting a holistic approach, collaborating with other healthcare professionals, and integrating emotional education into training programs enable physiotherapists to navigate the emotional complexities of their profession and provide more comprehensive and effective care.

REFERENCES

1. Bailen, N. H., Green, L. M., & Thompson, R. J. Understanding Emotion in Adolescents: A Review of Emotional Frequency, Intensity, Instability, and Clarity. Emotion Review, 2019;11(1), 63–73.
2. Gross J. J. Emotion regulation: Conceptual and empirical foundations. In Gross J. J. (Ed.), Handbook of emotion regulation (p. 3–20). New York, NY: Guilford Press; 2014.
3. Papez JW. A proposed mechanism of emotion. Arch Neurol Psychiatry. 1937; 38:725–43.
4. Bhattacharyya KB. James Wenceslaus papez, his circuit, and emotion. Ann Indian Acad Neurol. 2017; 20:207–210.
5. LeDoux, J.E. "Emotion circuits in the brain". Annual Review of Neuroscience. 2000; 23(1): 155–184.
6. Ressler KJ. Amygdala activity, fear, and anxiety: Modulation by stress. Biol Psychiatry. 2010; 67(12):1117–9.
7. Phelps EA. Emotion and cognition: Insights from studies of the human amygdala. Annu Rev Psychol. 2006; 57:27–53.
8. Etkin A, Wager TD. Functional neuroimaging of anxiety: A meta-analysis of emotional processing in PTSD, social anxiety disorder, and specific phobia. Am J Psychiatry. 2007;164(10):1476–88.
9. Tyng CM, Amin HU, Saad MNM, Malik AS. The Influences of Emotion on Learning and Memory. Front Psychol. 2017; 8:1454.
10. Anand KS, Dhikav V. Hippocampus in health and disease: An overview. Ann Indian Acad Neurol. 2012;15(4):239–46.
11. Hinds JA, Sanchez ER. The Role of the Hypothalamus–Pituitary–Adrenal (HPA) Axis in Test-Induced Anxiety: Assessments, Physiological Responses, and Molecular Details. Stresses. 2022; 2(1):146–155.
12. Ulrich-Lai YM, Herman JP. Neural regulation of endocrine and autonomic stress responses. Nat Rev Neurosci. 2009;10(6):397–409.
13. Hiser J, Koenigs M. The Multifaceted Role of the Ventromedial Prefrontal Cortex in Emotion, Decision Making, Social Cognition, and Psychopathology. Biol Psychiatry. 2018;83(8):638–647.
14. Rolls ET, Cheng W, Feng J. The orbitofrontal cortex: Reward, emotion and depression. Brain Commun. 2020;2(2): fcaa196.
15. Uddin LQ, Nomi JS, Hébert-Seropian B, Ghaziri J, Boucher O. Structure and Function of the Human Insula. J Clin Neurophysiol. 2017;34(4):300–306.
16. Apps MA, Rushworth MF, Chang SW. The Anterior Cingulate Gyrus and Social Cognition: Tracking the Motivation of Others. Neuron. 2016;90(4):692–707.
17. Dfarhud D, Malmir M, Khanahmadi M. Happiness & Health: The Biological Factors- Systematic Review Article. Iran J Public Health. 2014;43(11):1468–77.
18. Lewis RG, Florio E, Punzo D, Borrelli E. The Brain's Reward System in Health and Disease. Adv Exp Med Biol. 2021; 1344:57–69.
19. Herat LY, Schlaich MP, Matthews VB. Sympathetic stimulation with norepinephrine may come at a cost. Neural Regen Res. 2019;14(6):977–978.
20. Kreibig S. D. Autonomic nervous system activity in emotion: A review. Biol. Psychol.2010; 84:394–421.
21. Porges SW. The polyvagal perspective. Biol Psychol. 2007;74(2):116–43.
22. Davami, M. H., Baharlou, R., Vasmehjani, A. A., Ghanizadeh, A., Keshtkar, M., Dezhkam, I., et.al. Elevated IL-17 and TGF-β serum levels: A positive correlation between T-helper 17 cell-related pro-inflammatory responses with major depressive disorder. Basic and Clinical Neuroscience. 2016; 7(2): 137–142.

Contd...

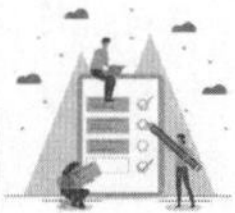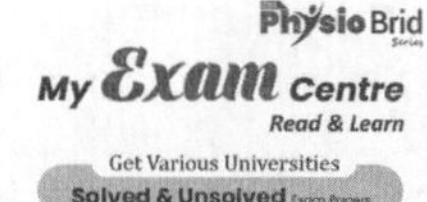

23. Gatchel, R. J., Peng, Y. B., Peters, M. L., Fuchs, P. N., & Turk, D.C. The biopsychosocial approach to chronic pain: Scientific advances and future directions. Psychological Bulletin. 2007; 133(4), 581–624.

24. Villemure, C., & Bushnell, M. C. Cognitive modulation of pain: How do attention and emotion influence pain processing? Pain.2002;95(3), 195–199.

25. Rhudy JL, Williams AE, McCabe KM, Nguyen MATV, Rambo P. Affective modulation of nociception at spinal and supraspinal levels. Psychophysiology. 2005; 42:579–587.

26. Russell, J. A.A circumplex model of affect. Journal of Personality and Social Psychology. 1980; 39: 1161–1178.

27. Barrett, L. F., Mesquita, B., Ochsner, K. N., & Gross, J. J. The experience of emotion. Annual Review of Psychology. 2007; 58: 373–403.

28. Davidson, R. J., Schwartz, G. E., Saron, C., Bennett, J., & Goleman, D. J. (1979, January). Frontal versus parietal EEG asymmetry during positive and negative affect. In Psychophysiology (Vol. 16, No. 2, p. 202–203). 40 West 20th street, New York, NY 10011-4211: Cambridge Univ Press.

29. Chakladar D.D., Chakraborty. S., EEG Based Emotion classification using "Correlation Based Subset Selection". Biologically Inspired Cognitive Architectures. 2018; 24: 98–106.

30. Posner J., Russell A.J., and Peterson B.S. The circumplex model of affect: An integrative approach to affective neuroscience, cognitive development, and psychopathology. Dev. Psychopathol. 2005; 17(3): 715–734.

31. Russell, J. A. Core affect and the psychological construction of emotion. Psychological Review. 2003;110(1): 145–172.

32. Gerber A.J., Posner J., Gorman D., Colibazzi T., Yu S., Wang Z., et al. An affective complex model of neural systems subserving valence, arousal, and cognitive overlay during the appraisal of emotional faces. Neuropsychologia. 2008; 46: 2129–2139.

33. Smith, C. A., & Lazarus, R. S. Appraisal components, core relational themes, and the emotions. Cognition & Emotion. 1993; 7(3-4): 233–269.

34. Horvers A, Tombeng N, Bosse T, Lazonder AW, Molenaar I. Detecting Emotions through Electrodermal Activity in Learning Contexts: A Systematic Review. Sensors (Basel). 2021;21(23):7869.

35. Khan T.H., Villanueva I., Vicioso P., Husman J. Exploring relationships between electrodermal activity, skin temperature, and performance during; Proceedings of the 2019 IEEE Frontiers in Education Conference (FIE); Covington, KY, USA. 16–19 October 2019; p. 1–5.

36. Thayer, J. F., & Lane, R. D.A model of neurovisceral integration in emotion regulation and dysregulation. Journal of Affective Disorders. 2000; 61(3): 201–216.

37. Thayer JF, Åhs F, Fredrikson M, Sollers JJ, Wager TD. A meta-analysis of heart rate variability and neuroimaging studies: Implications for heart rate variability as a marker of stress and health. Neuroscience and Biobehavioral Reviews. 2012;36(2):747–756.

38. Winkelmann T, Thayer JF, Pohlack S, Nees F, Grimm O, Flor H. Structural brain correlates of heart rate variability in a healthy young adult population. Brain Structure and Function. 2016:1–8.

39. Mather M, Thayer J. How heart rate variability affects emotion regulation brain networks. Curr Opin Behav Sci. 2018; 19:98–104.

40. Phan, K. L., et al. Functional neuroanatomy of emotion: A meta-analysis of emotion activation studies in PET and fMRI. NeuroImage. 2002; 16(2): 331–348.

Contd...

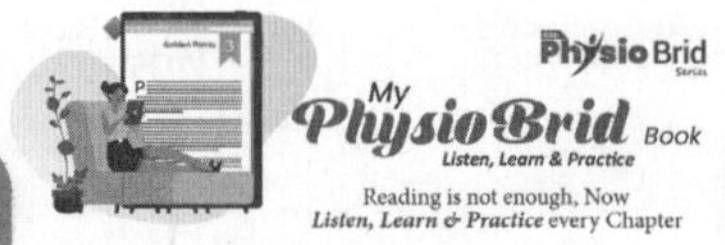

41. Calkins SD, Leerkes EM. Early attachment processes and the development of emotional self-regulation. In: Vohs KD, Baumeister RF, editors. Handbook of self-regulation: Research, theory and applications. 2. New York, NY: Guilford; 2010. p. 355–373.

42. Morris AS, Silk JS, Steinberg L, Myers SS, Robinson LR. The role of the family context in the development of emotion regulation. Social Development. 2007;16(2):361–388.

43. Stupica B, Sherman LJ, Cassidy J. Newborn irritability moderates the association between infant attachment security and toddler exploration and sociability. Child Development. 2011;82(5):1381–1389.

44. Kiff CJ, Lengua LJ, Zalewski M. Nature and nurturing: Parenting in the context of child temperament. Clinical Child and Family Psychology Review. 2011;14(3):251–301.

45. Thompson, R. A. Emotion regulation: A theme in search of definition. Monographs of the Society for Research in Child Development. 1994; 59(2-3): 25–52.

46. Carver LJ, Vaccaro BG. 12-month-old infants allocate increased neural resources to stimuli associated with negative adult emotion. Dev Psychol. 2007; 43(1):54–69.

47. Buhler-Wassmann AC, Hibel LC. Studying caregiver-infant co-regulation in dynamic, diverse cultural contexts: A call to action. Infant Behav Dev. 2021; 64:101586.

48. Feldman, R. Parent–infant synchrony: Biological foundations and developmental outcomes. Current Directions in Psychological Science. 2007; 16(6): 340–345.

49. Cassidy J, Jones JD, Shaver PR. Contributions of attachment theory and research: A framework for future research, translation, and policy. Dev Psychopathol. 2013; 25(4 Pt 2):1415–34.

50. Maciejewski DF, van Lier PAC, Branje SJT, Meeus WHJ, & Koot HM. A 5-year longitudinal study on mood variability across adolescence using daily diaries. Child Development. 2015; 86:1908–1921.

51. Morris AS, Silk JS, Steinberg L, Myers SS, & Robinson LR. The role of the family context in the development of emotion regulation. Social Development. 2007; 16:361–388.

52. McRae K, Gross JJ, Weber J, Robertson ER, Sokol-Hessner P, Ray RD, … & Ochsner KN. The development of emotion regulation: An fMRI study of cognitive reappraisal in children, adolescents and young adults. Social Cognitive and Affective Neuroscience. 2012; 7:11–22.

53. Neumann A, van Lier PAC, Gratz KL, & Koot HM. Multidimensional assessment of emotion regulation difficulties in adolescents using the difficulties in emotion regulation scale. Assessment. 2010; 17:138–149.

54. Suveg C, & Zeman J. Emotion regulation in children with anxiety disorders. Journal of Clinical Child and Adolescent Psychology. 2004; 33(4):750–759.

55. Young KS, Sandman CF, Craske MG. Positive and Negative Emotion Regulation in Adolescence: Links to Anxiety and Depression. Brain Sci. 2019; 9(4):76.

56. Xiaoyu La, Chunhua Mb, Yongfeng Mb. "Three pills" (cognitive reappraisal × social support × cognitive flexibility) and their impact on ADHD symptoms in early adolescence: Synergistic or compensatory effect? Personality and Individual Differences. 2023; 211: 112246.

57. Denham, S. A., et al. Emotional development in early childhood. Handbook of Early Childhood Development Research and Its Impact on Global Policy. 2012; 2: 143–170.

58. Eisenberg, N., et al. Prosocial development. Handbook of Child Psychology: Social, Emotional, and Personality Development. 2006; 3: 646–718.

59. Carstensen LL. The influence of a sense of time on human development. Science. 2006; 312:1913–1915.

Contd...

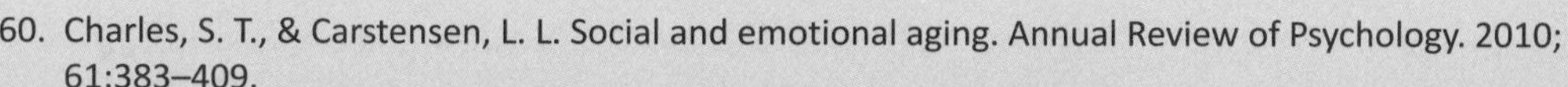

60. Charles, S. T., & Carstensen, L. L. Social and emotional aging. Annual Review of Psychology. 2010; 61:383–409.

61. Carstensen, L. L. Social and emotional patterns in adulthood: Support for socioemotional selectivity theory. Psychology and Aging. 1992; 7(3): 331–338.

62. Troy AS, Shallcross AJ, Brunner A, Friedman R, Jones MC. Cognitive reappraisal and acceptance: Effects on emotion, physiology, and perceived cognitive costs. Emotion. 2018;18(1):58–74.

63. Gross, J. J. The emerging field of emotion regulation: An integrative review. Review of General Psychology. 1998; 2(3): 271–299.

64. Gross, J. J., and John, O. P. Individual differences in two emotion regulation processes: Implications for affect, relationships, and well-being. J. Pers. Soc. Psychol. 2003; 85:348–362.

65. Sheppes, G., et al. Emotion regulation choice: A conceptual framework and supporting evidence. Journal of Experimental Psychology: General, 2015; 144(1): 35–45.

66. Troy, A. S., et al. Self-esteem and responses to social feedback: Evidence for a sociometer mechanism. Journal of Personality and Social Psychology. 2007; 92(6): 1065–1076.

67. Stanisławski K. The Coping Circumplex Model: An Integrative Model of the Structure of Coping with Stress. Front Psychol. 2019; 10:694

68. Aldao, A., et al. Emotion regulation strategies across psychopathology: A meta-analytic review. Clinical Psychology Review. 2010; 30(2): 217–237.

69. Zale EL, Ditre JW. Pain-Related Fear, Disability, and the Fear-Avoidance Model of Chronic Pain. Curr Opin Psychol. 2015; 5:24–30.

70. Alexanders, J., Anderson, A., & Henderson, S. Musculoskeletal physiotherapists' use of psychological interventions: A systematic review of therapists' perceptions and practice. Physiotherapy. 2015;101(2): 95–102.

71. Dickson, A., Knussen, C., & Flowers, P. Exploring the rehabilitation experience of patients admitted to hospital following a stroke: A qualitative study. Disability and Rehabilitation. 2017; 39(26): 2683–2692.

72. McCurley JL, Funes CJ, Zale EL, Lin A, Jacobo M, Jacobs JM, et. al. Preventing Chronic Emotional Distress in Stroke Survivors and Their Informal Caregivers. Neurocrit Care. 2019;30(3):581–589.

73. Monaco S, Renzi A, Galluzzi B, Mariani R, Di Trani M. The Relationship between Physiotherapist and Patient: A Qualitative Study on Physiotherapists' Representations on This Theme. Healthcare (Basel). 2022; 10(11):2123.

74. Besley, J., Kayes, N. M., & McPherson, K. M. Assessing therapeutic relationships in physiotherapy: Literature review. New Zealand Journal of Physiotherapy. 2011; 39(2): 81–91.

75. Kinney, M., McDermott, K., & Hines, N. Emotional intelligence and therapeutic alliance in physiotherapy: A narrative review. New Zealand Journal of Physiotherapy. 2018; 46(1): 43–50.

76. Gribble, N., Ladlow, P., & Kemper, C. The effects of emotional intelligence and empathy on clinician-patient relationship in physiotherapy. Physiotherapy Theory and Practice. 2019; 35(8):757–765.

77. Nicholls, D. A., & Gibson, B. E. The body and physiotherapy. Physiotherapy Theory and Practice. 2010; 26(8):497–509.

78. Gard, G., Gyllensten, A.L. The Importance of Emotions in Physiotherapeutic Practice. Physical Therapy Reviews. 2000; 5(3):155–160

79. Jack K, McLean SM, Moffett JK, Gardiner E. Barriers to treatment adherence in physiotherapy outpatient clinics: A systematic review. Man Ther. 2010; 15(3):220–8.

Contd...

80. Mahmood. A., Nayak. P., Deshmukh. A., English. C., Manikandan N., John Solomon N., et al. Measurement, determinants, barriers, and interventions for exercise adherence: A scoping review. Journal of Bodywork & Movement Therapies. 2023; 33: 95e105

81. Essery, R., Geraghty, A. W., Kirby, S., & Yardley, L. Predictors of adherence to home-based physical therapies: A systematic review. Disability and Rehabilitation. 2017; 39(6):519–534.

82. Lennon O, Ryan C, Helm M, Moore K, Sheridan A, Probst M, Cunningham C. Psychological Distress among Patients Attending Physiotherapy: A Survey-Based Investigation of Irish Physiotherapists' Current Practice and Opinions. Physiother Can. 2020 Summer;72(3):239–248.

83. Kozlowski D, Hutchinson M, Hurley J, Rowley J, Sutherland J. The role of emotion in clinical decision making: an integrative literature review. BMC Med Educ. 2017;17(1):255.

84. Langridge, N., Roberts, L., & Pope, C. The clinical reasoning processes of extended scope physiotherapists assessing patients with low back pain. Manual Therapy. 2015; 20(6):745–750.

85. Gribble, N., Kemper, C., & Portney, L. G. The effects of an emotional intelligence training program on physiotherapy students' emotional intelligence, empathy, and communication skills. Physiotherapy Theory and Practice. 2021; 37(6):681–692.

86. Stratton, T. D., Kerr, J., & Greenfield, B. Emotional labor in physiotherapy: A qualitative study of physiotherapists' experiences and perceptions. Physiotherapy Theory and Practice. 2021; 37(8):911–921.

87. Besley, J., Kayes, N. M., & McPherson, K. M. The impact of emotional disclosure on therapeutic alliance and patient outcomes in physiotherapy: A pilot study. Physiotherapy ResearchInternational. 2020; 25(1): e1819.

88. Klaber Moffett J. A., Richardson P.H. The Influence of the Physiotherapist-Patient Relationship on Pain and Disability. Physiother. Theory Pract. 1997; 13:89–96.

89. Essery, R., Geraghty, A. W., Yardley, L., & Stanford, N. Feasibility and acceptability of an emotion-focused intervention for patients undergoing physiotherapy for chronic musculoskeletal conditions: A pilot study. Physiotherapy Research International. 2022; 27(2): e1876.

90. Roberts, L., Wilson, M., & Pope, C. Development and evaluation of a mobile app for emotional support in physiotherapy rehabilitation: A randomized controlled trial. Journal of Medical Internet Research. 2023; 25(4): e29517.

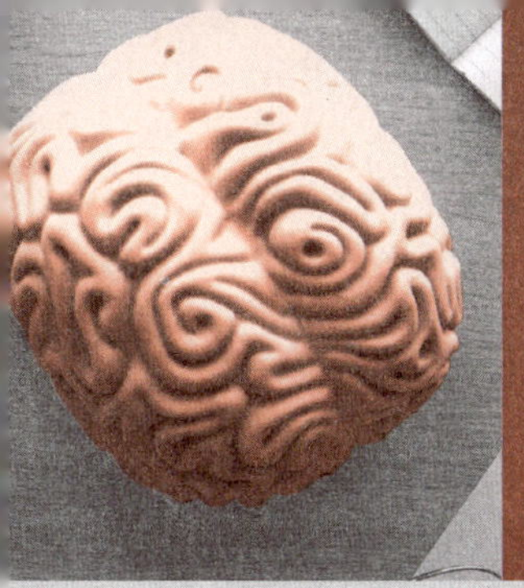

STUDENT ASSIGNMENT

LONG ANSWER QUESTIONS

1. Explain the neurobiological mechanism of emotions, including the role of the limbic system and its components in emotion processing.
2. Discuss the various theories of emotions, highlighting their strengths and weaknesses.
3. Describe the physiological mechanisms of emotions, including the role of the autonomic nervous system and neuroendocrine pathways.
4. Discuss the implications of emotion regulation strategies for mental health and well-being, differentiating between adaptive and maladaptive strategies.
5. Explain the role of emotions in physiotherapy practice, addressing how emotions impact patients' perspectives, therapeutic intervention, adherence, and clinical decision-making.

SHORT ANSWER QUESTIONS

1. Write about the neurobiology of emotions.
2. Define Cannon-Bard theory of emotion.
3. Define Russell's two-dimensional model of emotion.
4. Write a note on electrodermal activity.
5. Mention the benefits and challenges of integrating emotional intelligence training into physiotherapy education programs.
6. What is the concept of emotional barriers to treatment adherence?
7. What is the role of emotions in shaping patient experiences and expectations during physiotherapy rehabilitation?

MULTIPLE CHOICE QUESTIONS

1. **Which of the following is NOT a common emotion experienced by patients undergoing physiotherapy?**
   a. Fear
   b. Anxiety
   c. Frustration
   d. Indifference
2. **A physiotherapist notices that a patient seems anxious and hesitant during treatment sessions. Which emotional competency would be most helpful in this situation?**
   a. Self-awareness
   b. Self-regulation
   c. Empathy
   d. Emotional intelligence

3. **A patient has been struggling with adherence to their home exercise program. Which of the following emotional factors could be a potential barrier?**
    a. Hope
    b. Motivation
    c. Fear
    d. Empowerment

4. **A physiotherapist notices that a patient's pain behaviors seem to be influencing his clinical decision-making process. What could be a potential risk in this situation?**
    a. Emotional dissonance
    b. Lack of empathy
    c. Emotional burnout
    d. Overconfidence

5. **Which of the following statements about emotional intelligence (EI) in physiotherapy is TRUE?**
    a. EI is irrelevant in physiotherapy practice
    b. High EI can enhance therapeutic relationships and patient-centered care
    c. EI training is unnecessary for physiotherapists
    d. EI only matters for patients, not for physiotherapists

6. **Which of the following statements about emotional disclosure in physiotherapy is TRUE?**
    a. Emotional disclosure has no impact on therapeutic relationships or patient outcomes.
    b. Physiotherapists should actively discourage emotional disclosure from patients.
    c. Higher levels of emotional disclosure are associated with stronger therapeutic alliances.
    d. Emotional disclosure is only relevant for patients with mental health conditions.

7. **Which of the following is NOT a potential benefit of addressing emotions in physiotherapy practice?**
    a. Improved patient adherence
    b. Enhanced therapeutic relationships
    c. Increased job satisfaction for physiotherapists
    d. Faster physical recovery times

8. **Which of the following factors influencing individual differences in emotion regulation?**
    a. Personality traits
    b. Self-esteem
    c. Coping styles
    d. All of these

9. **Which of the following neurotransmitter do not impact emotions?**
    a. Serotonin
    b. Dopamine
    c. Cortisol
    d. Norepinephrine

10. **Which of the following is the emotion triggered sympathetic response?**
    a. Decreased digestive activity
    b. Rapid heart rate
    c. Dilation of pupils
    d. All of these

ANSWER KEY

1. d	2. c	3. c	4. a	5. b	6. c	7. d	8. d
9. c	10. b						

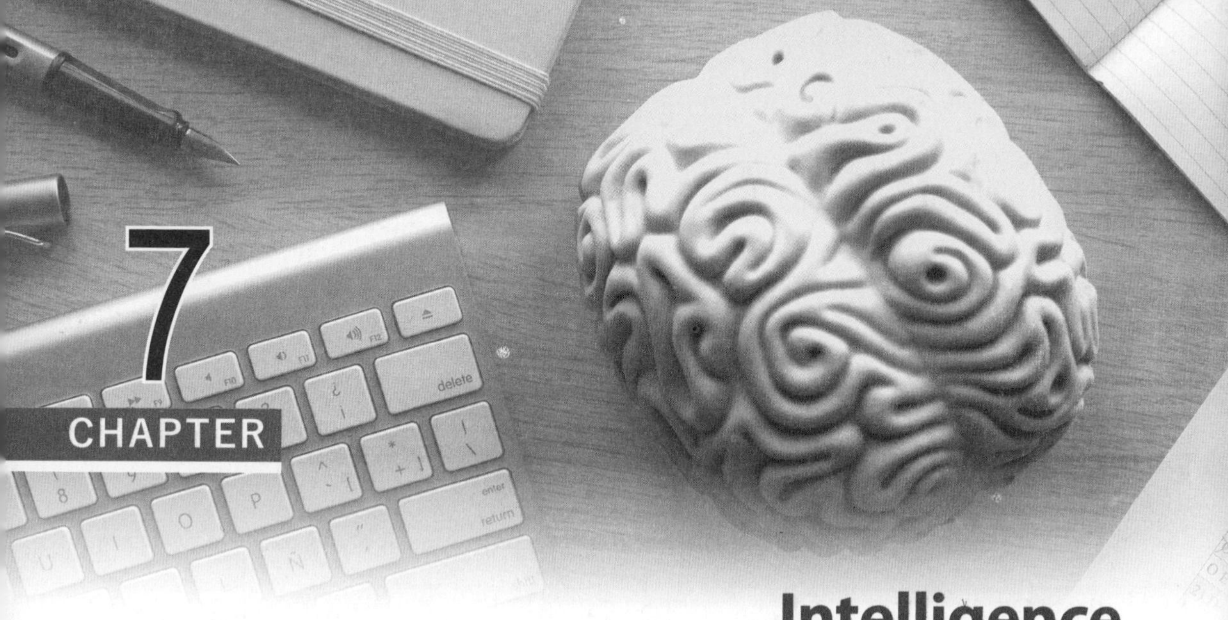

CHAPTER 7

Intelligence

Riya Kalra, Sushma K C, Kanu Goyal, Manu Goyal

LEARNING OBJECTIVES

After the completion of the chapter, the readers will be able to:
- Define intelligence and explore its various domains, moving beyond traditional academic performance to encompass a broader ability to understand and adapt to the environment.
- Examine the diverse theories of intelligence proposed by key researchers such as Spearman, Thorndike, Thurstone, Gardner, and Sternberg, and understand the implications of these theories for understanding human cognitive abilities.
- Investigate the neurological basis of intelligence, including the roles of the prefrontal cortex and the amygdala, and how brain imaging techniques have advanced our understanding of the biological basis of intelligence.
- Analyze the influence of intelligence on psychological and musculoskeletal health management, including diagnosis, treatment planning, therapeutic compliance, and outcomes.
- Explore recent advancements in artificial intelligence and cognitive technologies, such as generative Artificial Intelligence (AI), machine learning, reinforcement learning, and neurotechnology, and their implications for human cognitive enhancement.

CHAPTER OUTLINE

- Introduction
- Neurological Foundation
- Theories
- Types
- Assessment
- Impact on Mental and Physical Health
- Recent Advancement

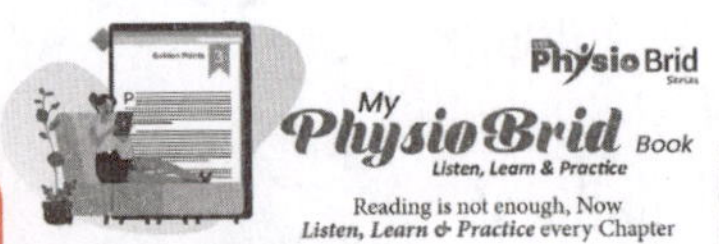

KEY TERMS

Adaptation: It is the process of adjusting to new conditions or environments.

Artificial intelligence (AI): It refers to the simulation of human intelligence in machines that are programmed to think like humans and mimic their actions.

Cognition: It refers to the mental processes involved in acquiring knowledge and understanding through thought, experience, and the senses.

Cognitive technologies: These are tools and systems designed to enhance human cognitive abilities.

Emotional intelligence or emotional quotient (EQ): It refers to the ability to recognize, understand, manage, and utilize emotions effectively.

Generative AI: It refers to artificial intelligence models that can generate new content, such as text, images or music, that is similar to human-created content.

Intelligence: It is the ability to perceive or deduce information, retain it as knowledge, and apply it to adapt effectively within a given environment.

Neurological foundations: It refers to the biological and neural processes that underpin cognitive functions.

Reinforcement learning: It is a type of machine learning that focuses on training models to make decisions by rewarding good behaviors and penalizing bad ones.

Treatment outcome: It refers to the results or effects of a particular treatment or intervention.

INTRODUCTION

Intelligence is characterized by the capability to observe or deduce information and store it as knowledge, which can be utilized in adaptive actions within a particular context or environment.[1] The phrase gained widespread recognition in the early 20th century, and the majority of psychologists agree that intelligence may be divided into distinct domains or competencies.[2,3]

The term intelligence has its roots in the Latin nouns *intelligentsia* or *intellēctus*, which are derived from the verb *intelligere*, signifying to grasp or understand. Thoroughly researched in humans and across diverse academic realms, intelligence has also been noted in non-human creatures and even plants. However, there remains contention about the extent to which these forms of life genuinely manifest intelligence.[4,5]

There is ongoing debate about the definition of intelligence, with differing viewpoints on its capabilities and whether it is possible to measure it.[6] The Wall Street Journal released an opinion piece titled "Mainstream Science on Intelligence" in 1994. The dispute over the book "The Bell Curve", which advocated altering policy based on alleged connections between intellect and race, prompted this. Of the 131 researchers invited to sign, 52 accepted the declaration, while 48 openly declined. The rest remained neutral. Intelligence was described as, "A very general mental capability that involves the ability to reason, plan, solve problems, think abstractly, comprehend complex ideas, learn quickly, and learn from experience. It is not merely book learning, a narrow academic skill or test-taking strategies. Rather, it reflects a broader and deeper capability for understanding our surroundings— 'catching on', 'making sense' of things or 'figuring out' what to do."[7]

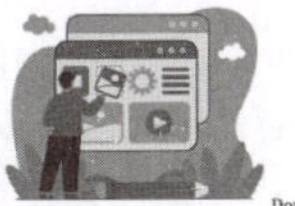

165

Besides those definitions, psychology and learning researchers also have suggested the following definitions of intelligence described in Table 7.1.

Table 7.1: Definitions of intelligence

Researchers	Proposed definitions of intelligence
David Wechsler	The overall ability of an individual to act with intention, think logically, and interact effectively with his surroundings.[8]
William Salter and Robert Sternberg	Purposeful adaptive behavior.
Reuven Feuerstein	The unique ability of humans to modify or adjust their cognitive functioning to satisfy the changing requirements of various life circumstances.[9]
Lloyd Humphreys	The result of gathering, committing knowledge to memory, retrieving, blending, contrasting, and using knowledge and conceptual abilities in novel situations.

The ability to receive or deduce information, retain it as knowledge, and deploy it to modify behavior in specific circumstances is the standard definition of intelligence.[2] This includes a variety of mental skills such as logical thinking, strategizing, resolving issues, conceptual thinking, understanding intricate concepts, and gaining knowledge through experience. Intelligence is not just about how well someone does in school or their grades. It is really about how well a person can understand things and adjust to different situations.[10, 11]

NEUROLOGICAL FOUNDATION

The concept of intelligence, especially in relation to brain anatomy, involves a complex interplay between cognitive processes and neural structures. Numerous studies have investigated the anatomical correlates of intelligence, illustrating the intricate connections between brain structure and cognitive function. Intelligence extends beyond what traditional IQ tests measure, engaging a broader neural network, with significant emphasis on the prefrontal cortex (PFC) and other brain regions.[12]

Recent research in neurobiology emphasizes the importance of a balanced interaction between the brain's rational and primitive minds for improving learning and thinking processes. The rational mind, situated in the neocortex, is crucial for planning, learning, memory, and making ethical distinctions. In contrast, the primitive mind, linked to the amygdala, governs basic emotions such as anger and fear. Effective information processing involves harmony between these two aspects of the brain, forming the basis of emotional intelligence.[13] The amygdala uses stored emotional memories to evaluate new information for potential threats or opportunities, comparing it with past experiences. During stress, the amygdala initiates a crisis response, releasing hormones, like cortisol, which can hinder cognitive functions, like focus and memory. The inhibitory connection between

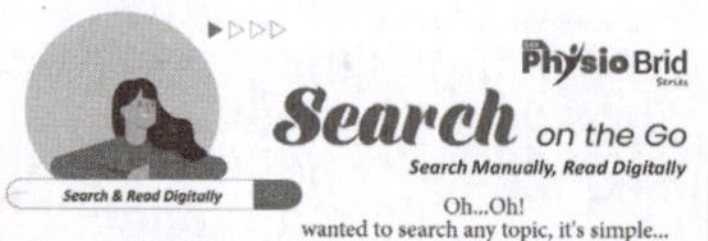

the prefrontal lobes and the amygdala is essential for self-control, adaptability, and maintaining calm in crisis situations.[14]

Advanced brain imaging techniques, such as MRI, have been utilized to examine the associations between brain volume, specific regional measurements, and intelligence, providing insights into the biological foundations of human cognitive abilities. Studies on the anatomical networks of the brain show that increased intelligence is linked to more effective information transfer in the brain, underscoring the critical role that the structural architecture of the brain plays in cognitive function.

Moreover, the efficiency of neural communication and the integration of various brain regions appear to play a pivotal role in enhancing intellectual capabilities, suggesting that intelligence is a product of both the structure and functionality of the brain. These discoveries underscore the complexity of intelligence, emphasizing the need to understand the neural bases of cognitive processes for a comprehensive understanding of human intelligence.[12]

THEORIES

The study of intelligence is characterized by a diversity of theories, each proposing distinct perspectives and assumptions, often conflicting with preceding ones. These theories, ranging from psychometric approaches to cognitive and biological perspectives, present varied understandings of intelligence, leading to ongoing debate and evolution within the field. Despite their differences, these theories collectively contribute to our comprehension of the multifaceted nature of intelligence, emphasizing its complexity and challenging researchers to integrate diverse viewpoints for a comprehensive understanding.

Faculty Theory

The Faculty Theory, prevalent during the 18th and 19th centuries, posits that the mind comprises distinct faculties such as reasoning, memory, discrimination, and imagination, which are believed to be independent and trainable through rigorous practice. However, this theory faced criticism from experimental psychologists who refuted the notion of separate and autonomous faculties within the brain, highlighting evidence that contradicted such claims.[15]

One Factor/UNI Factor Theory

It posits that consolidating all abilities into a single concept of general intelligence or 'common sense' assumes a perfect correlation among them, ignoring the reality of individual strengths in different areas and contradicting the widely acknowledged diversity in human skills.[15]

Spearman's Two-Factor Theory

Charles Spearman developed the theory in 1904 that intellectual abilities are composed of two elements: A general ability, termed the 'G' factor, and specific abilities, known as the 'S' factor.

Spearman suggested that the 'G' factor represents an inherent, universally applicable capability, with higher levels correlating to greater life achievements. Conversely, the 'S' factor is shaped by environmental factors and varies depending on the activity undertaken by an individual.[16]

Thorndike's Multifactor Theory

Thorndike rejected the concept of a singular General Ability, instead proposing that each mental task draws upon a combination of various skills. He described intellect in terms of four qualities:

1. Level, signifying the degree of complexity of activities that can be solved;
2. Range, which represents the quantity of assignments at a specific degree of difficulty;
3. Area, representing the breadth of situations to which an individual can respond;
4. Speed, indicating the rapidity of response to stimuli.[17]

Thurstone's Theory

Thurstone's perspective on intelligence differs from the perspective of both Thorndike and Spearman. He argues that intelligence isn't governed by a single overarching factor or a multitude of specific ones. Instead, he suggests that various mental operations cluster together based on common primary factors, each contributing to different facets of intelligence. Several fundamental components of intelligence reasoning, verbal, number, space, memory, and word fluency represent discrete skills.[12]

Structure of Intelligence Model by Guilford

In order to analyze each intellectual endeavor by its content, the mental process employed, and the final product, Guilford presented a three-dimensional model of intelligence. He divided the content into behavioral, symbolic, auditory, visual, and semantic categories. The following categories applied to the operations: Evaluation, divergent, convergent, memory recording, retention, and cognition. The categories used to group products were units, courses, and connections, systems, modifications, and ramifications. This model, which takes into account all of the components of intellectual tasks, provides a thorough comprehension of them.[18]

Hierarchical Theory of Vernon

Spearman's two-factor theory and Thurstone's multiple-factor theory are connected by Vernon's intelligence model. According to Spearman, the primary cause of individual differences is the "G" factor or general intelligence. It is ranked highest. Substantial group components constitute the following level, including practical, mechanical, spatial, and physical skills and verbal-numerical-educational skills. Minor group factors comprise the ones that are subsets of the major group factors and are found beneath them. Base-level intelligence or the 'S' factor, was first identified by Spearman as well.

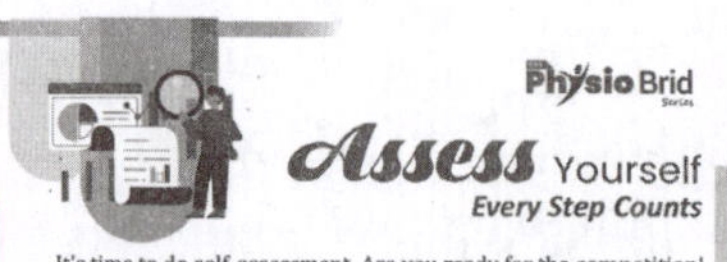

From 1969 onward, Vernon explored the roles of environmental and genetic factors in intellectual development. He concluded that about 60% of individual differences in intelligence are genetic and found evidence suggesting genetic involvement significant variances in average cognitive abilities between racial categories.[12]

Multiple Intelligences Theory of Gardner

Eight different categories of intelligence are proposed by Howard Gardner in "Frames of Mind" (1983): linguistic, spatial, artistic, bodily-kinesthetic, interpersonal, intrapersonal, mathematical and ecological (Fig. 7.1). Beyond conventional IQ tests, he contends that these various intelligences are vital.[19]

Intelligence Theory of Triarchic

In 1985, the triarchic theory of intelligence was discovered by Robert Sternberg, which supplemented elements absent from Gardner's theory. Sternberg described intelligence as the capacity to attain success based on personal standards and the sociocultural environment. His theory divides intelligence into three components: (1) Analytical, (2) Creative, and (3) Practical.[20, 21]

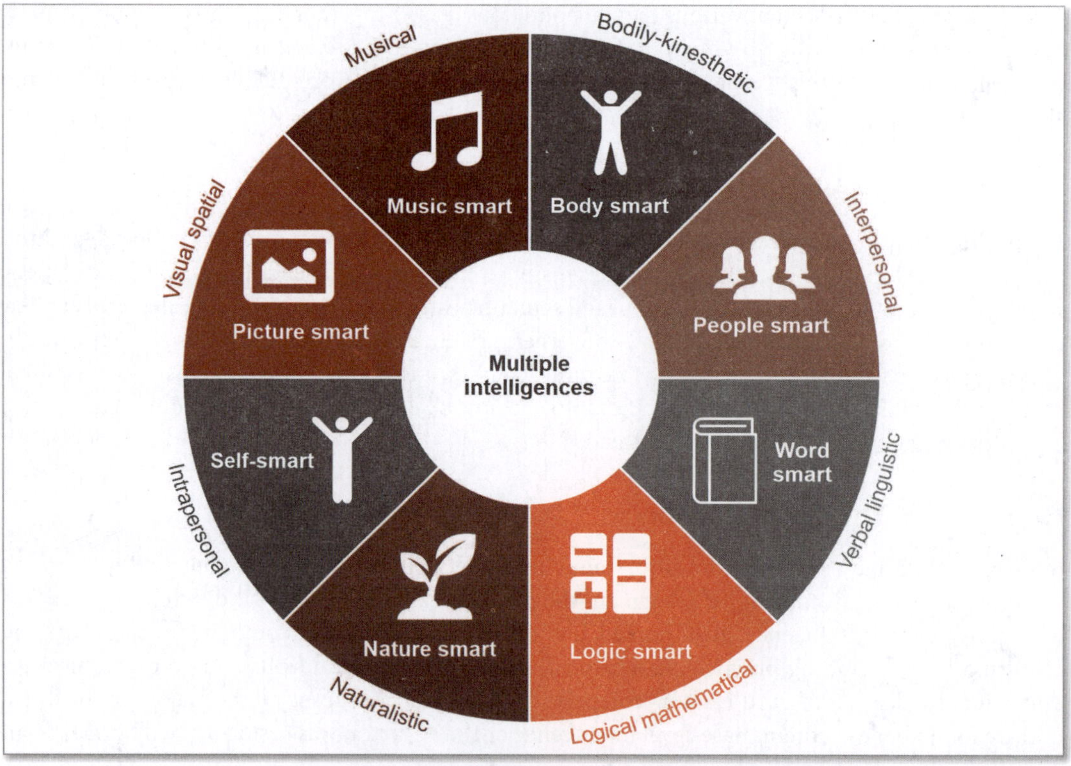

Fig. 7.1: Types of multiple intelligences as per the theory of Gardner

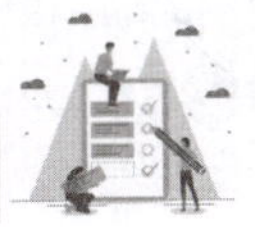
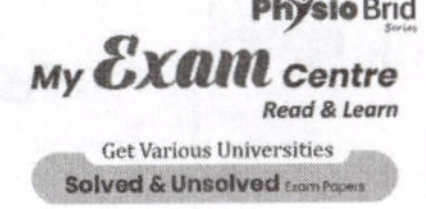

Anderson's Cognitive Development Theory

Anderson contends that the cognitive structures of humans are finely tuned to tackle the challenges presented by their environment. According to his viewpoint, discovering the optimal solution to environmental problems is akin to revealing the mechanism inherent within the architecture itself. This approach, termed 'Rational Analysis', factors in environmental information, agent objectives, and fundamental assumptions regarding computational cost to derive an optimal behavioral function. This function can subsequently undergo empirical testing, with adjustments made to assumptions if discrepancies arise. In contrast, Simon's perspective posits that assumptions about the architecture play a pivotal role in rational analysis, often carrying out the majority of analytical work.[12]

Structural Theory of Eysenck

Three neurological markers of intelligence were identified by Eysenck which involves average evoked potential, scrutiny time, and reactivity. Average evoked potential is a term used to describe the complexity of mental wave patterns, whereas reaction time and inspection time are measurable behaviors. Brighter individuals typically exhibit faster and more consistent reaction times and shorter inspection times. Moreover, their average evoked potential, assessed through electroencephalogram readings, displays greater intricacy compared to individuals with lower intelligence.[12]

Ceci's Biological Theory

Ceci (1990) posits the existence of multiple cognitive potentials that are innate and define the limits of cognitive functions. The opportunities and challenges that exist in a person's surroundings are closely linked to these potentials. He emphasizes the significance of context in showcasing cognitive abilities, which includes factors like domain-specific knowledge, personality traits, motivation, and educational background. This context may manifest in mental, social or physical dimensions.[22]

Emotional Intelligence Theory

Goleman (1995) listed the following components of emotional intelligence:

- **Knowing one's emotions:** Recognizing and understanding personal emotions.
- **Managing emotions:** Regulating emotions, especially in tough situations.
- **Motivating oneself:** Using emotions to set and pursue goals despite obstacles.
- **Recognizing emotions in others:** Empathizing and understanding others' emotions.
- **Handling relationships:** Skillfully navigating social interactions and managing emotions.

These abilities help individuals navigate social and personal interactions effectively.[23]

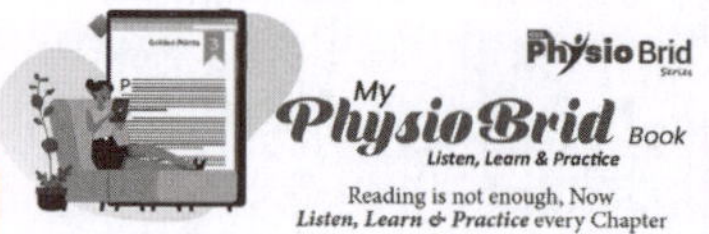

TYPES[24, 25]

- **Logical-mathematical intelligence**
  - **Description:** This refers to the capacity to apply logic to problems, carry out mathematical operations, and conduct scientific investigations.
  - **Characteristics:** Strong reasoning skills, problem-solving abilities, and the capacity to think abstractly.
- **Linguistic intelligence**
  - **Description:** The capacity to use words effectively, whether in speaking, writing or reading.
  - **Characteristics:** Proficiency in languages, good at storytelling, and skilled in reading comprehension and writing.
- **Spatial intelligence**
  - **Description:** The capacity for three-dimensional perception.
  - **Characteristics:** Good at visualizing objects, spatial judgment, and recognizing patterns.
- **Musical intelligence**
  - **Description:** The ability to perceive, compose, record, and analyze music.
  - **Characteristics:** Sensitivity to rhythm, pitch, meter, tone, and melody.
- **Physical-kinesthetic intelligence**
  - **Description:** The ability to skillfully control one's physical body and handle objects effectively.
  - **Characteristics:** Competent with their hands, whether creating or fixing things, and adept at physical pursuits-like sports or dance.
- **Interpersonal intelligence**
  - **Description:** The ability to understand and interact effectively with others.
  - **Characteristics:** Excellent at interpersonal communication, compassion, and perceiving other people's intentions, state of mind, and aspirations.
- **Self-awareness intelligence**
  - **Description:** The ability to comprehend self and value one's emotions, fears, and drives.
  - **Characteristics:** High self-awareness, introspective, and self-motivated.
- **Naturalistic intelligence**
  - **Description:** The ability to recognize and categorize plants, animals, and other aspects of nature.
  - **Characteristics:** Interest in biology, good at recognizing patterns in nature, and sensitivity to natural phenomena.
- **Existential intelligence**
  - **Description:** The capacity to think critically about the meaning of life, the universe, and existence.

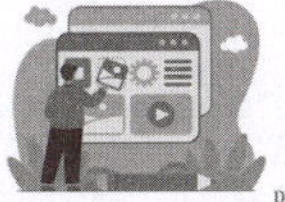
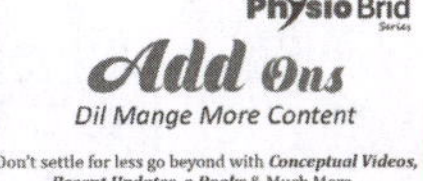

- **Characteristics:** Philosophical thinking, curiosity about the big questions of life, and reflective thinking.
- **Fluid intellect**
    - **Description:** The capacity to solve novel problems, recognize patterns, and reason abstractly and swiftly.
    - **Characteristics:** Problem-solving, logical thinking, and the ability to understand complex relationships.
- **Crystallized intellect**
    - **Description:** The capacity to apply experience and acquired information.
    - **Characteristics:** Using vocabulary, general knowledge, and expertise acquired over time.
- **Emotional intelligence (EI)**
    - **Description:** The ability to recognize, understand, manage, and utilize emotions effectively.
    - **Characteristics:** Social abilities, autonomy, empathetic thinking and mindfulness of emotions.

ASSESSMENT

Intelligence can be assessed through psychological tests. Alfred Binet (1875–1911) was the first psychologist to devise an intelligence test. Intelligence tests can be classified into two broad categories, (Fig. 7.2) namely:

1. Individual tests
2. Group tests

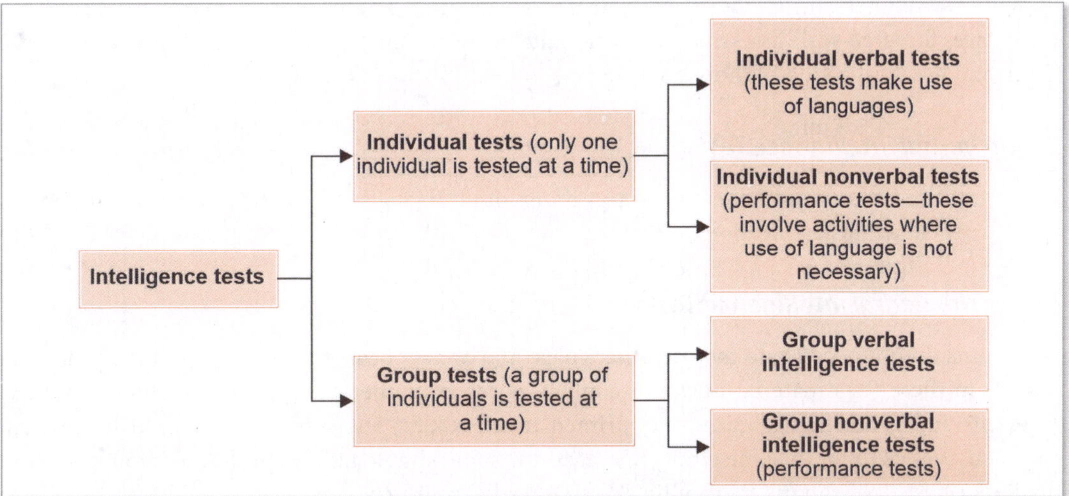

Fig. 7.2: Classification of intelligence tests

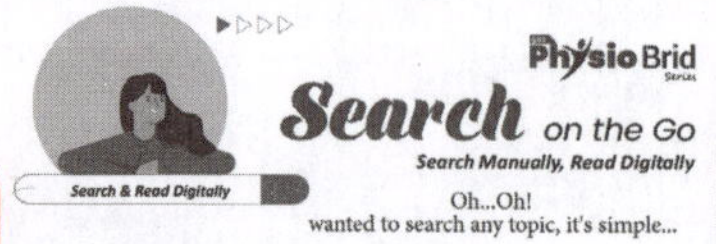

Individual Tests

These tests, such as the Stanford-Binet Intelligence Scale and Wechsler Adult Intelligence Scale (WAIS), are administered one-on-one, providing detailed insights into an individual's cognitive abilities. They allow examiners to observe nonverbal cues and problem-solving approaches, making them ideal for clinical, educational, and diagnostic purposes. However, they are time-consuming, resource-intensive, and require skilled professionals for administration.

Individual Verbal Tests

These tests are conducted on one individual at a time. These tests make use of languages. For example, Stanford-Binet Scale.

Individual Performance Tests

The complete nonverbal or nonlanguage tests of intelligence for testing an individual at a time fall into this category. These tests involve the manipulation of objects (e.g., picture arrangement, picture completion, block design, etc.) with minimum use of paper and pencil. Instructions are generally given by demonstrations and gestures. These tests are conducted on infants, mentally retarded, foreigners and those who do not understand language in which the tests are conducted. Example: Bhatia's Battery of Performance Test.

Group Tests

Tests like Raven's Progressive Matrices and the Cognitive Abilities Test (CogAT) assess multiple individuals simultaneously. They are efficient, cost-effective, and commonly used in schools and workplaces for large-scale assessments. While suitable for screening and trend analysis, they lack the depth and personalization of individual tests.

Group Verbal Intelligence Tests

These tests use language and are applied to a group of individuals at a time. Examples: Army Alpha Test, Army General Classification Test.

Group Nonverbal Intelligence Tests

These tests do not necessitate the use of language and are applicable to the group of individuals at a time. In these tests material does not contain words or numerical figures. It contains pictures, diagrams and geometrical figures, etc. printed in a booklet. The subject is required to perform such activities as to fill in some empty spaces, draw some simple figures, point out similarities and dissimilarities, etc. Examples: Army Beta Test, Raven's Progressive Matrices Test. Refer to Table 7.2 to understand the difference between individual and group tests.

Table 7.2: Comparison between individual and group tests

Individual tests	Group tests
These tests are conducted on one individual at a time. Hence, they are not economical in terms of time, labor and money	A group of children can be tested at the same time, hence economical
These tests are applicable for both adult and children	These tests cannot be administered to young children below the age of 10 years
These tests bring the tester and child closer and establish a better relationship between the two	Personal contact between the two is not possible

Uses

- Intelligence testing is used to forecast an individual's learning potential within a course of study.
- Intelligence tests assist in classifying students so that the instructor is aware of each student's potential for learning.
- Intelligence tests aid in distinguishing between gifted and slow learners so that distinct training approaches can be used for each of these two learning styles.
- Intelligence tests are utilized in the selection process for admission to various academic programs, as well as in the granting of scholarships and career counseling.
- Intelligence tests are employed in the hiring process for various positions.
- Tests of intelligence can also be helpful in child guidance. With their assistance, we can identify the children's academic deficiencies or other learning challenges.

Limitations

- Mathematically speaking, intelligence cannot be measured. Intelligence cannot guarantee that a person will succeed academically or professionally.
- Intelligence offers little insight into the person's temperament, feelings, morals or character—all of which are crucial to comprehending an individual's personality.

> **MUST KNOW**
>
> The concept of Intelligence Quotient (IQ) is a measure used to assess a person's cognitive abilities relative to others. It is derived from standardized tests designed to evaluate various aspects of intelligence, including logical reasoning, problem-solving skills, verbal comprehension, and mathematical abilities.
>
> - **Definition and calculation:**
> **IQ score:** Traditionally, an IQ score is calculated by dividing an individual's mental age (determined by test performance) by their chronological age and then multiplying the result by 100. However, modern IQ tests use a standard scoring system where the average IQ is set at 100, with a standard deviation of 15.
> **Example:** If a 10-year-old child performs at the level typical of a 12-year-old (mental age of 12), his/her IQ would traditionally be calculated as $(12/10) \times 100 = 120$.

Contd...

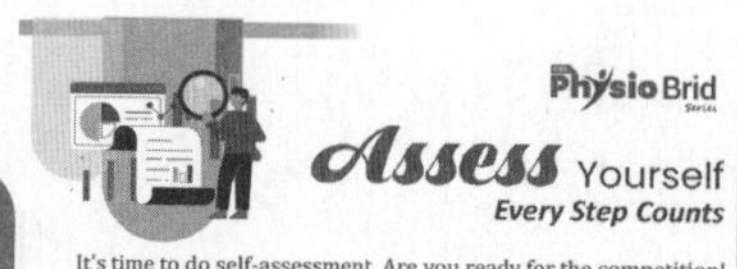

- **Distribution of IQ scores:**

  Normal distribution: IQ scores are typically distributed along a bell curve (normal distribution). Most people (about 68%) score within one standard deviation of the average (85–115).

- **Categories:**
  - **Below 70:** Intellectual disability.
  - **85–115:** Average intelligence.
  - **Above 130:** Considered gifted or highly intelligent.

- **Components of IQ tests:**
  - **Verbal comprehension:** Assesses vocabulary, comprehension, and verbal reasoning.
  - **Perceptual reasoning:** Measures nonverbal and fluid reasoning, such as solving puzzles and understanding patterns.
  - **Working memory:** Evaluates short-term memory and the ability to manipulate information mentally.
  - **Processing speed:** Tests how quickly an individual can process simple or routine information.

- **Interpretation and use:**
  - **Educational placement:** IQ scores are often used to identify students who may need special education services or who are eligible for gifted programs.
  - **Clinical diagnosis:** Used in the diagnosis of intellectual disabilities, cognitive impairments, and sometimes in assessing neurological conditions.
  - **Research:** In psychology and sociology, IQ scores are studied to understand human intelligence, its heritability, and its relation to various life outcomes, such as academic and job performance.

- **Limitations and criticisms:**
  - **Cultural bias:** Some IQ tests have been criticized for cultural bias, as they may favor individuals from certain cultural or linguistic backgrounds.
  - **Narrow scope:** IQ tests primarily measure certain types of cognitive abilities, particularly those related to academic skills. They do not fully capture creativity, emotional intelligence, practical problem-solving or social intelligence.
  - **Fixed versus Malleable:** There is ongoing debate about whether IQ represents a fixed trait or whether it can change over time with education, training, and environmental influences.

Tools

Wechsler Adult Intelligence Scale (WAIS)

- **Overview:** Developed by David Wechsler, the WAIS is one of the most widely used intelligence tests for adults.
- **Versions:** Currently, the WAIS-IV is the most recent version.
- **Components:** The test includes subtests that assess verbal comprehension, perceptual reasoning, working memory, and processing speed.
- **Purpose:** Used to assess overall intelligence and cognitive strengths and weaknesses.

Wechsler Intelligence Scale for Children (WISC)

- **Overview:** This scale is also developed by David Wechsler, the WISC is designed for children aged 6–16 years.

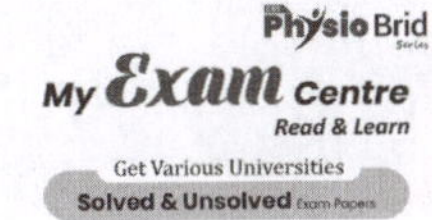

- **Versions:** The WISC-V is the latest version.
- **Components:** Similar to the WAIS, it assesses verbal comprehension, visual-spatial skills, fluid reasoning, working memory, and processing speed.
- **Purpose:** Commonly used in educational settings to identify learning disabilities and giftedness.

Stanford-Binet Intelligence Scales

- **Overview:** The Stanford-Binet test is one of the oldest intelligence tests, originally developed by Alfred Binet and later revised at Stanford University.
- **Versions:** The latest version is the Stanford-Binet 5 (SB5).
- **Components:** It includes five factors: Fluid reasoning, knowledge, quantitative reasoning, visual-spatial processing, and working memory.
- **Purpose:** Used across a wide age range (2–85+ years) to assess general intelligence.

Raven's Progressive Matrices

- **Overview:** A nonverbal intelligence test developed by John C Raven.
- **Components:** The test consists of multiple-choice questions where the individual must identify the missing piece in a series of patterns.
- **Purpose:** Measures abstract reasoning and is often considered a good measure of 'G' or general intelligence, especially in multicultural and nonverbal populations.

Cattell's Culture Fair Intelligence Test

- **Overview:** Designed by Raymond Cattell, this test aims to measure intelligence independent of cultural background.
- **Components:** The test includes nonverbal tasks, such as pattern recognition, sequences, and classification.
- **Purpose:** Used to minimize cultural and language biases in intelligence testing.

Woodcock-Johnson Tests of Cognitive Abilities

- **Overview:** The Woodcock-Johnson is a comprehensive set of tests used to measure general intellectual ability, specific cognitive abilities, and academic achievement.
- **Components:** It includes subtests that assess various cognitive domains such as auditory processing, visual processing, long-term retrieval, and processing speed.
- **Purpose:** Often used in educational settings to diagnose learning disabilities and to assess cognitive strengths and weaknesses.

Kaufman Assessment Battery for Children (KABC)

- **Overview:** Developed by Alan and Nadeen Kaufman, the KABC is designed for children aged 3–18 years.

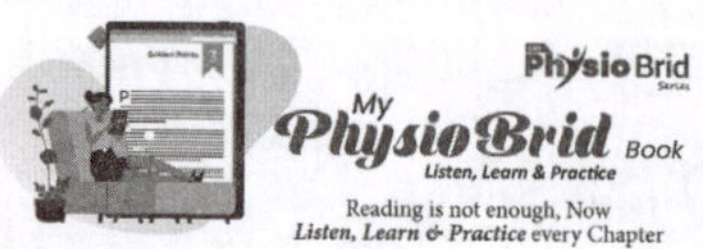

- **Components:** The test includes subtests that measure sequential processing, simultaneous processing, learning, and planning abilities.
- **Purpose:** Used to assess cognitive development in children and to identify learning disabilities and giftedness.

Universal Nonverbal Intelligence Test (UNIT)

- **Overview:** The UNIT is a completely nonverbal test designed to assess intelligence without relying on language.
- **Components:** The test includes tasks that involve memory, reasoning, and problem-solving using visual and spatial stimuli.
- **Purpose:** Particularly useful for individuals with language barriers, hearing impairments or those from diverse cultural backgrounds.

Differential Ability Scales (DAS)

- **Overview:** A battery of cognitive and achievement tests for children aged 2 years 6 months to 17 years 11 months.
- **Components:** The DAS measures cognitive abilities across several domains, including verbal, nonverbal, and spatial reasoning.
- **Purpose:** Commonly used in educational settings to assess cognitive abilities and diagnose learning disabilities.

Cognitive Assessment System (CAS)

- **Overview:** Based on the Planning, Attention, Simultaneous, Successive (PASS) theory of intelligence, the CAS assesses cognitive processing in children.
- **Components:** The test includes tasks that assess the four cognitive processes: Planning, attention, simultaneous processing, and successive processing.
- **Purpose:** Used to evaluate cognitive strengths and weaknesses, particularly in children with learning and attention difficulties.

Peabody Picture Vocabulary Test (PPVT)

- **Overview:** A test of receptive vocabulary for children and adults.
- **Components:** The individual is shown a series of pictures and asked to select the one that best represents a word spoken by the examiner.
- **Purpose:** Although primarily a vocabulary test, it is often used as a quick measure of verbal intelligence.

Bayley Scales of Infant and Toddler Development

- **Overview:** Designed for children between 1 month and 42 months of age.

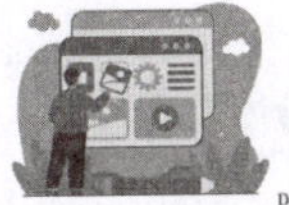

- **Components:** The test assesses cognitive, language, motor, social-emotional, and adaptive behavior.
- **Purpose:** Used to identify developmental delays and to guide early intervention strategies.

IMPACT ON MENTAL AND PHYSICAL HEALTH

Psychological

Intelligence plays a significant role in the management of psychological patients, impacting both the diagnosis and treatment processes. Higher cognitive abilities can aid in better understanding and compliance with therapeutic interventions, while lower cognitive functioning might require tailored approaches for effective treatment.

- **Diagnosis and assessment:** Intelligence influences the diagnostic process by helping clinicians understand the cognitive strengths and weaknesses of patients. It aids in differentiating between various psychological disorders, especially those with overlapping symptoms. For instance, neuropsychological assessments often include intelligence testing to inform the diagnostic process.[26]
- **Treatment planning:** Intelligence levels can guide the development of personalized treatment plans. Patients with higher intelligence might benefit from more cognitively demanding therapeutic approaches such as cognitive-behavioral therapy (CBT), which requires active participation and complex problem-solving skills. On the other hand, patients with lower intelligence may need simpler, more structured interventions.[27]
- **Therapeutic compliance:** Cognitive abilities influence how well patients understand and adhere to treatment regimens. Higher intelligence is generally associated with better comprehension of therapeutic instructions and adherence to prescribed treatments, enhancing outcomes.[28]
- **Outcome prediction:** Intelligence can be a predictor of treatment outcomes. Patients with higher intelligence may show better overall improvement due to their ability to engage with therapy more effectively and apply learned strategies outside the therapeutic context.[29]
- **Adaptation of therapeutic approaches:** Clinicians need to adapt therapeutic approaches based on the cognitive abilities of their patients. For example, therapy for patients with intellectual disabilities might focus more on behavioral techniques and the use of visual aids to facilitate understanding.[30]

In conclusion, intelligence significantly influences the management of psychological patients by affecting diagnosis, treatment planning, compliance, and outcomes. Tailoring interventions to match the cognitive abilities of patients can enhance therapeutic effectiveness and improve overall mental health outcomes.

Musculoskeletal

Intelligence can play a critical role in the management of musculoskeletal problems by influencing the understanding, adherence, and outcomes of treatment protocols. This can be seen in various aspects such as patient education, rehabilitation strategies, and self-management practices.

- **Patient education:** Higher intelligence levels can facilitate better understanding of musculoskeletal conditions and the importance of treatment plans. Educated patients are more likely to comprehend the necessity of specific exercises, postures, and ergonomics, which can prevent further injury and promote healing.[31]

- **Adherence to rehabilitation:** Cognitive abilities can impact a patient's ability to follow complex rehabilitation protocols. Patients with higher intelligence might find it easier to remember and adhere to prescribed exercises, leading to better recovery outcomes. Adherence to rehabilitation is crucial for the successful treatment of musculoskeletal problems.[32]

- **Self-management:** Intelligence can influence a patient's capability to engage in self-management of his musculoskeletal condition. This includes understanding his condition, recognizing symptoms, and knowing how to modify activities to reduce pain and avoid exacerbation of the injury. Effective self-management can significantly reduce the burden on healthcare systems and improve the quality of life for patients.[33]

- **Outcome prediction:** Intelligence might predict how well patients respond to treatments. Those with higher intelligence might utilize coping strategies more effectively and adhere to treatment plans more diligently, resulting in better clinical outcomes.[34]

- **Customization of therapy:** Clinicians may need to tailor their therapeutic approaches based on the cognitive abilities of their patients. For instance, simpler, more straightforward instructions and support might be required for patients with lower intelligence, ensuring they can follow through with the rehabilitation process effectively.[35]

Physio CORNER

Intelligence plays a significant role in the physiotherapeutic management of patients, influencing various aspects of assessment, treatment planning, patient adherence, and outcomes.

- **Assessment and diagnosis:** Intelligence can aid physiotherapists in assessing a patient's cognitive capacity to understand and participate in the treatment process. Cognitive assessments help tailor communication and instructional methods to suit the patient's level of understanding, ensuring effective diagnosis and treatment planning.[36]

- **Patient education:** Higher levels of intelligence can facilitate better understanding of the physiological basis of their conditions and the rationale behind specific therapeutic exercises. This understanding can motivate patients to engage more fully in their rehabilitation programs.[37]

- **Adherence to treatment plans:** Intelligence influences a patient's ability to follow complex rehabilitation protocols and maintain consistency in his exercises. Patients with higher cognitive abilities may find it easier to remember and adhere to prescribed regimens, which can enhance treatment outcomes.[38]

- **Self-management and coping strategies:** Patients with higher intelligence are often better at self-managing their conditions. They can apply problem-solving skills to modify activities and manage pain, reducing dependency on healthcare providers and improving long-term outcomes.[39]

- **Customization of therapy:** Understanding a patient's cognitive abilities allows physiotherapists to customize their therapeutic approaches. For patients with lower cognitive abilities, therapists may use simpler instructions, visual aids, and more frequent follow-ups to ensure comprehension and adherence.[40]

- **Outcome prediction:** Intelligence can be a predictor of how well patients respond to physiotherapy. Those with higher intelligence are likely to benefit more from treatments due to better understanding, adherence, and application of therapeutic strategies in their daily lives.[41]

CASE STUDY

Use of Intelligence Assessment in Physiotherapy

Emily Johnson is a 12-year-old girl diagnosed with spastic diplegia, a form of cerebral palsy that primarily affects the muscles of the lower body. She has been receiving physiotherapy since early childhood to improve her mobility, balance, and muscle strength. Emily is in a mainstream school but has been struggling academically, particularly with tasks that require sustained attention, problem-solving, and language comprehension.

Given these academic difficulties and the potential impact of cognitive factors on her physiotherapy outcomes, her neurologist referred her for an intelligence assessment to better understand her cognitive profile and how it might influence her rehabilitation.

Intelligence Assessment
- **Test administered:** Wechsler Intelligence Scale for Children (WISC-V)

Domains Assessed
- **Verbal comprehension:** Assesses verbal reasoning and concept formation.
- **Visual-spatial:** Measures spatial reasoning and visual-motor integration.
- **Fluid reasoning:** Evaluates the ability to solve novel problems.
- **Working memory:** Assesses short-term memory and attention.
- **Processing speed:** Measures the speed of processing simple or routine information.

Assessment Results
- **Overall IQ score:** 85 (Low Average range)
- **Verbal comprehension:** 78 (Borderline)
- **Visual-spatial:** 92 (Average)
- **Fluid reasoning:** 80 (Low Average)
- **Working memory:** 75 (Borderline)
- **Processing speed:** 90 (Average)

Interpretation
The results of the WISC-V indicate that Emily has overall cognitive abilities in the Low Average range, with specific weaknesses in verbal comprehension and working memory. These cognitive challenges could be contributing to her academic struggles and might also affect her ability to fully engage with and benefit from physiotherapy.

Impact on Physiotherapy
- **Challenges identified:**
  - **Instruction comprehension:** Emily's lower verbal comprehension may make it difficult for her to understand complex instructions or the reasoning behind certain exercises.
  - **Memory and attention:** Her weak working memory and attentional challenges might hinder her ability to remember multi-step exercises or maintain focus during sessions.
  - **Motivation and engagement:** Struggles with cognitive tasks could lead to frustration or reduced motivation in therapy, impacting her overall progress.

Contd...

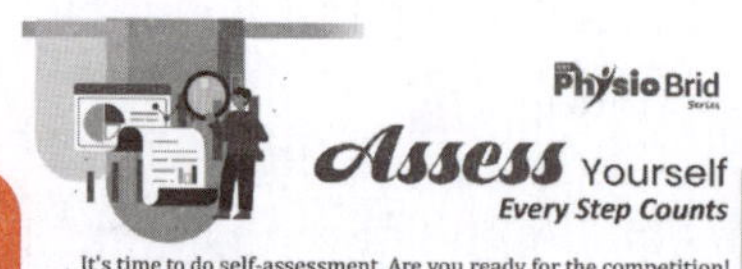

Adaptations in Physiotherapy Plan

- **Simplified instructions:**
  - Use simple, clear language when explaining exercises.
  - Break down complex tasks into smaller, manageable steps.
  - Use visual aids and demonstrations to complement verbal instructions.
- **Repetition and reinforcement:**
  - Increase the use of repetition in teaching new exercises to enhance learning and retention.
  - Provide frequent reminders and cues during sessions to help Emily stay on track.
- **Incorporating interests:**
  - Incorporate activities that Emily enjoys (e.g., playing with a therapy ball or engaging in interactive games) to increase her motivation and participation.
  - Use games that also stimulate cognitive functions, such as memory or attention, in a fun and engaging way.
- **Family involvement:**
  - Engage Emily's parents in the therapy process, teaching them how to reinforce exercises at home.
  - Provide the family with written or visual guides for home exercises to support Emily's learning and memory.
- **Shorter, focused sessions:**
  - Consider shorter, more frequent therapy sessions to match her attention span and reduce cognitive fatigue.
  - Use a variety of activities within each session to keep Emily engaged and prevent boredom.

Outcome

After implementing the adapted physiotherapy plan, Emily showed improved engagement in her sessions. She became more consistent in performing her exercises, both in the clinic and at home. Her balance and strength improved, and she became more confident in her mobility. The collaboration between the physiotherapist, family, and school ensured that Emily received comprehensive support, addressing both her physical and cognitive needs.

Conclusion

The use of intelligence assessment in Emily's case provided valuable insights that guided the development of a more tailored and effective physiotherapy plan. By understanding her cognitive strengths and weaknesses, the physiotherapist was able to adapt her approach, improving Emily's overall therapy experience and outcomes. This case illustrates the importance of a multidisciplinary approach in managing complex conditions like cerebral palsy, where cognitive factors can significantly influence rehabilitation success.

Intelligence significantly impacts the physiotherapeutic management of patients by influencing their ability to understand, adhere to, and benefit from treatment protocols. Personalized physiotherapy approaches based on cognitive abilities can enhance patient outcomes and overall effectiveness of rehabilitation.

RECENT ADVANCEMENT

Recent advancements in the field of intelligence, particularly artificial intelligence (AI) and human cognitive enhancement, have seen significant progress. These advancements are transforming various industries and aspects of daily life.

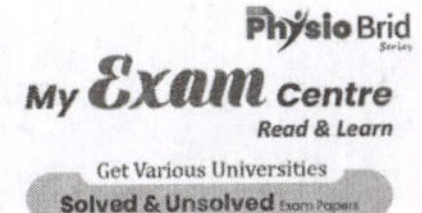

Artificial Intelligence and Machine Learning

- **Generative AI:** Technologies like OpenAI's GPT-4 and other large language models have advanced significantly, enabling more sophisticated natural language processing and generation. These models are used in various applications, from customer service to creative writing and medical research.[42]

- **AI in healthcare:** AI is increasingly used for evaluating diseases, patient outcome prediction and customizing treatment plans. For example, machine learning algorithms can analyze medical images with high accuracy, sometimes surpassing human performance in specific diagnostic tasks.[43]

- **Reinforcement learning:** Recent improvements in reinforcement learning have led to AI systems that can master complex tasks with minimal human intervention. For instance, DeepMind's AlphaFold has revolutionized protein folding predictions, significantly impacting biological and medical research.[44]

Neurotechnology and Cognitive Enhancement

- **Brain-Computer Interfaces (BCIs):** BCIs have seen remarkable progress, which enables direct interaction between the brain and external application and also this technology assists individuals with disabilities regain movement or communicate more effectively.

- **Neurostimulation techniques:** Technical advancements such as Transcranial Electromagnetic Stimulation and transcranial direct current stimulation (tDCS) are currently utilizing for enhancing cognitive abilities and treating neurological disorders, like depression and epilepsy.[45]

- **Cognitive computing:** Cognitive computing systems, like IBM Watson leverage AI to process and assess data, providing and supporting decision-making in fields such as healthcare, finance, and legal services.[46]

Artificial Intelligence Ethics and Governance

As AI technologies become more integrated into society, there is a growing focus on ethical considerations and governance frameworks to ensure responsible development and deployment. This includes addressing biases in AI algorithms, ensuring transparency, and protecting privacy.[47]

Quantum Computing and Artificial Intelligence

The intersection of quantum computing and AI is an emerging field with the ability to solve issues that are currently impossible for classical computers. Quantum AI could revolutionize fields such as cryptography, optimization, and complex system.[48]

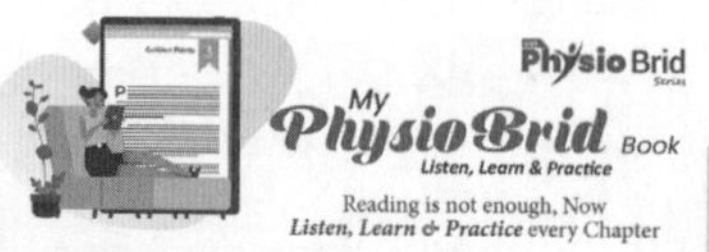

SUMMARY

- Intelligence encompasses the ability to receive information, retain it as information, and apply it to alterable behaviors within various contexts. It includes diverse cognitive skills which includes reasoning, problem-solving, and learning from experience.
- Originating in the early 1900s, the study of intelligence has evolved through numerous theories, from Spearman's theory to Gardner's multiple intelligences and Sternberg's theory, each highlighting different aspects of cognitive abilities.
- The concept remains complex and controversial, with debates on its definition and measurement. Intelligence is observed not only in humans but also in animals and plants, though the latter is contentious.
- It plays a critical role in fields like psychology, where it affects diagnosis, treatment, and outcomes in both psychological and musculoskeletal conditions. Advances in understanding the neurological basis of intelligence, alongside innovations in artificial intelligence (AI) and cognitive enhancement technologies, are transforming various sectors.
- Recent developments in AI, such as generative models and healthcare applications, coupled with progress in neurotechnology like brain-computer interfaces, highlight the rapid evolution and significant impact of intelligence research on society.

REFERENCES

1. Sharma, R. R. Emotional Intelligence from 17th Century to 21st Century: Perspectives and Directions for Future Research. Vision, 2008; 12(1): 59–66.
2. White, Margaret B. & Hall, Alfred E. An overview of intelligence testing. Phi Delta Kappa International, 1980; 58(4): 210–216
3. Buxton, Claude E. Influences in Psychology: Points of View in the Modern History of Psychology. Academic Press, 1985; 232: 1447–1448.
4. Goh, C.-H., Nam, H.G. and Park, Y.S. Stress memory in plants: A negative regulation of stomatal response and transient induction of rd22 gene to light in abscisic acid-entrained Arabidopsis plants. The Plant Journal, 2003; 36 (2): 240–255.
5. Volkov AG, Carrell H, Baldwin A, Markin VS. Electrical memory in Venus flytrap. Bioelectrochemistry, 2009; 75(2):142–147.
6. Legg, S., & Hutter, M. A Collection of Definitions of Intelligence. Artificial General Intelligence, 2007; 157:17–24.
7. Gottfredson, L. S. Mainstream science on intelligence: An editorial with 52 signatories, history and bibliography [Editorial]. Intelligence, 1997; 24(1): 13–23.
8. Wechsler, D. The Measurement of Adult Intelligence. 3rd Edition, the Williams & Wilkins Company, Baltimore, MD; 1944.
9. Tzuriel, David. Mediated Learning Experience and Cognitive Modifiability. Journal of Cognitive Education and Psychology, 2013; 12: 59–80.
10. Tirri, Kirsi & Nokelainen, Petri. Measuring Multiple Intelligences and Moral Sensitivies in Education, 2011; 5: 15–36.

Contd...

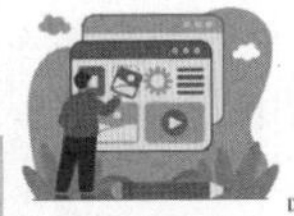
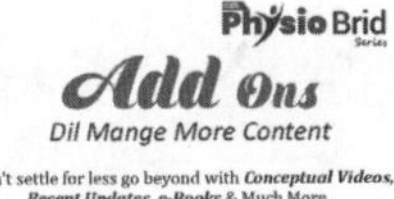

11. Stanek, Kevin & Ones, Deniz. Taxonomies and Compendia of Cognitive Ability and Personality Constructs and Measures Relevant to Industrial, Work and Organizational Psychology. The SAGE Handbook of Industrial, Work and Organizational Psychology, 2018; 366–407.

12. Berry W. Two Minds: There is no greater violence that ends violence, and no greater bigness with which to solve the problems of bigness. PROGRESSIVE-MADISON, 2002; 66(11):21–9.

13. LeDoux JE. The emotional brain: The mysterious underpinnings of emotional life. Simon and Schuster. 1998.

14. Wolkowitz OM, Reus VI, Weingartner H, Thompson K, Breier A, Doran A, Rubinow D, Pickar D. Cognitive effects of corticosteroids. The American journal of psychiatry, 1990; 147(10): 1297–303.

15. Pal, H.R., Pal, A., Tourani, P., Smith, Hilgard, C.D., Thorndike, E P, H., & Balasubramanian, D. THEORIES OF INTELLIGENCE. Everyman's Science, 2005; 3:181–186.

16. Spearmen, C. General intelligence objectively determined and measured. American Journal of Psychology, 1904; 15, 107–197.

17. Thorndike RM, Cunningham GK, Thorndike RL, Hagen EP. Measurement and evaluation in psychology and education. Macmillan Publishing Co, Inc; 1991.

18. Guilford JP. The nature of human intelligence. McGrawhill Book Co, 1967.

19. Gardner, H. The theory of multiple intelligence. Annals Of Dyslexia,1987; 37: 19–35.

20. Sternberg, R. J. Beyond IQ: A triarchic theory of human intelligence. Penguin Books, 1985.

21. Sternberg, R. J. The concept of intelligence and its role in lifelong learning and success. American psychologist, 1997; 52 (10): 1030.

22. Ceci SJ. Contextual trends in intellectual development. Developmental Review. 1993;13(4):403–35.

23. Goleman, D. Emotional Intelligence. New York: Bantam, 1995.

24. Davis K, Christodoulou J, Seider S, Gardner HE. The theory of multiple intelligences. Davis, K., Christodoulou, J., Seider, S., & Gardner, H. The theory of multiple intelligences. In RJ Sternberg & SB Kaufman (Eds.), Cambridge Handbook of Intelligence. 2011:485–503.

25. Cavas B, Cavas P. Multiple intelligences theory—Howard Gardner. Science Education in Theory and Practice: An Introductory Guide to Learning Theory. 2020:405–18.

26. Lezak MD, Howieson DB, Bigler ED, Tranel D. Neuropsychological assessment. 5th ed. Oxford: Oxford University Press; 2012.

27. Sternberg RJ, Grigorenko EL. Intelligence and culture: How culture shapes what intelligence means, and the implications for a science of well-being. Philos Trans R Soc Lond B Biol Sci. 2006;361(1475):2054–2064.

28. Kazdin AE. Treatment adherence and therapeutic change: An empirical examination of the guidelines for enhancing therapeutic gains. J Consult Clin Psychol. 1990;58(6):849–854.

29. Gottfredson LS. Intelligence: Is it the epidemiologists' elusive "fundamental cause" of social class inequalities in health? J Pers Soc Psychol. 2004;86(1):174–199.

30. Matson JL, Turygin NC, Beighley JS, Rieske RD, Matson ML. Applied behavior analysis in the treatment of autism spectrum disorder: Recent developments. In: Matson JL, editor. Applied behavior analysis. New York: Springer; 2015. p. 255–267.

31. Hall A, Tenenbaum G, Axtell R, et al. The role of cognitive processes in the perception of pain in sport. J Sports Sci. 2005;23(9):949–960.

Contd...

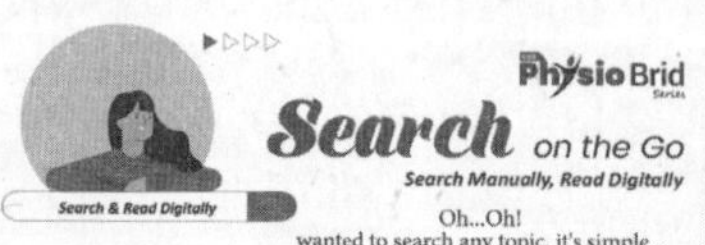

32. Campbell R, Evans M, Tucker M, Quilty B, Dieppe P, Donovan JL. Why don't patients do their exercises? Understanding non-compliance with physiotherapy in patients with osteoarthritis of the knee. J Epidemiol Community Health. 2001;55(2):132–138.

33. Lorig KR, Holman H. Self-management education: history, definition, outcomes, and mechanisms. Ann Behav Med. 2003;26(1):1–7.

34. Turner JA, Franklin G, Turk DC. Predictors of chronic disability in injured workers: A systematic literature synthesis. Am J Ind Med. 2000;38(6):707–722.

35. Dixon KE, Keefe FJ, Scipio CD, Perri LM, Abernethy AP. Psychological interventions for arthritis pain management in adults: A meta-analysis. Health Psychol. 2007;26(3):241–250.

36. Williams MA, Soiza RL, Jenkinson AM, Stewart A. EXercising with Computers in Later Life (EXCELL) - pilot and feasibility study of the acceptability of the Nintendo® WiiFit in community-dwelling fallers. BMC Res Notes. 2010;3:238.

37. Hall AM, Maher CG, Latimer J, Ferreira ML, Lam P. A systematic review of the effectiveness of cognitive-behavioral therapy for musculoskeletal pain. Clin J Pain. 2009;25(6):528–536.

38. Jack K, McLean SM, Moffett JK, Gardiner E. Barriers to treatment adherence in physiotherapy outpatient clinics: A systematic review. Man Ther. 2010;15(3):220–228.

39. Lorig KR, Holman HR. Self-management education: History, definition, outcomes, and mechanisms. Ann Behav Med. 2003;26(1):1–7.

40. Sluijs EM, Kok GJ, van der Zee J. Correlates of exercise compliance in physical therapy. Phys Ther. 1993;73(11):771–786.

41. Nicholas MK, Molloy AR, Tonkin LE, Beeston L. Manage Your Pain: Practical and Positive Ways of Adapting to Chronic Pain. Sydney: ABC Books; 2000.

42. Topol EJ. High-performance medicine: The convergence of human and artificial intelligence. Nat Med. 2019;25(1):44–56.

43. Senior AW, Evans R, Jumper J, et al. Improved protein structure prediction using potentials from deep learning. Nature. 2020;577(7792):706–710.

44. Wolpaw JR, Wolpaw EW. Brain-Computer Interfaces: Principles and Practice. 2nd ed. Oxford University Press; 2020.

45. Brunoni AR, Moffa AH, Fregni F, Palm U, Padberg F, Blumberger DM. Transcranial direct current stimulation for acute major depressive episodes: meta-analysis of individual patient data. Br J Psychiatry. 2016;208(6):522–531.

46. Ferrucci D, Levas A, Bagchi S, Gondek D, Mueller ET. Watson: Beyond Jeopardy! Artif Intell. 2013;199-200:93–105.

47. Jobin A, Ienca M, Vayena E. The global landscape of AI ethics guidelines. Nat Mach Intell. 2019;1(9):389–399.

48. Biamonte J, Wittek P, Pancotti N, Rebentrost P, Wiebe N, Lloyd S. Quantum machine learning. Nature. 2017;549(7671):195–202.

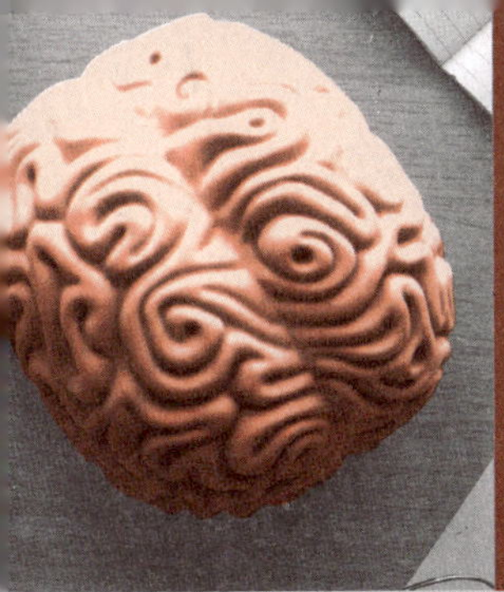

LONG ANSWER QUESTIONS

1. Define intelligence and discuss how its conceptualization has evolved over time. Highlight key theories and their proponents, including the contributions of Spearman, Thorndike, Thurstone, Gardner, Sternberg, and others.

2. Examine the neurological foundations of intelligence. What role do specific brain regions, such as the pre-frontal cortex and the amygdala, play in cognitive processes associated with intelligence?

3. Discuss how brain imaging techniques have advanced our understanding of the biological basis of intelligence.

4. Analyze the impact of intelligence on psychological treatment outcomes.

5. How do cognitive abilities influence diagnosis, treatment planning, therapeutic compliance, and adaptation of therapeutic approaches?

6. Discuss the relationship between intelligence and musculoskeletal health management.

7. How do cognitive abilities affect patient education, adherence to rehabilitation protocols, self-management practices, and overall treatment outcomes in musculoskeletal problems?

8. Explore the recent advancements in artificial intelligence (AI) and their implications for human cognitive enhancement.

9. How are technologies like generative AI, machine learning, reinforcement learning, and brain-computer interfaces transforming various sectors, particularly healthcare?

10. Evaluate the various types of intelligence proposed by Gardner's Theory of Multiple Intelligences and other models.

11. How do the different types of intelligence (e.g., logical-mathematical, linguistic, spatial, emotional) manifest in real-world settings, and what implications do they have for education and personal development?

12. Discuss the significance of emotional intelligence (EQ) as described by Goleman. What are its components, and how do they influence personal and professional success?

13. Critically assess the role of intelligence in the management of psychological distress.

14. How does understanding a patient's cognitive abilities help clinicians tailor their interventions, and what challenges might arise when working with patients of varying intelligence levels?

15. Investigate the implications of different intelligence theories on educational practices.

16. How can educators use insights from theories such as Gardner's Multiple Intelligences or Sternberg's triarchic theory to develop effective teaching strategies that cater to diverse learners?

17. Analyze the ethical and societal implications of advancements in neurotechnology and cognitive enhancement.

18. How do these technologies challenge our traditional understanding of intelligence and its measurement? What potential benefits and risks do they pose to individuals and society as a whole?

SHORT ANSWER QUESTIONS

1. What is intelligence?
2. State the various theories influenced our understanding of intelligence.
3. What are the key domains of intelligence?
4. How does intelligence influence health and therapy?
5. What are the neurological foundations of intelligence?
6. What are some recent advancements in AI?
7. What ethical considerations arise from AI advancements?
8. How does emotional intelligence differ from cognitive intelligence?
9. What is the role of brain-computer interfaces (BCIs) in cognitive enhancement?
10. Provide examples of how higher and lower intelligence levels can affect clinical practice.
11. How do you assess intelligence?

MULTIPLE CHOICE QUESTIONS

1. **What is the general capability described by the "Mainstream Science on Intelligence"?**
   a. Book learning and academic skills
   b. A very general mental capability that includes reasoning, planning, and problem-solving
   c. Specific technical skills
   d. Physical strength and agility

2. **Which theory of intelligence includes the 'G' factor and 'S' factors?**
   a. Thurstone's Primary Mental Abilities Theory
   b. Spearman's Two-Factor Theory
   c. Gardner's Theory of Multiple Intelligences
   d. Sternberg's Triarchic Theory of Intelligence

3. **Who proposed the theory of Structural Cognitive Modifiability?**
   a. Robert Sternberg
   b. David Wechsler
   c. Reuven Feuerstein
   d. Howard Gardner

4. **Which of the following is not one of Gardner's eight distinct types of intelligence?**
   a. Linguistic
   b. Logical-mathematical
   c. Emotional
   d. Spatial

5. **According to Vernon's hierarchical theory, which level represents specific abilities?**
   a. Major group factors
   b. Minor group factors
   c. 'G' factor
   d. 'S' factor

6. **Which intelligence theory suggests that intelligence is the result of processing and retrieving information to use in new contexts?**
   a. David Wechsler's theory
   b. Lloyd Humphreys' theory
   c. Anderson's theory of cognitive development
   d. Sternberg's triarchic theory

7. **What aspect does Eysenck's structural theory focus on in relation to intelligence?**
   a. Reaction time, inspection time, and average evoked potential
   b. Multiple intelligences including musical and bodily-kinesthetic
   c. Emotional intelligence such as managing emotions and motivating oneself
   d. Practical intelligence or "street smarts"

8. **Ceci's biological theory emphasizes the importance of which factor in showcasing cognitive abilities?**
   a. Genetic factors alone
   b. Environmental challenges and opportunities
   c. Reaction time and inspection time
   d. Book learning and academic performance

9. **Which recent advancement in artificial intelligence is known for mastering complex tasks with minimal human intervention?**
   a. Generative AI
   b. AI in healthcare
   c. Reinforcement learning
   d. Cognitive computing

10. **What is the main purpose of brain-computer interfaces (BCIs)?**
    a. Enhancing physical strength
    b. Enabling direct communication between the brain and external devices
    c. Improving book learning skills
    d. Managing emotional intelligence

Note

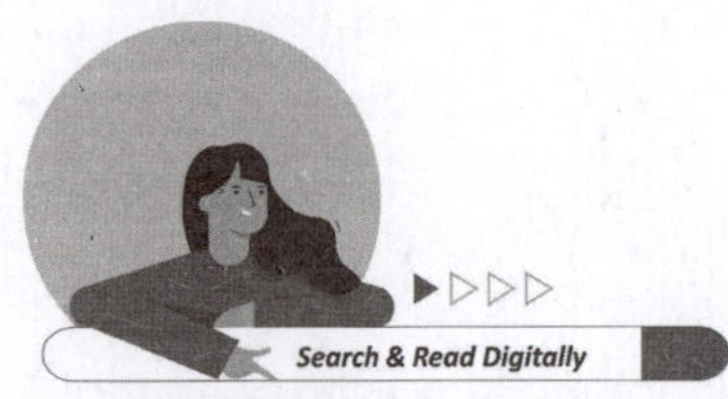

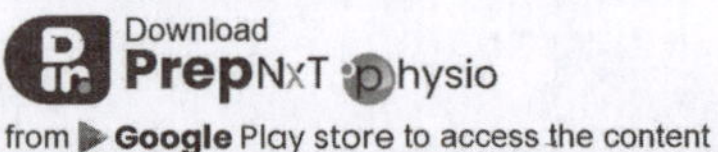

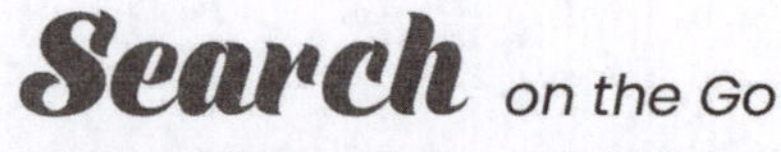

CBS Physio Brid Series

Search on the Go

Search Manually, Read Digitally

- Mapping of the most important topics from the Book at one place with one-click search
- Get Important topics of the book at one click

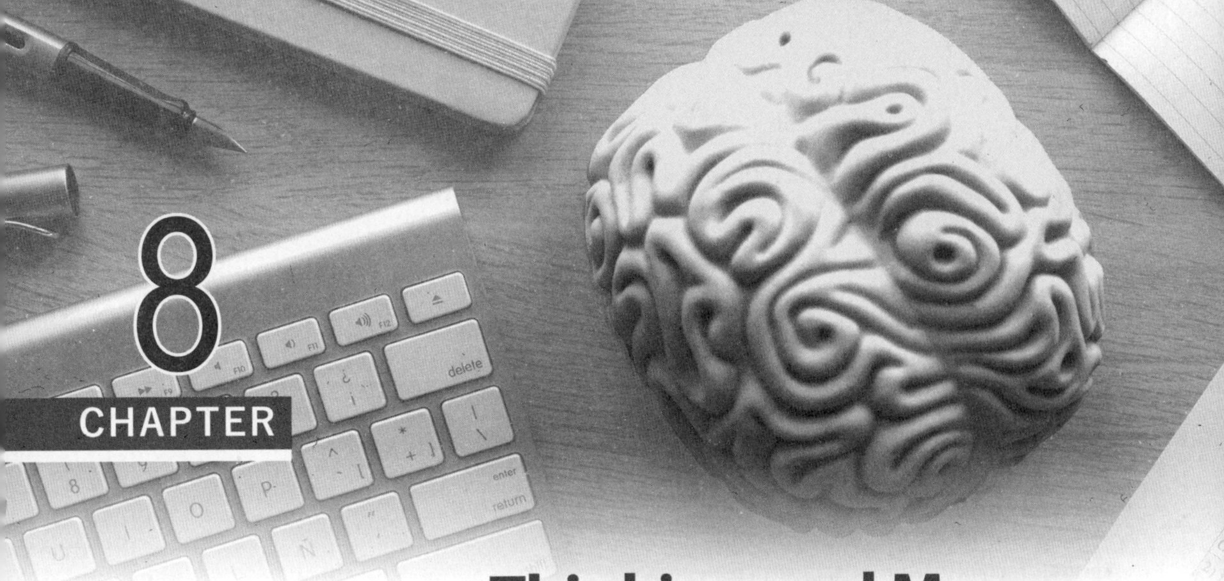

8

CHAPTER

Thinking and Memory

Manu Goyal, Kanu Goyal, Prateek Sharda

LEARNING OBJECTIVES

After the completion of the chapter, the readers will be able to:
- Understand the neurobiology of thinking and memory.
- Identify the types of the thinking and memory.
- Understand the development of the thinking process.
- Describe the role of thinking and memory in physiotherapy practice and their implications.
- Learn about the recent advancements in enhancing thinking and memory.

CHAPTER OUTLINE

- Introduction
- Thinking
- Theories
- Types of Thinking
- Implications in Clinical Practice
- Improvement Strategies
- Problem Solving
- Memory

- Types of Memory
- Stages of Memory
- Factors Influencing Memory
- Models of Memory
- Memory Assessment
- Memory Building Techniques
- Practical Aspect

KEY TERMS

Active learning techniques: Methods that involve direct engagement in learning activities to enhance understanding and retention.

Analytical thinking: The process of breaking down a whole into its parts to study them and their relationships.

Cerebral cortex: The outer layer of the brain responsible for various cognitive functions including thinking, reasoning, and decision-making.

Convergent thinking: A critical thought process that finds a single answer to a problem through logical reasoning.

Creative thinking: The ability to generate innovative and novel solutions.

Critical thinking: The objective analysis and evaluation of information.

Divergent thinking: A cognitive method aimed at generating multiple solutions, associated with creativity.

Dual-process theory (DPT): A theory that divides cognitive processes into two types: Type 1 (fast and intuitive) and Type 2 (slow and reflective).

Episodic memory: Stores personal experiences.

Explicit memory: Conscious recall of knowledge and experiences.

Heuristics: Mental shortcuts or rules of thumb used to simplify problem-solving.

Implicit memory: Unconscious retention of past experiences.

Logical thinking: Finding sensible solutions based on facts rather than emotions.

Long-term memory (LTM): Storage of information over extended periods.

Long-term potentiation (LTP): A cellular mechanism underlying synaptic plasticity and memory formation.

Memory: The ability to retain and recall information over time.

Metacognitive strategies: Techniques that involve the awareness and understanding of one's own thought processes.

Neural networks: Connections between neurons that enable the processing and transmission of information.

Neurobiology of thinking: The study of the biological mechanisms in the brain that underlie thinking processes.

Neuroplasticity: The brain's ability to adapt and reorganize in response to experiences and training.

Neurotransmitters: Chemical messengers in the brain that facilitate communication between neurons.

Neurotransmitter systems: Systems that regulate synaptic transmission and plasticity, including dopamine, glutamate, and acetylcholine.

Piaget's theory of cognitive development: A theory that outlines how children develop intellectual abilities and critical thinking skills from infancy to adulthood.

Priming: Facilitation of processing due to prior exposure.

Procedural memory: Memory for skills and procedures.

Semantic memory: Stores general knowledge and facts.

Short-term memory (STM): Temporary storage of information for immediate processing.

Subcortical structures: Brain regions beneath the cerebral cortex that play significant roles in cognitive processes, such as memory formation and emotional processing.

INTRODUCTION

Thinking and memory are important processes in psychology that help with problem-solving, decision-making, and learning. Thinking allows people to analyze situations, find solutions, and adapt to challenges, while memory helps store and recall information to learn from past experiences.

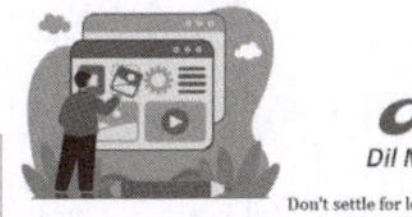

These processes also play a key role in managing emotions, building relationships, and responding to social situations. They are especially useful in areas like education, therapy, and rehabilitation, supporting learning and recovery. Thinking and memory are substantial components of human cognitive actions and effective communication. The current chapter describes the neurobiology of thinking and memory. The various theories of thinking and memory have been described. The chapter also highlights the types of thinking and memory, along with the memory assessment tests. The role of physiotherapy practice in enhancement of memory has been discussed.

THINKING

Thinking encompasses a variety of cognitive processes that involve acquisitions, processing, storage, and retrieval of information.[1] It involves several mental activities, including perceptions, memory, attention, language, motor skills, executive functioning, problem-solving and decision making.[2]

Neurobiology

Neurobiology is crucial to understand the neurobiology of thinking in order to comprehend the underlying mechanism of cognitive processes and its implications toward an effective clinical decision-making.

Neuroanatomy

The cerebral cortex and the subcortical structures play an important role in thinking and other cognitive functions such as reasoning, problem-solving, language and decision-making. Table 8.1 describes the various cortical and subcortical structures and their functions.

Table 8.1: Cerebral cortex and subcortical structures responsible in thinking[3]

Cerebral cortex		
Sl. no.	**Structure**	**Function**
1.	Frontal lobe	• Executive functions • Planning, decision-making, problem-solving • Pre-frontal cortex (DLPFC & ACC) and working memory
2.	Parietal lobe	• Spatial awareness • Attention • Sensory integration
3.	Temporal lobe	• Language processing • Memory formation • Auditory perception
4.	Occipital lobe	• Visual processing

Contd...

Subcortical structures		
Sl. no.	**Structure**	**Function**
1.	Hippocampus	Memory formation and consolidation
2.	Amygdala	• Emotional memory • Emotional processing
3.	Basal ganglia	• Procedural learning • Habit formation • Action selection

Abbreviations: ACC, anterior cingulate cortex; DLPFC, dorsolateral prefrontal cortex

Neurophysiology

The physiological processes underlying thinking involve complex interactions between neurons, neurotransmitters, and various brain regions. Table 8.2 highlights the various neurophysiological aspects in thinking.

Table 8.2: Neurophysiological aspects in thinking

Sl. no.	Neurophysiological aspect	Roles
1.	• Neurotransmitters • Glutamate • GABA • Dopamine • Serotonin • Acetylcholine	• Excitatory transmission • Inhibitory transmission • Reward, motivation, attention • Mood regulation • Memory, attention, learning
2.	Neural networks and connectivity	• Distributed processing and neural networks • Functional connectivity and integration • Structural connectivity and white matter tracts
3.	Neuroplasticity	• Experience—dependent plasticity • Learning and memory formation • Rehabilitation and recovery

Abbreviation: GABA, Gamma-aminobutyric acid

THEORIES

Dual-Process Theory

This theory is popular to divide types of cognitive processes into two distinct clusters, Type 1 (fast and intuitive process) and Type 2 (slow and reflective one).[4,5] Table 8.3 describes the various features of Dual-Process Theory (DPT).

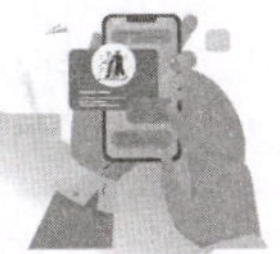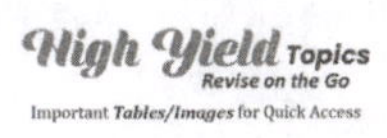

Table 8.3: Features of dual-process theory[6]

Sl. no.	DPT type	Features
1.	Type 1	Unconscious, implicit, automatic, low effort, rapid, high capacity, default, holistic, perceptual, evolutionary old, follows evolutionary rationality, shared with animals, nonverbal, modular, associative, domain-specific, contextualized, pragmatic, parallel, stereotypical, independent of general intelligence, independent of working memory.
2.	Type 2	Conscious, explicit, controlled, high effort, slow, low capacity, inhibitory, analytic, reflective, evolutionarily recent, follows individual rationality, uniquely human, linked to language, fluid intelligence, rule based, domain general, abstract, logical, sequential, egalitarian, heritable, linked to general intelligence, limited by working memory capacity.

The problem of this theory is to unite these two types and it is hypothesized that Type 1 processes rely on embodied prediction; whereas, Type 2 processes rely on symbolic—classical cognition.

Piaget's Theory of Cognitive Development

This theory focuses on how children develop intellectual abilities and critical thinking skills from infancy to adulthood. His stages of cognitive development outline (Fig. 8.1) how thinking evolves in complexity over time. Table 8.4 describes the excerpts about stages of cognitive development.

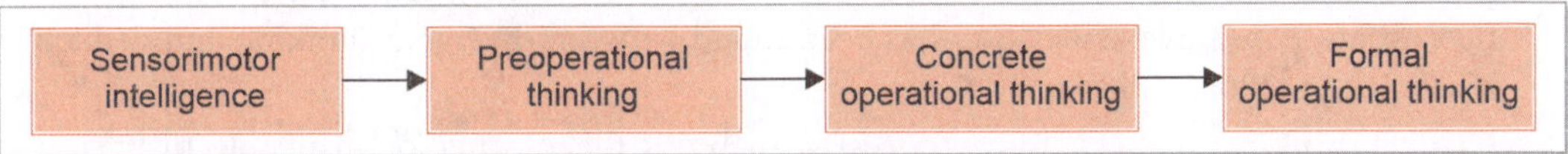

Fig. 8.1: Cognitive development stages

Table 8.4: Description on stages of cognitive development[7]

Sl. no.	Stage	Age range	Features
1.	Sensorimotor	0–2 years	• Discovering relationships between bodies and environment. • Coordination between sensory and motor responses. • Development of object permanence. • Usage of language for demands and cataloging.
2.	Preoperational	2–7 years	• Use of symbolic thought and language. • Learn to imitate and pretend to play. • Characterized by egocentrism. • Strong imagination and intuition.
3.	Concrete operational	7–11 years	• Use of logical thinking, inductive reasoning for problem solving. • Understanding of time, space and quantity and its applications.
4.	Formal operational	11 years and older	• Abstract logical reasoning. • Theoretical, hypothetical and counterfactual thinking. • Applications of learned concepts from one context to another. • Strategic planning becomes feasible.

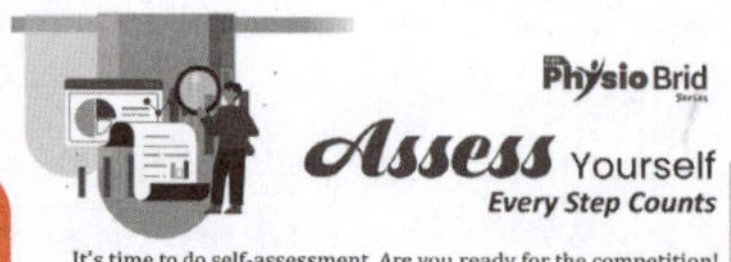

TYPES OF THINKING

Figure 8.2 delineates the various common types of thinking.

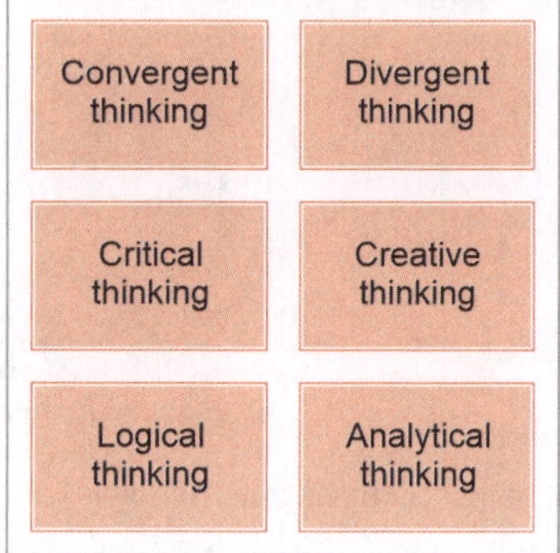

Fig. 8.2: Various types of thinking

1. **Convergent thinking:** It is a form of a critical thought process which finds out a single answer to a problem through logical reasoning and by evaluation of several possibilities and free from ambiguity. It results in the building of existing knowledge and put emphasis on speed, precision, logic and recognizes familiar and accumulating information.[8] It is an essential instrument to make decisions in high pressure scenarios in daily life.

2. **Divergent thinking:** It is a cognitive method aimed at generating multiple correct solutions. It is associated with key characteristics of creativity such as fluency and flexibility.[9] It is involved in generation of multitude of ideas by breaking the problem into several parts to gain insights on the mental task. It includes brainstorming, mapping of subject, artwork, free writing and meditation. Excessive divergent thinking is associated with counterproductivity as seen in mental problem, like schizophrenia. By promoting an active and open approach, it can produce positive therapeutic results such as coping mechanisms and reduction of anxiety and depression. A positive association has been found between divergent thinking and deductive reasoning in school children.[10]

3. **Critical thinking:** It is a cognitive process of analyzing the information in an objective manner, utilizing several skills to evaluate, conceptualizing and synthesizing information. It is based on universal intellectual values such as clarity, precision, relevance and fairness. It refines beliefs based on experience in continuous fashion, problem identification, information gathering, data interpretation, and drawing conclusions. It is a lifelong endeavor aimed at enhancing reasoning abilities, overcoming biases and contributing to a more rational society.

4. **Creative thinking:** It is also known as creative problem-solving. It is the ability to generate innovative and novel answers to questions. The key characteristics of it are analytical skills, innovation and collaboration. Lateral thinking, brainstorming, mind mapping are the ways to enhance creative thinking. Convergent and divergent thinking are the two typical modes of creative thinking.[11]

5. **Logical thinking:** It provides sensible solutions based on the facts rather than emotions by means of application of reasoning strategies and analyzing the situations and scenarios. It is crucial for learning, communication, decision-making, problem-solving and critical thinking.[12, 13] It can be developed by techniques such as—practice conditional statements, through engagement in creative activities, learning new skill, use of picture cards. It has shown that logical thinking acts as a moderator between predictor and outcome variable.[14]

6. **Analytical thinking:** It is a process of breakdown of whole entity into individual portions and later to study these fragments and their associations. It consists of three aspects—differentiating,

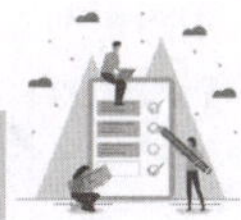
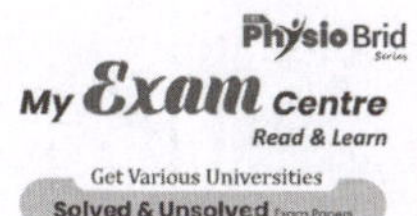

organizing and attributing respectively.[15] Various strategies can be employed to develop and enhance analytical skills such as observation of the surroundings by engagement of mind; book reading; learning how things work; asking questions; playing brain games; rationalizing decisions; beginning with clear framework; interdisciplinary analysis; engagement in active strategies.

IMPLICATIONS IN CLINICAL PRACTICE

Diagnostic Reasoning

Diagnostic reasoning involves understanding of neurological processes contributing toward clinical reasoning. It encompasses various forms, including pattern recognition, pathological reasoning, hypothetico-deductive (HD) reasoning.[16] The predictive brain model in diagnostic reasoning emphasizes the brain's adaptive, generative, energy-frugal, context-sensitive, probabilistic, and predictive nature in guiding diagnostic processes.[17] The nature of predictive processes across different contexts are shown in Figure 8.3.

The brain areas or neural correlates associated with pattern recognition form of diagnostic reasoning are temporal cortex, hippocampus and

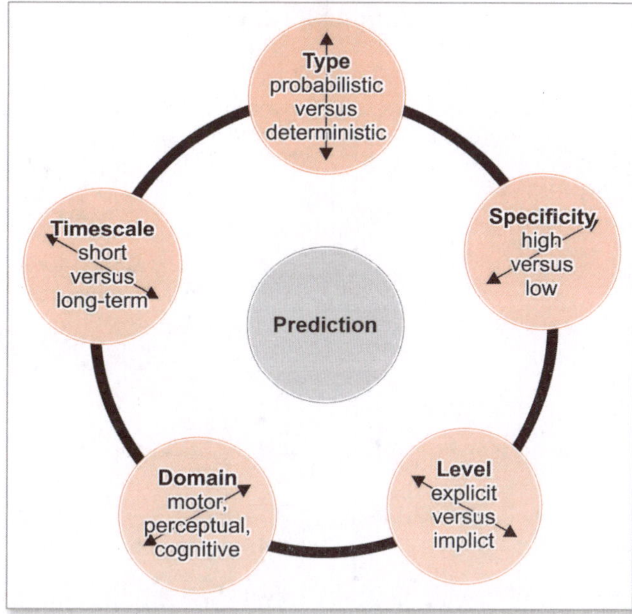

Fig. 8.3: Predictive processes[18]

basal ganglia, that are responsible for retrieval of previously learned information.[19] To identify patterns of symptoms in prompt way and matching them to probable diagnosis, an experienced clinician relies on pattern recognition.[20] Availability bias is a common limitation of pattern recognition that results in ignorance of lesser common diagnosis.[21] The process of HD reasoning involves formulation and testing of hypothesis through a systematic evaluation of patient information and evidence.[22] The neural correlates associated with it are prefrontal cortex, parietal cortex and anterior cingulate cortex.[19]

Treatment Decision-Making

Treatment decision-making involves various cognitive strategies and considerations that include data gathering, interpretation and evaluation to select an evidence-based decision as shown in the Figure 8.4. It includes several analyses to reach up to an appropriate decision making toward patient care.

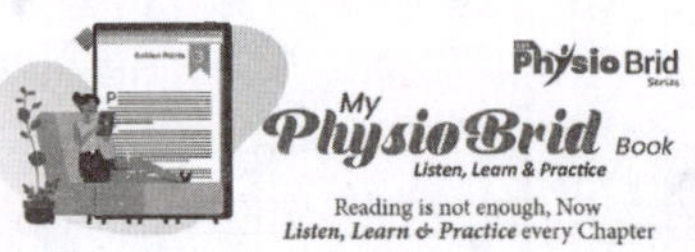

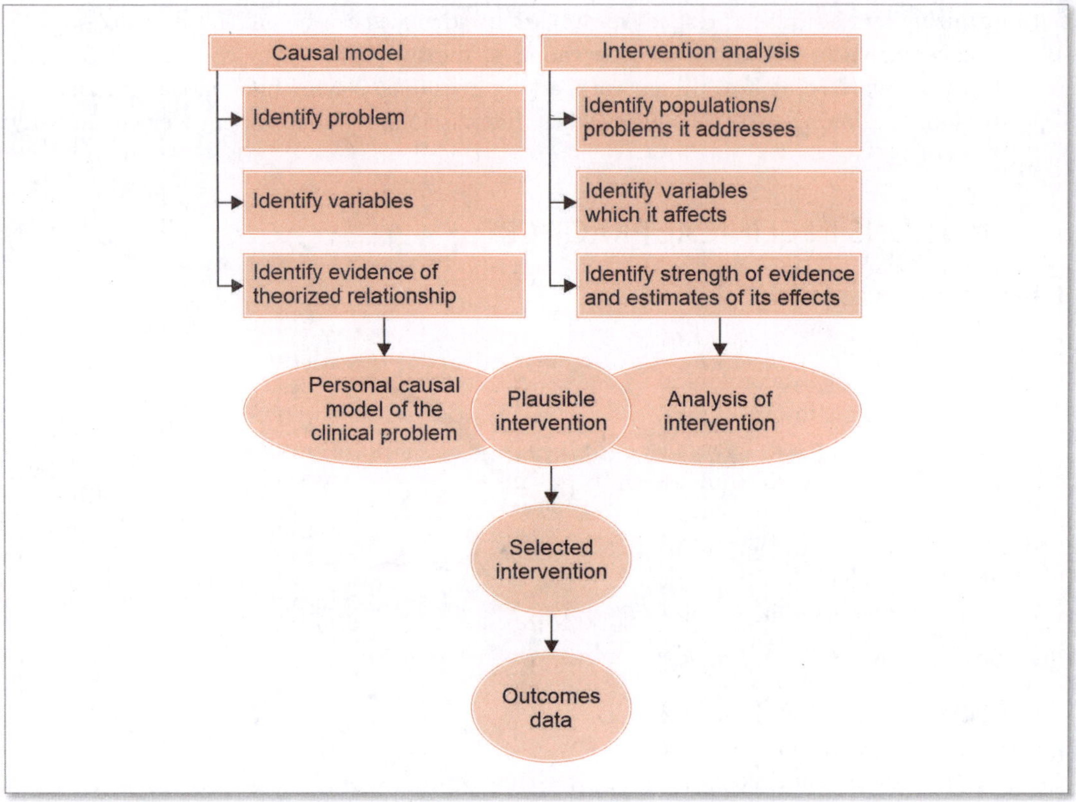

Fig. 8.4: Intervention selection process steps[23]

- **Risk assessment and benefit-risk analysis:** It involves emotional influences and shared decision-making. Emotion can influence risk assessment with amygdala playing a crucial role in it.[22] Adherence to treatment and outcomes can be improved by consideration of patient's preferences in decision-making.[24]

- **Evidence-based decision-making:** Integration of scientific evidence in form of latest research findings, clinical practice guidelines, and evidence-based recommendations into treatment decisions can improve patient outcomes.[20]

Clinical Reasoning

Clinical reasoning is a process by which the healthcare professionals collect cues, process the information, reach to an understanding of patient problem, plan and implement treatment protocols, evaluate outcomes, and reflection upon learning from the process. Figure 8.5 delineates the several types of clinical reasoning processes.

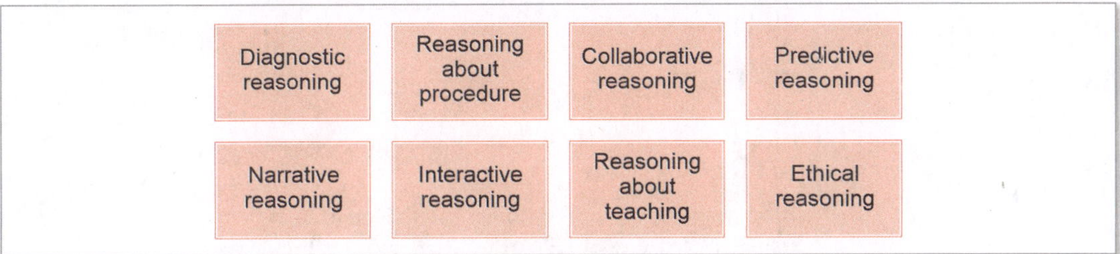

Fig. 8.5: Types of clinical reasoning

IMPROVEMENT STRATEGIES

The improvement in thinking skill is crucial for enhancement of cognitive performance, decision-making abilities, problem-solving capabilities and overall intellectual engagement. Various strategies have been proposed and studied to enhance different aspects of thinking, ranging from metacognitive strategies to cognitive training techniques.

Active Learning Techniques

Active learning techniques involve the direct engagement/participation in the tasks through discussions, problem-solving, case studies and demonstrations. The following strategies bolster the active learning techniques:

Problem-Based Learning

This approach encourages learners to solve complex, real-world problems, promoting deeper understanding and active engagement. Problem-based learning (PBL) is based upon the philosophy that the learning can be considered "constructive, self-directed, collaborative and contextual activity".[25] It is a small group teaching method that combines the knowledge acquisition with the origin of attitudes and generic skills as mentioned in the Table 8.5. Figure 8.6 displays the various steps of PBL. To define learning objectives, from the problem scenario, PBL uses several triggers (Table 8.6). In essence, PBL is an effective teaching learning method to impart education and it encourages the users to set their own learning goals.

Table 8.5: Generic skills and attitudes[26]

• Teamwork	• Cooperation
• Listening	• Appreciating colleagues' view
• Chairing a group	• Critical analysis of literature
• Recording	• Self-directed learning
• Use of resources	• Presentation skills

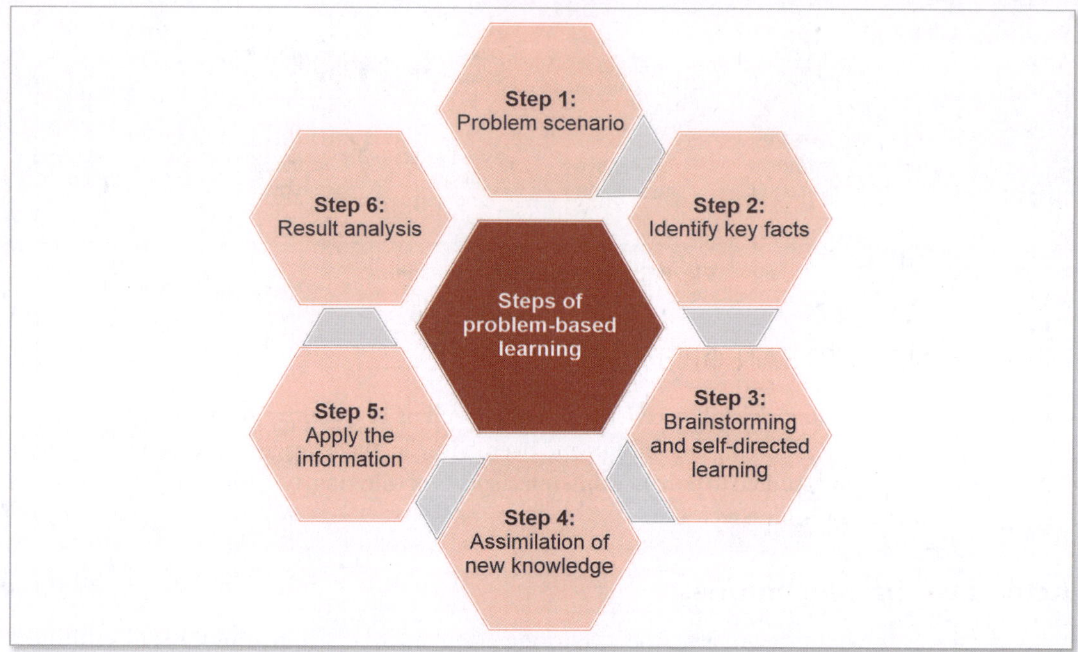

Fig. 8.6: Steps of problem-based learning

Table 8.6: Triggers for problem-based learning scenario in clinical settings[26]

• Photographs	• Family history
• Video clips	• A real or simulated environment
• Secondary data	• Excerpt from journal article
• Paper-based clinical scenarios	

Collaborative Learning (CL)

Working in groups enhances critical thinking by exposing individuals to diverse perspectives. For professional practice and training, understanding of an effective strategic collaborative learning is essential.[27] Collaboration is a mutual engagement in a coordinated fashion to achieve a common goal relating to the joint activity of participants.[28] Figure 8.7 reflects the various strategies of collaborative learning.

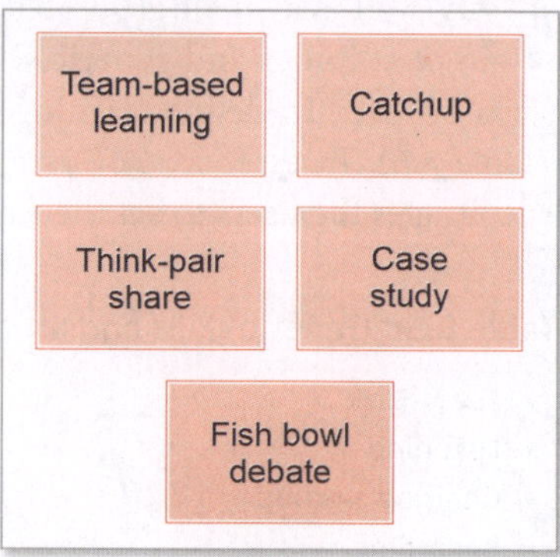

Fig. 8.7: Strategies of collaborative learning

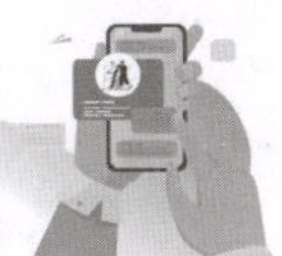
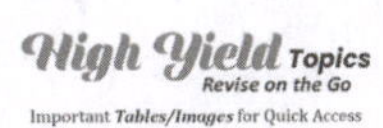

Metacognitive Strategies

Metacognition is the awareness and understanding of one's own thought processes. It involves planning, monitoring, and evaluating one's understanding and performance. The eight pillar model of metacognition as proposed by Drigas and Mitsea[29] is displayed in Figure 8.8 and is described below:

1. **Learning theory:** It integrates one's knowledge about cognition and its regulation. It was developed by John Flavell in the 1970s. He proposed four classes of metacognition:

    i.   Metacognitive knowledge

    ii. Metacognitive experiences

    iii. Tasks or goals

    iv. Strategies or activities.[30]

    It emphasizes the role of self-regulation and self-awareness in learning.

2. **Applying theory:** It can help learners gain awareness and control over thinking processes to learn more efficiently. By applying the principles of metacognition, one can enhance learning and problem-solving abilities.

3. **Self-observation:** It makes an individual to monitor their own progress, identify their strengths and weaknesses, and make ways to improve their performance.[31] It is of utmost importance in self-directed learning, where one can participate actively and thus promote awareness about thinking processes and empowerment toward learning. It improves learning outcomes and knowledge transfers to newer contexts as documented by the researchers.[31]

4. **Self-regulation:** It involves the ability to control and manage cognitive processes to achieve learning goals. The three main phases of self-regulated learning are:

    i.   Forethought (planning and goal setting)

    ii. Performance (actual learning tasks)

    iii. Self-reflection (evaluating and adjusting).

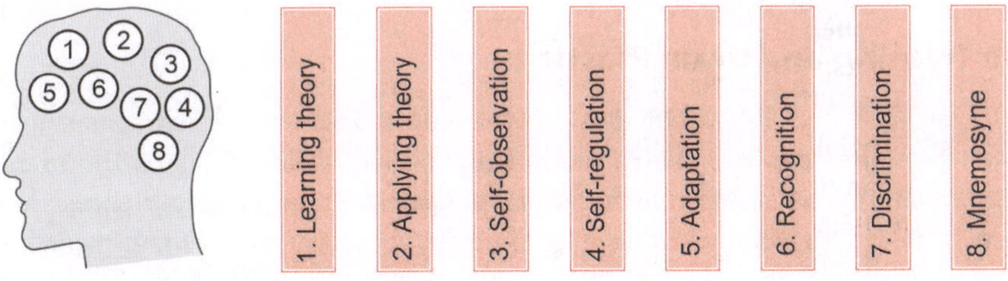

Fig. 8.8: The eight pillars of metacognition

5. **Adaptation:** It involves the ability to adjust and modify one's metacognitive strategies and skills in response to changing task demands or contexts.[32, 33] The key aspects of it includes:
   - Selecting and applying an appropriate metacognitive strategy to enhance performance on a task.
   - Adjusting metacognitive knowledge about one's strengths, weaknesses and the effectiveness of different strategies.
   - Regulating and controlling one's cognitive processes to optimize learning and problem-solving.
   - Transferring metacognitive skills learned in one context to new scenarios.

6. **Recognition:** It refers to the understanding of the patterns behind one's own thought processes. It is essential for effective learning and decision-making.

7. **Discrimination:** It refers to the ability to accurately assess one's own cognitive processes and performance, even in the absence of reliable first-order decision accuracy. It has implications for understanding the cognitive architecture underlying decision-making and self-awareness.

8. **Mnemosyne:** It refers to the "remembering of your real holistic total self and identity." It allows an individual to monitor and control their memory operations, i.e., memory capabilities and limitations.[29]

Self-Questioning

Encouraging learners to question their own knowledge and approach helps identify gaps in understanding. The key benefits of using this strategy are—encouraging metacognition, promoting deeper understanding, enhancing problem-solving skills and facilitating decision-making, improving learning and retention, developing self-awareness and self-regulation. Some examples of self-questioning prompts for decision making are:

- What are the potential outcomes of the treatment interventions? How do they align with the goals of rehabilitation?
- What are the potential risks and benefits of the intervention option? How can one mitigate the risks?

Cognitive Training and Brain Plasticity

Cognitive plasticity is defined as an individual internal potential under peculiar contextual scenarios.[34] The capacity to acquire cognitive skills/functions is known as plasticity.[35, 36] The brain possesses remarkable plasticity, allowing it to reorganize and adapt in response to experiences and training.[37] This plasticity can occur at different levels, including changes in metabolism, grey matter structure, white matter integrity, and functional brain activities such as EEG-derived biomarkers and resting-state functional connectivity (FC).[38] Building cognitive reserve through cognitive stimulation and training can potentially enhance thinking abilities and resilience against cognitive decline.[39] Cognitive training research has focused on improving cognitive processes such as processing

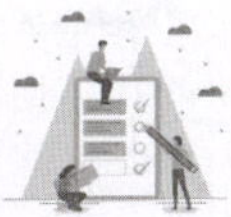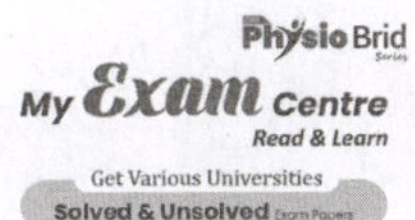

speed, inhibition, inductive reasoning, spatial orientation, episodic memory, fluid intelligence, and executive functioning.[34, 38] Cognitive training has been associated with increased grey matter volume and cortical volume in regions such as the prefrontal cortex, which is critical for executive control and fluid abilities.[40] Table 8.7 highlights various cognitive training techniques to improve thinking abilities.

Table 8.7: Cognitive training techniques

Technique	Description
Working memory technique	Engaging in activities that challenge and exercise working memory, such as dual n-back tasks and complex span tasks, can improve working memory capacity and fluid intelligence.[41]
Attention and processing speed training	These programs enhance the efficiency of attentional resource allocation and processing speed, decisive for various cognitive tasks and activities.[42]
Multimodal cognitive training	Cognitive-based computer training, physical exercises and noninvasive brain stimulation has been shown to enhance executive functions, planning and problem-solving, working memory.[43]

Mindfulness and Stress Reduction

These strategies enhance thinking abilities particularly in context to cognitive flexibility and self-regulation. Mindfulness reduces stress by allowing individuals to observe their thoughts and emotions without judgment, developing emotional regulation and better relaxation. Table 8.8 displays several key points:

Table 8.8: Key points of mindfulness

Key aspects	Description
Mindfulness-based stress reduction (MBSR)[44]	It reduces the relative weight of initial intuitions and facilitates deliberate thinking by improving cognitive reflection test scores.[45]
Cognitive reflection test scores (CRT)	It assesses the ability to override automatic responses and engage in more deliberate and analytical thinking.[45]
Mindfulness and self-compassion	It involves treating oneself with kindness and understanding.

Stress reduction techniques can mitigate the negative impact of stress on cognitive performance.[46]

PROBLEM SOLVING

Problem-solving is a cognitive process that involves identifying, analyzing, and solving problems. It is a fundamental skill in various aspects of life, from everyday challenges to complex professional tasks. Effective problem-solving often requires the application of strategies or techniques to reach a solution efficiently.

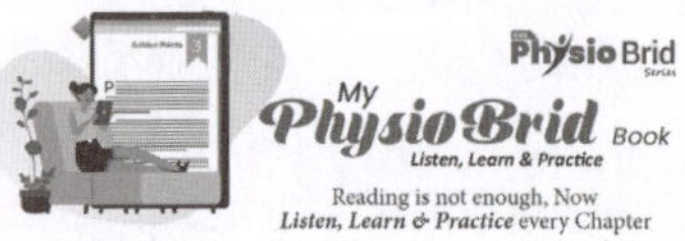

Algorithms

An algorithm is a step-by-step procedure or set of rules designed to solve a specific problem or perform a particular task. Figure 8.9 delineates the characteristics of an algorithm.

- **Divide and conquer algorithms:** Divide and Conquer is a problem-solving paradigm that involves breaking a complex problem into smaller subproblems, solving each subproblem independently, and then combining the solutions to obtain the final solution. It is widely used in various domains, including sorting algorithms (e.g., Merge Sort, Quick Sort), multiplying large numbers, and solving recurrence relations. The common examples using this approach are Strassen's algorithm for matrix multiplication, Karatsuba algorithm for fast multiplication of large numbers.

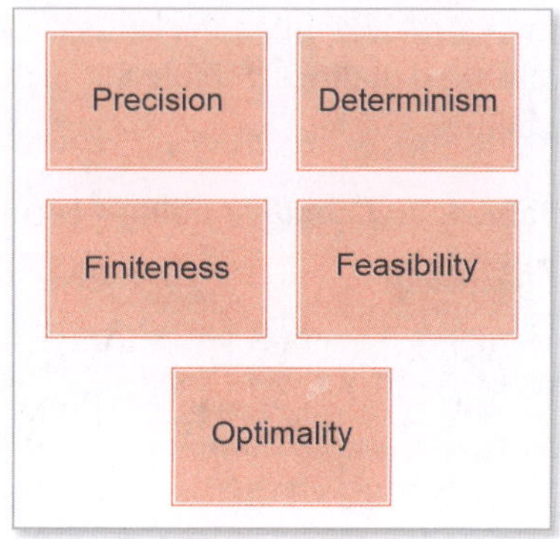

Fig. 8.9: Characteristics of algorithm

- **Dynamic programming algorithms:** It is a technique for solving complex problems by breaking them down into simpler subproblems, solving each subproblem once, and storing the solutions for later use, avoiding redundant calculations. It is widely used in optimization problems, such as the Knapsack Problem, Longest Common Subsequence, and Shortest Path problems.
- **Greedy algorithms:** It follows the principle of making locally optimal choices at each stage, with the hope of finding a global optimum solution. These are used in various optimization problems, such as scheduling, graph theory, and resource allocation problems, e.g., Huffman coding.

Heuristics

Heuristics are mental shortcuts or rules of thumb that simplify problem-solving by reducing the amount of information and cognitive effort required. Unlike algorithms, heuristics do not guarantee a solution and may lead to errors or suboptimal outcomes. However, they are valuable in situations where time and resources are limited, allowing individuals to make quick decisions based on incomplete information. Figure 8.10 delineates the characteristics of heuristics.

- **Hill climbing heuristic:** Hill climbing is a local search algorithm that starts with an initial solution and iteratively moves to a better solution in the neighborhood until no further improvements are possible. Hill climbing is used in various optimization problems, such as the Traveling Salesman Problem, scheduling problems, and machine learning tasks like training neural networks.

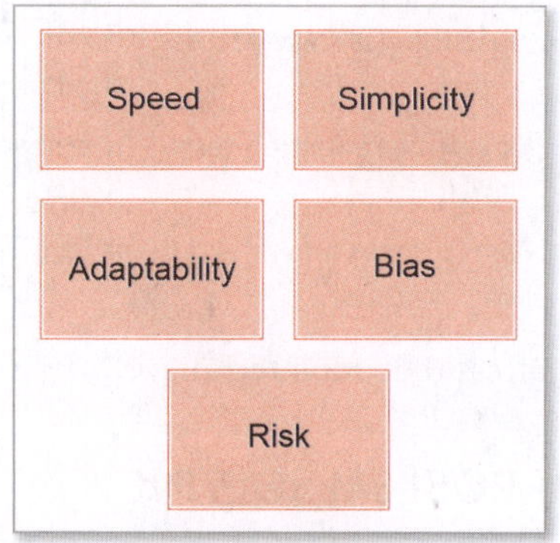

Fig. 8.10: Characteristics of heuristics

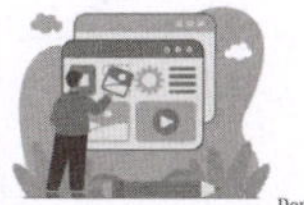

- **Simulated annealing heuristic:** Simulated annealing is a probabilistic technique that incorporates a controlled cooling schedule to escape local optima and explore the search space more thoroughly. It is widely used in various optimization problems, such as circuit design, protein folding, and scheduling problems.

MEMORY

Memory is a dynamic and complex process that allows individuals to retain and recall information over time.[47] It refers to the cognition processes involved in encoding of sensory input, the storage of encoded information and, the retrieval of stored information upon requirement.[48] It is influenced by various factors including attention, perception, emotion, and thinking strategies.

Neurobiology

It involves exploring the intricate neural mechanisms underlying the encoding, storage, and retrieval of information within the brain. Memory processes rely on the coordinated activity of various brain regions and neural circuits, each contributing to different aspects of memory formation and consolidation.

> **MUST KNOW**
>
> - **Hippocampus:** New memory formation
> - **Diencephalon:** Relaying and processing sensory information
> - **Midbrain:** Contributes in overall cognitive and motor tasks

Neuroanatomy

- **Hippocampus:** The hippocampus plays a central role in the formation and consolidation of declarative memories, including episodic and semantic memories.[49, 50] It is crucial for encoding new information and integrating it into existing memory networks. The hippocampus also supports spatial navigation and contextual memory processes.[51]
- **Amygdala:** The amygdala is involved in the processing of emotional memories and the modulation of memory consolidation. It plays a crucial role in encoding emotionally significant events and assigning emotional valence to memories, thereby influencing their subsequent retrieval and emotional salience.[52–54]
- **Prefrontal cortex:** The prefrontal cortex, particularly the dorsolateral prefrontal cortex (DLPFC) and ventromedial prefrontal cortex (vmPFC), is involved in executive functions, working memory, and the control of memory retrieval processes.[55] It modulates attention, cognitive control, and decision-making, influencing memory encoding and retrieval strategies.[56]
- **Medial temporal lobe:** The medial temporal lobe, including structures such as the hippocampus, entorhinal cortex, and perirhinal cortex, is critical for memory consolidation and the formation of long-term declarative memories.[57] It is involved in the transformation of short-term memories into stable long-term representations.[58]

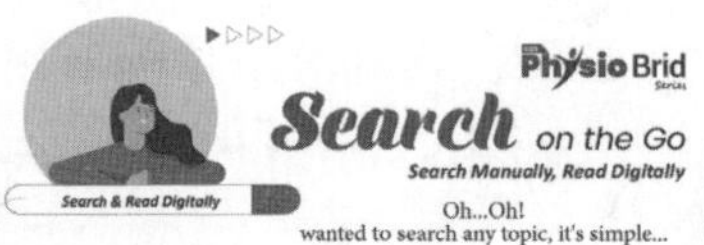

Physio CORNER

Exercise has a profound impact on memory and overall cognitive function. Here are several ways in which regular physical activity can enhance memory:

- **Increased blood flow to the brain:**
  - **Improved oxygen and nutrient delivery:** Exercise increases heart rate, which boosts blood flow to the brain. This improved circulation ensures that the brain receives more oxygen and nutrients, essential for optimal brain function.
  - **Neurovascular health:** Enhanced blood flow helps maintain the health of blood vessels in the brain, reducing the risk of vascular-related cognitive decline.

- **Neurogenesis (Growth of new neurons):**
  - **Hippocampal neurogenesis:** The hippocampus, a brain region crucial for memory formation, is one of the few areas in the brain where new neurons can grow throughout life. Regular aerobic exercise, such as running or swimming, stimulates the production of brain-derived neurotrophic factor (BDNF), a protein that supports the growth, survival, and differentiation of new neurons in the hippocampus.
  - **Enhanced memory formation:** The increase in new neurons in the hippocampus improves the brain's ability to form, retain, and recall memories.

- **Enhanced synaptic plasticity:**
  - **Strengthened neural connections:** Exercise promotes synaptic plasticity, which refers to the ability of synapses (the connections between neurons) to strengthen or weaken over time. This plasticity is crucial for learning and memory. Enhanced synaptic plasticity means that the brain can more effectively encode and retrieve information.
  - **Improved long-term potentiation (LTP):** LTP is a process that strengthens the connections between neurons, and it is essential for learning and memory. Exercise has been shown to enhance LTP, making it easier to learn and remember new information.

- **Reduction in inflammation and oxidative stress:**
  - **Anti-inflammatory effects:** Chronic inflammation can damage brain cells and impair memory. Exercise reduces systemic inflammation and helps maintain the health of brain cells, which is important for preserving memory.
  - **Decreased oxidative stress:** Exercise increases the production of antioxidants, which protect brain cells from oxidative stress (damage caused by free radicals). Lower oxidative stress helps preserve memory and cognitive function over time.

- **Improved mood and stress reduction:**
  - **Reduction in cortisol levels:** Chronic stress and elevated levels of the stress hormone cortisol can impair memory and lead to cognitive decline. Exercise helps regulate cortisol levels, reducing stress and its negative impact on memory.
  - **Enhanced mood:** Exercise stimulates the release of endorphins and other neurotransmitters like serotonin and dopamine, which improve mood and reduce anxiety and depression. Better mood and lower stress levels contribute to better memory performance.

- **Improved sleep quality:**
  - **Enhanced memory consolidation:** Exercise can improve the quality and duration of sleep. Sleep is crucial for memory consolidation, the process by which short-term memories are transformed into long-term memories. Regular physical activity helps ensure that you get enough deep sleep, during which memory consolidation occurs.

Contd...

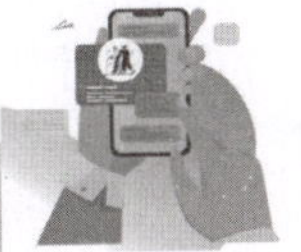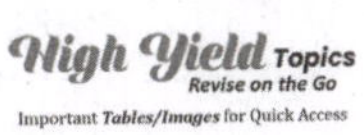

- **Regulation of sleep patterns:** Exercise helps regulate circadian rhythms, leading to more consistent and restful sleep patterns, which are vital for memory retention.
- **Cognitive reserve and brain resilience:**
  - **Increased cognitive reserve:** Cognitive reserve refers to the brain's ability to improvise and find alternative ways of functioning when faced with challenges like aging or disease. Regular exercise contributes to building cognitive reserve, which helps protect against age-related memory decline.
  - **Brain resilience:** Exercise helps the brain become more resilient to damage and age-related changes, reducing the risk of conditions like dementia that impair memory.
- **Stimulation of neurotransmitter production:**
  - **Increased levels of neurotransmitters:** Exercise boosts the production of neurotransmitters like acetylcholine, which is important for learning and memory. Higher levels of these neurotransmitters support better communication between neurons and improve memory processes.

Conclusion

Exercise enhances memory through a combination of biological, neurological, and psychological mechanisms. By increasing blood flow, promoting neurogenesis, enhancing synaptic plasticity, reducing inflammation, improving mood, and boosting sleep quality, exercise provides a comprehensive boost to cognitive health and memory function. Regular physical activity is thus a key factor in maintaining and improving memory across the lifespan.

Neurophysiology

- **Neural networks and pathways:**
  - **Hippocampal-diencephalic-midbrain circuit:** This circuit encompasses reciprocal connections between the hippocampus, thalamus, and midbrain structures, such as the substantia nigra (SN) and ventral tegmental area. It plays a crucial role in memory consolidation and reward-related learning processes.[59]
  - **Default mode network (DMN):** The default mode network, consisting of interconnected brain regions including the medial prefrontal cortex, posterior cingulate cortex, and hippocampus, is implicated in self-referential processing, autobiographical memory, and the resting-state brain activity associated with memory consolidation.[60] DMN bolsters the episodic memory in cognitively unimpaired older individuals.[61]

> **MUST KNOW**
>
> **Default mode network (DMN) supports:**
> - Memory formation
> - Memory retrieval
> - Memory consolidation
> - Memory disturbances
> - Memory and self-reference

- **Molecular mechanisms:**
  - **Long-term potentiation (LTP):** LTP is a cellular mechanism underlying synaptic plasticity and memory formation. It involves the strengthening of synaptic connections between neurons in response to repeated stimulation, leading to enhanced synaptic transmission and the consolidation of memory traces.[62, 63]

- **Neurotransmitter systems:** Modulation of synaptic transmission and synaptic plasticity underlying memory processes is done by neurotransmitter systems, including dopamine, glutamate, acetylcholine. They regulate the strength and efficacy of neuronal connections involved in memory encoding, consolidation, and retrieval.[64]

TYPES OF MEMORY

In the context of psychology, memory is a complex process involving multiple stages and types. Figure 8.11 shows different types of memory.

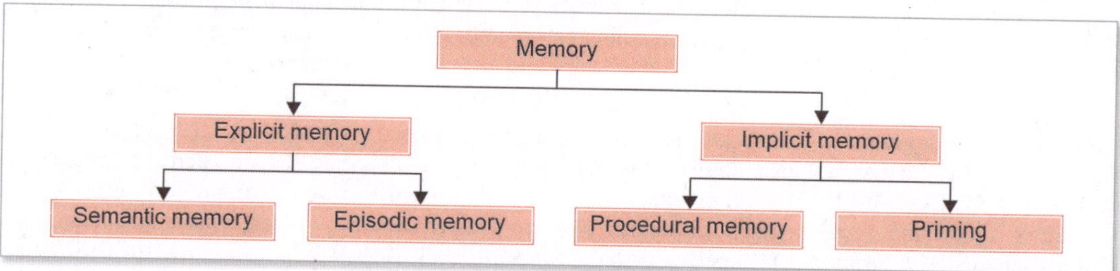

Fig. 8.11: Types of memory

Explicit Memory

Explicit memory is also known as declarative memory. It involves conscious recall of knowledge and experiences.

- **Semantic memory:** It stores general knowledge and factual information such as vocabulary, concepts and facts.
- **Episodic memory:** It stores personal experiences and events, such as autobiographical memories of specific times and places.

Implicit Memory

Implicit memory is also known as nondeclarative memory. It refers to the unconscious retention and influence of past experiences on present behavior and performance.

- **Procedural memory:** Memory for knowledge of skills and procedures and their execution.
- **Priming:** Facilitation of processing due to prior exposure.

STAGES OF MEMORY

The Atkinson and Shiffrin three-stage model of memory outlines the following stages:

1. **Sensory memory:** The beginning stage where sensory information is stored for a succinct period, usually less than a second. This stage helps in processing and retaining sensory information.

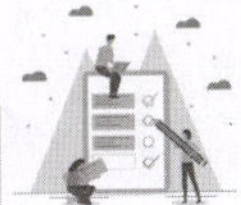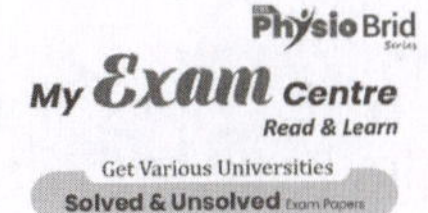

- **Iconic memory:** It refers to the sensory memory responsible for visual information. It allows individuals to retain visual images for a brief duration, typically less than one second.

- **Echoic memory:** It refers to the sensory memory responsible for auditory information. It enables individuals to retain auditory stimuli, such as spoken words or sounds, for a short period, typically up to a few seconds.

2. **Short-term memory (STM):** It is also known as working memory, temporarily stores information for immediate processing and manipulation. It has limited capacity and duration, typically holding information for up to 20–30 seconds unless rehearsed or transferred to long-term memory.

> **MUST KNOW**
>
> **Millers law:**
> - Also known as Magical Number Seven, Plus or Minus Two
> - Average person can hold seven items in their working memory.

3. **Long-term memory (LTM):** Long-term memory is the system responsible for the storage of information over extended periods, ranging from minutes to a lifetime. It has virtually unlimited capacity and can retain vast amounts of knowledge and experiences.

LTM includes:

- Explicit memory
- Implicit memory
- This model highlights how information flows through and is processed in these three distinct stages to form and retain memories.

FACTORS INFLUENCING MEMORY

Memory, as a cognitive function, is influenced by a variety of factors that can either enhance or impair the ability to encode, store, and retrieve information. Here are the key factors influencing memory from a psychological perspective:

- **Attention and focus:**
  - **Selective attention:** Memory is highly dependent on the level of attention given to information at the time of encoding. If attention is divided or distracted, encoding is less effective, leading to weaker memory formation.
  - **Sustained attention:** The ability to maintain focus over time also affects memory. Prolonged attention during learning improves the depth of encoding, making it easier to recall information later.

- **Emotion:**
  - **Emotional arousal:** Emotionally charged events tend to be remembered more vividly and accurately than neutral events. This is because emotions trigger the release of stress hormones like adrenaline and cortisol, which can enhance memory consolidation.
  - **Mood congruence:** The emotional state during encoding and retrieval can influence memory. People tend to recall information better when their mood at retrieval matches their mood during encoding (mood-congruent memory).

- **Repetition and practice:**
    - **Rehearsal:** Repeated exposure to information through rehearsal strengthens memory traces. Techniques like spaced repetition, where information is reviewed at increasing intervals, are particularly effective in enhancing long-term memory.
    - **Overlearning:** Continuing to practice information even after it has been initially learned can further consolidate it, making it more resistant to forgetting.
- **Association and context:**
    - **Contextual cues:** Memory is often influenced by the context in which information is learned. Context-dependent memory suggests that recalling information is easier when the context at retrieval matches the context at encoding.
    - **State-dependent memory:** Similar to context, the internal state (such as mood, environment or physiological condition) during encoding can affect recall. For instance, information learnt while in a particular mood is more easily recalled when the individual is in the same mood again.
- **Organization and chunking:**
    - **Organization:** Information that is well-organized and structured is easier to encode and recall. Organizing information into categories, hierarchies or using mnemonic devices can significantly enhance memory.
    - **Chunking:** Grouping individual pieces of information into larger, meaningful units (chunks) helps to overcome the limitations of short-term memory, making it easier to remember complex information.
- **Sleep:**
    - **Memory consolidation:** Sleep plays a critical role in consolidating memories. During sleep, especially during rapid eye movement (REM) and slow-wave sleep, the brain processes and integrates newly learned information, transferring it from short-term to long-term memory.
    - **Sleep deprivation:** Lack of sleep impairs the ability to form new memories and consolidate existing ones, leading to memory deficits.
- **Stress and anxiety:**
    - **Acute stress:** Moderate levels of acute stress can enhance memory, particularly for emotionally relevant information. However, excessive stress can have the opposite effect, disrupting encoding and recall.
    - **Chronic stress:** Long-term stress and anxiety can impair memory by affecting the hippocampus, a brain region essential for memory formation. High levels of cortisol, a stress hormone, can damage neural connections in the hippocampus over time.
- **Age:**
    - **Developmental stage:** Memory abilities change across the lifespan. Children and young adults tend to have stronger memory capabilities due to more robust neural plasticity. Memory typically declines with age, particularly in older adults, as cognitive processes slow down and neurodegenerative changes occur.

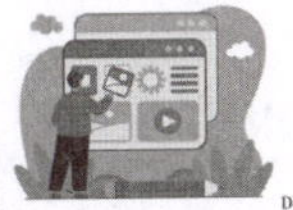

- **Age-related memory decline:** Age-related factors, such as changes in the brain's structure (e.g., hippocampal shrinkage) and function, can lead to difficulties with both short-term and long-term memories.
- **Cognitive load:**
  - **Information overload:** The amount of information processed at one time can impact memory. When the cognitive load is too high, it becomes difficult to encode all information effectively, leading to poorer recall.
  - **Working memory capacity:** The capacity of working memory or the ability to hold and manipulate information in mind over short periods, can influence how well information is remembered. Individuals with greater working memory capacity can handle more complex tasks and encode information more effectively.
- **Nutrition and health:**
  - **Diet:** Nutrition affects brain health and memory. Diets rich in antioxidants, healthy fats, and nutrients like omega-3 fatty acids, vitamins, and minerals are associated with better cognitive function and memory.
  - **Exercise:** Regular physical activity promotes neurogenesis (growth of new neurons) and improves memory by enhancing brain plasticity and reducing inflammation.
  - **Medical conditions:** Conditions such as depression, diabetes, and cardiovascular disease can negatively impact memory. Additionally, neurodegenerative diseases like Alzheimer's directly impair memory function.
- **Substance use:**
  - **Alcohol:** Excessive alcohol consumption can lead to memory impairments, particularly affecting short-term memory and the ability to form new memories (a phenomenon known as blackout).
  - **Drugs:** Certain drugs, especially those that are psychoactive, can alter memory processes. For example, benzodiazepines can impair memory encoding and retrieval, while stimulants may temporarily enhance certain aspects of memory.
- **Social and environmental factors:**
  - **Social interaction:** Engaging in social activities and maintaining social connections can boost memory, particularly in older adults. Social interaction stimulates cognitive processes and provides emotional support, which is beneficial for memory.
  - **Environmental enrichment:** Environments rich in stimuli, such as learning new skills, exposure to varied experiences, and engaging in mentally challenging activities, can enhance memory and protect against cognitive decline.
- **Motivation and interest:**
  - **Personal relevance:** Information that is personally relevant or interesting to the individual is more likely to be remembered. The level of motivation to remember something also influences how effectively it is encoded and recalled.

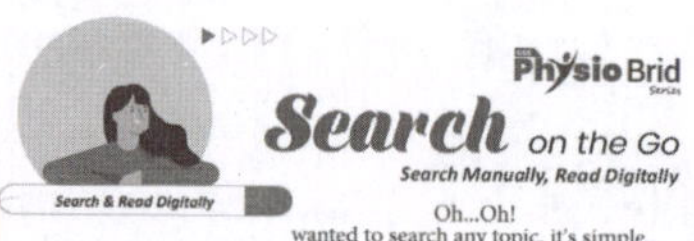

- **Goal-oriented learning:** When learning is tied to specific goals or outcomes, individuals are more likely to engage deeply with the material, leading to better memory retention.

Memory is a complex cognitive function influenced by a variety of factors, ranging from biological and psychological to social and environmental. Understanding these factors can help in developing strategies to improve memory and mitigate memory-related challenges. Factors influencing memory are given in Table 8.9.

Table 8.9: Factors influencing memory

Extrinsic factors	Intrinsic factors
• Meaningfulness of material • Amount of material • Time required to vocalize response • Distractions	• Age • Maturity • Will to learn • Interest and attention • Intelligence • Rest and sleep • Medical conditions

MODELS OF MEMORY

These frameworks are required to better understand the mechanism of memory processing and storage in the human brain. There are several models that have been developed to explain different aspects of memory:

- **Atkinson-Shiffrin Model (1968)[65]:** It is often referred to as "modal model" and has three distinct components:
    i. **Sensory store:** Where sensory information initially enters memory.
    ii. **Short-term store (Working memory):** Temporary holding of information; it allows for manipulation and rehearsals.
    iii. **Long-term store:** Indefinite storage of memory.
- **Levels of processing model (Craik – Lockhart)[66]:** It provides a set of oriented attitudes purely from memory input or encoding end. Two types of levels of processing have been described:
    i. **Shallow processing:** Focuses on superficial features of information.
    ii. **Deep processing:** Involves deeper semantic processing and further expressive acquaintances.
- **Baddeley's model of working memory[67]:** It is a multimodal system with individual function. It depicts as the following in the brain.
    - **Central executive:** Prefrontal cortex manages attention and regulates the flow of message.
    - **Phonological loop:** Broca's and Wernicke's area process auditory information.
    - **Episodic buffer:** Parietal lobe stores information related to particular event.
    - **Visuospatial sketchpad:** Occipital Lobe processes visual and spatial information.

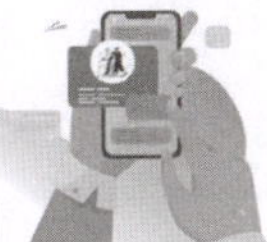
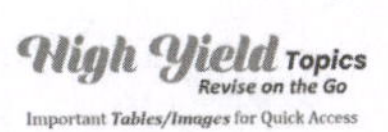

- **Serial-parallel independent model of memory:**
  - **Serial processing:** Processing of information in a sequential fashion.
  - **Parallel processing:** Simultaneous processing of multiple pieces of information.
- **Memory NEoStructural Inter-Systemic model (MNESIS)[68]:** It comprises five memory systems, highlighting interactions between semantic and episodic memory systems.

MEMORY ASSESSMENT

Memory assessment typically measures different aspects and types of memory. The common memory tests are shown in the Figure 8.12.

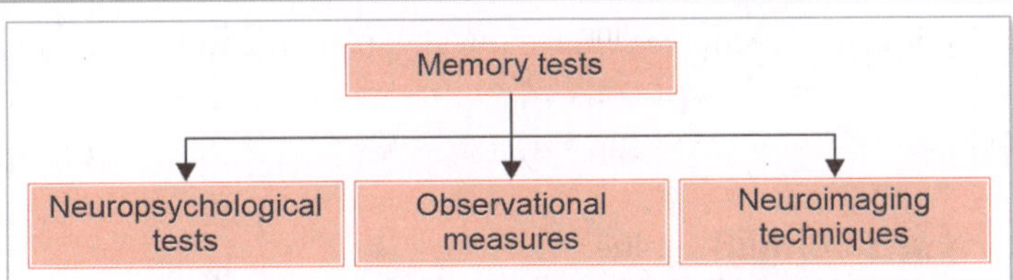

Fig. 8.12: Standardized memory assessment tests

Neuropsychological Tests

It includes:

- **Wechsler Memory Scale (WMS)[69]:** It assesses various aspects of memory function, including verbal, visual and working memory respectively.

  WMS consists of:
  - Digit span
  - Logical memory
  - Visual reproduction
- **California Verbal Learning Technique (CVLT)[70]:** It assesses verbal learning and memory by presenting a list of words for immediate recall, followed by delayed recall and recognition trials.
- **Rivermead Behavioral Memory Test (RBMT)[71]:** It assesses memory abilities relevant to everyday function.

  RBMT consists of:
  - Story recall
  - Face recognition
  - Route finding

Observational Measures

Observational measures include qualitative assessment of memory function by providing valuable insights into functional memory abilities.

- **Cognitive assessment of memory and problem solving (CAMPS)[72]:** It assesses memory and problem-solving abilities in everyday situations, such as preparation of meals and management of finances. It is used to identify cognitive impairments, to diagnose conditions such as dementia, traumatic brain injuries, to guide treatments and rehabilitation protocols.

- **Direct observation of functional abilities (DOFA)**[73]: It is used to assess functional abilities by observing individuals performing their activities of daily living. It is particularly useful in individuals with Parkinson's disease.

Neuroimaging Techniques

Functional Magnetic Resonance Imaging (fMRI) and Positron Emission Tomography (PET) provide insights into the neural correlates of memory function. The use of fMRI & PET has contributed to better understanding of memory processes and its related disorders, such as Alzheimer's disease.

Physio CORNER

Memory can be impaired in various medical conditions, affecting different aspects of memory, such as short-term, long-term, and working memory. Below are some key medical conditions where memory impairment is commonly observed:

Condition	Features
1. Alzheimer's disease	• **Type:** Neurodegenerative disease. • **Memory impact:** Alzheimer's is characterized by progressive memory loss, starting with short-term memory and eventually affecting long-term memory and other cognitive functions. Patients often struggle with remembering recent events, names, and places, while older memories may be preserved longer. • **Associated symptoms:** Confusion, disorientation, language difficulties, and impaired reasoning.
2. Dementia (Other forms)	• **Types:** Includes vascular dementia, Lewy body dementia (LBD), frontotemporal dementia, etc. • **Memory impact:** Each type of dementia affects memory differently. For example, vascular dementia may cause sudden memory lapses due to strokes or blockages in blood vessels, while frontotemporal dementia may initially affect behavior and language before memory. • **Associated symptoms:** Depending on the type, symptoms can include difficulties with problem-solving, planning, judgment, and language.
3. Traumatic brain injury (TBI)	• **Type:** Physical injury to the brain. • **Memory impact:** TBI can cause both retrograde amnesia (loss of pre-injury memories) and anterograde amnesia (inability to form new memories). The severity and location of the injury determine the extent of memory loss. • **Associated symptoms:** Cognitive impairments, emotional disturbances, headaches, and physical disabilities.

Contd...

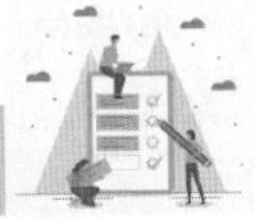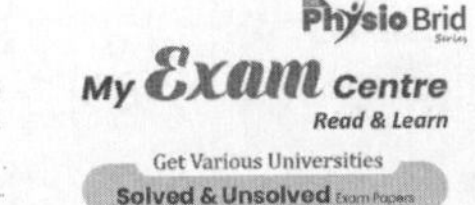

Condition	Features
4. Stroke	• **Type:** Disruption of blood flow to the brain. • **Memory impact:** Strokes can lead to memory loss, particularly if the areas of the brain involved in memory, such as the hippocampus or frontal lobes, are affected. Memory impairment can be specific to the type of information, such as verbal or visual memory. • **Associated symptoms:** Depending on the stroke's location, symptoms may include paralysis, speech difficulties, vision problems, and impaired cognitive functions.
5. Epilepsy	• **Type:** Neurological disorder characterized by recurrent seizures. • **Memory impact:** Repeated seizures, especially those originating in the temporal lobes (where the hippocampus is located), can impair memory. Postictal confusion (confusion following a seizure) often includes memory lapses. • **Associated symptoms:** Seizures, mood swings, and cognitive impairments.
6. Parkinson's disease	• **Type:** Neurodegenerative disorder. • **Memory impact:** Parkinson's disease can lead to memory problems, particularly in the later stages. Memory impairment is often related to difficulties with retrieval and working memory rather than encoding. • **Associated symptoms:** Motor symptoms such as tremors, rigidity, and bradykinesia, as well as cognitive decline and mood disorders.
7. Multiple sclerosis (MS)	• **Type:** Autoimmune disease affecting the central nervous system. • **Memory impact:** MS can lead to memory problems, particularly with working memory and short-term memory. These issues are often related to the cognitive fatigue that MS patients experience. • **Associated symptoms:** Physical symptoms like muscle weakness and coordination issues, as well as cognitive symptoms like attention deficits and executive function impairments.
8. Depression	• **Type:** Mood disorder. • **Memory impact:** Depression is associated with difficulties in concentrating, retaining information, and recalling memories. Memory issues in depression are often related to reduced motivation and attention, impacting both short-term and long-term memory. • **Associated symptoms:** Persistent sadness, fatigue, loss of interest, and changes in sleep and appetite.
9. Anxiety disorders	• **Type:** Mental health conditions including generalized anxiety disorder (GAD), panic disorder, etc. • **Memory impact:** Chronic anxiety can impair memory, particularly working memory, due to constant distraction and hyperarousal. The stress associated with anxiety can also affect the ability to encode and retrieve memories. • **Associated symptoms:** Excessive worry, restlessness, irritability, and physical symptoms like increased heart rate.

Contd...

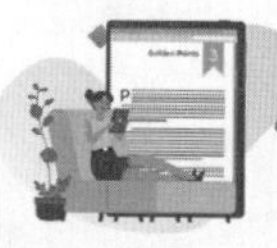
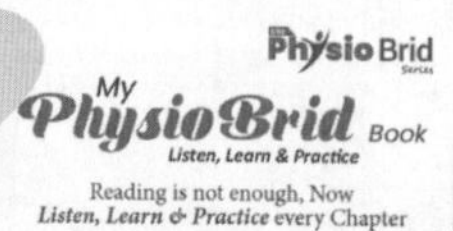

Condition	Features
10. Schizophrenia	• **Type:** Severe mental disorder characterized by delusions, hallucinations, and cognitive impairments. • **Memory impact:** Schizophrenia often involves impairments in working memory, episodic memory (recalling personal experiences), and executive functions. Patients may have difficulty organizing and retrieving memories. • **Associated symptoms:** Hallucinations, delusions, disorganized thinking, and impaired social functioning.
11. Substance abuse	• **Type:** Chronic use of drugs or alcohol. • **Memory impact:** Long-term substance abuse, particularly of alcohol (leading to conditions like Wernicke-Korsakoff syndrome), can cause significant memory impairments. These can include blackouts, difficulty forming new memories, and long-term cognitive decline. • **Associated symptoms:** Dependency, withdrawal symptoms, and social and occupational impairments.
12. Hypothyroidism	• **Type:** Endocrine disorder. • **Memory impact:** An underactive thyroid gland can lead to memory problems, particularly with short-term memory. The cognitive effects of hypothyroidism are thought to be reversible with proper treatment. • **Associated symptoms:** Fatigue, weight gain, depression, and cold intolerance.
13. Chronic fatigue syndrome (CFS)	• **Type:** Complex disorder characterized by extreme fatigue. • **Memory impact:** Individuals with CFS often experience "brain fog", which includes memory lapses, difficulty concentrating, and impaired executive function. • **Associated symptoms:** Severe, unexplained fatigue, sleep disturbances, and pain.
14. Sleep disorders	• **Type:** Includes conditions like insomnia, sleep apnea, and narcolepsy. • **Memory impact:** Poor sleep quality, especially lack of REM sleep, can impair memory consolidation, leading to difficulties in both short-term and long-term memory. • **Associated symptoms:** Excessive daytime sleepiness, mood disturbances, and cognitive impairments.
15. Nutritional deficiencies	• **Type:** Deficiencies in vitamins and minerals, such as vitamin B_{12}. • **Memory impact:** Deficiencies, especially in vitamin B_{12}, can lead to memory problems and cognitive decline. Severe deficiencies may result in conditions like Wernicke-Korsakoff syndrome, characterized by significant memory impairments. • **Associated symptoms:** Fatigue, weakness, neurological symptoms, and anemia.

Contd...

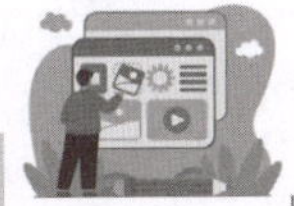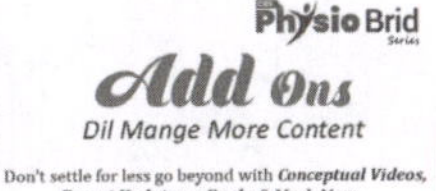

Condition	Features
16. Infectious diseases	• **Type:** Infections that affect the brain, such as meningitis, encephalitis or HIV-associated neurocognitive disorder (HAND). • **Memory impact:** Infections of the central nervous system can lead to acute or chronic memory impairments, depending on the severity and location of the infection. • **Associated symptoms:** Fever, headaches, confusion, and neurological deficits.
17. Brain tumors	• **Type:** Abnormal growth of brain cells. • **Memory impact:** Tumors, depending on their location in the brain, can impair memory by disrupting normal brain function. Tumors in the temporal lobe, where the hippocampus is located, are particularly likely to affect memory. • **Associated symptoms:** Headaches, seizures, vision problems, and cognitive changes.

MEMORY BUILDING TECHNIQUES

Memory building techniques are enhancement strategies and practices for memory encoding, storage and retrieval. The memory building techniques highlighted below are proven to be effective in memory enhancement across different population and ages.

- **Cognitive stimulation therapy (CST):** Engaging in structured activities like puzzles, word games, and group discussions to enhance cognitive function.

- **Reminiscence therapy:** Using photos, music or familiar objects to trigger past memories and improve mood.

- **Memory aids:** Utilizing tools such as sticky notes, calendars, labeled objects, and voice assistants to support memory recall.

- **Spaced repetition:** Reviewing information at increasing intervals over time to strengthen long-term retention.

- **Visualization and association:** Creating mental images or linking new information to existing knowledge, such as the Method of Loci (memory palace).

- **Chunking:** Breaking large pieces of information into smaller, manageable units for better recall (e.g., grouping numbers in a phone number).

- **Mnemonics:** Using acronyms, rhymes or phrases to encode information (e.g., "PEMDAS" for math operations).

- **Repetition and routine:** Reinforcing information and maintaining consistent daily routines to reduce cognitive load and confusion.

- **Sensory stimulation:** Triggering recall through familiar smells, sounds or tactile objects.

- **Errorless learning:** Teaching new skills or information by minimizing mistakes during practice to strengthen correct recall pathways.

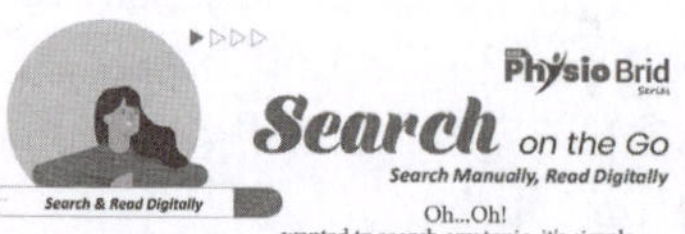

- **Elaborative rehearsal:** Connecting new information to existing knowledge by asking "how" and "why" to deepen understanding.
- **Active recall:** Testing oneself frequently instead of passively reviewing notes to strengthen memory pathways.
- **Mindfulness and relaxation techniques:** Reducing stress through deep breathing, meditation or yoga to enhance focus and memory retention.
- **Sleep optimization:** Consolidating memories through adequate and quality sleep, with naps aiding memory retention.
- **Physical exercise:** Engaging in regular aerobic exercise to improve blood flow to the brain and enhance cognitive health.
- **Healthy diet:** Consuming brain-boosting foods like omega-3-rich fish, leafy greens, nuts, and berries to support cognitive health.
- **Storytelling and teaching:** Explaining what you have learned to someone else to reinforce understanding and recall.
- **Music therapy:** Listening to familiar songs or melodies to stimulate emotional and cognitive responses.
- **Technology support:** Using apps like Anki, Quizlet, Lumosity or MindMate for memory-focused exercises and reminders.
- **Memory journaling:** Writing down important information repeatedly to reinforce learning and memory retention.
- **Social interaction:** Participating in group activities and meaningful conversations to stimulate cognition and maintain mental well-being.
- **Occupational therapy:** Developing strategies to compensate for memory challenges and maintain daily functioning.
- **Pharmacological interventions:** Using medications like Donepezil or Memantine to slow cognitive decline, particularly in dementia.

MUST KNOW

- **Mnemonics:** Acronyms and acrostics
- **Visualization and imagery:** Method of Loci or memory palaces
- **Chunking:** Grouping by meaning and recoding
- **Spaced repetition:** Spaced learning and flashcards

PRACTICAL ASPECT

Physiotherapy plays a significant role in enhancement of memory, typically in individuals with dementia or mild cognitive impairments. Memory improvement is due to several mechanisms after physiotherapy as described below.

- **Maintaining Familiar Movement Patterns:** It can aid in retaining procedural memory related to motor skills. This is achieved by ensuring therapeutic atmosphere, providing consistency and familiarity allowing patients to perform movements they are accustomed to.[74]

- **Exercise and physical activity:** Aerobic exercises (AE) have proven to be beneficial in enhancement of memory performance. AE stimulate the production of brain-derived neurotrophic factor (BDNF), responsible for growth of neurons and promotion of synaptic plasticity.[75]

- **Functional training:** Exercises mimicking activities of daily living in individuals with dementia can improve their memory skills and enhance their quality of life.[76]

CASE STUDY

Patient Details
Name: Margaret Thompson
Age: 78 years
Gender: Female
Occupation: Retired school teacher
Living situation: Resides with her husband, who is her primary caregiver

Chief Complaint
Progressive memory declines over the past 2 years, impacting daily functioning and straining family relationships.

Presenting Symptoms
- **Short-term memory impairment:**
  - Frequent forgetting of recent conversations.
  - Repeatedly asking the same questions.
- **Difficulty with daily tasks:**
  - Forgetting appointments.
  - Misplacing items regularly.
- **Cognitive and functional decline:**
  - Challenges in maintaining independence in daily activities.
- **Social and emotional impact:**
  - Remains socially active but increasing memory issues have caused stress within her marital relationship.

Additional Information
Despite her memory challenges, Margaret enjoys gardening, reading, and spending time with her grandchildren. Her family is concerned about the impact of her memory loss on her safety and overall quality of life. They have sought professional intervention to explore strategies for improving her memory and preserving her cognitive abilities.

Contd...

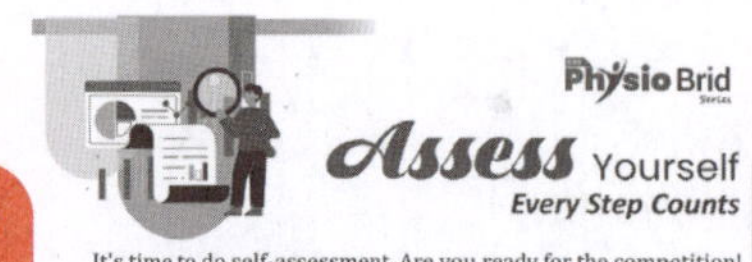

Assessment

Before starting the intervention, Margaret underwent a comprehensive cognitive assessment using standardized tools, such as the Mini-Mental State Examination (MMSE) and the Montreal Cognitive Assessment (MoCA). These assessments confirmed a diagnosis of mild-to-moderate Alzheimer's disease, with particular deficits in short-term memory, attention, and executive functioning.

Intervention Plan: Memory Improvement Strategies

- **Cognitive stimulation therapy (CST):**
  - **Objective:** To engage Margaret in mentally stimulating activities that target memory, language, and executive functioning, helping to slow cognitive decline and improve memory.
  - **Sessions:** Twice-weekly group sessions, each lasting 45–60 minutes, over a 14-week period.
  - **Activities:**
    - *Word games and puzzles:* Activities like word searches, crossword puzzles, and memory matching games to stimulate verbal memory and recall.
    - *Discussion groups:* Conversations on various topics, such as current events or Margaret's personal interests, to encourage memory retrieval and social interaction.
    - *Orientation exercises:* Tasks that involve recalling the date, time, and place, to reinforce temporal and spatial orientation.

- **Memory aids and external strategies:**
  - **Objective:** To help Margaret compensate for memory loss by using external aids and strategies that support daily functioning.
  - **Tools:**
    - *Memory notebook:* A daily planner where Margaret records important information, such as appointments, tasks, and reminders. This notebook also includes a section for journaling, where she can write about her day to reinforce memory through reflection.
    - *Medication management:* A pill organizer labeled with days of the week, coupled with alarm reminders on her phone, to ensure she takes her medication on time.
    - *Visual cues:* Placing labels on cabinets and drawers around the house to help Margaret find items more easily.

- **Errorless learning:**
  - **Objective:** To help Margaret learn and retain new information by minimizing errors during the learning process, thus reducing frustration and reinforcing correct responses.
  - **Techniques:**
    - *Step-by-step guidance:* When teaching new tasks or routines, Margaret was guided through each step without being given the opportunity to make errors. For example, if learning a new phone number, she would be provided with prompts and support until she could recall it correctly without mistakes.
    - *Spaced retrieval:* Margaret practiced recalling information over gradually increasing intervals of time. For example, she would learn a name and then be asked to recall it after 1 minute, 5 minutes, 15 minutes, and so on.

- **Reminiscence therapy:**
  - **Objective:** To stimulate memory by encouraging Margaret to recall and talk about past experiences, which can strengthen cognitive connections and improve mood.

Contd...

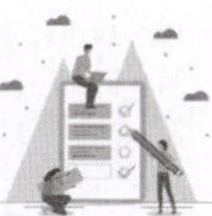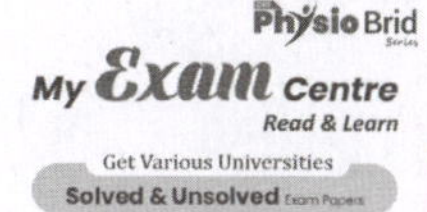

- **Sessions:** Weekly individual sessions with a therapist, focusing on specific themes, such as childhood memories, important life events, and family history.
- **Activities:**
  - *Photo albums:* Reviewing old photographs and discussing the events and people in them.
  - *Music therapy:* Listening to and singing along with music from Margaret's past, which has been shown to evoke strong memories and emotional responses.

- **Physical activity and lifestyle modifications:**
  - **Objective:** To enhance brain health and memory through regular physical activity, a balanced diet, and stress reduction.
  - **Exercise program:** Margaret was encouraged to participate in daily walks and light exercise routines designed to improve circulation and overall cognitive health.
  - **Diet:** Emphasis was placed on a Mediterranean diet rich in fruits, vegetables, whole grains, and healthy fats, which are linked to better cognitive functioning.
  - **Sleep hygiene:** Establishing a consistent sleep routine to ensure Margaret gets enough restorative sleep, which is essential for memory consolidation.

Outcomes and Progress

- **Improvement in memory function:** Margaret demonstrated noticeable improvements in recalling daily activities and managing her appointments. Her short-term memory showed some stabilization, and she became more confident in completing daily tasks independently.
- **Increased use of compensatory strategies:** Margaret became proficient in using her memory notebook and visual cues around the house. These external aids helped her reduce forgetfulness and manage her day-to-day activities more effectively.
- **Enhanced quality of life:** The cognitive stimulation and reminiscence therapies had a positive impact on Margaret's mood and self-esteem. She reported feeling more engaged and less anxious about her memory lapses. Her husband also noted that she seemed more content and socially active.
- **Maintained social connections:** The group sessions in Cognitive Stimulation Therapy provided Margaret with social interaction opportunities, which not only helped with her memory but also kept her socially connected and emotionally supported.
- **Slowing of cognitive decline:** Follow-up assessments using the MMSE and MoCA showed that Margaret's cognitive scores remained stable, indicating that the interventions helped slow the progression of memory decline.

Conclusion

This case study illustrates the effectiveness of a multi-faceted approach to improving memory in a patient with mild-to-moderate dementia. By combining cognitive stimulation therapy, the use of memory aids, errorless learning techniques, reminiscence therapy, and lifestyle modifications, Margaret was able to maintain her memory and cognitive functions, enhancing her quality of life and daily independence.

This approach highlights the importance of early intervention and the use of personalized strategies to address memory issues in dementia, offering hope for individuals and families dealing with this challenging condition.

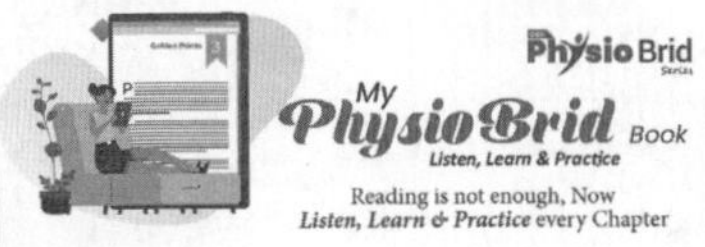

SUMMARY

- As integrated cognitive processes, thinking and memory play a vital role in the understanding and processing of an information. Both are essential for clinical reasoning, decision-making, problem-solving and framing the long-term and short-term goals toward the rehabilitation of the patients. Exercises and stress reduction methods are useful in enhancing the memory and sharpening the thinking processes.
- The chapter mentions the intricate neurobiological mechanisms that form the cognitive process of thinking. It highlights the significant roles played by various brain regions, including the cerebral cortex and subcortical structures such as the hippocampus, amygdala, and basal ganglia. The interplay between neurons and neurotransmitters, along with the concepts of neural networks and neuroplasticity, is discussed in detail, providing a solid foundation for understanding the physiological basis of thinking.
- Two prominent theories of thought are examined: The Dual-Process Theory (DPT) and Piaget's Theory of Cognitive Development. DPT distinguishes between fast, intuitive thinking (Type 1) and slow, reflective thinking (Type 2), while Piaget's theory outlines the stages of cognitive development from infancy to adulthood, illustrating how thinking evolves in complexity.
- The chapter further classifies thinking into several types, each with distinct characteristics and applications. Convergent thinking focuses on finding a single, logical solution to a problem, divergent thinking encourages the generation of multiple creative solutions, critical thinking involves the objective analysis and evaluation of information, and analytical thinking involves breaking down complex problems into manageable parts. The importance of each type in various contexts, including clinical practice, is highlighted.
- The practical applications of thinking in physiotherapy are discussed, emphasizing the significance of diagnostic reasoning, treatment decision-making, and clinical reasoning. These cognitive processes are crucial for effective patient care, and the document provides insights into how healthcare professionals can leverage them to enhance clinical outcomes.
- The chapter explains about memory, exploring its neurobiological foundations, types, stages, and models. The key brain regions involved in memory formation and consolidation are detailed, including the hippocampus, amygdala, prefrontal cortex, and medial temporal lobe. The mechanisms of long-term potentiation and the role of neurotransmitter systems in memory processes are also discussed.
- Memory is categorized into explicit (declarative) and implicit (nondeclarative) types, with further sub-types such as semantic, episodic, procedural, and priming. The stages of memory, from sensory memory through short-term memory to long-term memory, are explained, providing a clear framework for understanding how information is processed and stored in the brain.
- Several models of memory are explored, including the Atkinson-Shiffrin Model, Levels of Processing Model, Baddeley's Model of Working Memory, and the Serial-Parallel Independent Model of Memory. These models offer different perspectives on how memory functions, contributing to a deeper understanding of the complexities of memory processes.
- The chapter discusses various methods for assessing memory, including neuropsychological tests, observational measures, and neuroimaging techniques. It also highlights the role of physiotherapy in enhancing memory, particularly in individuals with dementia or mild cognitive impairments. Techniques such as maintaining familiar movement patterns, exercise, and functional training are discussed as effective strategies for memory improvement.

Contd...

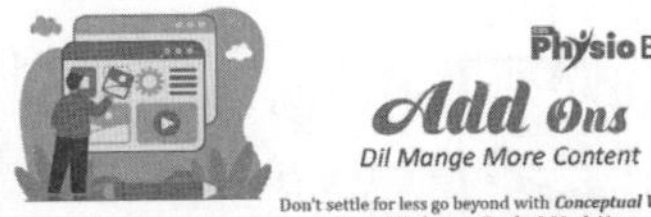

- In conclusion, the chapter talks about the importance of thinking and memory in both everyday life and professional practice, particularly in the field of physiotherapy. By understanding the neurobiological foundations, different types, and practical applications of these cognitive processes, healthcare professionals can enhance their clinical reasoning, decision-making, and overall patient care. The advancements in cognitive training and the integration of physiotherapy interventions offer promising avenues for improving cognitive functions and quality of life.

REFERENCES

1. Lawlor P. G. The panorama of opioid-related cognitive dysfunction in patients with cancer: A critical literature appraisal. Cancer. 2002; 94:1836–1853.

2. Gellman M., Rick Turner J. (eds). Encyclopedia of Behavioral Medicine. 2013; New York, NY: Springer.

3. Rosenbloom M. H., Schmahmann J.D., Price B.H. The Functional Neuroanatomy of Decision-Making. J Neuropsychiatry Clin Neurosci. 2012; 24 (3): 266–277.

4. Kahneman, D. Thinking, Fast and Slow. 2011; New York, NY: Farrar, Strauss, Giroux

5. Evans, J., and Stanovich, K. Dual-Process theories of higher cognition: Advancing the debate. Perspect. Psychol. Sci. 2013; 8: 223–241

6. Bellini-Leiti S.C. Dual Process Theory: Embodied and Predictive; Symbolic and Classical. Front. Psychol. 2022; 13:805386

7. Malik F., Marwaha R. Cognitive Development. Treasure Island (FL): StatPearls Publishing; 2024.

8. Cropley A., In praise of convergent thinking. Creativity Research Journal. 2006; 18(3):391–404

9. Guilford J. P., The Structure of Intellect. Psychological Bulletin. 1956; 53:267–93.

10. De Chantal PL., Gagnon-St-Pierre E., Markovits H., Divergent Thinking Promotes Deductive Reasoning in Preschoolers. Child Development. 2019; 91 (4): 1–16.

11. Brophy, D. R. Comparing the attributes, activities, and performance of divergent, convergent, and combination thinkers. Creativity Research Journal. 2001; 13: 439–455.

12. Widodo, S. A., & Turmudi, T. Guardian Student Thinking Process in Resolving Issues Divergence. Journal of Education and Learning. 2017; 11(4): 432–438.

13. Juhanda, A., Rustaman, N. Y., & Wulan, A. R. The profile of logical thinking biology prospective teachers. In Journal of Physics: Conference Series, 2019; 1157(2). IOP Publishing.

14. Punia P., Malik R., Bala M., Phor M., Chander Y. Relationship between Logical Thinking, Metacognitive Skills, and Problem-Solving Abilities: Mediating and Moderating Effect Analysis. Polish Psychological Bulletin. 2023; 53 (4): 243–253.

15. Krathwohl D R. A Revision of Bloom' s Taxonomy: Theory Pract. 2002; 41: 37–41.

16. Díaz Guzmán J. Razonamiento diagnóstico en neurología. Errores más comunes [Diagnostic reasoning in neurology. An analysis of the more frequent errors]. Neurologia. 2003;18 Suppl 2:3–10.

17. Lim T.K. The predictive brain model in diagnostic reasoning. The Asia Pacific Scholar. 2021; 6(2): 1–8.

18. Bubic A., von Cramon D.Y., Schubotz R.I. Prediction, cognition and the brain. Frontiers in Human Neuroscience. 2010; 4(25): 1–15.

19. Van der Linden, D., Duncker, D., & Petrides, M. The neuroanatomical correlates of clinical reasoning across the continuum of training. Journal of Cognitive Enhancement. 2016;1(2):141–151.

Contd...

20. Norman, G. R., Monteiro, S. D., Sherbino, J., Ilgen, J. S., Schmidt, H. G., & Mamede, S. The causes of errors in clinical reasoning: Cognitive biases, knowledge deficits, and dual process thinking. Academic Medicine. 2017; 92(1): 23–30.

21. Croskerry, P. Clinical cognition and diagnostic error: Applications of a dual process model of reasoning. Advances in Health Sciences Education. 2009; 14(1): 27–35.

22. Marcum, J.A. The role of emotions in clinical reasoning and decision making. Journal of Medicine and Philosophy. 2012; 37(6): 501–519.

23. Benfield A, Krueger RB. Making Decision-Making Visible-Teaching the Process of Evaluating Interventions. Int J Environ Res Public Health. 2021;18(7):3635.

24. Engel, A. K., Maye, A., Kurthen, M., & König, P. Where's the action? The pragmatic turn in cognitive science. Trends in Cognitive Sciences. 2013; 17(5): 202–209.

25. Dolmans, W. De Grave, I. Wolfhagen, C.P.M. van der Vleuten. Problem-based learning: future challenges for educational practice and research. Med Educ. 2005; 39 (7): 732–741

26. Wood F.D. ABC of learning and teaching in medicine Problem based learning. BMJ. 2003; 326: 328–330.

27. Graesser, Arthur C., Stephen M. Fiore, Samuel Greiff, Jessica Andrews-Todd, Peter W. Foltz et.al. Advancing the Science of Collaborative Problem Solving. Psychological Science in the Public Interest. 2018; 19: 59–92

28. Détienne, Françoise, Michael Baker, and Jean-Marie Burkhardt. Perspectives on Quality of Collaboration in Design. CoDesign. 2102; 8: 197–99

29. Drigas. A., Mitsea E. The 8 Pillars of Metacognition. International Journal of Emerging Technologies in Learning. 2020; 15(21): 162–77.

30. Flavell, J. H. Metacognition and cognitive monitoring: A new area of cognitive-developmental inquiry. American Psychologist. 1979; 34: 906–911

31. Craig, K., Hale, D., Grainger, C. et al. Evaluating metacognitive self-reports: Systematic reviews of the value of self-report in metacognitive research. Metacognition Learning. 2020; 15: 155–213.

32. Questienne L, Van Opstal F, van Dijck JP, Gevers W. Metacognition and cognitive control: behavioral adaptation requires conflict experience. Q J Exp Psychol (Hove). 2018;71(2):411–423.

33. Commodari E, La Rosa VL, Sagone E, Indiana ML. Interpersonal Adaptation, Self-Efficacy, and Metacognitive Skills in Italian Adolescents with Specific Learning Disorders: A Cross-Sectional Study. Eur J Investig Health Psychol Educ. 2022;12(8):1034–1049.

34. Willis S.L., Schaie K.W. Cognitive training and plasticity: Theoretical perspective and methodological consequences. Restor Neurol Neurosci. 2009; 27(5): 375–389.

35. Jones S, Nyberg L, Sandblom J, Stigsdotter Neely A, Ingvar M, Petersson K, et al. Cognitive and neural plasticity in aging: General and task-specific limitations. Neurosci Biobehav Rev. 2006; 30:864–871.

36. Mercado E. Neural and cognitive plasticity: From maps to minds. Psychol Bull. 2008; 134:109–137.

37. Lövdén, M., Bäckman, L., Lindenberger, U., Schaefer, S., & Schmiedek, F. A theoretical framework for the study of adult cognitive plasticity. Psychological Bulletin. 2010; 136(4): 659–676.

38. Park DC, Bischof GN. The aging mind: Neuroplasticity in response to cognitive training. Dialogues Clin Neurosci. 2013;15(1):109–19.

39. Barulli, D., & Stern, Y. Efficiency, capacity, compensation, maintenance, plasticity: Emerging concepts in cognitive reserve. Trends in Cognitive Sciences. 2013; 17(10): 502–509.

40. Nguyen L., Murphy K., Andrews G. Cognitive and neural plasticity in old age: A systematic review of evidence from executive functions cognition training. Ageing Research Reviews. 2019; 53 (8): 100912.

Contd...

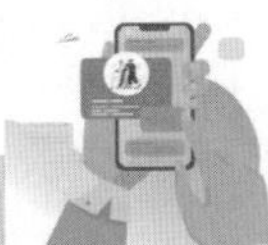
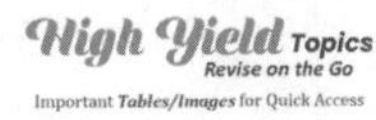

41. Au, J., Sheehan, E., Tsai, N., Duncan, G. J., Buschkuehl, M., & Jaeggi, S. M. Improving fluid intelligence with training on working memory: A meta-analysis. Psychonomic Bulletin & Review. 2015; 22(2): 366–377.

42. Ball, K., Berch, D. B., Helmers, K. F., Jobe, J. B., Leveck, M. D., Marsiske, M. et. al. Effects of cognitive training interventions with older adults: A randomized controlled trial. JAMA. 2002; 288(18): 2271–2281.

43. Ward, N., Paul, E., Watson, P. et al. Enhanced Learning through Multimodal Training: Evidence from a Comprehensive Cognitive, Physical Fitness, and Neuroscience Intervention. Sci Rep. 2017; 7: 5808

44. Sanilevici M, Reuveni O, Lev-Ari S, Golland Y, Levit-Binnun N. Mindfulness-Based Stress Reduction Increases Mental Wellbeing and Emotion Regulation During the First Wave of the COVID-19 Pandemic: A Synchronous Online Intervention Study. Front Psychol. 2021.

45. Lachaud L, Jacquet B, Bourlier M, Baratgin J. Mindfulness-based stress reduction is linked with an improved Cognitive Reflection Test score. Front Psychol. 2023; 14:1272324.

46. Mrazek, M. D., Franklin, M. S., Phillips, D. T., Baird, B., & Schooler, J. W. Mindfulness training improves working memory capacity and GRE performance while reducing mind wandering. Psychological Science. 2013; 24(5): 776–781.

47. Zlotnik G, Vansintjan A. Memory: An Extended Definition. Front Psychol. 2019; 10:2523.

48. Squire L. R. Memory and brain systems: 1969–2009. J. Neurosci. 2009; 29: 12711–12716.

49. Tulving E, Markowitsch HJ. Episodic and declarative memory: Role of the hippocampus. Hippocampus. 1998;8(3):198–204.

50. Wiltgen BJ, Zhou M, Cai Y, Balaji J, Karlsson MG, Parivash SN, Li W, Silva AJ. The hippocampus plays a selective role in the retrieval of detailed contextual memories. Curr Biol. 2010; 20(15):1336–44.

51. Eichenbaum H. The role of the hippocampus in navigation is memory. J Neurophysiol. 2017;117(4):1785–1796.

52. McGaugh JL. The amygdala modulates the consolidation of memories of emotionally arousing experiences. Annu Rev Neurosci. 2004; 27:1–28.

53. Phelps EA, LeDoux JE. Contributions of the amygdala to emotion processing: From animal models to human behavior. Neuron. 2005;48(2):175–87.

54. Paz, R. & Pare, D. Physiological basis for emotional modulation of memory circuits by the amygdala. Curr. Opin. Neurobiol. 2013; 23: 381–386.

55. Nejati V, Majdi R, Salehinejad MA, Nitsche MA. The role of dorsolateral and ventromedial prefrontal cortex in the processing of emotional dimensions. Sci Rep. 2021;11(1):1971.

56. Friedman NP, Robbins TW. The role of prefrontal cortex in cognitive control and executive function. Neuropsychopharmacology. 2022;47(1):72–89.

57. Dickerson, B., Eichenbaum, H. The Episodic Memory System: Neurocircuitry and Disorders. Neuropsychopharmacology. 2010; 35: 86–104.

58. Jeneson A, Squire LR. Working memory, long-term memory, and medial temporal lobe function. Learn Mem. 2011;19(1):15–25.

59. Aggleton JP, O'Mara SM, Vann SD, Wright NF, Tsanov M, Erichsen JT. Hippocampal-anterior thalamic pathways for memory: Uncovering a network of direct and indirect actions. Eur J Neurosci. 2010;31(12):2292–307.

60. Raichle ME. The brain's default mode network. Annu Rev Neurosci. 2015; 38:433–47.

61. Huo L, Li R, Wang P, Zheng Z, Li J. The Default Mode Network Supports Episodic Memory in Cognitively Unimpaired Elderly Individuals: Different Contributions to Immediate Recall and Delayed Recall. Front Aging Neurosci. 2018; 10:6.

Contd...

62. Takeuchi T, Duszkiewicz AJ, Morris RG. The synaptic plasticity and memory hypothesis: encoding, storage and persistence. Philos Trans R Soc Lond B Biol Sci. 2013;369(1633):20130288.

63. Goto A. Synaptic plasticity during systems memory consolidation. Neuroscience Research. 2022; 183: 1–6.

64. Bazzari AH, Parri HR. Neuromodulators and Long-Term Synaptic Plasticity in Learning and Memory: A Steered-Glutamatergic Perspective. Brain Sci. 2019;9(11):300.

65. Wixted J.T. Atkinson and Shiffrin's (1968) influential model overshadowed their contemporary theory of human memory. Journal of Memory and Language. 2024; 136: 104471

66. Craik F, Lockhart R. Levels of processing: A framework for memory research. J Verbal Learn Verbal Behav. 1972; 11:671–684.

67. Chai WJ, Abd Hamid AI, Abdullah JM. Working Memory From the Psychological and Neurosciences Perspectives: A Review. Front Psychol. 2018; 27 (9): 401.

68. Eustache F., Viard A., Desgranges B. The MNESIS model: Memory systems and processes, identity and future thinking. Neuropsychologia. 2016; 87: 96–109.

69. Wechsler, D. Wechsler Memory Scale®-Fourth Edition (WMS-IV). Pearson Assessment, 2009.

70. Delis, D.C., Kramer, J.H., Kaplan, E., and Thompkins, B.A.O. CVLT: California Verbal Learning Test – adult Version: Manual. New York, NY: Psychological Corporation. 1987.

71. B.A., Cockburn, J. and Baddeley, A. Rivermead Behavioural Memory Test. Thames Valley Test Company, London. 1985.

72. Bahar-Fuchs A, Clare L, Woods B. Cognitive training and cognitive rehabilitation for persons with mild to moderate dementia of the Alzheimer's or vascular type: A review. Alzheimers Res Ther. 2013;5(4):35.

73. De Oliveira GSR, Bressan L, Balarini F, Jesuino E Silva RS, Brito MMCM, Foss MP, Santos-Lobato BL, Tumas V. Direct and indirect assessment of functional abilities in patients with Parkinson's disease transitioning to dementia. Dement Neuropsychol. 2020;14(2):171–177.

74. Yokogawa M, Taniguchi Y, Yoneda Y. Qualitative research concerning physiotherapy approaches to encourage physical activity in older adults with dementia. PLoS One. 2023;18(7): e0289290.

75. Ferrer-Uris B, Ramos MA, Busquets A, Angulo-Barroso R. Can exercise shape your brain? A review of aerobic exercise effects on cognitive function and neuro-physiological underpinning mechanisms. AIMS Neurosci. 2022;9(2):150–174.

76. Pahlavani HA. Exercise therapy to prevent and treat Alzheimer's disease. Front Aging Neurosci. 2023; 15:1243869.

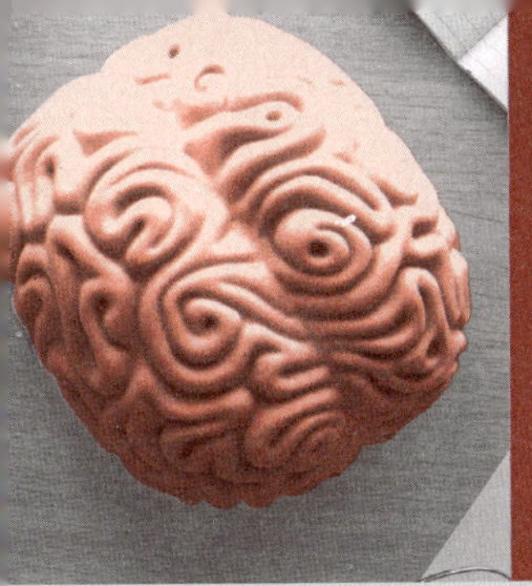

LONG ANSWER QUESTIONS

1. Compare and contrast the different types of memory, discussing their characteristics and functions.
2. Explain the thinking in problem solving.
3. Describe the types of memory assessment.
4. Describe the various strategies to enhance different aspects of thinking.
5. Explain the types of thinking and their implication in the clinical practice.

SHORT ANSWER QUESTIONS

1. Write a note on active learning techniques.
2. Define neurobiology of memory.
3. What are the stages of cognition development?
4. Enlist the characteristics of an algorithm.
5. Write about the Baddeley's process of working memory.
6. What are the steps of problem-based learning?
7. Write briefly about the role of physiotherapy in memory enhancement.
8. Define neuroplasticity.
9. Differentiate between convergent thinking and divergent thinking.
10. What are the features of dual process theory?

MULTIPLE CHOICE QUESTIONS

1. **Which brain structure plays a key role in memory formation and consolidation?**
   - a. Amygdala
   - b. Prefrontal cortex
   - c. Hippocampus
   - d. Basal ganglia
2. **Sensory memory is responsible for briefly retaining which type of information?**
   - a. Semantic
   - b. Visual
   - c. Procedural
   - d. Episodic
3. **Which memory enhancement technique involves organizing information into smaller, manageable units?**
   - a. Chunking
   - b. Mnemonics
   - c. Visualization
   - d. Spaced repetition

4. **Which physiotherapy intervention has been linked to improvements in cognitive function, including memory?**
   a. Hydrotherapy
   b. Massage therapy
   c. Exercise therapy
   d. Electrotherapy

5. **What type of memory is responsible for storing personal experiences and events?**
   a. Semantic memory
   b. Procedural memory
   c. Episodic memory
   d. Implicit memory

6. **Mnemonics primarily aid in which memory process?**
   a. Encoding
   b. Storage
   c. Retrieval
   d. Consolidation

7. **How many pillars of metacognition are there?**
   a. 6
   b. 7
   c. 8
   d. 9

8. **Which of the following is not the characteristic of an algorithm?**
   a. Precision
   b. Bias
   c. Finiteness
   d. Optimality

9. **What is the age range for concrete operational stage of cognition development?**
   a. 0–2 years
   b. 2–7 years
   c. 7–11 years
   d. >11 years

10. **Neuroplasticity refers to the brain's ability to:**
    a. Form new neurons
    b. Adapt and reorganize
    c. Strengthen synaptic connections
    d. All of these

ANSWER KEY

1. c	2. b	3. a	4. c	5. c	6. a	7. c	8. b
9. c	10. d						

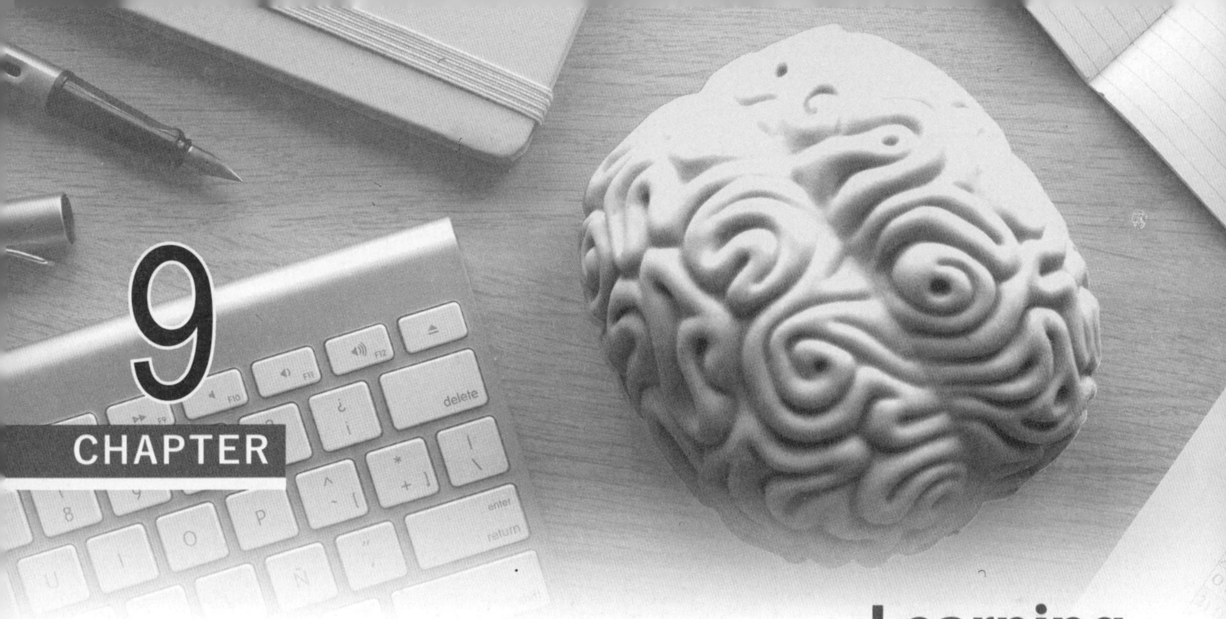

Learning

Neha Sharma, Rittu Sharma

LEARNING OBJECTIVES

After the completion of the chapter, the readers will be able to:

- Explain the five major learning theories: Behaviorism, cognitivism, constructivism, connectivism, and humanism.
- Discuss how each theory influences teaching methods and learning outcomes in clinical and research settings.
- Describe various types of learning, including observational, cognitive, verbal, serial, and implicit learning.
- Provide examples of how each type of learning applies in educational and clinical contexts.
- Define common learning disabilities such as dyslexia, dyscalculia, and dysgraphia.
- Discuss the impact of these disabilities on learning processes and the associated psychological and social deficits.
- Explain the concept of e-learning and its effectiveness in education.
- Discuss the myths and challenges associated with e-learning, particularly in the post-COVID-19 era.
- Describe the importance of the clinical learning environment in shaping learning experiences.
- Identify the strengths, limitations, and challenges of clinical teaching.

CHAPTER OUTLINE

- Introduction
- Learning Process
- Paradigms of Learning
- Theories of Learning
- Types of Learning
- Factors Facilitating Learning
- Clinical Learning Environment
- E-Learning
- Learning Disability

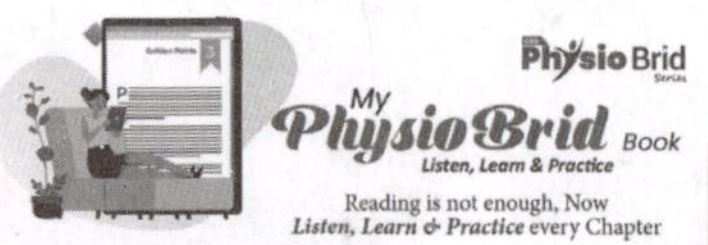

KEY TERMS

Behaviorism: A learning theory that focuses on observable actions and their consequences, emphasizing the importance of linking sensory stimuli and responses.

Clinical learning environment (CLE): The physical and interpersonal setting where clinical education takes place, influencing how knowledge, skills, and values are acquired and applied.

Cognitive learning: Learning that involves the acquisition and processing of information based on existing knowledge.

Cognitivism: A theory that explains learning as an internal process of information processing and cognitive restructuring.

Connectivism: A theory that emphasizes learning through the formation of connections and networks, both internally and externally.

Constructivism: A learning theory that posits learning as a process of building new ideas based on existing knowledge and experiences.

E-Learning: Learning facilitated by electronic resources, such as computers and the internet.

Humanism: A learning theory that views learning as a natural desire for self-actualization and personal growth.

Implicit learning: Learning that occurs without conscious effort or awareness.

Learning disabilities: A group of conditions that affect the ability to acquire, process, and understand information, including dyslexia, dyscalculia, and dysgraphia.

Motivation: The driving force that initiates and sustains learning activities, including intrinsic and extrinsic motivation.

Observational learning: Learning that occurs through observing the actions of others.

Perceptual learning: The improvement in the ability to interpret sensory information through experience.

Reinforcement: The process of strengthening a desired behavior through positive or negative consequences.

Verbal learning: Learning that occurs through the use of words and language.

INTRODUCTION

Learning is a behavior change in a human being which results due to previous experience. Learning theories helps an individual in acquiring, processing, retaining, and recalling knowledge during the important phases of learning.[1]

Motivation also helps in initiating the process of learning, which also acts as a booster and finally help in achieving the desired target of goal. Learning was first introduced by Plato, who was the ancient Greek philosopher.[2, 3] According to him, learning is a passive process where the knowledge is already inculcated in an individual since birth, and any further information acquired during the experiences are merely a recollection of experiences and knowledge that soul of a human already holds. John Locke, an English philosopher and physician proposed another statement that human beings are born without having innate knowledge, and according to him knowledge is gained through experiences with the environment. This statement is also known as *"Blank Slate Theory"*.[4]

LEARNING PROCESS

- Learning process always involves and occurs through past experiences (Fig. 9.1).

- Repeated prior experience after doing some particular activity in a structured way leads to formation of habit.

- Learning causes permanent behavioral changes in an individual. These changes must be distinguished as these are neither permanent nor can be learned.

- Learning process consists of a series of psychological events.

- It is an in-fact process, which is not similar to performance. Performance is a response or action taken by an individual against a particular environmental stimulus.

> **MUST KNOW**
>
> Learning is a process which always occurs based on experiences, behavior, and psychological events.

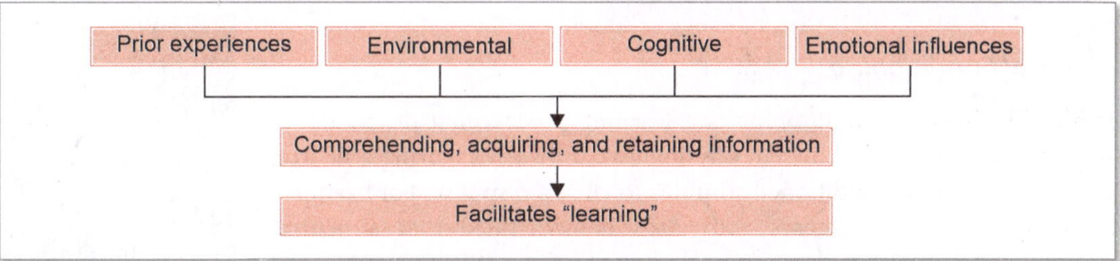

Fig. 9.1: Learning process

PARADIGMS OF LEARNING

There are many ways in which learning takes place. Conditioning is easiest type of it, in which a given environmental cue becomes effective in producing an outcome. Conditioning are of two types; classical conditioning and operant conditioning.[6]

Classical conditioning is also known as unconscious learning in which learning process occurs through relationship between an unconditioned stimulus, and a neutral stimulus. Pavlov's classic experiment with dogs is the perfect example of classical conditioning. Operant conditioning is also known as instrumental conditioning.[7] In this, a relationship is made between a behavior of an individual and a consequence of that behavior whether that is positive or negative. In operant conditioning, a reward of particular activity causes increase in behavioral change while failure or punishment in that particular activity leads to decrease in behavioral change.[4, 5]

THEORIES OF LEARNING

A total of five learning theories,[5, 8] globally accepted are:

1. Behaviorism

2. Cognitivism

3. Constructivism

4. Connectivism

5. Humanism

Behaviorism

Learning occurs through linking sensory stimuli and responses. Behaviorism theory focuses on actions which can be observed, under the conditions they are performed, and the strengthening of desired behaviors. Performance of an individual increases after the learning process, and an establishment of a specific new behavior is the outcome of learning. In this an individual should have good knowledge to start up the proper learning environment, and also to elicit the correct responses from the learners/students.

Classical Conditioning

Principle: Classical conditioning is a learning process first described by Ivan Pavlov (Fig. 9.2), a Russian physiologist. It involves pairing a neutral stimulus with an unconditioned stimulus to elicit a response. For example, Pavlov's famous experiments with dogs demonstrated that a neutral stimulus, like a bell, could be associated with food (the unconditioned stimulus) to eventually produce a conditioned response (salivation) even when the bell was rung without food being presented (Fig. 9.3).

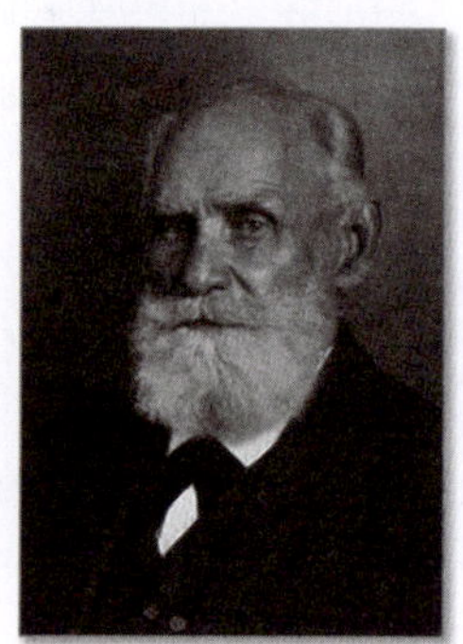

Fig. 9.2: Ivan Pavlov

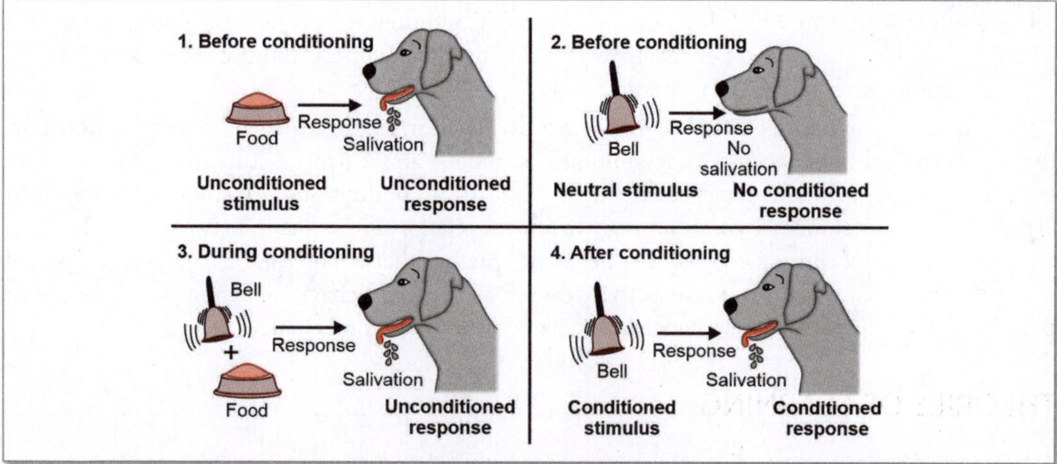

Fig. 9.3: Classical conditioning experiment

In this process:

- **Unconditioned stimulus (US)**: A stimulus that naturally triggers a response (e.g., food).
- **Unconditioned response (UR)**: The automatic response to the unconditioned stimulus (e.g., salivation when food is presented).
- **Conditioned stimulus (CS)**: A previously neutral stimulus that, after being associated with the unconditioned stimulus, triggers a similar response (e.g., the bell).
- **Conditioned response (CR)**: The learned response to the conditioned stimulus (e.g., salivation in response to the bell alone).

Classical conditioning demonstrates how associations between stimuli can shape behavior, and it has applications in various fields including psychology, education, and therapy.

Example: Pavlov's dogs learned to salivate (conditioned response) at the sound of a bell (conditioned stimulus) after the bell was repeatedly paired with food (unconditioned stimulus).

Operant Conditioning

Principle: Operant conditioning is a learning principle developed by B F Skinner (Fig. 9.4), which focuses on how behaviors are influenced by their consequences. In this process, behaviors are either encouraged or discouraged based on the rewards or punishments that follow them.

Key components of operant conditioning include:

- **Reinforcement**: Increases the likelihood of a behavior being repeated.
  - **Positive reinforcement:** Providing a rewarding stimulus after a behavior (e.g., giving a treat for good behavior).
  - **Negative reinforcement**: Removing an unpleasant stimulus after a behavior (e.g., stopping a loud noise when a button is pressed).
- **Punishment:** Decreases the likelihood of a behavior being repeated.
  - **Positive punishment:** Adding an unpleasant stimulus after a behavior (e.g., extra chores for breaking a rule).
  - **Negative punishment:** Removing a pleasant stimulus after a behavior (e.g., taking away a toy for misbehavior).

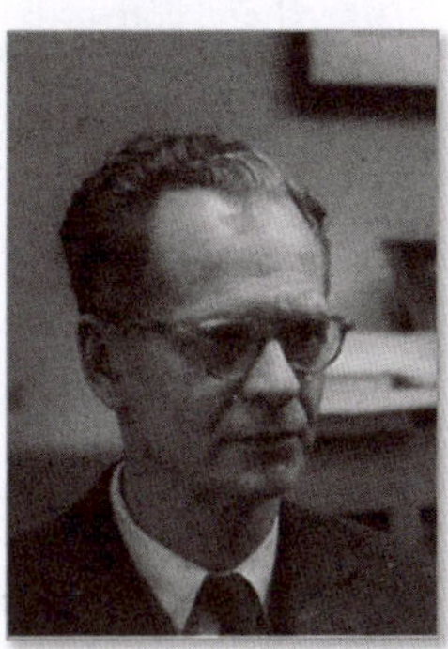

Fig. 9.4: B F Skinner

Example: A child learns to clean his room to receive praise from parents (positive reinforcement) or to avoid being scolded (negative reinforcement).

Skinner's operant conditioning chamber (also called a Skinner Box) was designed to teach rats how to push a lever (Fig. 9.5). This behavior is not natural to rats, so operant conditioning with positive and negative reinforcement were performed in order to teach the behavior.

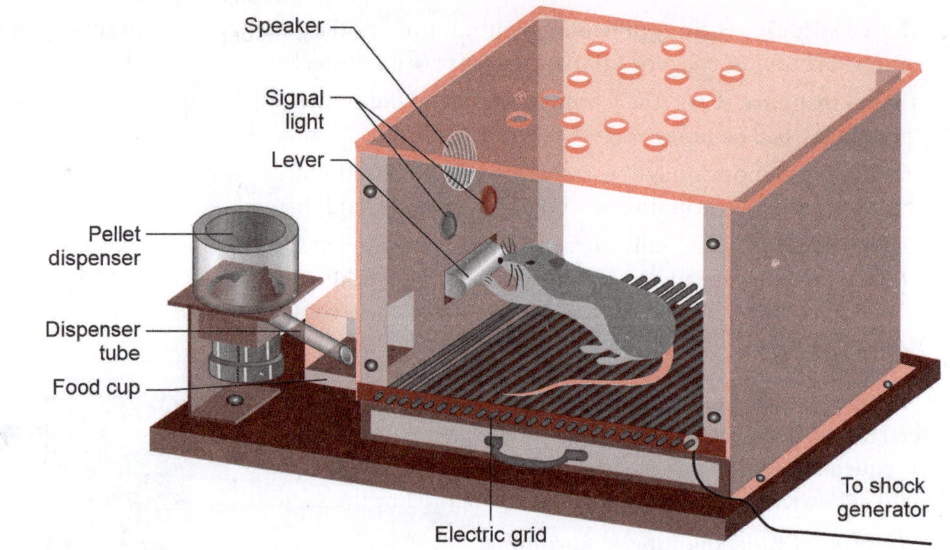

Positive reinforcement: A rat was awarded food when he pressed the lever.

Negative reinforcement: A rat was able to turn off electric shocks produced by the floor by pressing the lever.

Fig. 9.5: Skinner box experiment

Table 9.1 shows the distinction between classical and operant conditioning.

Table 9.1: Differences between classical and operant conditioning

	Classical conditioning	Operant conditioning
Pioneers	• Ivan Pavlov • John B Watson	• Edward Thorndike • B F Skinner
Major terms	• Neutral stimulus (NS) • Unconditioned stimulus (UCS) • Conditioned stimulus (CS) • Unconditioned response (UCR) • Conditioned response (CR) • Conditioned emotional response (CER)	• Reinforcers (primary and secondary) • Reinforcement (primary and secondary) • Punishment (positive and negative) • Shaping • Reinforcement schedules (continuous and partial)
Example	Cringing at the sound of a dentist's drill	A baby cries and someone picks it up

Contd...

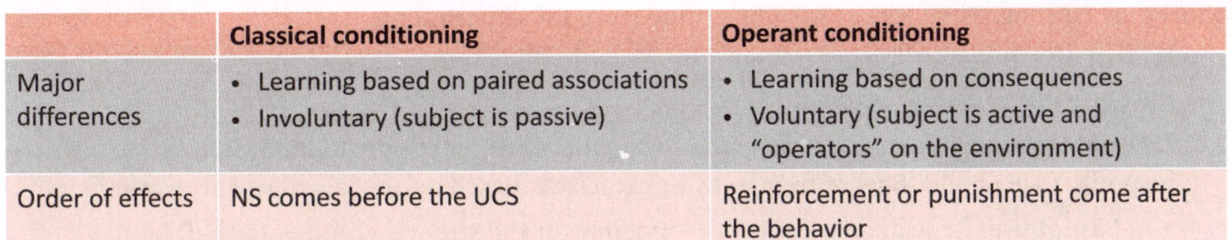

	Classical conditioning	**Operant conditioning**
Major differences	• Learning based on paired associations • Involuntary (subject is passive)	• Learning based on consequences • Voluntary (subject is active and "operators" on the environment)
Order of effects	NS comes before the UCS	Reinforcement or punishment come after the behavior

Trial and Error Method of Learning

Principle: Thorndike's trial and error method of learning, developed by Edward Thorndike, is a foundational concept in educational psychology. It describes how individuals learn to solve problems through a process of experimenting with various actions and learning from the outcomes.

Key aspects of this method include:

- **Trial and error**: An individual attempts different responses to a problem until they find one that works. For example, a cat might try various ways to escape from a puzzle box and eventually, it finds out the way to solve the puzzle box (Fig. 9.6).

- **Law of effect**: This principle states that behaviors followed by satisfying outcomes are more likely to be repeated, while behaviors followed by unpleasant outcomes are less likely to be repeated. In other words, successful actions are reinforced, and unsuccessful ones are discarded.

- **Learning through success**: As individuals make repeated attempts and receive feedback on their actions, they gradually learn which strategies are effective and which are not, leading to more efficient problem-solving over time.

Example: A student studies hard and receives good grades, reinforcing the behavior of studying.

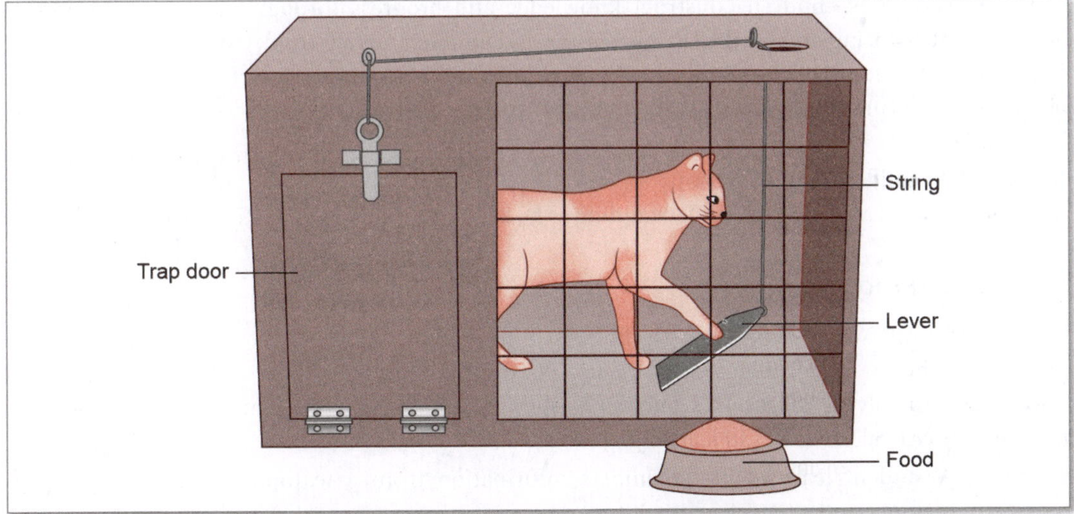

Fig. 9.6: Experiment conducted by Thorndike

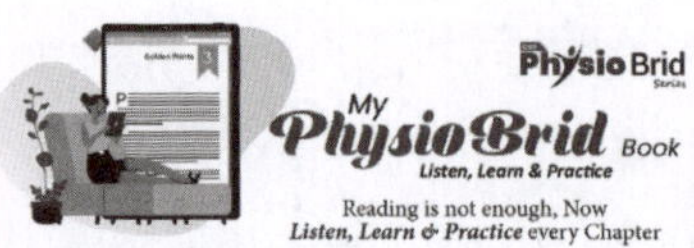

Thorndike had suggested three laws of learning from the experiment:

1. **Law of effect:** Any response followed by reward will be strengthened. Any response, which is unsuccessful, will be weakened.
2. **Law of frequency:** There is a direct relationship between repetition and the strength of stimulus-response (S-R) bond. Law of frequency or exercise is based on the law of use or disuse.
   - **Law of use:** Repeated task shows a tendency for the strengthening of the S-R bond.
   - **Law of disuse:** Unrepeated tasks shows a tendency for the weakening of the S-R bond.
3. **Law of recency:** Any activity, which is learnt, recently has an advantage of being repeated once again because of fresh experience.

Cognitivism

This theory of learning, based on the work of Jean Piaget, a Swiss psychologist, states that learning occurs through the internal processing of information by an individual, rather than merely as a response to external environmental stimuli. Learning also occurs through the processing of information, and organizing it structurally within a domain of previous acquired information. Theory of cognitivism puts emphasis on the thought process of an individual, with a focus on metacognition, where an individual thinks about their own thinking. Behavioral change in this occurs after the inner workings of thinking which occurs based on the new information received. This type of learning process involves both acquisition and reorganization of cognitive entities.

Piaget's Theory of Cognitive Development

Principle: Piaget's theory of cognitive development was developed by Swiss psychologist Jean Piaget and it explains how children construct knowledge and progress through four stages of mental development, focusing on how they think, reason, and understand the world. Cognitive development occurs in four stages: (1) Sensorimotor, (2) Preoperational, (3) Concrete operational, and (4) Formal operational. Learning is a process of adaptation, involving assimilation and accommodation of new information.

Example: A child learns to classify objects (e.g., animals) by building on prior knowledge (assimilation) and adjusting his understanding as he encounters new information (accommodation).

Information Processing Theory

Principle: George Miller, a cognitive psychologist and computer scientist, developed the Information Processing Theory. According to the theory, learning is similar to how a computer processes information, involving stages like encoding, storage, and retrieval. Attention, perception, and memory are critical processes in learning.

Example: A student learns and remembers information from a textbook by encoding it into long-term memory and later retrieving it for an exam.

Social Learning Theory

Social learning theory bridges behaviorism and cognitivism by emphasizing the role of observational learning, imitation, and modeling in learning.

Principle: Albert Bandura's social learning theory emphasizes that people learn behaviors, attitudes, and emotional reactions through observing and imitating others. This theory highlights the role of social influences and modeling in the learning process.

Key points:

- **Observational learning:** Bandura posits that people can learn new behaviors by watching others, rather than through direct experience. For example, children might imitate behaviors they see on television or in their family environment.

- **Modeling:** The process involves observing and replicating the actions of role models. Effective models are often those who are perceived as similar, competent or successful.

- **Attention, retention, reproduction, motivation**: Bandura identified these four key processes in observational learning:

    i. **Attention:** To learn, one must pay attention to the model.

    ii. **Retention:** Remembering the observed behavior is crucial for later reproduction.

    iii. **Reproduction:** The ability to replicate the observed behavior.

    iv. **Motivation:** The willingness to reproduce the behavior, which can be influenced by rewards, punishments or perceived self-efficacy.

- **Self-efficacy:**
    - *Example*: A child learns to solve a puzzle by watching a parent or teacher doing it first and then trying it himself.

Concept of Self-Efficacy

Principle: A key concept in Bandura's theory, self-efficacy refers to an individual's belief in their own ability to succeed. This belief influences their motivation and persistence. An individual's belief in his ability to succeed in specific situations influences his behavior and learning. Higher self-efficacy leads to greater effort and persistence in learning tasks.

Example: A student who believes he can master mathematical concepts is more likely to engage with challenging problems and can through difficulties.

Constructivism

The theory of constructivism states that learning in an individual happens by establishing new ideas based on existing previous knowledge, and experiences gained from the environment. Two prominent figures in constructivism are Jerome Bruner and Lev Vygotsky. The theory of constructivism also focuses on the internal thinking of an individual but does not make assumptions

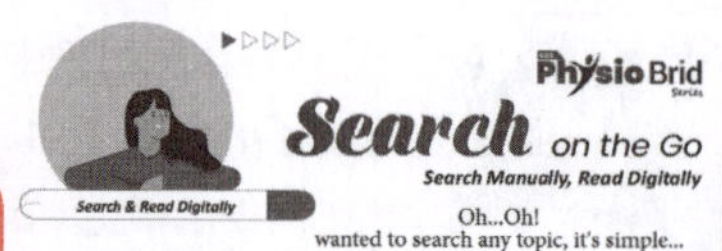

like theory of cognitivism, that how the connections or links will be made between one thought and another thought. Learning based on making connections, and establishing creative ideas from previous experiences and knowledge creates mental preparations. These mental preparations are subjective in nature, and every human being is having a unique construction of knowledge.

Principle: Learners actively construct their own understanding and knowledge of the world, building on their experiences and interactions. Learning is a social process, influenced by cultural and contextual factors.

Example: A student learns more effectively through hands-on activities and collaboration with peers, guided by a teacher (scaffolding).

Connectivism

The theory of connectivism states that learning process occurs through the formation of connections and links between each other, as well as their hobbies, roles, and other different aspects of life. Learning is the ability which transverse and construct these methods. The theory of connectivism also works based on the theory of cognitivism, but the difference is that, learning not only resides within an individual, but also spreads across the networks of individuals. According to this, knowledge can reside outside the individual but learning through connectivism focuses on organizing and locating information structurally that may be controlled by an individual. George Siemens and Stephen Downes are proponents of this idea.

Principle: Connectivism is a relatively recent theory that emphasizes the role of social and cultural context in learning. It asserts that learning occurs through networks and is facilitated by technology, especially in the digital age.

Key Concepts

- **Learning networks**: Connections formed with people and information sources.
- **Diversity of opinions**: Essential for learning; exposure to differing perspectives enhances understanding.
- **Knowledge management**: Ability to identify, organize, and interpret information is crucial.

Humanism

The theory of humanism is closely related to the theory of connectivism. It states that learning is a strong natural desire with an ultimate target of achieving self-actualization. A state where an individual feels that all his or her physical, emotional, and cognitive needs have been fulfilled. A learning style is the way of an individual likes to absorb, process, comprehend, and retain a new collection of information. There are seven types of learning styles in psychology. These are physical, logical, social, solitary, visual, aural, and verbal.[9]

Maslow's Hierarchy of Needs

Principle: Abraham Maslow proposed Maslow's hierarchy of needs. Learning and self-actualization occur when basic needs (physiological, safety, love/belonging, esteem) are met. The individuals reach their full potential and engage in meaningful learning after fulfilling their basic needs.

Example: A student struggling with basic needs like food and safety may find it difficult to focus on learning until those needs are addressed.

Rogers' Experiential Learning

Principle: Carl Rogers developed the concept of experiential learning. Learning is most effective when it is self-initiated, experiential, and relevant to the learner's interests. Teachers should create a supportive environment that fosters self-directed learning.

Example: A student learns best when allowed to explore topics of personal interest, with the teacher acting as a facilitator rather than a director.

Implications in Clinical Practice, Research and Teaching[5, 8]

Learning theories play a very important role in physiotherapy clinical practice, research and teaching. It helps physiotherapy professors, and clinicians to have clear knowledge of physiotherapy skills, and how to apply these skills in treating patients, teaching students, and guiding them in their research interests. Learning theories correlate with each other, and also with teaching, clinical practice, and research methods in physiotherapy.

- **Behaviorism:** In this, the teacher needs to be active, should have good knowledge base to start up the proper and effective learning environment so that learner/student should find out the solution to the query raised by the teacher.
- **Cognitivism:** In this, the role of teacher is in designing and structuring the content of learning material.
- **Connectivism:** In this, teacher provides guidance to the learners/students related to their study fields and also toward outside their focus.
- **Constructivism:** In this, teacher is a facilitator, who provides guidance to the students which helps provides to the students/learners to bring a unique set of prior experiences to get the knowledge they are acquiring.
- **Humanism:** Humanism focuses on the student/learner's capability, potential, and autonomy where teacher encourage students/learners to be self-directed.

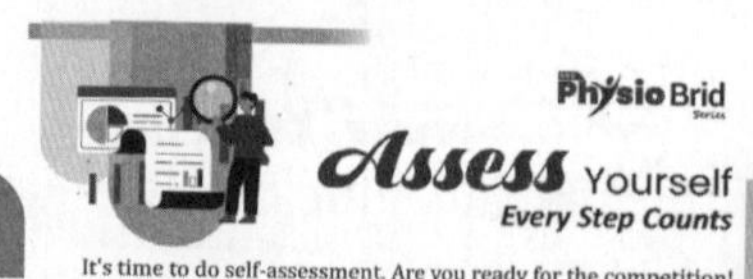

Physio CORNER

Constraint-Induced Movement Therapy (CIMT) is a specialized rehabilitation approach designed to improve motor function in individuals with motor impairments, such as those following a stroke. The therapy focuses on enhancing the use of a constrained limb (often the affected limb) through intensive practice and repetition. Here is an overview of the physiological mechanisms involved in CIMT:

- **Neuroplasticity:**
  - **Definition:** Neuroplasticity refers to the brain's ability to reorganize itself by forming new neural connections.
  - **Mechanism:** CIMT leverages neuroplasticity by promoting the reorganization of brain areas responsible for motor control. Intensive use of the affected limb encourages the brain to adapt and rewire itself, often leading to improved motor function.
- **Motor cortex activation:**
  - **Definition:** The motor cortex is a region of the brain involved in planning, controlling, and executing voluntary movements.
  - **Mechanism:** CIMT involves repetitive and task-specific training, which increases the activation of the motor cortex associated with the affected limb. This enhanced cortical activation is crucial for improving motor skills and strength in the constrained limb.
- **Strengthening and coordination:**
  - **Definition:** Strengthening refers to increasing muscle strength, while coordination involves the ability to use muscles together effectively.
  - **Mechanism:** By intensively practicing tasks with the affected limb, CIMT helps strengthen muscles and improve coordination. The increased use of the limb leads to muscle adaptation, improved control, and more effective execution of movements.
- **Reduction of learned non-use:**
  - **Definition:** Learned non-use is a phenomenon where individuals avoid using their affected limb due to perceived ineffectiveness or difficulty.
  - **Mechanism:** CIMT directly addresses learned non-use by constraining the unaffected limb, forcing the patient to rely on the affected limb for daily activities. This process reduces the tendency to neglect the affected limb and encourages its functional use.
- **Enhancement of functional skills:**
  - **Definition:** Functional skills are abilities that enable an individual to perform daily activities effectively.
  - **Mechanism:** CIMT involves practicing functional tasks that mimic real-life activities. This task-oriented approach helps in the development of skills necessary for everyday activities, enhancing overall functional independence.
- **Feedback and adaptation:**
  - **Definition:** Feedback involves receiving information about performance, which can be used to improve skill execution.
  - **Mechanism:** During CIMT, continuous feedback from therapists and self-monitoring help individuals refine their movements and adjust their strategies. This feedback loop is essential for motor learning and adaptation.

Constraint-Induced Movement Therapy utilizes several physiological mechanisms to improve motor function. It promotes neuroplasticity and motor cortex activation, strengthens muscles, enhances coordination, reduces learned non-use, and improves functional skills. The therapy's focus on intensive, task-specific practice and constraint of the unaffected limb drives these physiological changes, leading to better motor outcomes and increased functional independence for individuals with motor impairments.

Role in Clinical and Communication Delivery[5, 8]

- **Behaviorism:** It is useful in clinical and communication skills.
- **Cognitivism:** In this process, the new information related to the clinical course are recommended, and then processed internally to generate new ideas which further improves the structure of knowledge.
- **Constructivism:** In this, the students/learners need to grasp the core concepts of basic health sciences or subjects related to their area of interests, so that they could establish the connections of clinical aspects relevant to their field.
- **Connectivism:** The learning process in connectivism is similar to constructivism. In this, learning occurs through the process of forming connections between existing previous knowledge, and innate qualities of an individual. This approach of learning is appropriate in that kind of areas of health sciences which requires appropriate knowledge between different health areas. This type of learning is very much in trend in the time of digital age.
- **Humanism:** In this approach, a teacher allows learner/students to learn subject by themselves who desires for more information. Learning is innate, and having goal of self-actualization in an individual.

Refer to Figure 9.7 to understand the importance of learning theories in research and clinical teaching.

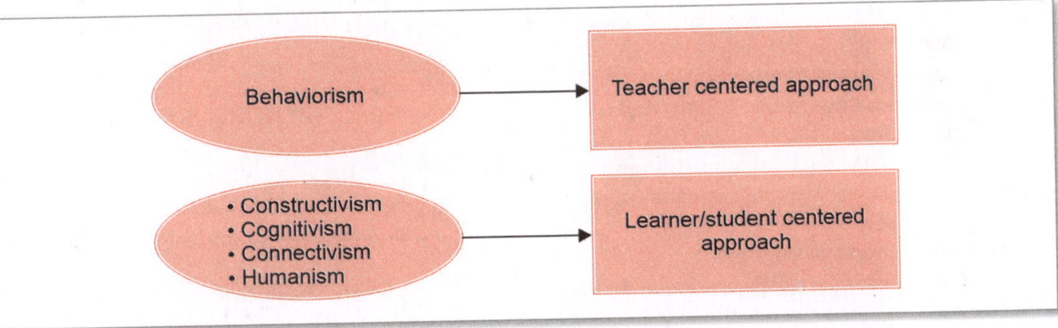

Fig. 9.7: Importance of learning theories in research and clinical teaching

CASE STUDY

Motor Learning with Constraint-Induced Movement Therapy (CIMT) in Stroke

Patient Profile
- **Name:** Emily Johnson
- **Age:** 45 years
- **Diagnosis:** Chronic Stroke, left-sided hemiparesis
- **Duration post-stroke:** 18 months
- **Primary issue:** Significant motor impairment and reduced use of her affected left arm.

Contd...

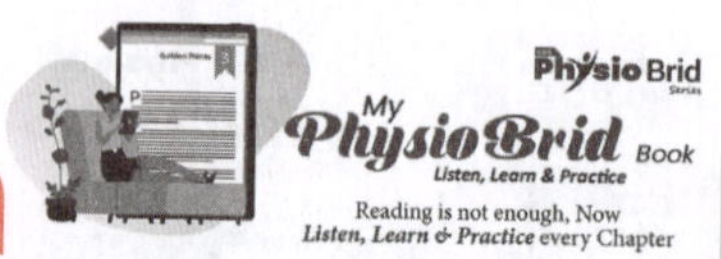

Treatment Plan

- **Intervention:** Constraint-Induced Movement Therapy (CIMT)
- **Duration:** 6 weeks
- **Frequency:** 6 hrs/day, 5 days a week
- **Components:**
  - **Constraint:** Emily's unaffected right arm is restrained using a sling or mitt.
  - **Task-oriented training:** Intensive, repetitive practice of tasks using the affected left arm.
  - *Shaping:* Gradual progression of task difficulty to encourage functional improvement.

Psychological Impact

- **Increased motivation and self-efficacy:**
  - **Observation:** Emily initially showed reluctance and frustration due to previous failed attempts at therapy. However, as she began to see gradual improvements in her ability to perform daily tasks, her motivation increased.
  - **Impact:** The progressive nature of CIMT and visible improvements boosted Emily's confidence in her ability to regain functionality. This was reflected in her increased engagement and persistence in therapy sessions.
- **Emotional resilience and adaptation:**
  - **Observation:** The intensive nature of CIMT led to both physical and emotional challenges. Emily experienced moments of discouragement, particularly when progress seemed slow.
  - **Impact:** Psychological support, including counseling and encouragement from therapists, helped Emily develop resilience. She learned to manage her frustrations better and remained committed to her therapy goals.
- **Reduction in learned non-use:**
  - **Observation:** Prior to CIMT, Emily had unconsciously avoided using her affected arm, relying heavily on her unaffected side.
  - **Impact:** CIMT forced Emily to use her affected arm for daily tasks, gradually reducing the learned non-use behavior. This shift in behavior was accompanied by a positive change in her self-perception, seeing herself as more capable person.
- **Social interaction and support:**
  - **Observation:** Emily's participation in group therapy sessions, where she interacted with other stroke survivors undergoing CIMT, provided additional emotional support and motivation.
  - **Impact:** The social aspect of the therapy provided a sense of community and understanding, which was crucial for emotional well-being. Peer support helped Emily stay motivated and reduced feelings of isolation.

Outcome

After 6 weeks of CIMT, Emily showed significant improvements in the motor function of her affected arm. She was able to perform more complex tasks independently and reported higher satisfaction with her daily activities. Psychologically, Emily demonstrated increased self-efficacy, emotional resilience, and a more positive outlook on her recovery.

Constraint-Induced Movement Therapy not only facilitated significant motor improvements in Emily's affected arm but also had a profound psychological impact. The therapy enhanced her motivation, resilience, and self-efficacy, contributing to a more holistic recovery process. The integration of psychological support alongside physical therapy played a critical role in Emily's overall progress and well-being.

TYPES OF LEARNING

Observational Learning

Learning in this takes place by observing activities occurring in the surroundings. This form of learning was also known as imitation. By observing society's behavior, individuals can learn social learning. In many such situations, a person does not know how to react in society, but it could become possible just by observing behavior of other individuals and imitate their behavior, this process is known as "modeling", which is also a form of learning. The role of modeling, and the role of consequences are two major aspects of observational learning, and contribute toward behavioral change.[8, 10, 11]

Behavioral change can occur through observation which is incidental in nature and occurs in the context of environmental activities. Observing superiors, inspiring, and likeable persons, and then emulating their behavior is an example of observational learning. By observation, children learn how to behave in society. The way to perform activities of daily living such as dressing, combing hairs, buttoning shirts, and tying shoes laces are learned through others, and also considered examples of observational learning. This type of learning also helps in personality development among children. Social behaviors such as showing aggressiveness, politeness, diligence, and indolence in the behavior, all can be acquired through observational learning method.[8, 10, 11]

> **MUST KNOW**
>
> Children are the best example of modeling. Whatever they learn, always gather information from their parents, and society just by observing them.

Cognitive Learning

Cognitive learning focuses on the existing knowledge of the learner which they apply and learn new things to enhance their brain's capability. It involves two types of learning, namely: (1) Insight learning and (2) Latent learning.[1, 10, 12, 13, 14]

Wolfgang Köhler's concept of learning by insight, developed through his work with chimpanzees, emphasizes a form of problem-solving that occurs suddenly rather than through gradual trial and error (Fig. 9.8). Köhler's research demonstrated that animals, and by extension humans, can experience sudden realizations or "insights" into solutions to problems.

Key points:

- **Köhler's experiments:** Köhler conducted experiments with chimpanzees, such as using tools to reach bananas that were out of reach. He observed that the chimps often solved the problem by suddenly realizing how to use objects in novel ways, rather than through random attempts.[12]
- **Gestalt theory:** Köhler's work is associated with Gestalt psychology, which emphasizes the holistic nature of perception and problem-solving. Insight learning reflects a reorganization of cognitive processes to perceive the problem and solution in a new way.[8, 12]

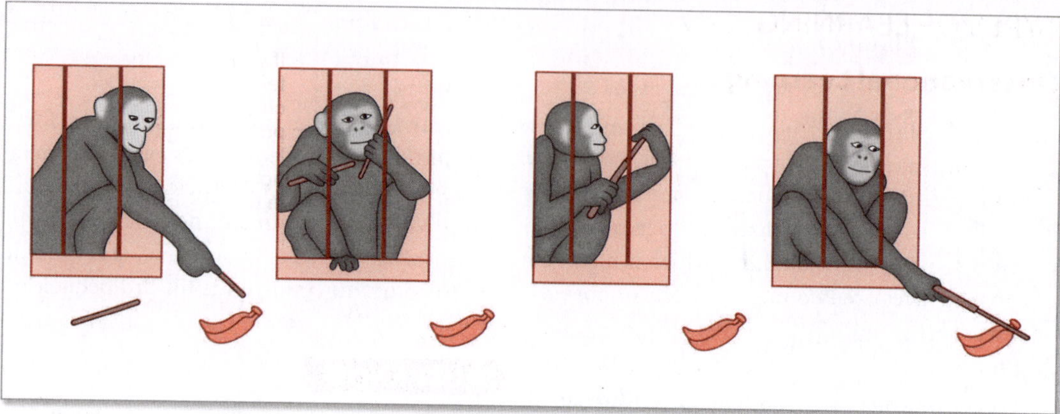

Fig. 9.8: Köhler's experiment

Köhler's insights into problem-solving highlight the capacity for sudden cognitive breakthroughs and the ability to reorganize information for effective problem resolution.

- **Insight learning:** According to Köhler, the process in which solution to a problem becomes suddenly clear is known as insight learning. Sudden solution to a problem is a key to insight learning. Example of insight learning is: A question is asked from a student/learner and they are not able to answer that particular question in 5–10 minutes, but suddenly an answer appears.[1, 12, 13] Insight learning tells that learning not only occurs by the number of events of conditions associated between environmental cue and its related outcome but also having a cognitive association between its initiation and its end.[1, 12, 13]

- **Latent learning:** In latent learning, an individual learns a new learning but does not perform it unless reinforcement is provided for demonstrating it. Latent learning does not comply with constraints of behaviorism, as in this learning is occurring in that way which is not observable until there is a reason to demonstrate it. Example: Children learn activities of daily living such as cooking, driving a car, etc., by watching the actions of their parents but they only demonstrate it later when the learned material is needed in action.[1, 12, 13]

Domain-Based Learning

The following types of learning are domain-based learning (Fig. 9.9):

- Verbal learning
- Motor learning
- Affect learning
- Cognitive learning
- Skill learning

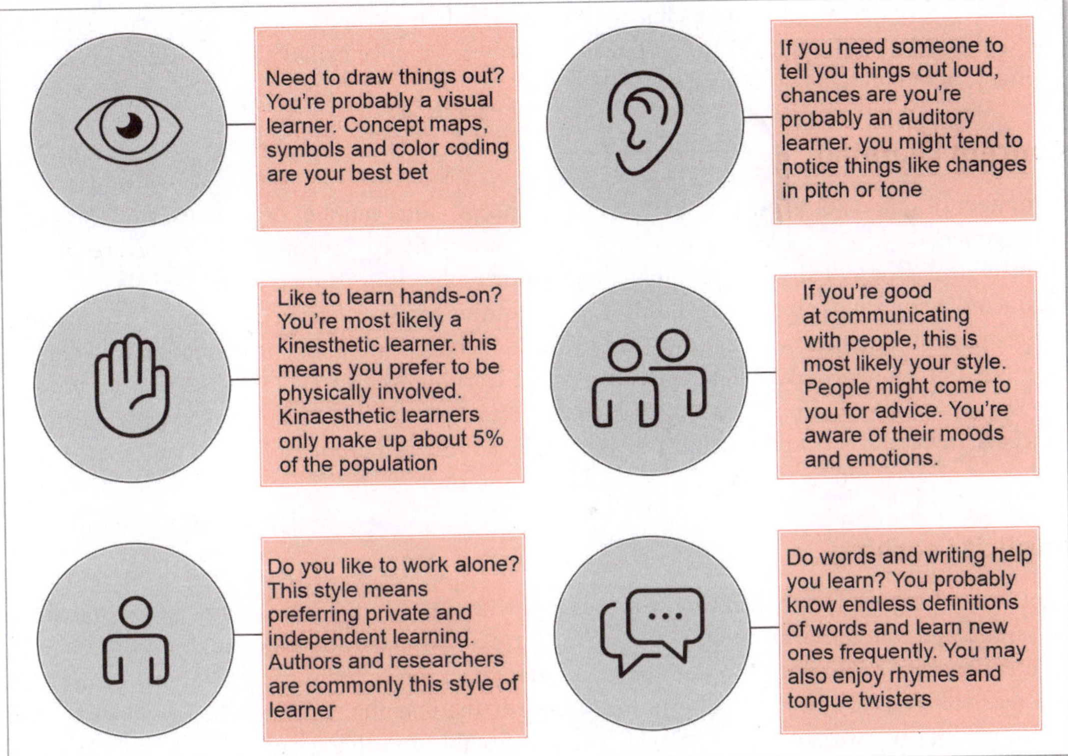

Fig. 9.9: Types of domain-based learning

Verbal Learning

Learning which occurs by using variety of familiar words, syllables, unfamiliar words, paragraphs, and sentences is known as verbal learning. This the most human-friendly type of learning.

- **Paired-associative learning** is one of the methods used in verbal learning. In this, firstly a list of paired associates are prepared, and then the first word of a pair is used as a "stimulus", and another word of the pair is used as a "response". This type of learning is used when an individual wants to learn a foreign language.[10, 14]
- **Serial learning**, is another type of verbal learning. In this method of learning, an individual first learns the list of verbal items consisted of most familiar words, syllables, and least familiar words, and then he presents the entire list of items in same order, as it is mentioned in the list.[10, 14]

Skill Learning

The ability to perform assigned complex task properly, smoothly, and clearly is known as skill learning. Driving a car, navigating a ship or preparing a food all are perfect examples of skill learning.

It also involves exercising and practicing one particular activity. When an individual keeps practicing one skill or activity, his performance gradually increases. 'Practice makes a man perfect' is a perfect saying, which represents skill learning.[11, 15]

Concept Learning

A number of objects or events is referred to as 'concept'. Total number of animals, fruits or other environmental objects are examples of concepts. A specific feature of an object or creature or event which is observed or discriminated with other objects is known as concept learning.[6, 13] Characteristics such as size, shape, number, color and texture are known as features.[3] Connecting the features of an object with another and forming a concept may vary from simple to complex. Two types of concepts are mainly used in concept learning, they are: (1) Artificial concepts and (2) Natural concepts. Those concepts which are clear, precise and firm are known as artificial concepts. In natural concepts, the features are usually not defined properly. Natural concepts include biological objects, and human remnants such as houses, clothes, etc.[6, 13]

Implicit Learning

Implicit learning is a type of learning which occurs without an individual's or a person's awareness. Perceptual and conceptual priming are the two main types of implicit learning. The ability to recognize different external cues which is accountable to cause alteration in brain perception processing, this process is referred to as perceptual priming. Whereas, the potential to access the knowledge about understanding of particular context which is accountable for alteration within brain structure, who processes sematic information. Examples of implicit learning are category/concept learning and sequence learning. Generally, implicit learning and memory appear together which reflects the manner of working of different regions of brain who are specialized areas for processing various types of learning and its information. It also refers to learning something without intention to learn a particular activity. It involves a permanent modification of an individual's activity occurring from its interaction with external stimuli in the absence of intention of someone about the learning end and its methods. Learned activity in implicit learning can be performed rapidly and automatically. Implicit learning is having four main properties, they are: (1) Processing information by unconscious mode, (2) Obtained information is displayed through abstract representation, (3) Incidental nature of learning, and (4) Independent attentional resources. Implicit learning has been used in many skill activities such as learning a foreign language, and motor-social skills.[13, 16, 17]

Collective Learning

Collective learning is a cumulative process which results in establishing information based on social interactions. Such information should be in the form of structure, routines, norms, approaches, and strategies that guide action plan. In this, learning occurs because of interactions of various mechanisms where one person is sharing knowledge with another person. It is mostly used in

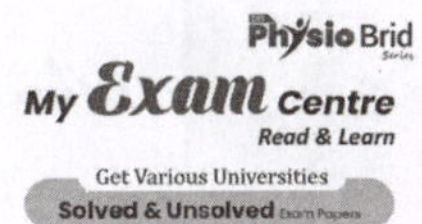

organization theory, psychology, and sociology. It helps in formation of values and identities by means of social interactions. It helps in intellectual social academic development. It also helps in developing comprehensive understanding of concepts related to the specific areas of interests. Examples of collective learning are: Conducting academic classes of students on Zoom meetings, Google meet, and another social platform. This type of learning was very successful and helpful at the time of COVID-19 pandemic. It helps in sharing experiences between each other and also to collaborate with each other to solve problem, and solution to the problem.[18, 19]

Statistical Learning

Statistical learning is defined as wide set statistical tools used for understanding the data. There are two types of statistical learning, namely: (1) Supervised statistical learning, and (2) Unsupervised statistical learning.[20, 21]

Supervised Statistical Learning

Supervised statistical learning comprises creating a statistical model which predicts, estimates, and provides output-based inputs. Supervised statistical learning is followed in the fields of medicine, business, and astrophysics.[20, 21]

Unsupervised Statistical Learning

In unsupervised statistical learning, there is no supervising output but inputs are present. Also, a student cannot learn relationship and structures from the defined statistical data.[20, 21]

> **MUST KNOW**
>
> Concept learning, collective learning and statistical learning are used in research and methodology. A good researcher should have in-depth knowledge of these three types of learning.

e-learning

e-learning is defined as a learning system based on structured teaching with the help of electronic resources, libraries, databases, and social platforms is known as e-learning. The major components of e-learning are use of computers, and internet. Nowadays, e-learning through computer and internet is very much in trend. With the help of e-learning, transferring of knowledge and skills along with delivery of information to large number of recipients became very easier. This method of e-learning is very time saving and eco-friendly in nature.[22, 23] e-learning is described in more detail later in this chapter.

Perceptual Learning

Perceptual learning refers to the improvement in our ability to interpret sensory information, such as what we see, hear, feel, taste or smell, through experience. Furthermore, they are not just coincidental but instead serve a purpose, such as enhancing sensitivity to subtle or unclear stimuli.[24]

A significant advancement in grasping perceptual learning is the discovery that it entails altering how sensory information is represented in the brain.[31] Consequently, perceptual learning is not solely about honing attention to detect unique stimulus attributes or refining sensory processing due to heightened alertness.[25, 26]

Mechanism

Enhanced performance on perceptual tasks through practice or training is well-documented, yet the exact mechanisms behind perceptual learning remain a topic of debate.[24] Training typically boosts performance across various visual tasks, with some learning being specific to factors like retinal location, spatial frequency or orientation of stimuli. The specificity observed, particularly about retinal location and stimulus attributes, is suggested to signify neural plasticity within fundamental visual processing mechanisms.[26]

Unique Features

Enhancements in perceptual task performance resulting from training may not necessarily signify perceptual learning. Similar effects on performance can also be shown from other forms of learning, such as those involving task rules, associations, and strategies. Contrary to these more advanced learning styles, it involves increased sensitivity that is unaffected by nonperceptual elements such as motor, cognitive or other. As a result, reductions in the strength of stimulus, clarity or time needed to reach a particular accuracy level are commonly used to evaluate perceptual learning.[26] By using signal detection theory on such data, one may differentiate between perceptual sensitivity changes and other factors, such as decision biases. It is important to differentiate between perceptual learning and higher-level task learning, particularly for nonhuman subjects, by identifying these sensitivity changes without corresponding performance changes for readily perceived stimuli acquiring task rules *via* experimentation. Moreover, perceptual learning frequently—though not always—relates to the precise stimulus configuration that was employed during training, such as the position and orientation of visual stimuli in a task that tests texture discrimination.[24, 25]

Perceptual learning poses challenges due to its occurrence across diverse conditions, likely reflecting a wide array of neural alterations. Studies have shown that perceptual learning occurs in a variety of sensory modalities and is associated by alterations in different sensory pathways. Moreover, there might be considerable variations in the mechanisms and features of perceptual learning within each modality, especially when it comes to two aspects: (1) Reward processing and (2) Attention.[24, 25]

Attention to a specific task or relevant sensory feature appears crucial for certain forms of perceptual learning. However, under certain conditions, perceptual learning can occur in some situations even in the absence of concentrated attention on the characteristic, however, it may not be as strong as it is when attention is focused on it. Thus, paying attention can either support or improve perceptual learning.[24]

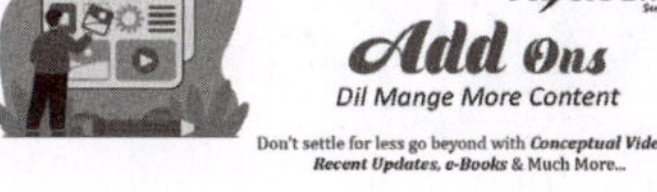

Similarly, reward can facilitate certain forms of perceptual learning. For instance, learning of a visual feature can occur with the provision of rewards, even in the absence of focused attention on that feature.[24] It is thought that rewards-driven modifications to perceptual judgments underlie other types of visual perceptual learning. The dopaminergic system, which is essential to other forms of reinforcement learning and can influence how tones are represented in the auditory cortex during perceptual learning, is probably involved in these changes. Active research areas include the prevalence of such reward-related mechanisms in perceptual learning and their interactions with attentional systems.[25]

Models

Models serve as valuable tools for testing of learning and plasticity theories, allowing for the examination of difficult patterns found in empirical literature.[25] Modules for sensory representation, decision-making, learning, and potentially attention, reward, and feedback systems are all commonly included in comprehensive models. Noise or variability in the system's internal responses is a further crucial aspect.[26] The accuracy of performance relies heavily on distinguishing signal from internal noise. Computational models predict behavioral outcomes by processing stimuli inputs and detailing the computations performed in each module.[24]

FACTORS FACILITATING LEARNING

Factors which are responsible for facilitating learning are continuous and partial reinforcement, motivation, and preparedness for learning.[4]

Continuous and Partial Reinforcement

When a reward is provided every time a desired behavior occurs, it is continuous reinforcement learning technique. While in partial reinforcement a reward is given for a desired behavior occasionally.[4]

Motivation

Motivation is a mental and physiological state which allows an individual to act for fulfilling his needs. It energizes an individual to function optimally for achieving his targets. Motivation is a prerequisite of learning. It has two types namely, intrinsic motivation, and extrinsic motivation. Learning things by enjoying the particular activity or having interests in learning some particular activity is known as intrinsic motivation. Activity which provides the means for activating other goals related to another goal is known as extrinsic motivation.[2, 3]

Preparedness for Learning

Human beings can learn associations which are genetically embedded in them because they are gifted with genetic preparedness. Every species has variations in there sensory, motor and response behavior.

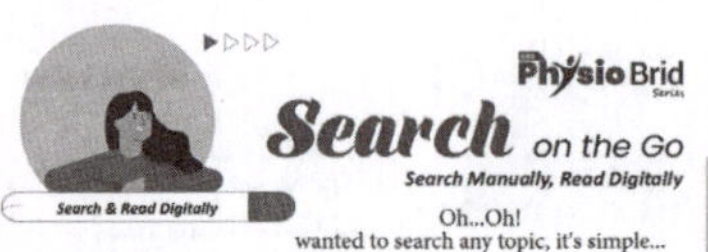

A particular type of associative learning is easy for human beings, and apes because they are gifted with genetic preparedness but these associative learnings are extremely difficult for other species such as reptiles (snakes and chameleon), and mammals (cats and rats). Species for that genetic preparedness are not having much potential, they can learn specific tasks with only great difficulties and resistance.[4]

MUST KNOW

Various factors which influence learning

Factor	Description	Examples
Cognitive factors	Influences related to mental processes involved in learning.	Memory capacity, problem-solving skills, attention.
Motivational factors	Elements that drive an individual's desire to learn and persist.	Intrinsic motivation, extrinsic rewards, goal-setting.
Emotional factors	Emotional states that impact the learning process.	Stress, anxiety, self-esteem, emotional support.
Social factors	Interactions and relationships that influence learning.	Peer influence, teacher support, family environment.
Environmental factors	External conditions and settings where learning takes place.	Classroom environment, access to resources, physical space.
Cultural factors	Cultural background and values that affect learning processes and content.	Language, cultural norms, educational practices.
Developmental factors	Stage of cognitive and emotional development that affects learning abilities.	Age, developmental milestones, readiness for learning.
Health factors	Physical health conditions that impact learning capabilities.	Chronic illnesses, nutritional status, fatigue.
Educational factors	Aspects of the education system and instructional methods that influence learning.	Teaching methods, curriculum design, assessment strategies.
Technological factors	Availability and use of technology in the learning process.	Access to computers, educational software, online resources.
Personal factors	Individual characteristics and preferences that affect learning.	Learning style, prior knowledge, cognitive strengths and weaknesses.
Experiential factors	Previous experiences and practical exposure that impact learning.	Hands-on practice, real-world applications, past learning experiences.

CLINICAL LEARNING ENVIRONMENT

The clinical learning environment's (CLE) design significantly impacts trainees and educators, influencing how they acquire and apply knowledge, skills, and values.[27] Despite being dynamic, the physical CLE is often perceived as static. Interpersonal factors, such as social dynamics and personnel roles, also shape learners' and educators' experiences within the physical environment.[28] However, there is scarce literature on how educators and trainees can effectively utilize clinical spaces for education during active patient care.

The CLE plays a crucial role in shaping learners' perceptions, impacting aspects such as supervision, feedback, autonomy, and psychological safety. Physical spaces within the CLE encompass formal classrooms, conference rooms, and informal areas like corridors and lounges, with a focus on patient care settings. These spaces are part of larger clinical units, buildings, and institutions.[28] While buildings are designed to endure for over 50 years, the layout of clinical units may evolve over decades, and furnishings and equipment within them can change frequently.[27]

Strengths

The CLE offers numerous advantages. It also addresses real-world challenges within the professional aspect, enhancing motivation through active engagement. Teachers serve as role models for professional thinking, behavior, and attitudes. It uniquely integrates the teaching and learning of professional skills.[27] However, despite its potential strengths, clinical teaching often faces criticism for inconsistency, insufficient intellectual stimulation, and a disorganized approach.

Challenges

- Time constraints.
- Balancing competing demands: Clinical, administrative, and research responsibilities.
- In essence, while clinically-based education is theoretically sound, its effectiveness is often hindered by implementation challenges.[27]
- Opportunistic nature complicates planning efforts.
- More students led to a significant demand on resources.
- Decreased patient availability due to shorter hospital stays, patient frailty, and consent refusals.
- Insufficient resources and support.
- Clinical settings may not be conducive to teaching.
- Inadequate rewards and recognition for educators.
- Unclear objectives and expectations.
- Emphasis on memorization over problem-solving skills and attitudes.
- Instruction often too advanced for learners' level.
- Passive learning rather than active engagement.
- Insufficient supervision and feedback.
- Limited opportunities for reflection and discussion.
- Use of humiliation as a teaching method.

- Failure to obtain informed consent from patients.
- Disregard for patient privacy and dignity.

Clinical Learning Patterns

Learning style is a learner's/student's accordant way of using and responding to the environmental cue related to learning.[4] It is a way in which learner/student understands process, and retains information. There are two types of learning styles namely: (1) Relational style, and (2) Analytical style.[29, 30]

Relational Style

In this, learner/student perceives information in small parts of the whole context, and exhibits intuitive thinking. Also, gaining knowledge related to human context, social content which are mostly having experimental relevance. In this, a learner/student focuses on task-oriented concerning non-academic areas. Student/learner is having a good memory for verbally-presented ideas.[29, 30]

Analytical Style

In this, a student/learner focuses on a total context in detail. This type of style exhibits sequential and structured thinking. This type of style produces good memory for abstract ideas. Analytical style is mostly found in school and college environments. This type of style mostly focusses on task-oriented concerning academic activities.[29, 30]

E-LEARNING

The psychology of e-learning explores how psychological principles and theories can enhance online learning experiences by understanding how learners process, retain, and apply information in digital environments. Key aspects include managing cognitive load to avoid overwhelming learners, utilizing intrinsic and extrinsic motivators to drive engagement, and encouraging self-regulation for autonomy and self-directed learning. It also emphasizes the importance of social learning through peer interactions and collaborative tools, personalization to cater to individual learning preferences, and providing timely, constructive feedback to reinforce learning. By applying these principles, e-learning can become more effective, engaging, and inclusive.

Method of Delivery

Just as constructing a bridge relies on engineering principles, effective learning should be grounded in the psychology of learning. However, there is often a significant gap between practice and theory in training and education.[31] Many educators lack sufficient training in learning psychology. In corporate training, instructors are frequently drawn from other areas of the organization or possess

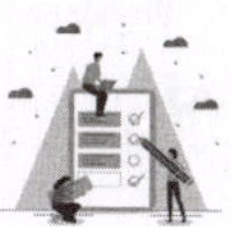
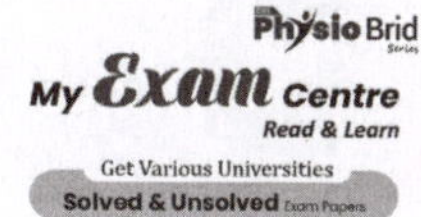

expertise in the subject matter without adequate training in learning psychology or instructional design. Similarly, in medical education, clinicians and lecturers are often experts in their field but lack formal training in teaching methods or learning psychology.[27]

Psychology has seen shifts from behaviorism to cognitive psychology and, more recently, to constructivism. Behaviorism focuses on conditioning responses to stimuli, primarily through external reinforcement.[32] Cognitive psychology delved deeper into internal cognitive factors in learning, while social constructivism has advanced our understanding of how learners construct knowledge as they learn.[33]

> **MUST KNOW**
>
> **Behaviorism → Cognitive Psychology → Constructivism**
>
> Behaviorism focuses on conditioning responses to stimuli, primarily through external reinforcement. Cognitive psychology delved deeper into internal cognitive factors in learning, while social constructivism has advanced our understanding of how learners construct knowledge as they learn.

Despite significant advancements in the psychology of learning, particularly in understanding how learning occurs and how it can be enhanced, medical education has often lagged in incorporating these changes.[33] Research findings are frequently poorly disseminated and seldom applied in practice. Much of the theoretical framework in training and education could be characterized as trendy and lacking empirical support.[32]

In practice, training remains heavily influenced by behaviorist theory, focusing on external factors, and neglecting internal cognitive processes. This one-sided perspective is exemplified by the joke about two behaviorists, highlighting the disregard for subjective experiences. Traditional training methods still center around teachers delivering content in classrooms, treating learners as passive recipients rather than active, motivated, and complex constructors of knowledge, as revealed by the psychology of learning.[32]

The conventional classroom-based approach often resembles a "sheep-dip" experience, which is profoundly behaviorist in its design, delivery, and evaluation. As the psychology of learning has evolved to become more learner-centric, so has the delivery of education. There are noticeable discrepancies between learner-centric theories in the psychology of learning and the behaviorist practices commonly found in educational settings.[27]

- Overreliance on one-way communication ('tell' mode)
- Inadequate assessment of prerequisites
- Limited attention to fostering motivation
- Insufficient cognitive engagement
- Common occurrence of cognitive overload
- Predominance of mass training over distributed learning
- Lack of reinforcement

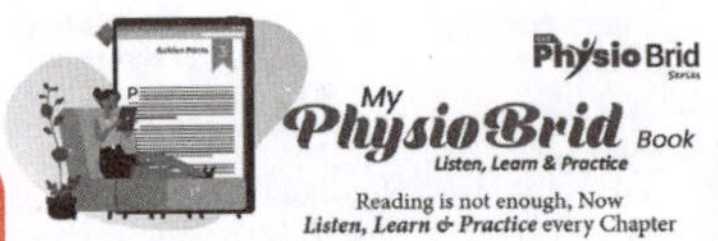

E-Learning versus Traditional Methods

Post-treatment test scores indicate that learners exhibit greater learning outcomes with computer-based instruction compared to traditional teaching methods.[31]

Research literature in training, conducted by Fletcher and Tobias, it is asserted that learners demonstrate greater learning outcomes through computer-based instruction compared to traditional teaching methods. This claim is supported by specific studies conducted by Willett (1983), Kulik (1994), and Fletcher et al. (1999). One contributing factor to this enhanced effectiveness is the heightened level of engagement facilitated by interactivity in computer-based instruction. This increased participation leads to greater cognitive engagement and, consequently, improved retention. In essence, active participation enhances retention.[31, 33]

Furthermore, the self-paced nature of computer-based learning contributes to higher retention rates, as learners can digest the content at their own speed, rather than being dictated by the pace of a teacher in a classroom setting. Learners have the flexibility to pause, review, repeat, and integrate the learning into their existing knowledge structures, a feature not readily available in traditional classrooms.[34, 35]

However, the effectiveness of computer-based instruction is contingent upon the quality of the content design. It is likely that the quality of text, audio, graphics, animation, and video in computer-based instruction surpasses that of traditional training environments. For example, using videos or pictures of real patients exhibiting these symptoms could greatly enhance teaching methods such as balloon angioplasty or recognizing symptoms of schizophrenia.[34, 35]

Comparison of Time

Learners interact with computer-based training when they are provided with the same learning materials as those who are using other methods.[34, 35] Tobias and Fletcher, in their research survey, also support the notion that learners using computer-based instruction typically experience time savings ranging from 30% to 60%.[33]

This accelerated rate of learning is caused by several reasons. First of all, when learners are immediately exposed to images and other media, the pace and quality of the presentation are greatly accelerated. This is in contrast to traditional techniques, when learners are often presented with slow and low-quality images on charts or overhead projectors. Furthermore, the self-paced aspect of computer-based training reduces needless waiting for group members to catch up or have questions answered, which speeds up the learning process.[33]

Coping with Different Types of Learners

Any given course will encompass a diverse group of learners with varying backgrounds, experiences, personalities, and motivations. A traditional classroom setting may only cater to a portion of this audience, often resulting in a mismatch between the course content and individual learner needs.

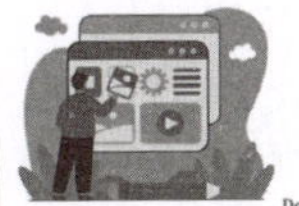

Without proper diagnosis before the course, educators can only make educated guesses about which learners will benefit most.[34]

Learners may find the course either too fast or too slow, too broad or too narrow in focus, and either relevant or irrelevant to their needs. Teachers struggle to address the diverse needs within the group, as the classroom typically operates on a supply-based model rather than catering to individual demand.[33, 34] This overlooks a fundamental principle in the psychology of learning: that individual learner's matter, and his unique needs must be accommodated.

Empowering learners with greater responsibility for their learning is key to addressing these challenges. Conducting a thorough needs analysis before the course can ensure better-targeted training, reducing wasted effort and failure. E-learning, with its self-paced nature and ability to customize learning paths based on prerequisites, holds promise for more targeted and successful learning experiences.[33, 34]

Determining a learner's readiness for a particular learning task can be achieved through simple pretests, which can be conveniently administered online. These pretests provide individuals and their mentors with a clear understanding of their current knowledge level. Ongoing assessment, facilitated by online systems, allows for continuous monitoring of progress and adjustment of learning plans as needed.[33, 34] Furthermore, online platforms open possibilities for intelligent tutoring, where software can analyze users' learning behavior and make personalized recommendations to enhance effectiveness.

Challenges

Despite the advantages or benefits, e-learning also presents with a few challanges.

Motivation

Behaviorism overlooked the importance of internal motivation in learning, which research indicates plays a significant role – "we only learn when we want to". Learning is most effective when driven by personal goals rather than external factors. Self-reference, opportunities for reflection, and learner autonomy are key motivational factors, that facilitate faster learning. Thus, learning should be learner-centric, with teachers shifting from delivering knowledge to supporting learners. In e-learning, design should focus on individual relevance, reflective experiences, media choice, and a shift in the teacher's role toward learner support and motivation.[31]

Dropouts

When it comes to learner motivation, e-learning poses difficulties that can result in problems like dissatisfaction, high dropout rates, and boredom. This psychological aspect of the e-learning issue is critical because although e-learning may increase effectiveness, learner willingness to participate is not always assured.[31]

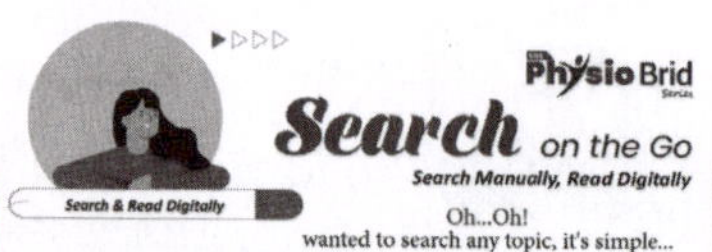

The traditional association of learning with classrooms and courses must be overcome, as learners have been conditioned to this model through years of classroom-based education. Dropout rates in e-learning are viewed differently; some argue that dropout is not necessarily a failure, but rather a natural part of flexible, learner-centric models.[34] Spaced learning, rather than fixed-time courses, is considered more effective, aligning with the constructivist approach to learning that emphasizes incremental steps and personalized mental models.[35]

Reward

An additional challenge is the perception of training as a reward, particularly with residential courses seen as opportunities for time off or enjoyable trips. While this may seem positive, it often leads to inefficient use of training budgets, with learners motivated more by perks than by learning. This expectation from training, where learning through e-learning method is viewed as a cost-effective measure rather than a valuable learning opportunity. To address this, organizations should emphasize personal benefits such as career advancement and job improvement to sell the value of e-learning.[35]

Appeal

Effective learning by means of traditional methods or e-learning methods, depends on cognitive engagement. While some classroom training remains lecture-based, e-learning's interactivity fosters higher retention through increased simulation and engagement. Meaningful content organization and personal relevance also bolster retention. Learners benefit from chunking information, self-referencing, and personalized learning experiences, all facilitated by e-learning's accessibility and flexibility. Metacognition or learning how to learn, remains underutilized but holds significant potential to enhance learning outcomes. Encouraging students to actively engage with content through generative techniques like note-taking and summarizing can further boost learning effectiveness.[35]

Learning Experience

Ebbinghaus's findings from 1885 emphasize the significance of distributed practice in learning. This approach, spread over time, enhances memory consolidation, and reduces fatigue effects compared to massed practice.[35] Analogous to medical slow-release mechanisms, learning benefits from regular, smaller doses are tailored to the learner's needs. Research conducted in 1914 supports the effectiveness of spaced learning over concentrated sessions. For instance, a study by Baddley and Longman in 1978 demonstrated superior learning outcomes when practice was spread over multiple days rather than condensed into a single session.[33] Besides improving retention, distributing learning sessions is more convenient for learners, aligning with their work patterns and providing on-demand access to learning.[34]

Realism

Reeves and Nass (1999) conducted psychological studies suggesting that people react socially and naturally to media, often treating computers as if they were people.[34] This phenomenon arises from our evolutionary background and the tendency to perceive anything that seems real as real. Here are key points from their research:

- **Consistency and conformity:** Media that align with social and physical rules are more enjoyable. Meeting human expectations fosters feelings of accomplishment and empowerment.

- **Arousal:** Emotional engagement at the beginning of an e-learning program enhances memory retention.

- **Politeness:** Interfaces should greet users and bid them farewell politely to enhance engagement.

- **Flattery:** Praise, even if insincere, can motivate learners. Negative feedback should be given sparingly and in conversational terms.

- **Negativity:** Negative experiences can grab attention and improve memory, but they should be used judiciously.

- **Interpersonal distance:** Close-up shots and point-of-view shots enhance attention and memory, especially in images of people.

- **Personality:** Consistent and strong personalities in media are preferred over mixed personalities.

- **Specialists and teams:** Testimonials from peers and experts influence learners. Emphasizing tasks as team efforts enhances engagement.

- **Voice and fidelity:** Audio quality is more important than image fidelity. Poor audio quality is psychologically unsettling.

- **Synchrony:** Unnatural timing and audio-video asynchrony disrupt learning. Meaningful animation is beneficial, but constant motion can be distracting.

These principles inform the design of effective e-learning experiences, focusing on engagement, interaction, and psychological comfort for learners.[34]

Lack of Tenacious Qualities

Short- and Long-Term Memory

Ebbinghaus's conducted study in 1885, "On Memory," demonstrated the rapid decline of learned content over time (Fig. 9.10).[36]

Most of the loss occurred within the first few minutes, highlighting the importance of transferring knowledge from short- to long-term memory. Despite over a century of research on memory models, many educators overlook this issue. Traditional classroom-based learning often

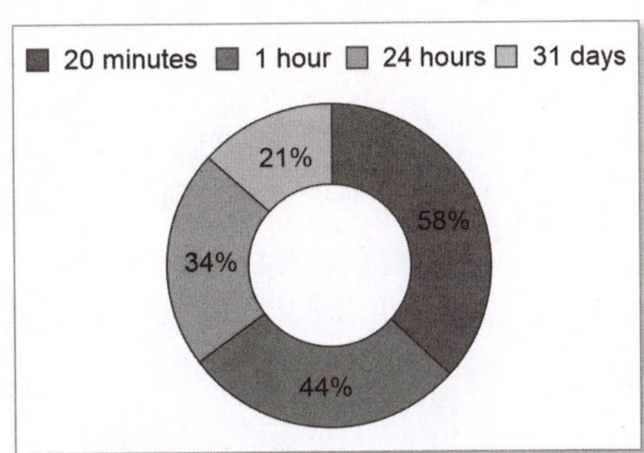

Fig. 9.10: Time-related decline in learning[36]

fails to reinforce learning effectively, leading to significant memory loss. Improving reinforcement methods could potentially increase learning productivity.

Reinforcement and Retention

"Sheep-dip training", often leaves learners to fend for themselves afterward. This approach neglects the importance of reinforcement in retaining knowledge, contradicting established theories of learning.[36] While theory emphasizes the transfer of knowledge from short- to long-term memory, practice often fails to reinforce learning effectively.

Courses are favored because they are self-contained and easy to administer, but they are rarely evaluated for their effectiveness. Immediate reinforcement of theory into practice is crucial for retention and behavioral change. Relying solely on courses may hinder behavioral change by prioritizing convenience for training providers over the needs of learners.[36]

E-learning's flexibility allows learning to be delivered on-demand, closely tied to real-world tasks, which enhances reinforcement through workplace practice. Learners can revisit material as needed, particularly for episodic skills. Additionally, the networked nature of e-learning enables various reinforcement events like emails, reminders, and synchronous experiences, further solidifying learning.[32]

LEARNING DISABILITY

Learning disabilities are a group heterogeneous conditions where there is a deficit in reading, writing, processing, and understanding language which further manifests as a difficulty to speak, write, spell, understand, and solve mathematical calculations (Fig. 9.11).[37, 38]

Reading Disability

Reading disability is also termed dyslexia. One of the most common type of learning disability is dyslexia, which accounts at least 80% of total learning disabilities. "Reading" requires, the ability to understand the relation that exists between alphabets and their associated sound, which is referred

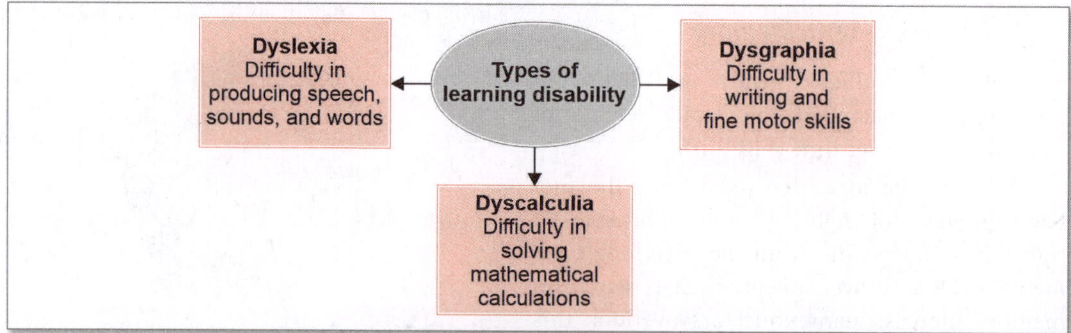

Fig. 9.11: Types of learning disabilities

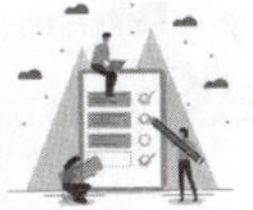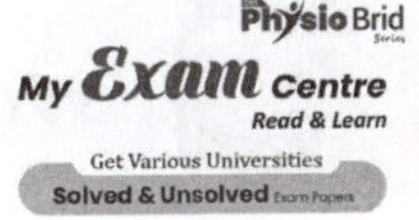

to as phonetics. It causes disruption in processing speech, sound of an individual, and also in words (phenomes). Children with dyslexia are having difficulties in fluency with reading which causes accurate reading skills but slow and full of efforts.[39, 40]

Dyscalculia

Dyscalculia is defined as in which a child is having difficulty in understanding or learning mathematical calculations. In this, a child is having difficulty in organizing problem, following multiple steps calculations, how to use different mathematical calculation signs while solving mathematical operations. Child with dyscalculia also having confusions while solving basic mathematical operations.[37, 41]

Dysgraphia

Dysgraphia is difficulty in writing despite through instruction. In this, a child is having inconsistent and illegible writing skills, confusion in alphabetical letters, mixing upper- and lower-case letters, writing on a line instead between the page lines. Child with dysgraphia is also having difficulty in fine motor skills such as trouble in holding pencil or pen, writing with pen or pencil, and inability to hold and using scissors.[38, 41]

Children with learning disabilities also having psychological problems. Mostly up to 30% of them experience behavioral and emotional problems. They are also hyperactive in nature. In children with learning disabilities, there is a strong association between in attentiveness and dyslexia.[38, 41]

SUMMARY

- Learning is a process which is a true result of past experience. Behaviorism, cognitivism, constructivism, connectivism, and humanism are the five learning theories.
- These theories help in teaching and learning methods in clinical and research setups.
- Among them, behaviorism is a teacher-centered approach while others are student or learner centered approaches.
- There are numerous types of learning, which helps in gaining knowledge and information in various different ways, and which we can imply in our physiotherapy clinical understanding, teaching, and research activities.
- Factors which facilitate learning are: continuous and partial reinforcement, motivation, and preparedness for learning.
- Types of learning styles are analytical style, and relational style.
- E-learning is nowadays very common, and mostly followed in the digital area after COVID-19. E-learning is having psychological myths which affects learning.
- Learning disabilities are those which hinders learning process at the beginning phase of life. Children are mostly affected and having difficulties in reading, writing, and understanding the context: Dysgraphia, dyslexia, and dyscalculia are three common types of learning disabilities.

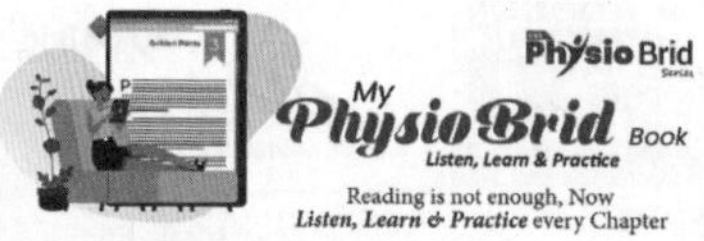

REFERENCES

1. Weinstein Y, Madan CR, Sumeracki MA. Teaching the Sience of Learning. Cogn Res Princ Implic. 2018;3(2):1–17.

2. Morris LS, Grehl MM, Rutter SB, Mehta M, Westwater ML. On what motivates us: A Detailed Review of Intrinsic v. Extrinsic Motivation. Psychol Med. 2022;52(10):1801–16.

3. Rea SD, Wang L, Muenks K, Yan VX. Students Can (Mostly) Recognize Effective Learning , So Why Do They Not Do It ? J Intell. 2022;10:1–28.

4. Whitehead AN. Laerning. In: Psychology. 2006. p. 1–146.

5. Badyal, Singh. Learning Theories: The Basics to Learn in Medical Education. Int J Appl Basic Med Res. 2017;7(1):S1–3.

6. Martin AJ. Educational Psychology and Student Learning: The Potential of Load Reduction Instruction for Exploring Surface and Deep Approaches to Learning. Psychol Educ Rev. 2019;43(1):23–7.

7. Nougaret S, Ferrucci L, Genovesio A. Neuroscience and Biobehavioral Reviews Role of the social actor during social interaction and learning in human- monkey paradigms. Neurosci Biobehav Rev [Internet]. 2019;102(March):242–50. Available from: https://doi.org/10.1016/j.neubiorev.2019.05.004

8. Pange J, Lekka A, Toki EI. Different learning theories applied to diverse learning subjects A pilot study. Procedia Soc Behjavoral Sci [Internet]. 2010;9:800–4. Available from: http://dx.doi.org/10.1016/j.sbspro.2010.12.237

9. Mercer S, Ryan S. Stretching the boundaries: language learning psychology. Palgrave Commun [Internet]. 2016;2(May):1–5. Available from: http://dx.doi.org/10.1057/palcomms.2016.31

10. 1Johnston C, Hayes LJ. Understanding Observational Learning: An Interbehavioral Approach. Anal Verbal Behav. 2011;27:191–203.

11. Han Y, Kamaruzaman S, Syed B, Ji L. Use of Observational Learning to Promote Motor Skill Learning in Physical Education: A Systematic Review. Int J Environ Res Public Health. 2022;19:1–18.

12. Adams NE. Bloom's taxonomy of cognitive learning objectives. J Med Libr Assoc. 2015;103(July):152–3.

13. Moreton E, Pater J. Phonological Concept Learning. Cogn Sci. 2017;41:4–69.

14. Schreiner T, Rasch B. Boosting vocabulary learning by verbal cueing during sleep. Cereb cortex. 2015;25(11):4169–79.

15. Fleischer P, Abbasi A, Fealy AW, Danielsen NP, Sandhu R, Raj PR, et al. Emergent Low-Frequency Activity in Cortico- Cerebellar Networks with Motor Skill Learning. ENEURO. 2023;10(February):1–12.

16. Seger CA. Implicit learning. Psycological Bull. 1995;115(2):163–92.

17. Musfeld P. Repetition learning is neither a continuous nor an implicit process. Psychol Cogn Sci. 2023;120(16):1–8.

18. Shirado H. Individual and collective learning in groups facing danger. Sci Rep [Internet]. 2022;12:1–13. Available from: https://doi.org/10.1038/s41598-022-10255-3

19. Collet J, Morford J, Lewin P, Sasaki T, Biro D, Morford J, et al. Mechanisms of collective learning: how can animal groups improve collective performance when repeating a task ? Philos Trans B. 2023;10:1–14.

20. Aslin RN. Statistical learning: A powerful mechanism that operates by mere exposure. Wiley Interdiscip Rev Cogn Sci. 2018;8:1–12.

21. Thiessen ED, Thiessen ED. What's statistical about learning? Insights from modeling statistical learning as a set of memory processes. Philos Trans B. 2017;5:1–10.

Contd...

22. Naciri A, Radid M, Kharbach A, Chemsi G. E-learning in health professions education during the COVID-19 pandemic: A Systematic Review. J Educ Eval Heal Prof. 2021;18:1–11.

23. Fuzzy HA, Study ANP, Faraz S, Ardestani M, Adibi S, Golshan A, et al. Factors Influencing the Effectiveness of E-Learning in. Healthcare. 2023;11:1–15.

24. Manuscript A. Perceptual learning: Toward a comprehensive theory. Annu Rev Psychol. 2015;66(Eagleman 2011):197–221.

25. Herzog MH, Cretenoud AF. What is new in perceptual learning? J Vis. 2017;17:1–4.

26. Wenger MJ, Rhoten SE. Perceptual Learning Produces Perceptual Objects. J Exp Psychol Learn Mem Cogn. 2021;46(3):1–41.

27. Benamer HTS, Alsuwaidi L, Khan N, Jackson L, Lakshmanan J, Ho SB, et al. Clinical learning environments across two different healthcare settings using the undergraduate clinical education environment measure. BMC Med Educ. 2023;23:1–7.

28. Alshammari T, Alqahtani S, Jumaan M Al, Gosling C, Beovich B, Williams B. The Perceptions and Expectations of the Clinical Learning Environment in Saudi Arabia: A Multidisciplinary Study. Clin Learn Environ. 2023;77(2):132–6.

29. Romanelli F, Bird E, Ryan M. Learning Styles: A Review of Theory , Application , and Best Practices. Am J Pharm Educ. 2009;73(1):1–5.

30. Mishra A, Gada P, Shah I. Learning styles Cavitatory tuberculosis in complex cyanotic heart disease. Natl Med J India. 2014;29(3):28–9.

31. Gaze CM. Popular psychological myths: A comparison of students' beliefs across the psychology major. J Scholarsh Teach Learn. 2014;14(2):46–60.

32. Ruczynski LIA, Pol MHJ Van De, Schouwenberg BJJW, Laan RFJM. Learning clinical reasoning in the workplace: A student perspective. BMC Med Educ [Internet]. 2022;1–8. Available from: https://doi.org/10.1186/s12909-021-03083-y

33. Guevara K, Fattah L, Ritt-olson A, Yin P ling, Litman L, Farouk SS, et al. Busting myths in online education: Faculty examples from the field. J Clin Transl Sci. 2021;(149):1–8.

34. Rodríguez-prada C, Orgaz C, Cubillas CP. Myths in psychology: Psychological Misconceptions Among Spanish Psychology Students. 2022;1–22.

35. Sibicky M, Klein CL, Embrescia E. Psychological Misconceptions and Their Relation to Students' Lay Beliefs of Psychological Misconceptions and Their Relation to Students' Lay Beliefs of Mind. Soc Teach Psychol [Internet]. 2021;(September 2020):1–7. Available from: https://doi.org/10.1177/0098628320959925

36. Murre JMJ, Dros J. Replication and Analysis of Ebbinghaus' Forgetting Curve. PLoS One. 2015;10(17):1–23.

37. Agostini F, Zoccolotti P. brain sciences Domain-General Cognitive Skills in Children with Mathematical Difficulties and Dyscalculia: A Systematic Review of the Literature. Brain Sci. 2022;12:1–34.

38. Chung PJ, Patel DR, Nizami I. Disorder of written expression and dysgraphia: Definition, diagnosis , and management. Transl Pediatr. 2020;9(3):46–54.

39. Seth F, Sunderdas G, College M, Edward K, Memorial VII. Specific Learning Disabilities in India: Current Situation and the Path Ahead. Indian Pediatr. 2022;59:367–70.

40. Hulme C, Snowling MJ. Reading disorders and dyslexia. Curr Opin Pediatr. 2017;28(6):731–5.

41. Fletcher JM, Grigorenko EL. Neuropsychology of Learning Disabilities: The past and the future. J Int Neuropsychol Soc. 2018;23:930–40.

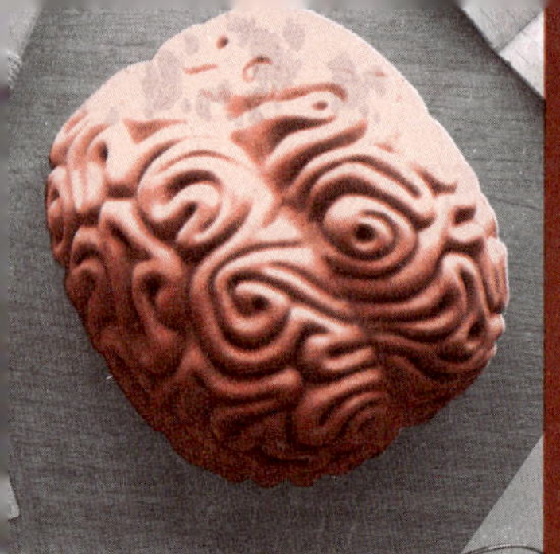

LONG ANSWER QUESTIONS

1. Explain in detail learning theories with examples.
2. Discuss learning disabilities and its types.
3. Discuss role of learning theories in physiotherapy teaching, clinicals and research.
4. Discuss in detail psychological need of e-learning.
5. Discuss strength and challenges of clinical learning environment.

SHORT ANSWER QUESTIONS

1. What is learning and styles of learning?
2. Enumerate challenges of clinical teaching.
3. Write about learning and its types.
4. Mention learning, and its uses in physiotherapy research.
5. Define e-learning and its uses in post COVID-19 era.

MULTIPLE CHOICE QUESTIONS

1. **Learning theory of "cognitivism" was proposed by:**
   a. John Locke
   b. Jean Piaget
   c. Jean Ayres
   d. None of these

2. **Dysgraphia is associated with:**
   a. Difficulty in reading
   b. Difficulty in writing
   c. Difficulty in speaking
   d. Difficulty in understanding

3. **What are the factors facilitating learning?**
   a. Motivation
   b. Continuous reinforcement
   c. Preparedness for learning
   d. All of these

4. **Theory which follows "self-actualization" is:**
   a. Connectivism
   b. Cognitivism
   c. Humanism
   d. Constructivism

5. **What are the methods used in verbal learning?**
   a. Serial learning
   b. Paired-associative learning
   c. None of these
   d. Both a and b

6. **How much decline of learned content in 1 hour?**
    a. 58%
    b. 44%
    c. 34%
    d. 21%

7. **Which one is the full form of CLE?**
    a. Continuing Legal Education
    b. Clinical Learning Environment
    c. Cutaneous Lupus Erythematous
    d. None of these

8. **Which factor is concerned in perceptual learning?**
    a. Attention
    b. Reward processing
    c. Both a and b
    d. None of these

9. **Learners using computer-based instruction experienced time savings ranging from:**
    a. 20–50%
    b. 30–60%
    c. 40–70%
    d. 50–80%

10. **Training boosts performance across various visual tasks, with some learning being specific to which factor?**
    a. Retinal location
    b. Spatial frequency
    c. Orientation of stimuli
    d. All of these

ANSWER KEY

| **1.** b | **2.** b | **3.** d | **4.** c | **5.** d | **6.** a | **7.** b | **8.** b |
| **9.** c | **10.** d | | | | | | |

Note

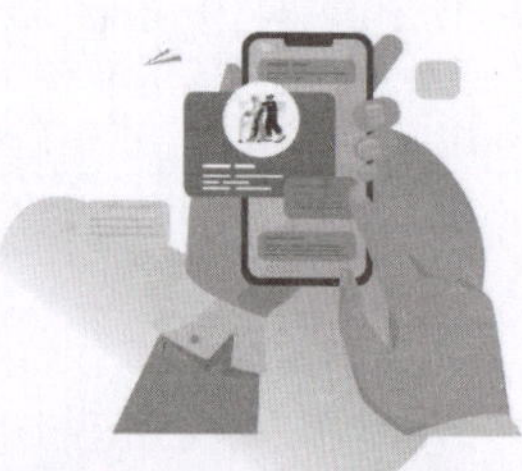
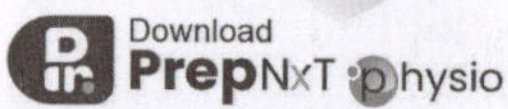

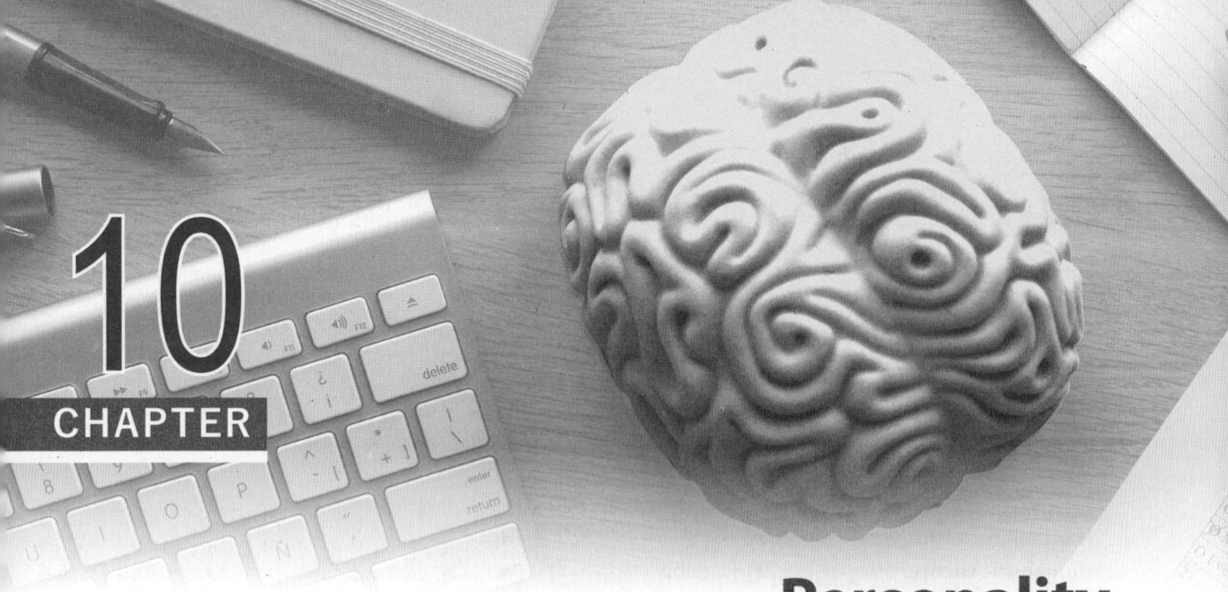

Personality

Hina Vaish

Hina Vaish

LEARNING OBJECTIVES

After the completion of the chapter, the readers will be able to:

- Define personality and explain its significance in understanding human behavior.
- Identify and describe the key traits and characteristics that make up an individual's personality.
- Explain the role of genetic, familial, societal, and personal experiences in shaping personality.
- Discuss how different life events and experiences can influence the development of personality traits.
- Describe the major theories of personality, including psychoanalytic, humanistic, and cognitive approaches.
- Explain the key concepts and principles underlying each theory and their contribution to understanding of personality.
- Understand the various methods used to assess personality, such as observation, objective tests, and projective tests.
- Describe the strengths and limitations of each assessment technique and its applicability in various contexts.
- Discuss the practical implications of personality theories and assessment techniques in clinical settings, particularly in physiotherapy.
- Explain how an understanding of personality can enhance the effectiveness of patient care and interpersonal relationships.
- Reflect on one's own personality traits and how that influences one's own behavior and interactions with others.
- Apply personality assessment techniques to evaluate others and understand their behavior patterns.

CHAPTER OUTLINE

- Introduction
- Definitions
- Characteristics
- Traits
- Factors Influencing Development of Personality
- Theories of Personality
- Assessment
- Practical Aspects
- Recent Advances

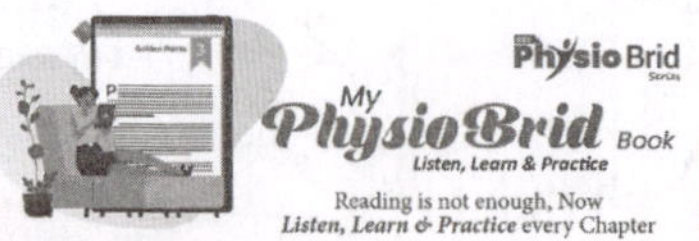

KEY TERMS

Cognitive theory: It emphasizes the process by which individuals organize their impressions of reality from sensations and perceptions.

Conscious: Mental activity (thinking, feelings, and memories) that can be accessed at any time.

Ego: Aspect of individuals' personality that represents themselves or the part of their personality that others can see.

Extrovert: Sociable, outgoing, active spontaneous, tough-minded people.

Heritability: Differences among people that is due to genetics.

Humanistic theory: It emphasizes individual's personal view of the world, self-concept, and push toward growth or self-actualization.

Id: Aspect of personality made up of our primitive instincts and drives, such as cravings for food, drink, and sex.

Ideal self: A psychological concept that describes a person's idealized version of themselves.

Introvert: Tender minded, reserved, passive, cautious and deep people.

Learning theory: This theory emphasizes that a person's behavior in any given circumstance is determined by the unique features of his past neuroticism.

Personality: It refers to ingrained characteristics and tendencies that lead people to think, feel, and act in particular ways on a regular basis.

Projective test: A method of evaluating personality in which subjects react to unclear cues to disclose feelings, impulses, and desires that are otherwise hidden.

Psychoanalytic theory: This theory highlights stages in development, a conflict amid pleasure seeking and reality demands; sexuality is the source for conflict and human growth.

Superego: Aspect of the personality that acts as the moral compass or conscience.

Traits: These are distinctive behavioral patterns.

Unconscious: Mental activity that we are not aware of or unable to access.

INTRODUCTION

The term "personality" is related to charm, charisma, and attractiveness. "He has a pleasant personality, but he is not smart". The word "personality" is used frequently.

A person's behavior that is consistent and broad in nature is referred to as his/her personality. It is a person's complete and comprehensive description.

A person's personality encompasses all their behavioral traits, including habits, ways of thinking, attitudes, and interests, as well as their individual viewpoint of life. It is the wholeness of a person. It encompasses one's temperament, as well as one's physical, mental, emotional, and behavioral characteristics.

This chapter goes into further detail on the definition, traits, theories, and evaluation of personality.

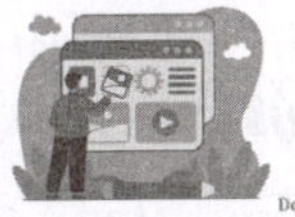

DEFINITIONS

The word personality originates from "persona", which means a mask worn by an actor.

Personality is what makes an individual unique. Psychologists define personality in different ways.

"Personality is the dynamic organization within the individual of those psychological systems, his characteristics, behaviors and thoughts."[1]
—*Gordon Allport, 1961*

"Personality is that which permits a prediction of what a person will do in a given situation."[2]
—*Cattell, 1950*

"Mind is divided into three components: *id*, *ego*, and *superego*, and that the interactions and conflicts among the components create personality."[3]
—*Freud, 1923/1949*

"Personality refers to deeply-ingrained patterns of behavior, which include the way one relates to, perceives and thinks about the environment and oneself."[4]
—*American Psychiatric Association, 1987*

A person's personality can be defined by his/her inner traits, behavioral traits or both. Every person has an exclusive form of continuing, lifelong traits, along with the way of connecting to other individuals and the environment. It is believed that the personality is enduring, steady, and hard to alter.

An individual's personality is what makes him unique. It encompasses an individual's distinct psychological traits that, over time, affect a range of recognizable behavior patterns (both overt and covert) in various contexts.

CHARACTERISTICS

- Self-consciousness is the main trait.
- Personality is a combination of environment and inheritance.
- A person's personality evolves *via* constant interaction with his surroundings. The formation of personality is influenced by a variety of experiences, social and cultural influences, and both.
- Personality is dynamic in nature.
- A personality constantly modifies its surroundings and internal existence. Tension and strain result from inadequate adjustment, and the person is always learning new adjusting patterns.
- Personality of each person is unique.
- Personality always aspires to achieve goals.
- The lives of all individuals have meaning, and they work hard to achieve their objectives. Each person's life is distinct and special.

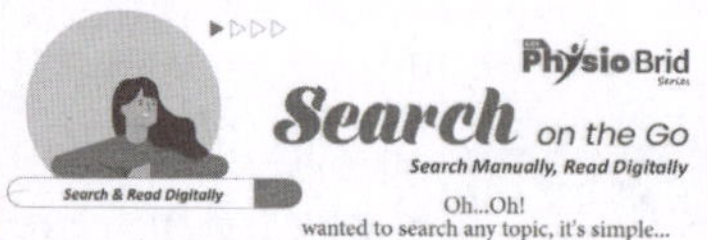

TRAITS

Traits are characteristic way of behaving. They are personal characteristics of an individual in different ways in different aspects.[5]

The traits are as follows:

- **Personal appearance:** A lot of emphasis is placed on a person's "looks", which encompass not only their complexion, height, and weight but also their attire, voice, and other unique personal traits. However, sometimes having good traits like helpfulness, friendliness, and kindness make up for a lack of beauty.

- **Intelligence:** It is the capacity to adapt to novel circumstances and solve problems. It is the capacity for learning and mental alertness. Although there are individual differences, for a balanced personality, intelligence is desired.

- **Emotions:** A healthy personality requires emotional maturity and stability.

- **Sociability:** By encouraging children to play in groups and share their belongings and experiences, the foundation of social solidarity is laid.

- **Ascendance-submission:** This characteristic denotes assertiveness. In most cases, those in lower social positions are ruled over and subject to those in higher positions.

- **Moral character:** This characteristic relates to social acceptance of whether a person has a balanced personality and is working toward a clear goal that will benefit their society.

FACTORS INFLUENCING DEVELOPMENT OF PERSONALITY

- **Genetic and growth factors:**
  - The child inherits the traits from parents through genetics. The way the nervous system, endocrine system, and body type function all affect personality.
  - Genetic disorders have an impact on personality. The child's personality may be influenced by the mother's health and illnesses during pregnancy. Parental habits like smoking or addiction during pregnancy can have an influence on child's personality and development.

- **Family, society and culture:**
  - A person's personality is greatly shaped by the family and social circles because they set the example for rewards and punishments.
  - Parents offer their children the closest possible social environment. As a result, a person begins to develop some of their fundamental personality traits, as early as, in childhood.
  - Every society has its own set of accepted and unacceptable behaviors and cultures, as well as ethical and other values, concepts of achievement, status, and prestige, as well as conventional values.

- **Personal experiences:**
  - The development of personality is also influenced by unique personal experiences. These experiences serve as the foundation for the distinctive features that make each person unique.

Severe illness, traumatic experiences, etc., are examples of negative experiences that can negatively affect personality development and prevent it from evolving freely and fully. In severe situations, they may also cause abnormalities in behavior.

> **MUST KNOW**
>
> **Personal experiences affect personality**
> - **Positive experiences** lead to better personality development
> - **Negative experiences** adversely affect the personality development

- On the other hand, positive elements that support a better development of personality include achievement, success, and exhilarating experiences.

THEORIES OF PERSONALITY

Type Approach

- **Hippocrates** paired body features with personality tempers.[6]
  - **Blood:** Sanguine nature, joyful and lively.
  - **Phlegm:** Phlegmatic nature, uninterested and sluggish.
  - **Black bile:** Melancholy nature, gloomy and perturbing.
  - **Yellow bile:** Choleric nature, short-tempered.
- **William Sheldon** associated physique to temperament.[7, 8]
  - **Endomorphic:** Fat, relaxed, friendly and fond of eating.
  - **Mesomorphic:** Well-built, strong, active and confident.
  - **Ectomorphic:** Slim, artistic and introvert.
- **Kretschmer classification**[9]
  - **Asthenic type:** Slender body, may suffer from schizophrenia.
  - **Pyknic type:** Round body, may suffer from manic-depressive illness.
  - **Athletic type:** Muscular, prone to epilepsy.
  - **Dysplastic type:** Are those who cannot be classified as any of the other three types.
- **Eysenck's three dimensions of personality (Fig. 10.1)**

  Eysenck suggested introversion-extroversion, emotional stability/neuroticism and psychoticism.[10]
  - Introverts are tender minded, reserved, passive, cautious and deep.
  - Extroverts are social, friendly, active, spontaneous, tough-minded people.

> **MUST KNOW**
>
> **Introverts and Extroverts**
> - **Introverts:** Socially withdrawn, inward turning, shy reserved, work alone, interested in themselves, thought oriented.
>   *Example:* Poets, philosophers, scientists, artists and others of such types of individuals belong to this group.
> - **Extroverts:** Sociable, outward-turning, friendly, action oriented, interested in the world around them.
>   *Example:* Politicians, social workers, lawyers, salesmen, etc., belong to this group.

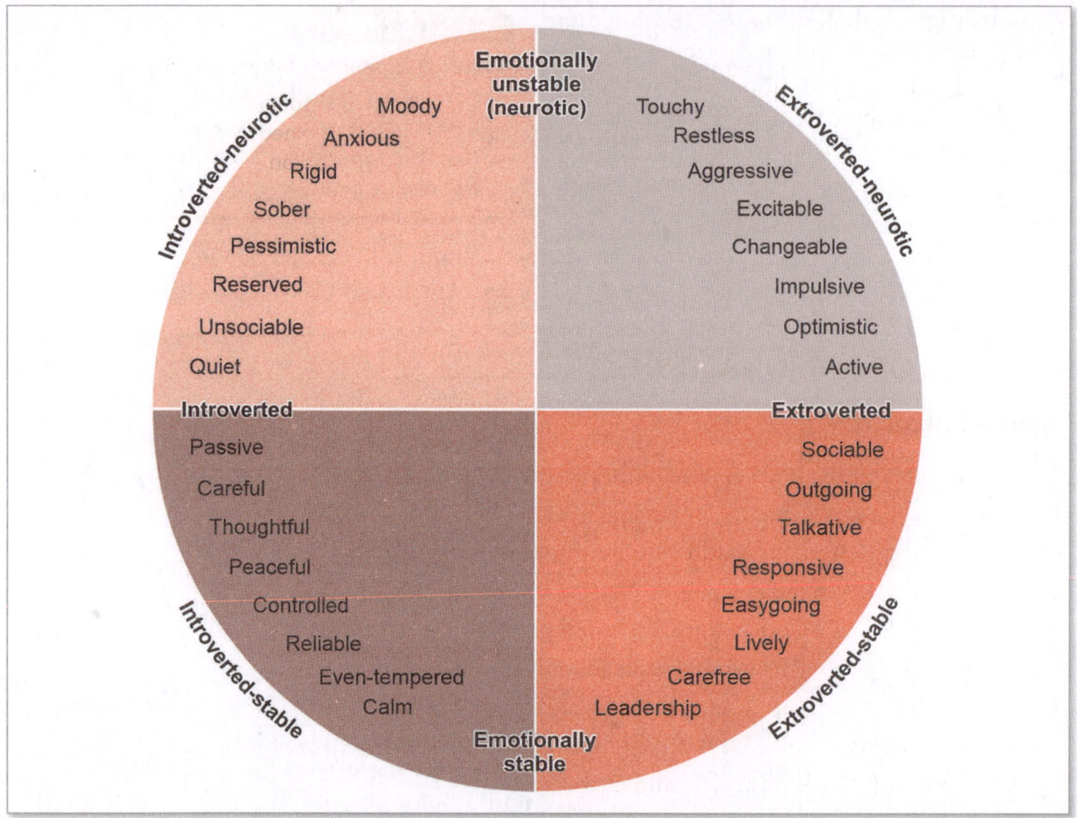

Fig. 10.1: Eysenck's three dimensions of personality

Most of the individuals are **ambiverts,** having extrovertism and introvertism in different proportions.

- **Neuroticism/emotional stability:** It is a person's affinity to be upset or emotional, while stability is the tendency to remain emotionally constant.
- **Psychoticism:** Persons who are high on this trait incline to have difficulty dealing with reality and may act antisocial, aggressive and nonempathetic.

Table 10.1 lists the differences between extrovert and introvert.

The Type A, B, C, and D Theory

Friedman and Rosenman proposed that individuals belong to one of the two basic types of personality, type A and type B;[11] a person with type C personality seems to lack emotions.[12] Type D is defined as distressed (Fig. 10.2).[13]

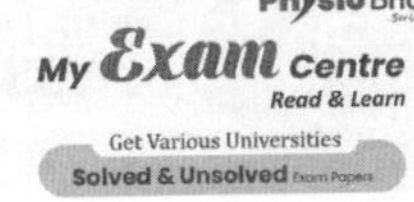

Table 10.1: Differences between extroverts and introverts

Dimension	Extroverts	Introverts
Social interaction	Thrive in social situations; enjoy being around people	Prefer solitary activities; may feel drained by prolonged social interaction
Energy source	Gain energy from external stimulation, especially social interactions	Gain energy from solitude and quiet reflection
Communication style	Outgoing, talkative, and expressive	Reserved, thoughtful, and more reflective in communication
Decision-making	Often make quick decisions and may prefer spontaneity	Tend to think things through carefully before making decisions
Work style	Prefer group work and collaboration; enjoy brainstorming sessions	Prefer working independently; may excel in focused, solitary tasks
Attention focus	Oriented toward the external environment and people	Oriented toward internal thoughts and ideas
Comfort zone	Comfortable with socializing and being the center of attention	Comfortable in solitude or with close, trusted friends
Response to stimuli	Seek out excitement and external stimulation	Prefer calm, controlled environments with less stimulation
Social network	Tend to have a wide circle of friends and acquaintances	Tend to have a smaller, close-knit group of friends
Learning preferences	Learn best through interaction, discussion, and hands-on activities	Learn best through observation, reading, and solitary study
Public speaking	More likely to enjoy public speaking and being in the spotlight	May find public speaking challenging and prefer not to be the center of attention
Behavior in groups	Often take charge in group settings and are seen as leaders	May take on a more passive or supportive role in groups
Approach to challenges	Often approach challenges with enthusiasm and a desire to engage with others	May prefer to tackle challenges independently or with careful planning
Recharging	Recharge by engaging in activities that involve others	Recharge by spending time alone or in quiet environments
Reaction to new situations	Eager to explore new opportunities and meet new people	May approach new situations with caution and prefer familiar settings

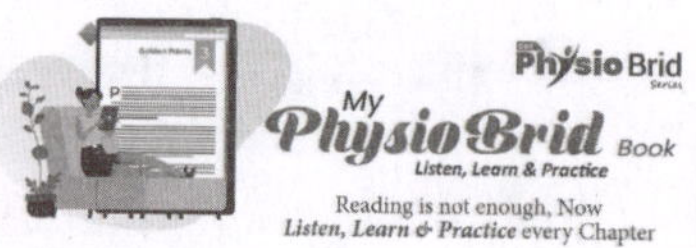

Type A personality
Hard-driving, competitive, live under constant pressure, seeks recognition and advancement and takes on multiple activities with deadlines to meet, alert, competent, performs tasks near their maximum capacity.
When put under stressful conditions he is likely to become hostile, impatient, anxious and disorganized.

Type B personality	**Type C personality**	**Type D personality**
Noncompetitive, easy going, placid, unflappable, work harder when given a deadline. Bear stress easily	Lacks emotions, does not usually affirm himself and wants to pacify others	Type D personality or the 'distressed' personality with negative affectivity and social inhibition

Fig. 10.2: Type A, B, C and D personality

Trait Approach to Personality

Gordon Allport's Trait Theory

Traits are the foundation of a person's personality and what makes them distinctive. Allport classified traits into three categories.[14]

1. **Cardinal traits:** A person arranges their life around certain characteristics known as cardinal traits. Power or success for others, as well as self-sacrifice for the greater good, may be involved. Not every individual acquires cardinal traits.

2. **Central traits:** These qualities, like honesty or conscientiousness, that are considered to be essential to a person.

3. **Secondary traits:** These are defined as less significant attributes, such as specific attitudes, preferences, and behavioral patterns, that are not essential to comprehension of a person's personality.

Raymond Cattell's Trait Theory

He proposed that there are two types of traits based on factorial analysis.[3, 15]

1. **Surface traits:** Characteristics that are prevalent and at the behavior level, such as trained, cultured, adventurous, carefree, kind, vigorous, energetic, friendly.

2. **Source traits:** Basic and are the roots of surface traits, such as balanced, frankness, optimism, intelligence, egotism, assertiveness, stubbornness, general emotional.

Though traits may appear to be unrelated to one another, there is a great deal of interaction between them in real behavior. Seldom does any particular behavior exhibit just one characteristic.

The Five-Factor Theory

The first version, called The Big Five, was introduced in 1963 by Warren Norman.[16] But only in 1990 it became popular with the work of R R McCrae and P T Costa, Jr., who called it as The Five Factor Theory (Fig. 10.3).[17]

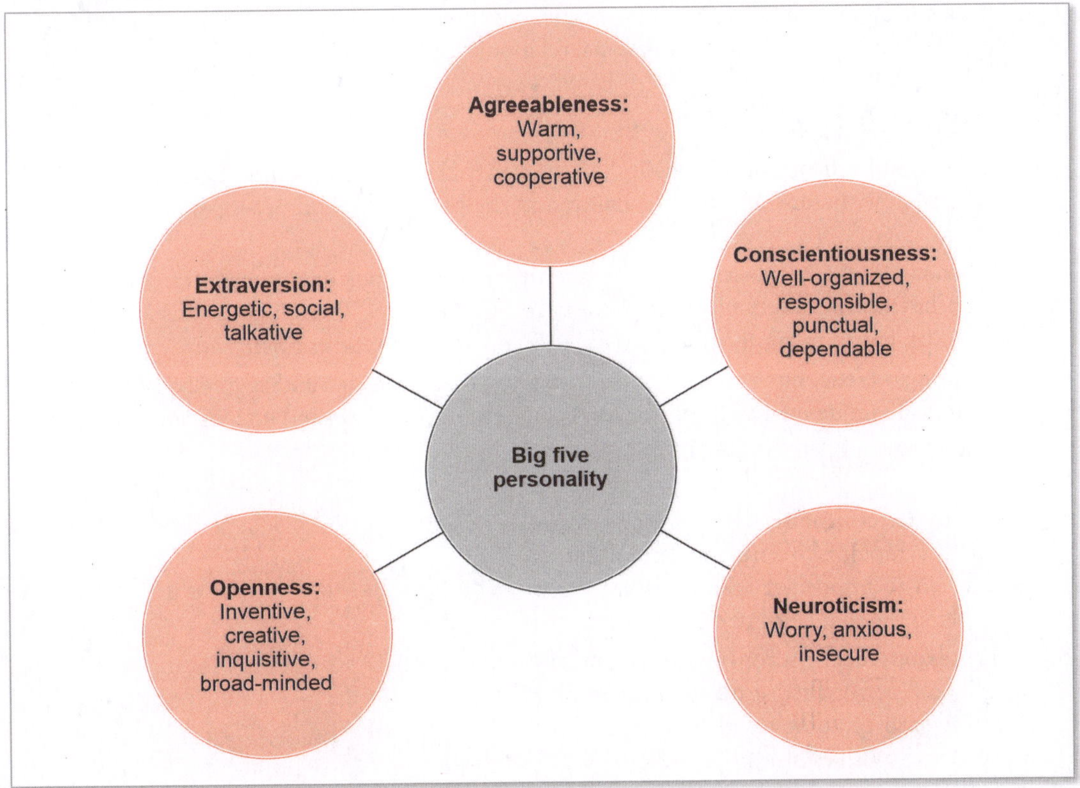

Fig. 10.3: Five factor theory

Psychodynamic Theories

Psychodynamic theories of personality emphasize the influence of unconscious processes, early childhood experiences, and internal conflicts on personality development. Sigmund Freud's Psychoanalytic Theory focuses on the interaction between the id (primitive desires), ego (rational mediator), and superego (moral conscience), as well as psychosexual stages of development.

MUST KNOW

Psychodynamic Theories
- Psychoanalytic theory by Freud
- Analytical psychology by Jung
- Individual psychology by Adler
- Psychoanalytic interpersonal theory by Horney
- Psychosocial theory by Erikson

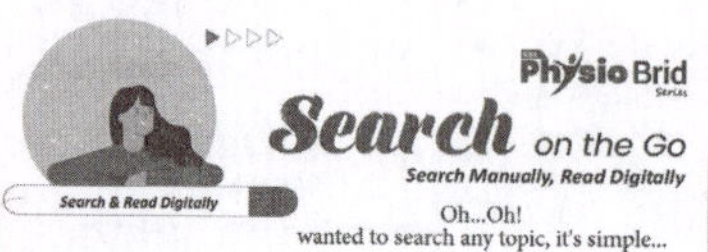

Carl Jung's Analytical Psychology highlights the collective unconscious and archetypes, while Alfred Adler's Individual Psychology emphasizes striving for superiority and the impact of social interest and birth order. Karen Horney's Interpersonal Psychoanalytic Theory explores the role of social and cultural factors, focusing on basic anxiety and coping strategies. Erik Erikson's Psychosocial Theory outlines eight stages of psychosocial development, each involving a key conflict shaped by individual growth and social influences. These theories collectively underscore the complexity of personality and the interplay of unconscious drives, social relationships, and life experiences.

Psychoanalytic Theory by Freud

The goals of Freud's theory of personality[3] are to clarify the nature of mind, the abnormal aspects of personality, how therapy affects personality, and the beginnings and progression of personality development.

Psychoanalytic theory places events within an individual's personality or intra-psychic events that drive behaviors or intentions to act, at the core of personality. These motivations are frequently conscious to us, but some motivations also function on an unconscious level.

According to Freud, our strongest desires are those that are sexual and aggressive. Our thoughts and behaviors are influenced by these desires through both conscious and unconscious processes.

Fundamental Concepts

- **Psychic determinants:** According to Freud, symptoms were meaningfully connected to important life events rather than being random (Fig. 10.4).

- **Early experience:** According to Freud, a person's personality grows continually from "womb to tomb", with all previous experiences shaping their current personality. These experiences have the greatest influence on the development of an individual's personality during infancy and early childhood.

- **Drive and instincts:** Human behavior was said to be driven by psychic energy that all people possess.

Initially, Freud suggested two theories. The first is known as ego or self-preservation (e.g., hunger, thirst) and

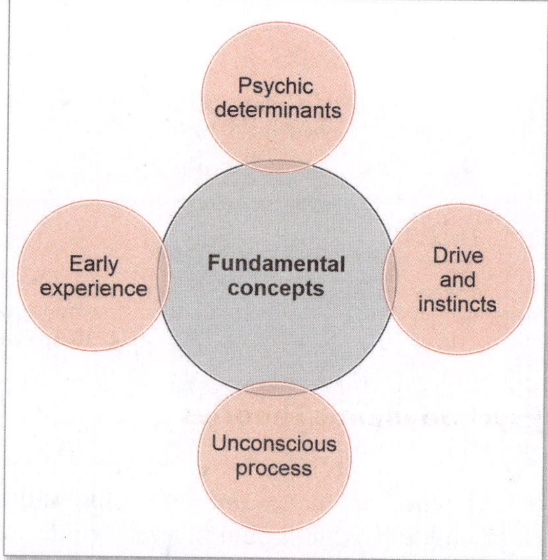

Fig. 10.4: Fundamental concepts underlying the psychodynamic approach

other is known as eros, which is linked to sexual desire and the maintenance of the species. He referred sexual cravings as "libido", which he saw as a mental force that drives individuals to engage in all sorts of sensory pleasure. Intense sexual urges must be satisfied promptly, either directly or indirectly, through dreams and fantasies.

Freud claimed that these broadly defined sexual drives function in infants as well and do not only manifest during puberty. According to Freud's dual theory of drive, almost all behavior is motivated by both the sexual and aggressive drives.

- **Unconscious processes**: Freud placed a very high value on the idea that human thought, feeling, and behavior are influenced by unconscious factors. He asserted that unconscious drives may influence our behavior. We might act without realizing why we are doing it or without easily accessing the real reason behind it. There is a clear reason for our conduct. Although, unconscious processes hide latent content from us, we are completely aware of everything we say, do, and perceive. Neurotic (anxiety-related) symptoms and nightmares, along with slips of the pen and tongue, are interpreted as occuring at the unconscious level of thinking and information processing. Freud claimed that these mistakes carry significance and meanings.

The Structure of Personality

According to Freud, personality variations result from the different ways that individuals addressed their basic needs. He proposed a never-ending conflict between the super ego and the id, elements of the personality, which is mediated by the ego, as the explanation for these disparities.

- **Id:** It is described as the personality's primal unconscious covenant or the stone home of essential urges. It conducts irrationally, acting on instinct, seeking expression and immediate fulfilment. The pleasure principle regulates the id, which is described as the unrestrained pursuit of enjoyment, particularly sexual, bodily, and emotional pleasures.
  - *Example:* Advertisements such as of clothing, cigarettes, vehicles, cosmetics that imply to viewers that using their products would enhance their appearance and make them seem more appealing reach straight to the id. They are driven by "pleasure principle" or gratification.
- **Superego:** It is the storehouse of an individual's values, which include moral views learned from society. The superego, which is essentially equivalent to the conscience, forms when a kid internalizes parental and other substantial adult prohibitions against socially unacceptable conduct. It is the inner voice. The superego also comprises the ego and a person's vision of the sort of person they should aspire to be.
  - *Example:* Advertisements of healthy food, self-care, and organic products which influence our best selves. The superego, which stands for the conscience, directs us. It works to combat the attraction and enticement of the id while keeping our best interests in mind (Fig. 10.5).

As a result, the superego, which represents society in the person, usually opposes the id, which represents survival. The id wishes to do what feels good, but the superego, based on the morals, insists on doing the 'right'. When the id and the superego disagree, the ego works out a compromise that at least somewhat satisfies both. When id and superego forces rise, it turns increasingly difficult for the ego to reach an optional compromise.

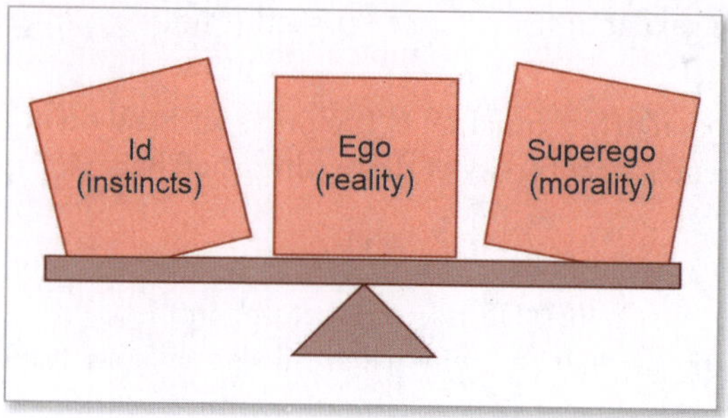

Fig. 10.5: The Id, ego, superego

Freud's Stages of Personality Development

Freud focused on both biological and sexual development. In his theory of child development, Freud established a succession of phases based on physical zones. He described the lips, arms, and genital parts as excitable zones. According to Freud, every human being passes through five stages. Problems encountered during any level of deprivation or overindulgence may result in fixation at that stage (Fig. 10.6).

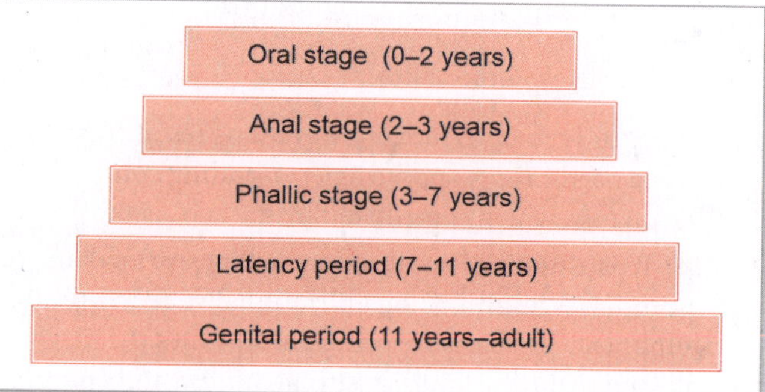

Fig. 10.6: Stages of personality development by Freud

- **Oral stage:** Infants get sexual pleasure *via* sucking and subsequently biting. Feeding and touch with mother will assist to make the mouth the center of pleasure throughout the first year.
  - Examples of problems encountered with associated person fixated at oral stage: Alcoholism, drug addiction, smoking, obesity, nail biting, and a lack of trust in other people.
- **Anal stage:** This stage happens when parents are instructing their child to use the toilet. According to psychoanalytic theory, the anal stage begins with pleasure from the ejection of feces.
  - Examples of problems encountered with associated person fixated at anal stage: Constipation, perfectionism, obsessive compulsive disorder.
- **Phallic stage:** The pleasure is derived by fondling the genitals. The youngster develops sexual emotions for the parent of the opposing sex. Freud referred to these thoughts and sensations as the Oedipus and Electra complexes in boys and girls, respectively. The sons strive to identify with and emulate their father. Boys mimic their father's behavior, regardless of its morality. Thus, the boys acquire a superego. Similarly, through association with their mother, females acquire a superego.

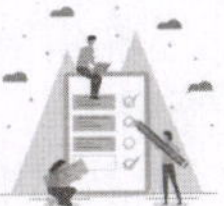
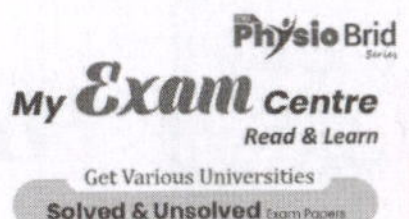

- Examples of problems encountered with associated person fixated at phallic stage: Sexual identity issues in general, homosexuality, transsexuality, and trouble submitting to authority.
- **Latency period:** Sexual interests are suppressed and remain latent until puberty. Period of gang development and intense gang loyalty. Boys cluster together and avoid females. Girls despised guys.
    - Examples of problems encountered with associated person fixated at latency stage: Inability to intellectualize; absence of motivation in school or job.
- **Genital period:** Young individuals begin to experience romantic attraction and emotional upheaval.
    - Examples of problems encountered with associated person fixated at genital stage: Frigidity, impotence, premature ejaculation, unsatisfactory relationships.

According to Freud, the first 6 years of a child's development impact what happens to it later in life.

Personality Dynamics

Freud's theories have profoundly impacted the field of modern psychology, with his concepts of the unconscious mind continuing to shape our understanding of human behavior and personality dynamics. According to Freud:

- **Mind:** Mind is a function of the body; it does not exist independently. It represents the aggregate of many mental processes or activities. Mental processes may be aware, unconscious or preconscious.
- **Conscious:** According to Freud, the conscious part of the mind is made up of mental activity that we are aware of, such as ideas, emotions, and sensations. It only works while the subject is awake.
- **Unconscious:** The unconscious is the greatest element of the mind. It encompasses our suppressed urges, unidentified anxieties and phobias, and a variety of other things. Material stored in the unconscious has a strong impact on our ideas and emotions (unconscious motivation). The preconscious, often known as the subconscious, is the area of the mind where thoughts and emotions are stored and largely forgotten. It also keeps certain inappropriate, distressing unconscious memories from entering the conscious consciousness. Materials from the subconscious can be brought to the conscious mind if the individual focuses on recollection. It leads the individual's sensible behavior.

Psychosocial Theory by Erikson

Erikson emphasized the social connections that are crucial at each stage of personality development. Erikson recognized eight phases, each representing a conflict or developmental challenge (Fig. 10.7 and Table 10.2).[18]

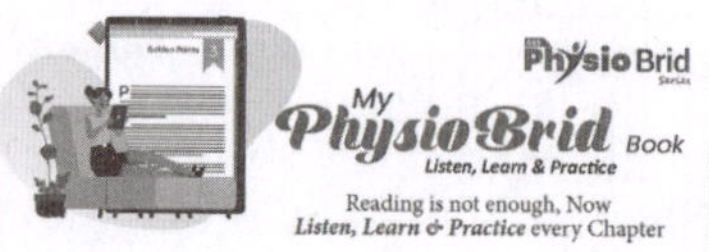

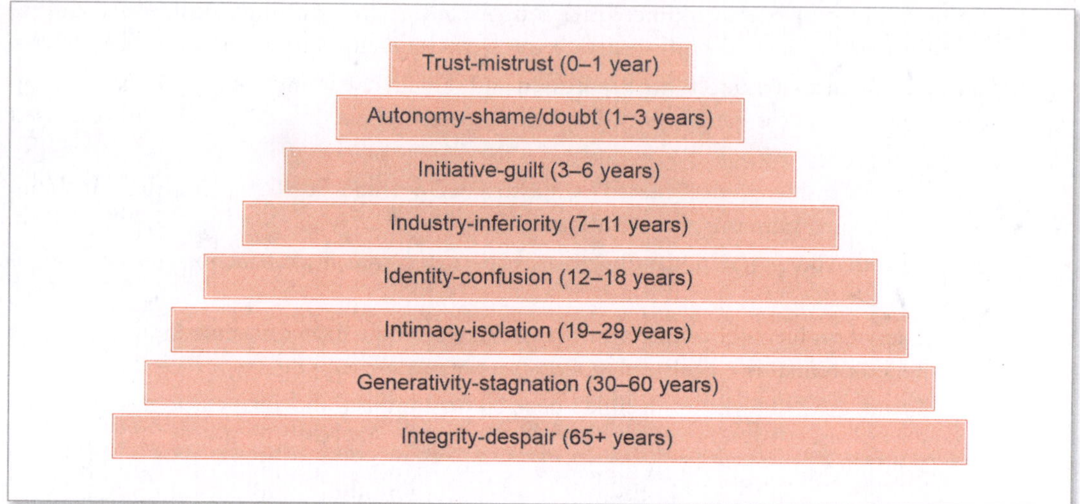

Fig. 10.7: Eight stages of Erikson's psychosocial theory

Table 10.2: Erikson's psychosocial stages of development

Stage	Basic conflict	Virtue	Description
Infancy 0–1 year	Trust versus mistrust	Hope	Trust (or mistrust) that basic needs, such as nourishment and affection, will be met
Early childhood 1–3 years	Autonomy versus shame/doubt	Will	Develop a sense of independence in many tasks
Play age 3–6 years	Initiative versus guilt	Purpose	Take initiative on some activities—may develop guilt when unsuccessful or boundaries overstepped
School age 7–11 years	Industry versus inferiority	Competence	Develop self-confidence in abilities when competent or sense or inferiority when not
Adolescence 12–18 years	Identity versus confusion	Fidelity	Experiment with and develop identity and roles
Early adulthood 19–29 years	Intimacy versus isolation	Love	Establish intimacy and relationships with others
Middle age 30–64 years	Generativity versus stagnation	Care	Contribute to society and be part of a family
Old age 65 onward	Integrity versus despair	Wisdom	Assess and make sense of life and meaning of contributions

CASE STUDY

Understanding Psychosocial needs during Rehabilitation

Patient Background

Name: Mr X

Age: 55 years

Condition: Recovering from a stroke

Medical history: Hypertension, Type 2 Diabetes, and mild depression

Current status: Limited mobility on the right side of the body, difficulty with speech (aphasia), and experiencing anxiety about returning to work and daily activities.

Mr X, a 55-year-old male, recently experienced a stroke, leading to physical impairments and a significant reduction in his ability to perform daily activities. As a result, he was referred to physiotherapy to regain mobility, improve his speech, and restore confidence in his daily functions. Erikson's stages of psychosocial development provide a useful framework for understanding how Mr X's psychological state might impact his recovery and how the physiotherapist can support his psychosocial needs during rehabilitation.

Application

1. **Stage: Generativity versus Stagnation (40–65 years)**
   - **Developmental challenge:** In this stage, individuals strive to contribute to society and support the next generation. Success leads to feelings of usefulness and accomplishment, while failure results in shallow involvement in the world and a sense of stagnation.
   - **Patient's context:** Mr X, who was an active professional and family man before his stroke, now faces the challenge of feeling irrelevant due to his sudden physical limitations. His anxiety about returning to work and fulfilling his familial and societal roles is heightened due to his condition.
   - **Physiotherapy intervention:**
     - **Goal setting:** The physiotherapist works with Mr X to set realistic, meaningful goals related to his recovery, such as gradually returning to work and participating in family activities.
     - **Involvement in therapy planning:** By involving Mr X in the planning of his rehabilitation program, the physiotherapist ensures that Mr X feels a sense of control and purpose in his recovery.
     - **Community engagement:** Encouraging Mr X to participate in group therapy sessions or community activities designed for stroke survivors can help him rebuild a sense of contribution and generativity.
     - **Progress monitoring:** Regularly reviewing progress with Mr X to reinforce his achievements and adjust goals to maintain his motivation and engagement in the therapy process.

2. **Stage: Integrity versus Despair (65 years and older)**
   - **Developmental challenge:** In this stage, individuals reflect on their life and either come away with a sense of integrity and fulfilment or feel despair over missed opportunities and regrets.
   - **Patient's context:** Although Mr X is only 55, his condition may prompt early reflections on life achievements and fears about the future. His physical limitations could lead to feelings of despair, especially if he believes his productive life is prematurely ending.
   - **Physiotherapy intervention:**
     - **Life review and reflection:** The physiotherapist can encourage Mr X to engage in discussions related to his life achievements and how his current efforts in rehabilitation are a continuation of his life's work.

Contd...

- **Positive reinforcement:** By highlighting small victories in his recovery, the physiotherapist can help Mr X maintain a sense of integrity, reassuring him that he is still contributing positively to his life and those around him.
- **Family involvement:** Involving Mr X's family in therapy sessions can help him see the positive impact of his rehabilitation on his loved ones, reinforcing his sense of purpose.

3. Addressing depression and anxiety
- **Erikson's theory relevance**: Erikson's stages emphasize the importance of resolving the psychosocial conflict of each stage. Unresolved issues in previous stages can manifest as depression and anxiety in adulthood.
- **Patient's context**: Mr X's mild depression and anxiety may stem from unresolved conflicts in earlier stages, such as issues with identity, autonomy or trust. These unresolved issues can hinder his motivation and progress in physiotherapy.
- **Physiotherapy intervention:**
  - **Emotional support:** The physiotherapist can provide emotional support and refer Mr X to a psychologist for deeper mental health interventions, if needed.
  - **Cognitive-behavioral strategies:** Implementing cognitive-behavioral techniques within therapy sessions to address negative thought patterns related to his recovery and self-worth.
  - **Building trust:** Establishing a strong therapeutic relationship can help address any underlying trust issues and promote a sense of security and hope in the rehabilitation process.

Outcome and Reflection

By integrating Erikson's stages of psychosocial development into Mr X's physiotherapy treatment, the physiotherapist can tailor interventions that address both his physical and psychological needs. This holistic approach can significantly enhance Mr X's motivation, emotional well-being, and overall recovery.

- **Short-term outcome:** Mr X shows gradual improvement in mobility and speech, and his participation in therapy increases as he feels more hopeful about his recovery.
- **Long-term outcome:** Over time, Mr X regains a significant degree of independence and is able to resume work on a part-time basis. His sense of purpose and connection to his community is restored, reducing feelings of stagnation and despair.

This case study illustrates how understanding the psychological stages of development can inform and enhance the effectiveness of physiotherapy, particularly in cases where psychological well-being is closely intertwined with physical recovery.

Carl Jung Theory

Carl Jung extended the idea of unconsciousness. For him, the unconscious contained essential psychological truths that all people share, not just the life experiences of an individual. The idea of the "collective unconscious" suggests that we are all predisposed to respond similarly to stimuli. According to Jung, a healthy integrated personality balances opposing forces within the individual, such as feminine sensitivity and masculine aggression. Jung added the necessity to create and the necessity to self-actualize—two equally potent unconscious instincts—to the primal urges of aggression and sex.

Jung claimed that universal archetypes represent the collective unconscious. Archetypes are indications, symbols or patterns of thought and/or behavior that we received from our ancestors.

According to Jung, these mythical pictures or cultural symbols are neither static nor stable. Instead, several distinct archetypes can overlap or mix at any time. Jung hypothesized several common archetypes to describe the unconscious mind.[19, 20]

Anima is represented by an idealized lady who drives men to partake in feminine activities.

- **Animus:** Woman's source of significance and power, which causes anger toward man while simultaneously increasing self-knowledge.
- **Hero:** Beginning with a modest birth and overcoming evil and death.
- **Persona:** The mask we wear to hide our true selves from the outer world.
- **Self:** The entire personality; the root of the overall mind.
- **Shadow:** The psyche's unethical and dark sides.
- **Trickster:** A youngster who seeks self-gratification by nasty and unfeeling behavior.
- **Wise old man:** Portrayed as a symbol of wisdom or understanding.

Learning Theories

This theory holds that a person's behavior in any given circumstance is determined by the unique features of his past. As a result, most of theorists believe that interactions between individuals and situations shape human personality.[21]

According to social learning theories, rewards and punishments have an impact on people's behavior and personalities, but differing behaviors do not necessarily indicate different motivations. They see humans as creatures of habit or reactionary tendencies that are shaped by the system.

As per the learning theories, individuals learn all sorts of actions in similar way as animals using classical and operant conditioning. If there are any distinctions, they are because human learning happens in more complicated environments. Human learning takes place in a social setting, and it is in this situation that person develops novel reactions to a range of circumstances.

The classical and instrumental conditioning have an impact on an individual's personality. Additionally, it acknowledges a unique kind of learning mechanism that goes by several names, including imitation, modelling, and observational learning. In this kind of learning, an individual picks up a response by witnessing other people respond in that way.

Dollard and Miller's Theory of Learning

The process of learning or habit formation is at the center of Dollard and Miller's theory formulation. They talk about this process's four main components:

1. **Drive:** It prompts an individual to act.
2. **Cues:** It indicates appropriate behavior, which will lessen drive.
3. **Response:** It is the behavior itself.
4. **Reinforcement or reward:** It eases drive tension, enhances the relationship between cues and response.

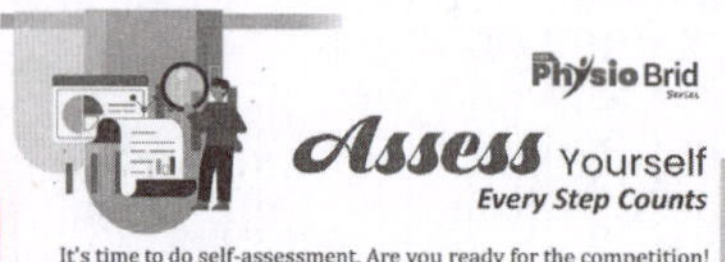

Cognitive Theories

There are significant individual variations in how people perceive any given external circumstance. The process by which individuals organize their impressions of reality from sensations and perceptions is emphasized by cognitive theories.

Individuals play in forming their own identities. People are not merely passive recipients of their surroundings; rather, they actively shape them, even though environments play a significant role in our lives. We evaluate options and choose the context in which we act and are acted upon.

Numerous personality theories emphasize the role of situational elements (social and environmental signals) and cognitive processes in determining behavior.[22]

Jean Piaget's Theory of Cognitive Development

Piaget's theory suggests that learning is a process of adaptation and organization. Children progress through four stages of cognitive development, each characterized by different abilities and ways of thinking.

Stages

1. **Sensorimotor stage (0–2 years):** Learning through sensory experiences and manipulating objects.
2. **Preoperational stage (2–7 years):** Development of language and symbolic thinking but lacking logical reasoning.
3. **Concrete operational stage (7–11 years):** Development of logical thinking about concrete events; understanding of conservation.
4. **Formal operational stage (12+ years):** Development of abstract and hypothetical reasoning.

Personal Construct Theory

George Kelly created the Personal Construct Theory, a theory that focuses primarily on how everyone actively constructs his world through cognition. He maintained that there are always various ways for people to define their current struggles or reconstruct their past. According to Kelly, a personal construct is an individual's perception of how two things are like one another and how they differ from a third. It emphasizes the individuality of every person's personality a great deal.

Humanistic Theory

Humanistic theories of personality are related with the person's individual view of the world, self-concept, and push in the direction of growth or self-actualization.

Roger's Self-Theory

Individuals must have the appropriate degree of overlap between their real and ideal selves, according to Carl Rogers' personality theory. The ideal self is who the person is now. Individuals aspire to be their ideal selves. Rogers believed that it is always difficult to achieve the appropriate level of considerable overlap between the real and ideal selves.[23]

Maslow's Self-Actualization Theory

Self-actualization refers to the ability to become the best version of oneself. Maslow framed his notion of self-actualization inside a hierarchy of needs (Fig. 10.8).[24] The hierarchy reflects five requirements, sorted from lowest to highest, as follows:

1. **Physiological needs** include food, drink, shelter, warmth, and sleep, all of which are necessary for survival.

2. **Safety needs** include the want to feel safe, stable, and fearful.

3. **Love and belongingness needs:** The need to belong socially through connections with friends and family.

4. **Esteem needs:** The need to experience both self-esteem based on one's accomplishments and talents, and acknowledgment and respect from others.

5. **Self-actualization needs** are the need to seek and realize one's unique potentials.

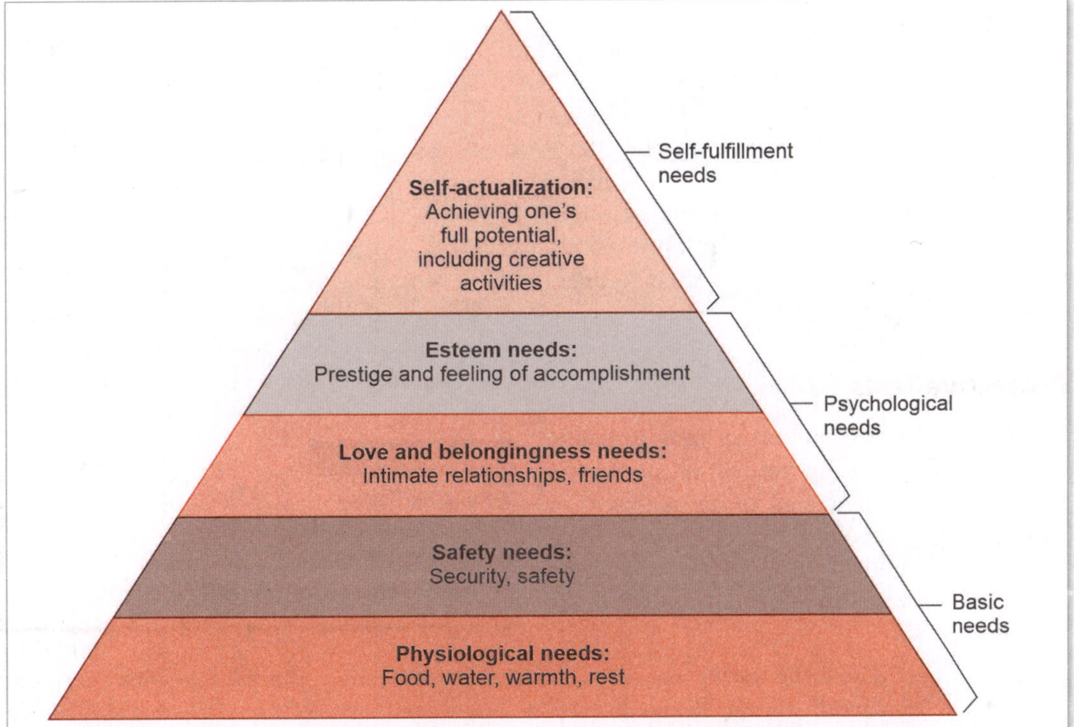

Fig. 10.8: Maslow's hierarchy of needs

ASSESSMENT

There are many ways of assessing personality as discussed here:[25, 26]

Observation and Rating

A popular technique for evaluating personality is to watch someone's behavior and then assign a score.

For instance, during an interview, the interviewers assess a person's personality on a scale from low to high based on how they see him behave. This approach is known as the rating method. Two methods exist for doing such a rating:

1. **Global approach:** A scale ranging from low to high efficacy is used to develop characteristics. It can be useful when time is limited and many individuals need to be assessed or when personality scores are just one of many considerations.

2. **Analytic approach:** Here, a variety of traits or qualities are evaluated separately in place of the entire personality, and these individual ratings are added together.

Objective Tests

Personality tests that adhere to objective guidelines and have a relatively simple scoring system are considered objective (Fig. 10.9).

Minnesota Multiphasic Personality Inventory (MMPI) is a popular objective assessment. The person taking the test responds to a series of questions regarding their feelings, ideas, and behaviors.

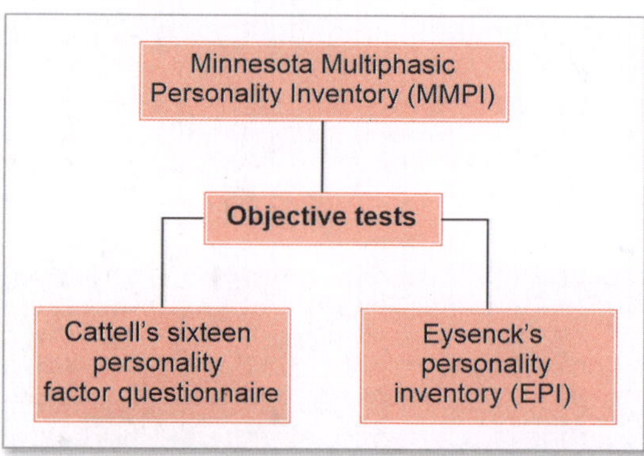

Fig. 10.9: Objective test of personality

Projective Tests

Psychologists employ projective tests to assess personality based on a related phenomenon. Things are often perceived by us not as they are, but rather as we are, especially when they are unclear or vague. When we give something meaning, we often project our personalities onto it.

MUST KNOW

Projective Tests
- Word association test
- Rorschach inkblot test
- Thematic apperception test

In a projective test, the test's purpose is concealed while a subject is presented with a series of intentionally ambiguous stimuli, like an abstract design, partial pictures, and drawings that can be interpreted in numerous ways.

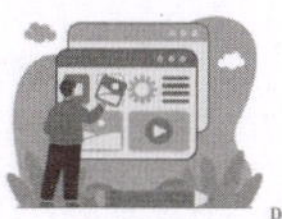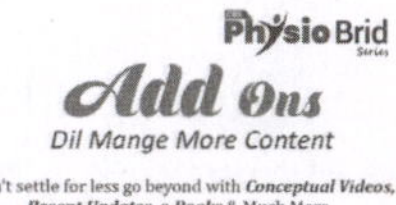

The individual might be asked to complete the drawings, tell tales about the drawings or explain the pattern. Due to the ambiguity of the stimuli, responses to them depend in part on the individual's contributions to the situation, specifically.

Psychoanalysts employed projective tests so that the results would disclose the patients' unconscious personality dynamics. For instance, to reveal fears and ideas that are emotionally charged.

Word Association Test

Carl Jung used word association with a list of frequently used words.

Example: When you hear the word "home", what comes to mind?

Rorschach Inkblot Test

Rorschach inkblot test was created by Hermann Rorschach and is a useful tool for examining the unconscious influences on personality and behavior. It is predicated on the idea that a person's entire personality is expressed in every performance they give. The subject of this is reacting to inkblots.

The first phase adopts free association and the second phase is inquiry. The responses are interpreted and analyzed as per significance of response. The subject responses may be scored in terms of three categories.

1. **Location:** Is the entire inkblot involved in the response or just a portion of it?
2. **Factors:** Is the subject reacting to the blot's texture, color or shape?
3. **Content:** What is the meaning of the answer? Such as plants and animals?

There are ten cards in the test. There are blots in black and white and colored ones. The subject is told to report everything they see on the inkblot card after looking at each inkblot individually (Fig. 10.10).

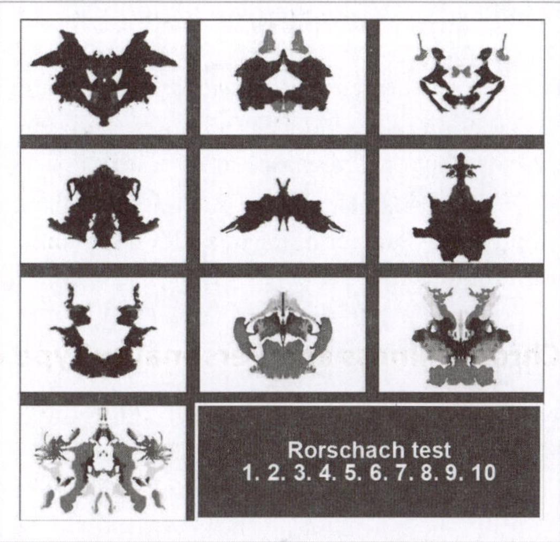

Fig. 10.10: Rorschach Inkblot test

Thematic Apperception Test

Thematic apperception test (TAT) was developed by American psychologists, Henry A Murray and Christiana Morgan in 1930. This test uses photographs of real-world scenarios. The thirty images are selected by the psychologist, who typically selects a set for each subject, based on which subjects are most likely to provide particularly pertinent information. In TAT, participants are asked to conjure up a narrative that describes what is happening, what has happened in the past, what is about to happen, and what the characters are feeling and thinking. Most people express their perception by identifying with one of the characters in the pictures. The interpretation and scoring system considers the story's protagonist, conflicts in the protagonist, theme, content, narrative style, the subject's attitude toward sex and authority, and emotion.

PRACTICAL ASPECTS

According to recent research, personality can be a reliable indicator of health and well-being.

Low Back Pain Outcomes and Personality Type of Patients

Higher degrees of disability appeared to be associated with higher kinesiophobia levels and lower overall physical therapy improvement in patients. Extrovert patients showed a weak therapeutic alliance with their therapist, whereas neurotic patients reported higher levels of improvement.[27]

Cardiovascular Disease and Personality Type of Patients

In most stressful situations, personality type A individuals have higher propensity than their type B counterparts. It was discovered that there was a substantial mean difference between the personality types for performance dimensions: teaching and training and relationships with co-workers.[28]

The present evidence proposes that personality characteristics may be linked with the development of cardiovascular diseases.[29]

Some personality traits such as optimism, openness to experience, and curiosity have been found to be protecting against development of cardiovascular diseases and therefore are called 'cardio protective' personality traits.[30]

Chronic Illness and Personality Type of Therapist

Research suggests that individuals with chronic illnesses who receive care from therapists who exhibit traits such as calmness, relaxation, security, and resilience report a higher decline in the complaints in comparison to those who receive care from therapists who exhibit less of these traits.[31]

Physio CORNER

- A physiotherapist can more accurately predict his/her own behavior and that of others if he/she had a good understanding of personality.
- To provide effective patient care, a physiotherapist should not only gain knowledge and skills but also cultivate a strong, endearing personality.
- In their work environments, physiotherapists collaborate with other medical professionals, and they are expected to exhibit specific behaviors and qualities.

Contd...

- A physiotherapist works with people of all ages. The emotional, sensitive, dependent, and demanding needs of their patients can be recognized by a skilled, perceptive physiotherapist.
- Physiotherapists may find it helpful to assess and manage their patients if they have a better understanding of the impact of personality traits in relation to the ailments (Fig. 10.11).

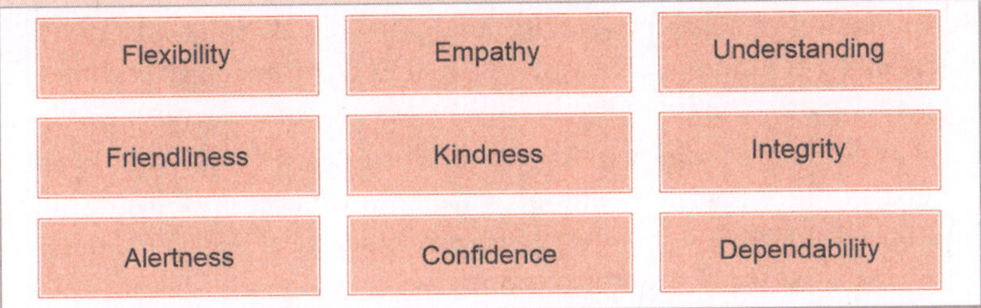

Fig. 10.11: Personal attributes a physiotherapist should possess

CASE STUDY

A Case Study on Bank Employees: Personality Traits and Work Engagement[32]

A study investigated the engagement and the big 5 personality traits among female employees, as well relationships of personality traits with work engagement. 150 female employees of three distinct banks were surveyed. The study's findings demonstrated a positive correlation between the personality traits and work engagement. While neuroticism was found to be negatively correlated with work engagement and its dimensions—vigor, dedication, and absorption, extroversion, agreeableness, conscientiousness, and openness correlated with work engagement.

CASE STUDY

A Case Study of Teachers: Personality Traits and Thinking Styles[33]

A study investigated the relationship of thinking styles with personality traits among teachers of Arab descent, who constitute a minority in Israel's Arab educational system. In addition to helping students develop their skills, teachers are crucial in helping them form their ideas, perspectives, and personality traits. Teachers' individual personalities and ways of thinking have a big impact on how well they perform in their roles as educationalists. The Arab minority in Israel's constituents resides in a contemporary society that nevertheless possesses distinct traditional elements. In all, 205 Arab educators took part in the research. The results of the study indicate that among teachers, thinking styles and personality traits were positively correlated.

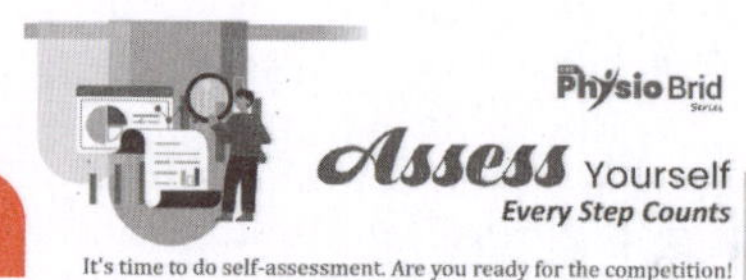

RECENT ADVANCES

An attempt has been made for personalizing psychological evaluation using the five-factor model.[34] To explain mental distress, the Enactivist Big-5 Theory of Personality considers the individual as well as the environment they live in. This comprehensive viewpoint, which has its roots in phenomenological philosophy, sees psychological dysfunction as defined by a diminished capacity to grasp reality. For example, someone with a high extroversion level would be distressed to be confined to a static environment because he/she thrives on exploring new possibilities.

The influence of certain personality traits on behavioral decision-making can either be enabling or inhibiting, and the influence of the same personality attributes on decisions made in behavior might differ.[35] As a result, an analysis of how personality traits affect behavioral decision-making has to take particular behavioral scenarios into account.

SUMMARY

- Personality, a concept that is central to understanding human behavior and interactions. Personality encompasses the unique and consistent patterns of thoughts, feelings, and behaviors that define an individual. It delves into the various aspects of personality, including its definition, traits, influencing factors, and theoretical frameworks. Additionally, it examines different methods for assessing personality, highlighting their relevance in both theoretical understanding and practical applications, particularly in clinical settings such as physiotherapy.

- Specific traits like personal appearance, intelligence, emotions, sociability, ascendance-submission, and moral character contribute to an individual's overall personality profile. Emphasis is placed on the uniqueness of each individual's personality and the dynamic nature of these traits, which evolve through constant interaction with the environment.

- Understanding the development of personality involves examining a range of factors. Genetic and growth factors, including the inheritance of traits from parents and the impact of genetic disorders, are discussed as foundational influences. The role of family, society, and culture in shaping personality is explored, highlighting how social norms, values, and experiences contribute to the formation of personality traits. Personal experiences, both positive and negative, are also identified as significant factors in personality development.

- The psychoanalytic theory, pioneered by Freud, focuses on the concepts of the id, ego, and superego, and the stages of personality development. Humanistic theories, including those of Rogers and Maslow, are explored, emphasizing the role of self-concept and self-actualization. Cognitive theories are also examined, highlighting the importance of how individuals perceive and interpret their experiences.

- Assessing personality involves a variety of methods, each with its own strengths and limitations. These include observation and rating methods, objective tests like the MMPI, and projective tests such as the Rorschach Inkblot test and the Thematic Apperception Test (TAT). These methods provide insights into both the conscious and unconscious aspects of personality, offering a comprehensive understanding of an individual's personality profile.

- The practical implications of understanding personality are discussed, with a focus on clinical settings, particularly physiotherapy. The unit highlights how knowledge of personality can enhance therapeutic relationships and patient care. It also discusses the importance of personality traits in effective communication and interpersonal relationships within the healthcare setting.

Contd...

- Personality is a complex and dynamic aspect of human behavior, influenced by a myriad of factors and understood through various theoretical frameworks. Personality is important in both theoretical and practical contexts. By understanding the various aspects of personality and the methods used to assess it, individuals can gain valuable insights into their own behavior and that of others, enhancing their ability to interact effectively in diverse settings.

REFERENCES

1. Allport, G. W. Pattern and growth in personality. Holt, Reinhart & Winston:1961
2. Cattell, R.B. Personality: A systematic, theoretical and factual study. New York: McGraw Hill:1950
3. Freud, S. (1923/1949). The ego and the id. London, England: Hogarth Press. (Original work published 1923)
4. Krishnamurthy K. Historical Perspectives on Personality – The Past and Current Concept: The Search is Not Yet Over. Archives of Medicine and Health Sciences.2018 6(1):180–186.
5. Diener E, Lucas RE, Cummings JA. .Personality Traits. In: Cummings JA & Sanders L. Introduction To Psychology University Of Saskatchewan. 2019
6. Merenda, PF. "Toward a Four-Factor Theory of Temperament and/or Personality". Journal of Personality Assessment.1987; 51 (3): 367–374.
7. Sheldon WH, Steven SS, & Tucker, WB. The varieties of human physique;1940.
8. Sheldon WA. Atlas of men, a guide for somatotyping the adult male at all ages;1954
9. Kretschmer E. Physique and Character: An Investigation of the Nature of Constitution and of the Theory of Temperament; with 31 Plates. London: Kegan Paul, Trench, Trubner;1925.
10. Eysenck HJ. The biological basis of personality. Springfield, IL, USA: Charles C. Thomas;1965
11. Friedman M, Roseman R. Type A behavior and your heart. In: Alfred A, editor. New York: Knopf; 1974
12. Greer S, Morris T. Psychological attributes of women who develop breast cancer: a controlled study. J Psychosom Res. 1975 Apr;19(2):147–53.
13. Kupper N & Denollet J. Type D Personality as a Risk Factor in Coronary Heart Disease: a Review of Current Evidence. Current Cardiology Reports, 2018;20(104):8.
14. Allport, GW. Concepts of trait and personality. Psychological Bulletin. 1927;24(5):284–293.
15. Cattell RB. The scientific analysis of Personality. Baltimore: Penguin Books;1965
16. Norman, WT. Toward an adequate taxonomy of personality attributes: Replicated factor 54 structure in peer nomination personality ratings. Journal of Abnormal and Social Psychology. 1963; 66:574–583.
17. McCrae, RR. & Costa, PT. Personality in adulthood. New York: Guilford Press;1990.
18. Orenstein GA, Lewis L. Eriksons Stages of Psychosocial Development. [Updated 2022 Nov 7]. In: StatPearls [Internet]. Treasure Island (FL): StatPearls Publishing; 2024 Jan-. Available from: https://www.ncbi.nlm.nih.gov/books/NBK556096/
19. Jung, C. G. The phenomenology of the spirit in fairy tales. The Archetypes and the Collective Unconscious.1948; 9(Part 1):207-254.
20. Jung, C. G. Collected works. Vol. 12. Psychology and alchemy;1953.
21. Gandhi MH, Mukherji P. Learning Theories. [Updated 2023 Jul 17]. In: StatPearls [Internet]. Treasure Island (FL): StatPearls Publishing; 2024 Jan-. Available from: https://www.ncbi.nlm.nih.gov/books/NBK562189/

Contd...

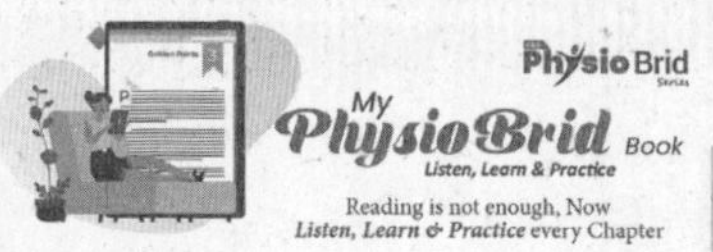

22. DiGiuseppe R., David D., & Venezia R. Cognitive theories. In J. C. Norcross, G. R. VandenBos, D. K. Freedheim, & B. O. Olatunji (Eds.), APA handbook of clinical psychology: Theory and research. American Psychological Association. 2016. p. 145–182.

23. Yao L, Kabir R. Person-Centered Therapy (Rogerian Therapy) [Updated 2023 Feb 9]. In: StatPearls [Internet]. Treasure Island (FL): StatPearls Publishing; 2024 Jan-. Available from: https://www.ncbi.nlm.nih.gov/books/NBK589708/

24. McLeod, S. A. Maslow's hierarchy of needs. 2018, May 21. Retrieved from https://www.simplypsychology.org/maslow.html

25. Wheeler MA, Archer RP. Personality Assessment In: Friedman HS. Encyclopedia of Mental Health (Second Edition), Academic Press.2016, p. 267-269.

26. McGrath RE, & Carroll E.J. The current status of "projective" "tests" In H. Cooper, P. M. Camic, D. L. Long, A. T. Panter, D. Rindskopf, & K. J. Sher (Eds.), APA handbook of research methods in psychology, Vol. 1. Foundations, planning, measures, and psychometrics. American Psychological Association. 2012, p 329–348.

27. Hanney WJ, Dhalla F, Kelly C, Tomberlin A, Kolber MJ, Wilson AT, Salamh PA. The Influence of Personality Type on Patient Outcome Measures and Therapeutic Alliance in Patients with Low Back Pain. NeuroSci. 2023; 4(3):186-194.

28. Friedman M, Roseman R. Type A behavior and your heart. In: Alfred A, editor. New York: Knopf; 1974.

29. Janjhua Y, Chandrakanta. Behavior of personality type toward stress and job performance: a study of healthcare professionals. J Family Med Prim Care. 2012 Jul;1(2):109-13.

30. Sahoo S, Padhy SK, Padhee B, Singla N, Sarkar S. Role of personality in cardiovascular diseases: An issue that needs to be focused too! Indian Heart J. 2018 Dec;70 Suppl 3(Suppl 3):S471-S477. doi: 10.1016/j.ihj.2018.11.003.

31. Buining EM, Kooijman MK, Swinkels IC, Pisters MF, Veenhof C. Exploring physiotherapists' personality traits that may influence treatment outcome in patients with chronic diseases: a cohort study. BMC Health Serv Res. 2015 Dec 16;15:558.

32. Bansal E, Bhushan P, Gupta G. Personality Traits and Work Engagement: A Case Study on Female Bank Employees in Banking Sector. Parikalpana - KIIT Journal of Management. 2020:72-82

33. Hussain & Abu J. 'Personality Traits and Thinking Styles: A Case Study of Arab Teachers as Members of a Minority in Israel.' American Journal of Educational Research. 2020;8(5): 325-331.

34. Yu Y, Zhao Y, Li D, Zhang J, Li J. The Relationship Between Big Five Personality and Social Well-Being of Chinese Residents: The Mediating Effect of Social Support. Front Psychol. 2021 Mar 5;11:613659.

35. Yan M, Zhang J, Ge P, Wu Y. Personality theory: New factors to incorporate in public decision-making in communities. Health Care Sci. 2023; 2:198–203.

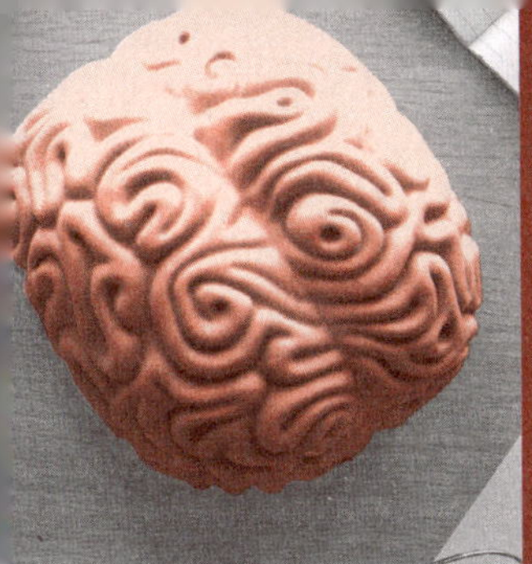

STUDENT ASSIGNMENT

LONG ANSWER QUESTIONS

1. Explain the theories of personality.
2. Explain Freud's psychoanalytic theory.
3. Explain factors influencing the development of personality and its characteristics.
4. Discuss the determinants of personality.
5. Explain the trait theory of personality. Discuss the various trait compositions necessary to have effective physiotherapist-patient relationship.
6. Describe the personality assessment techniques in detail.
7. Explain the importance of personality for physiotherapists.

SHORT ANSWER QUESTIONS

1. What do you understand by introvertism and extrovertism?
2. Write about development of personality.
3. Give two examples for projective tests of personality.
4. Define id, ego and superego.
5. Mention the characteristics of personality.
6. Write about Freud psychoanalytic theory.

MULTIPLE CHOICE QUESTIONS

1. **A set of comparatively stable dispositions, traits or qualities that lend some consistency to an individual's behaviors is referred to as:**
   a. Personality
   b. Trait
   c. Characteristic
   d. A genetic predisposition

2. **Which trait represents a range between extreme extroversion and extreme introversion?**
   a. Agreeableness
   b. Conscientiousness
   c. Openness
   d. Neuroticism

3. **Extraversion is a personality trait characterized by which of the following?**
   a. Low energy in social situations
   b. Reserved behavior
   c. Talkativeness
   d. Careful thinking before speaking

4. **Neuroticism is a personality trait characterized by:**
   a. Emotional instability
   b. Sociability
   c. Altruism
   d. Competitiveness

5. **Positive personality traits include:**
   a. Aggressiveness
   b. Arrogance
   c. Ambition
   d. Coldness

6. **Who emphasized the role of self-concept in personality?**
   a. Rogers
   b. Mischel
   c. Eysenck
   d. Alder

7. **What are the advantages of projective personality tests?**
   a. All people would score them the same
   b. Not transparent to the subject
   c. Less reliable
   d. Have lie scales

8. **Thematic Appreciation test was developed by:**
   a. Henry Murray and Christiana Morgan
   b. Roger
   c. Jung
   d. Freud

9. **According to _______________, individuals may be classified into two distinct personality dimensions: neuroticism/stability and extroversion/introversion.**
   a. Freud
   b. Hans Eysencks
   c. Carls Roger
   d. Carl Jung

10. **Collective unconsciousness is associated with:**
    a. Freud
    b. Roger
    c. Jung
    d. Alder

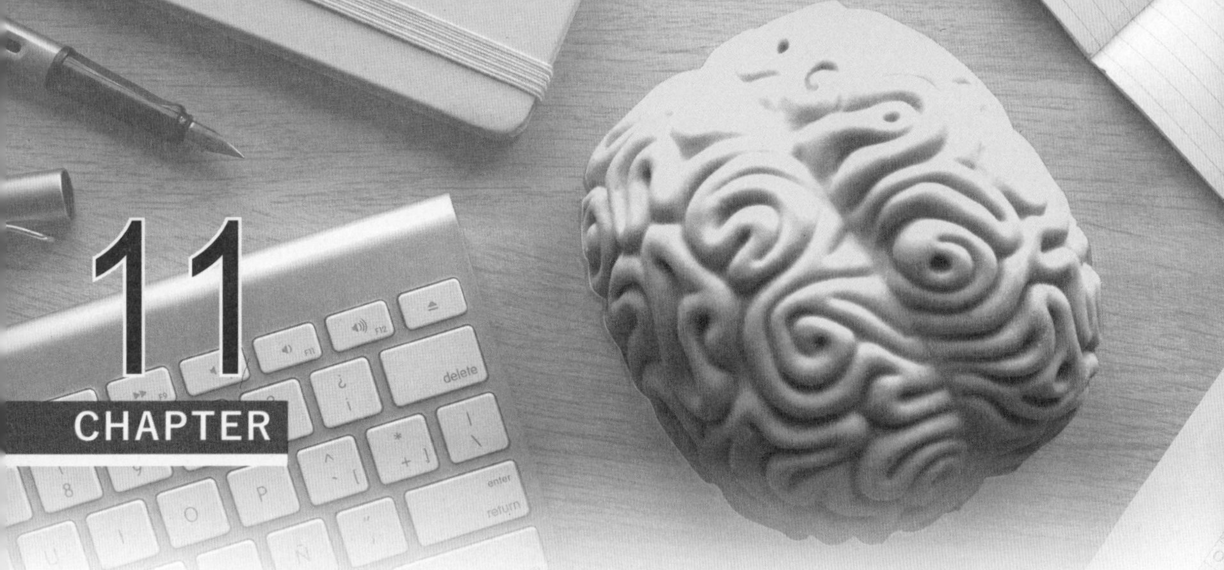

Defense Mechanisms of the Ego

Kajal Taneja

LEARNING OBJECTIVES

After the completion of the chapter, the readers will be able to:
- Understand the concept of defense mechanisms.
- Recognize the different classifications of defense mechanisms.
- Provide a detailed description of each defense mechanism, including its function and typical situations in which it may be employed.
- Illustrate each defense mechanism with practical, real-world examples.

CHAPTER OUTLINE

- Introduction
- Defense Mechanisms
- Clinical Application

KEY TERMS

Defense mechanisms: Unconscious mental processes that protect the ego from internal and external threats.

Projection: Attributing one's own unwanted feelings, qualities or desires to someone else to relieve tension and anxiety.

Psychological defense mechanisms: Specific strategies employed by the mind to cope with stress and maintain psychological stability.

Rationalization: Substituting an unacceptable unconscious motive with a conscious, socially acceptable motive.

Regression: Returning to an earlier stage of development in response to stress or threat, often exhibited through childlike behavior.

Sublimation: Channeling socially unacceptable impulses into socially acceptable behaviors or activities.

INTRODUCTION

The father of psychoanalysis, Sigmund Freud was the first person who began discussing defense mechanism related to functioning of mental apparatus structurally. He classified them as id, ego and superego. Later on, Anna Freud, his daughter continued her work in defining, as well as, analyzing this defense mechanism and came up with more than 10 defense mechanisms in 20th century. Thereafter, till date the count has been in increasing trend. The purpose of the ego, which is a coherent arrangement of functions, is to prevent pain by controlling or resisting the expression of primal urges to comply with external demands.[1]

DEFENSE MECHANISMS

According to Anna Freud, these defense mechanisms are "unconscious resources used by the ego" to reduce the internal stress. They are unconscious, as well as, involuntary mental processes. Every single person uses this mechanism to balance subjectivity and reality. They allude to a series of mental operations created in psychoanalytic theory to safeguard the integrity of the ego system (mind). Defense mechanisms guard against potentially dangerous external stimuli, as well as, internally generated threatening impulses and urges.[1]

Use of Defense Mechanisms

The effectiveness of a defense depends on its not being conscious. When the purpose of the defense is consciously understood, its value diminishes. It is then replaced by a new, cognitively more sophisticated defense. From teenage till middle age, the development of defense mechanisms occurs into more adaptive defenses. In elderly, this development gets inverted.[2]

There are certain unexpected clues which can be observed while interviewing a person to identify the defenses used. These clues are seen in effect, behavior, speech or in content, for example, looking away from a person during conversation, suddenly change of topic during conversation.[3]

Classification of Defense Mechanisms

Refer to Table 11.1 to understand the George Vaillant's four level classification of defense mechanisms:

Table 11.1: George Vaillant's four level classification of defense mechanisms[4]

Narcissistic	Immature	Neurotic	Mature
Denial	Acting out	Displacement	Altruism
Projection	Regression	Dissociation	Humor
Distortion	Passive-aggressive behavior	Reaction formation	Sublimation
Splitting	Schizoid fantasy	Repression	Anticipation
	Somatization	Isolation	Suppression

Contd...

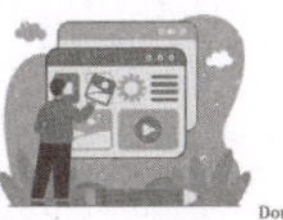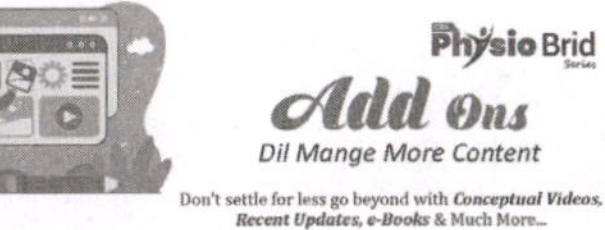

Narcissistic	Immature	Neurotic	Mature
	Introjection	Rationalization	Asceticism
	Hypochondriasis	Sexualization	
	Blocking	Intellectualization	

The important defense mechanisms seen in clinical settings are presented in the following MUST KNOW box.

MUST KNOW

Defense mechanisms used in various age groups

Period	Age group	Defense mechanisms
Oral	0–2 years	• Fixation • Compensation • Denial • Displacement
Habit training	1–3 years	• Conversion • Identification • Sublimation • Reaction formation • Introjection • Transference
Late childhood	3–6 years	• Repression • Rationalization • Regression
Latency period	6–12 years	Projection

Narcissistic-Psychotic Defenses

These are the earliest mechanisms to develop. They are seen in children and adult dreams or fantasies. Persons with psychosis also have these defenses.

Denial

When individuals deny the existence of anything that they find really unpleasant, they are denying reality. Denial is most helpful in situations of death, serious illness or something fearful and threatening.

For example:

• A patient refusing the impending death.

- Many old people refuse their decline in mental and physical powers as they advance in age.
- A middle-aged man who is a chronic alcoholic with liver failure may deny that alcohol is a problem for him.
- The excessive denial may lead to serious difficulties in health and lifestyle.

Projection

Projection is a way of attributing one's unwanted feelings, qualities or desires by shifting them on to someone else. It relieves tension and anxiety. For example, person who has the impulse to harm their brother often attribute that the brother wants to harm instead. A person is unfaithful to their spouse and accuses the spouse of infidelity. In schizophrenia, there might be delusion of persecution. Persons with this disorder use projection where they believe that their family members or strangers are trying to kill them, for example, by mixing poison in their food or keeping a check on them through cameras to kill them.

Immature Defenses

Acting Out

Acting Out is the expressing of an unconscious wish or impulse in the form of extreme behavior. It is used when the persons are not able to articulate their feelings. For example, instead of telling someone that one is angry with them, one might yell at them or throw something against wall. They may also engage in self-injurious behaviors such as cutting the forearm impulsively due to emotional pain.[4]

Regression

An individual starts behaving in a childlike manner whenever there is a threatful situation (i.e., behave in a less matured way). For example, facing the comparison with a younger sibling who performs better in school, 10-year-old may start to have toilet accidents, revert to babbling, demanding to be carried like a baby or suck their thumb. When life gets hectic or stressful, children and adults may regress to an earlier oral stage of development, such as biting nails or sucking their thumbs. Extreme forms and degrees of regression result in psychosis.

Passive-Aggressive Behavior

Passive-aggressive behavior is expression of anger or feelings of annoyance toward an object indirectly and ineffectively through passivity. Instead of showing hostile behavior visibly, people may choose to confuse others. Example, refusing to speak to someone. This behavior arises from not being able to express angry or frustrated feelings in direct and open manner. These people might not complete the assignments in a group on time.

Somatization

The psychic distress finds an outlet through manifestation of bodily symptoms. The symptoms are not traced to any physical cause. For example, an individual is going through a relationship breakup and somatization occurs through severe fatigue. An elderly grandfather who is stressed by the fights with his son may have unexplained pain in the body.

> **MUST KNOW**
>
> - Illness anxiety disorder (IAD), formerly known as hypochondriasis, is a syndrome characterized by extreme fear of having a major medical illness despite the presence of few or no symptoms. Individuals with IAD frequently consult doctors about symptoms they think are related to a health issue or may mistakenly think that minor symptoms are more dangerous than they actually are.
> - Even while there might not be a physical ailment, persons with IAD have very real worries, and their anxiety can seriously interfere with their ability to go about their everyday lives.

Fantasy or Daydreaming

It is disengagement with reality particularly when one faces troublesome situations in life. They withdraw into an imagined world and in that world, everything is possible which gives temporary satisfaction. One stops thinking about the current difficulties. It is a pleasant and may help them during the time of stress. For example, patients who are very ill may fantasize that when they recover, many good things will happen to them. Excessive daydreaming may lead to loss of contact with reality. It is seen in a psychotic disorder called schizophrenia.[4]

Neurotic Defenses

Repression

Repression is the basic to all other forms of defense mechanisms. There is a lot of psychic energy utilized in this defense mechanism and a sort of "burying alive" mechanisms. Repression is a process of unconscious forgetfulness of the unpleasant and conflict producing emotions and desires. If these experiences were to remain in the conscious, they would cause a person to feel ashamed, guilty and unworthy. According to R D Laing, "We forget and then forget that we forgot". The unconscious traumatic memories or urges may come up in the form of accidents, slips or neurotic symptoms such as anxiety when expressed. For example, Freudian slip of the tongue. Another example is if a child is sexually abused the child may not remember the abuse but that may be shown in the form of bed-wetting or refusal of food or anxiety symptoms in adulthood.

Reaction Formation

Unacceptable or threatening thoughts are dealt with by formation of opposite attitude, behavior or feelings. "The best defense is a good offense." For example, if the people are too humble, too concerned,

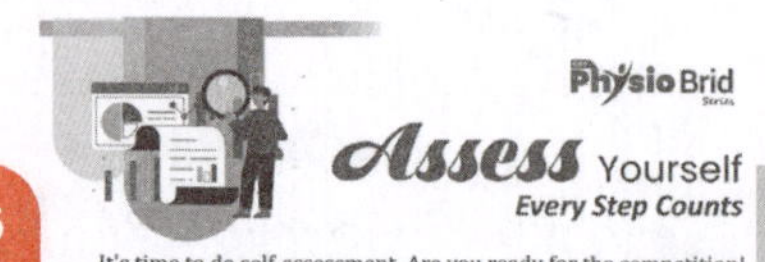

too loving or too harsh in their expression against topics such as alcoholism, homosexuality or child abuse, there is possibility that they are unconsciously having the exactly opposite feelings. For example, a person who dislikes their boss may hide their feelings by always being nice to them. A girl suffering from an eating disorder may often talk about others weight and makes fun of them. She may accuse others of having an eating disorder while hiding her own problem.

Rationalization

There is substitution of an unacceptable unconscious motive by a conscious motive that is acceptable. The justification of our tasks is given by making an excuse or giving alternate explanation. It is a defense mechanism in which an individual justifies their failures and socially unacceptable behavior by giving socially approved reasons. Rationalization is not lying.

For examples:

- Students who fail to crack an entrance exam may complain that hostel atmosphere is not favorable for study.
- A tense father who beats their child may rationalize that it is for the child's good.
- An employee who fails to get promotion may blame the employer's partiality. It is like a blanket to cover the human weakness. It operates in two forms.
    i. **Sour grapes:** (From Aesop's fable of Fox and Grapes)

       A young man who fails to get a beautiful wife may remark that a beautiful wife is a liability.
    ii. **Sweet lemon:** The individual justifies their lower achievements by pointing out their merits. A poor man may say, "He does not want to earn money" because "money is the root cause of many evils".

Intellectualization

This defense mechanism utilizes reasoning just like rationalization. It is the use of logic (intellectual abilities) in thinking or while talking, in order to distance oneself from an emotion or fearful situation. It helps an individual to focus on the external reality.

All healthcare workers including doctors, nurses or other medical workers often use the technique of detaching themselves from emotions through stating the facts or statements in a calm way to the patient. Example, if there is a patient who is terminally ill, the doctor may inform the family members in calm voice and discuss the management plan with them.

Displacement

In this, the affect or impulse does not get altered but the person substitutes a different displaced object, that is less conflictual than the original one. There is generalization or redirecting of a feeling or a response to an object onto another. The person utilizing this defense might not know that the expressed feeling was for someone else.

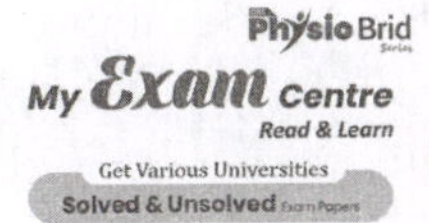

For example, a mother who is angry with her neighbor but cannot show it may beat her son for accidentally breaking a pot.

A teenager boy who is upset with the parents for not allowing him to go to a party alone might fight with the younger sibling displacing his anger.[4]

Identification

The person experiences the personal sense of fulfillment in the success and achievements of other people or groups. An individual to varied degrees, molds themselves into someone else. Parts of others are unconsciously adopted.

For examples:

- Hero worship is an obvious form of identification.
- An uneducated mother often takes her daughter's education as her own achievements.
- Individuals may burst into tears when the protagonist is shown mercilessly attacked by villains, while watching a film.
- Much of learning process in childhood is through identification.

It plays a major part in the process of formation of a child's personality and in the process of acculturation. If the object of identification is good, their effect on us will be constructive. One can't grow and mature completely by this without having our own identity.

Compensation

Compensation means giving up something to replace a loss or to make up for a defect. It is similar to nature's compensation—a blind person develops extraordinary keen hearing. When people are frustrated in their desires in one direction, they compensate for it by attaining success in other directions. For example, a student who is poor in academics may become the state champion in dancing.

Withdrawal

In situations of being criticized, ridiculed or disgraced on account of some prior unfortunate experience or failure, some people resort to withdrawal, for example, avoiding all the works assigned to a person. It is a protective device by which the person prevents further hurt and damage to their security by withdrawing from people. It may be temporary and makes no real friends. It is one of the dominant personality traits of the schizophrenics.[4]

Conversion/Dissociation

Conversion/dissociation is the channelizing of emotional conflicts to a physical symptom for which there is no underlying medical reason. Symptoms maybe in the form of inability to see, hear, walk or speak. For example, a student may develop fever during exam. A daughter who witnessed domestic violence at home by her father may wish to hit him. However, she could suddenly develop complete paralysis of her right arm, which would serve two purposes.

1. Resolve the conflict (inability to strike her father)
2. Bring her a great deal of attention and sympathy

A cross-sectional study on 102 adolescents revealed that girls use more of neurotic defenses such as repression, dissociation and reaction formation as compared to boys who employ undoing, isolation of affect and intellectualization.[5]

An 8-year longitudinal follow-up study on depressed adolescents has shown that the defenses of displacement, isolation, and reaction formation were independent predictors of adult diagnosis of personality disorders.[6]

Mature Defenses

They are mature mechanisms as they require a higher sense of emotional regulation. These help a person to accept the unpleasurable reality. They have a protective role and improve the chances of satisfaction in life and relationships. Feelings of pleasure and control get augmented with the use of these mature mechanisms. These defenses help to integrate conflicting emotions and thoughts, while still remaining effective.[7]

Altruism

These are the tasks done for the benefits of a larger group or society as a whole. It may involve disservice to oneself. There is compassion and desire to help others. For example, starting a nonprofit organization, dedicating oneself to a cause or advocating for social justice and equality. Another example, the parents of a child who died in an accident, decide to donate the organs of the child.

Suppression

Suppression is a defense mechanism in which a person chooses not to talk about certain unsolicited thoughts, experiences or feelings. These are kept away from awareness. We merely push such thoughts into the background that is our subconscious mind, where they are accessible to us whenever we wish to remember them. As it is conscious, it is not a defense mechanism in the strict sense. For example, someone witnesses a train accident and he pushes the feelings of fear on a side and helps other injured people. When asked about this incident, he may choose to avoid talking about it.

Humor

Overtly communicating unpleasant or stressful ideas and feelings that gives pleasure to others by emphasizing the amusing or ironic aspects of the conflict. Using comedy as a means of openly expressing feelings and ideas without causing discomfort to oneself or others. The rule is that it is done in a way that no unpleasant effect on others is produced. It relieves the stress of the person and yet focus on what is too terrible to be tolerated. For example, oncologists who treat cancer patients use humor that is helpful for building a good relationship with patients.

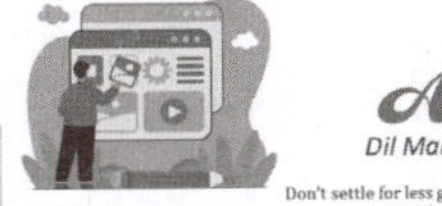
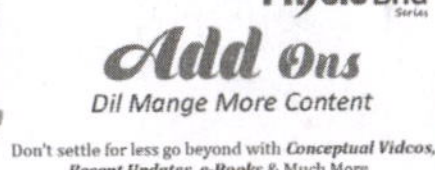

Sublimation

Channelizing of socially unacceptable impulses or wishes into behaviors that are more acceptable. It provides an outlet for these impulses. It represented the pinnacle of ego defense mechanism for Sigmund Freud. It consists of a redirection of impulses to socially valued activities and goals. Much of the cultural heritage, literature, music, and art are the product of sublimation.

For example:

- If a person has aggressive drives, they may take up karate to find a more socially acceptable way to channelize their aggression. It promotes a sense of accomplishment.
- A person who has the desire for being in charge with control and order, becomes a Chief Executive Officer (CEO) of a company.
- A writer may divert some of his impulses to kill others to the creation of a poem or novel, with the theme of killing thus indirectly satisfying his urge.[8]

CLINICAL APPLICATION

Recognition of the kind of defense mechanisms used by an individual and communicating about it with the members of the multidisciplinary team improves care of the patient. Psychotherapists using brief psychodynamic therapy notice that the increase in use of adaptive defense mechanisms is a slow process. It is noticed much later than the symptomatic improvement. Over the course, progress of patient's symptoms can be tracked by the treating therapist by observing the defensive functioning such as in patients with borderline personality disorder.[8–10]

Physio CORNER

Understanding ego defense mechanisms is crucial for physiotherapists, as these psychological processes can impact a patient's behavior, attitude, and response to treatment. Here are some important aspects that a physiotherapist should know:

- **Definition and purpose:**
  - **Ego defense mechanisms:** These are unconscious psychological strategies that individuals use to protect themselves from anxiety, stress, and uncomfortable emotions. They help maintain psychological stability and self-esteem.
  - **Purpose:** Defense mechanisms reduce the impact of stressful events or internal conflicts on an individual's conscious mind, enabling them to function more effectively.
- **Common defense mechanisms:**
  - **Denial:** Refusal to accept reality or facts, leading patients to ignore or reject the seriousness of their condition.
    - **Physiotherapy impact:** Patients might not adhere to treatment plans because they don't acknowledge the severity of their injury or condition.
  - **Repression:** Unconsciously blocking unpleasant thoughts or feelings from awareness.
    - **Physiotherapy impact:** Repressed emotions or trauma can manifest as physical symptoms, complicating the rehabilitation process.

Contd...

- **Rationalization:** Justifying behaviors or feelings with logical reasons, often avoiding the true explanation.
  - *Physiotherapy impact:* Patients might rationalize noncompliance with treatment by giving excuses that seem reasonable, but are actually avoiding deeper issues.
- **Projection:** Attributing one's own unacceptable thoughts or feelings to others.
  - *Physiotherapy impact:* Patients may project their frustrations or fears onto the therapist, creating barriers in the therapeutic relationship.
- **Displacement:** Redirecting emotions from a threatening target to a safer one.
  - *Physiotherapy impact:* Patients might express anger or frustration toward the therapist instead of addressing the real source of their emotions.
- **Regression:** Reverting to an earlier stage of development in response to stress.
  - *Physiotherapy impact:* Patients might exhibit childlike behavior or dependency, requiring a more supportive and nurturing approach in therapy.

- **Recognizing defense mechanisms in patients:**
  - **Behavioral clues:** Understanding patient behaviors that might indicate the use of defense mechanisms, such as avoidance of certain topics, inconsistent stories or unusual emotional responses.
  - **Communication:** Being attentive to how patients express themselves and respond to stressors during sessions can help identify when they are using defense mechanisms.

- **Therapeutic response:**
  - **Building trust:** Establishing a strong, trusting relationship with patients encourages them to feel safe and reduces the need for defense mechanisms.
  - **Patient education:** Gently educating patients about their behavior patterns without confronting them directly can help them gain insight.
  - **Empathy and support:** Offering empathy and understanding helps patients feel accepted, which can reduce their reliance on defensive behaviors.
  - **Referral to psychotherapy:** If defense mechanisms are significantly hindering progress, a referral to a psychologist or counselor may be necessary for more in-depth psychological intervention.

- **Impact on treatment compliance:**
  - **Understanding resistance:** Resistance to treatment might be a sign of underlying defense mechanisms at play. Recognizing this can help tailor approaches to improve compliance.
  - **Patient-centered approach:** Adapting treatment plans to accommodate the patient's psychological state, ensuring that his defense mechanisms are acknowledged and gently addressed.

- **Documentation and communication:**
  - **Documentation:** Keeping detailed notes on patient behaviors, responses, and any suspected defense mechanisms can help track progress and inform treatment adjustments.
  - **Team communication:** Sharing insights about a patient's use of defense mechanisms with other healthcare providers can help ensure a consistent, multidisciplinary approach to care.

- **Self-awareness for the therapist:**
  - **Reflective practice:** Being aware of one's own potential defense mechanisms and emotional responses during patient interactions is crucial. This helps in maintaining professional boundaries and providing the best care.

- **Cultural and individual differences:**
  - **Cultural sensitivity:** Understanding that defense mechanisms can vary across cultures and individuals, and being sensitive to these differences is important for effective therapy.

By understanding and addressing ego defense mechanisms, physiotherapists can enhance patient engagement, improve treatment outcomes, and foster a more supportive therapeutic environment.

CASE STUDY

Role of Physiotherapy in Conversion Disorder

Patient Background
- **Name:** Sarah Jones
- **Age:** 32 years
- **Occupation:** Administrative assistant
- **Presenting symptoms:** Sudden onset of unexplained weakness and paralysis in the left leg, with no underlying neurological cause found.
- **Medical history:** No significant physical illness, but recent stressful life events, including the death of a close family member and work-related stress.
- **Diagnosis:** Conversion disorder (functional neurological symptom disorder)

Context

Sarah Jones, a 32-year-old woman, presented with sudden weakness and paralysis in her left leg. After a comprehensive medical evaluation, no organic cause for her symptoms was identified. Given her recent exposure to significant stressors, she was diagnosed with conversion disorder, a condition where psychological stress manifests as physical symptoms.

Understanding Conversion Disorder

Conversion disorder is a mental health condition where psychological conflicts or stressors are converted into physical symptoms that affect voluntary motor or sensory functions. Common symptoms include paralysis, movement disorders, gait abnormalities, and sensory disturbances, often without a clear medical cause. While the symptoms are not intentionally produced, they can be debilitating and impact daily functioning.

Role of Physiotherapy in Treatment

Physiotherapy plays a crucial role in the management of conversion disorder by addressing the physical symptoms while considering the underlying psychological factors. The primary goals of physiotherapy in this context are to help the patient regain functional mobility, reduce disability, and support psychological well-being.

Intervention Plan
- **Initial assessment**
  - **Objective:** To evaluate Sarah's physical abilities, limitations, and identify any patterns in her movement that may be influenced by psychological factors.
  - **Approach:**
    - *Detailed physical examination:* Assess muscle strength, range of motion (ROM), gait analysis, and balance. The therapist noted inconsistencies in Sarah's weakness, such as variable strength during different parts of the assessment, which is often indicative of functional symptoms.
    - *Psychological screening:* Collaborate with a psychologist to screen for underlying anxiety, depression or other psychological factors contributing to her symptoms.
    - *Patient education:* Explain the nature of conversion disorder to Sarah, emphasizing that her symptoms, while not caused by physical illness, are real and can improve with treatment.
- **Establishing a therapeutic alliance**
  - **Objective:** Build trust and rapport with Sarah to ensure her active participation in therapy.

Contd...

- **Approach:**
  - *Empathy and understanding:* The physiotherapist took time to listen to Sarah's concerns, validating her experiences, and ensuring she felt heard and understood.
  - *Positive reinforcement:* Encourage small achievements and focus on progress rather than the severity of symptoms.
- **Gradual mobilization and functional retraining:**
  - **Objective:** To restore normal movement patterns and improve Sarah's functional independence.
  - **Approach:**
    - *Graded exercises:* Start with gentle, low-resistance exercises to improve muscle strength and endurance, gradually increasing intensity as Sarah's confidence in her abilities grew.
    - *Gait training:* Use parallel bars and supported ambulation to help Sarah relearn walking. Emphasis was placed on normalizing movement patterns and reducing any fear associated with movement.
    - *Functional tasks:* Integrate tasks that are meaningful to Sarah, such as walking to the mailbox or standing to make a cup of tea. This helped bridge the gap between therapy and daily life.
- **Cognitive-behavioral strategies:**
  - **Objective:** Address the psychological factors contributing to the physical symptoms.
  - **Approach:**
    - *Cognitive restructuring:* The physiotherapist worked with Sarah to identify and challenge any negative or catastrophic thoughts related to her symptoms, helping to reduce anxiety and fear associated with movement.
    - *Relaxation techniques:* Incorporate relaxation and mindfulness exercises to help Sarah manage stress, which may trigger or exacerbate her symptoms.
- **Multidisciplinary collaboration:**
  - **Objective:** Ensure comprehensive care by involving other healthcare professionals.
  - **Approach:**
    - *Psychological support:* Regular sessions with a psychologist trained in treating functional neurological disorders to address underlying emotional issues and provide cognitive-behavioral therapy (CBT).
    - *Medical monitoring:* Continuous collaboration with her primary care physician and neurologist to monitor her progress and rule out any emerging physical conditions.
- **Family involvement and education:**
  - **Objective:** Educate Sarah's family about conversion disorder and how they can support her recovery.
  - **Approach:**
    - *Family counseling:* Educate Sarah's family on the importance of supportive behavior and avoiding reinforcement of disability. Encourage them to be positive and patient, and to focus on her capabilities rather than her limitations.

Outcome

- **Short-term:** After a few weeks of physiotherapy, Sarah began to regain strength in her left leg. Her gait improved, and she started to walk short distances with minimal support. The use of cognitive-behavioral strategies helped reduce her fear of movement, and she reported feeling more confident in her ability to recover.

Contd...

- **Long-term:** Over several months, Sarah's symptoms significantly improved. She regained full mobility in her left leg and was able to return to work part-time. Her psychological well-being also improved, with reduced anxiety and better coping mechanisms for stress. Sarah continued to engage in both physiotherapy and psychological support to maintain her progress and prevent relapse.

Conclusion

This case study illustrates the effectiveness of physiotherapy in treating conversion disorder, particularly when combined with psychological interventions. By addressing both the physical and psychological aspects of the disorder, the treatment helped Sarah regain her functional abilities and improve her overall quality of life. The success of this approach highlights the importance of a holistic, patient-centered strategy in the management of conversion disorder.

SUMMARY

- The chapter delves into the fascinating realm of psychological defense mechanisms, a cornerstone of psychoanalytic theory. Pioneered by Sigmund Freud and further elaborated by his daughter, Anna Freud, defense mechanisms are understood as the mind's unconscious strategies to protect the ego from internal and external threats. These mechanisms operate beneath the surface of conscious awareness, playing a crucial role in how individuals cope with stress, anxiety, and the challenges of daily life.

- The chapter begins by outlining the historical context, tracing the development of defense mechanisms from Sigmund Freud's initial conceptualization to Anna Freud's detailed analysis and identification of over 10 distinct mechanisms. It highlights the ego's central role in managing the tension between primal urges and societal demands, emphasizing the importance of these mechanisms in maintaining mental stability and adapting to environmental pressures.

- The chapter classifies defense mechanisms into four broad categories: Narcissistic-psychotic, immature, neurotic, and mature, each reflecting different levels of psychological development and effectiveness in handling stress.

  i. **Narcissistic-psychotic defenses:** These are the earliest and most primitive mechanisms, often observed in children and individuals experiencing psychosis. They include denial, where individuals refuse to acknowledge unpleasant realities, and projection, where unwanted feelings or impulses are attributed to others.

  ii. **Immature defenses:** This category encompasses mechanisms that are less adaptive and more overt in their expression. Examples include acting out, where unconscious wishes are expressed through extreme behavior; regression, a retreat to childlike behavior in the face of stress; passive-aggressive behavior, indirect expression of anger; somatization, where psychological distress manifests as physical symptoms; and fantasy or daydreaming, an escape into an imagined world.

  iii. **Neurotic defenses:** These mechanisms are more refined but still serve to manage unacceptable thoughts and feelings. They include repression, the unconscious exclusion of traumatic memories or urges; reaction formation, where individuals adopt an opposite attitude to mask their true feelings; rationalization, the justification of actions with socially acceptable reasons; intellectualization, using logic to distance oneself from emotions; displacement, redirecting feelings toward a less threatening object; identification, adopting the qualities of others; compensation, achieving success in one area to make up for a failure in another; withdrawal, avoiding social interactions to protect oneself; and conversion/dissociation, manifesting emotional conflicts as physical symptoms.

Contd...

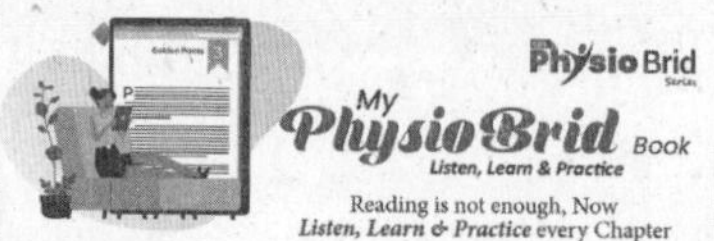

iv. **Mature defenses:** The most adaptive and effective mechanisms, they help individuals accept reality and improve life satisfaction. Altruism involves helping others for the benefit of society; suppression consciously keeps certain thoughts or feelings out of awareness; humor uses comedy to express stressful ideas; and sublimation channels unacceptable impulses into socially valued activities.

- Recognizing and understanding these defense mechanisms is crucial for therapeutic interventions, as they provide insight into an individual's coping strategies and psychological state. The chapter emphasizes that while defense mechanisms are inherently unconscious and often adaptive, they can become problematic if they prevent individuals from facing reality or lead to maladaptive behaviors.

- In conclusion, this chapter provides a comprehensive overview of defense mechanisms, illustrating how they operate and their significance in the human psyche. By understanding these mechanisms, we can better appreciate the complexities of human behavior and the mind's remarkable capacity for self-protection and adaptation.

REFERENCES

1. Cramer P. Defense mechanisms: 40 years of empirical research. Journal of Personality Assessment. 2015;97(2):114–22.

2. Diehl M, Chui H, Hay EL, Lumley MA, Gruhn, D, Labouvie-Vief G. Change in coping and defense mechanisms across adulthood: Longitudinal findings in a European American sample. Developmental Psychology. 2014;50(2):634–48.

3. Perry JC. Anomalies and specific functions in the clinical identification of defense mechanisms. J Clin Psychol. 2014;70(5):406–18.

4. William W, Meissner S.J, Classical Psychoanalysis. Kaplan and Sadock's Comprehensive Textbook of Psychiatry – 10th ed. Wolters Kluver; 2017:2219–28.

5. Di Giuseppe M, Gennaro A, Lingiardi V, Perry JC. The Role of Defense Mechanisms in Emerging Personality Disorders in Clinical Adolescents. Psychiatry.2019;82920:128–142.

6. Strandholm T, Kiviruusu O, Karlsson L, Miettunen J, Marttunen M. Defense Mechanisms in Adolescence as Predictors of Adult Personality Disorders. J Nerv Ment Dis. 2016;204(5):349–54.

7. Metzger J.A. Adaptive defense mechanisms: Function and Transcendence. J Clin Psychol. 2014; 70(5):478–488.

8. Zanarini MC, Weingeroff JL, Frankenburg FR. Defense mechanisms associated with borderline personality disorder. J Pers Disord. 2009;23(2):113–21.

9. Kramer U, Despland JN, Michel L, Drapeau M, de Roten Y. Change in defense mechanisms and coping over the course of short-term dynamic psychotherapy for adjustment disorder. J Clin Psychol. 2010; 66(12):1232–41.

10. Hersoug AG, Sexton HC, Hoglend P. Contribution of defensive functioning to the quality of working alliance and psychotherapy outcome. Am J Psychother. 2002; 56(4):539–54.

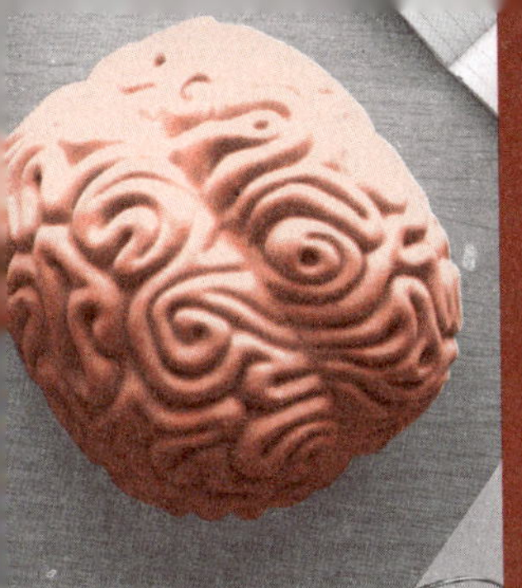

LONG ANSWER QUESTIONS

1. Explain defense mechanisms.
2. Discuss narcissistic-psychotic defense mechanisms.
3. Describe immature defense mechanisms.
4. Discuss neurotic defense mechanisms.
5. What are mature defense mechanisms? Explain with examples.

SHORT ANSWER QUESTIONS

1. Define defense mechanisms.
2. What do you understand by projection?
3. What is sublimation? Give an example.
4. What is reaction formation?
5. What is displacement?
6. What is somatization?

MULTIPLE CHOICE QUESTIONS

1. **According to psychoanalytic theory, defense mechanisms are considered to be:**
   a. Normal
   b. Pathological
   c. Immature
   d. Abnormal

2. **Who introduces a four-level classification of defense mechanisms?**
   a. Sigmund Freud
   b. Anna Freud
   c. George Valliant
   d. Robert Plutchik

3. **Defense mechanism that shifts sexual or aggressive impulse to a less threatening target is:**
   a. Dissociation
   b. Displacement
   c. Reaction formation
   d. Rationalization

4. **Dinesh's family members confront him regarding his excessive alcohol consumption 7 days a week, but he thinks he does not have a problem. Which is the defense mechanism employed?**
   a. Denial
   b. Repression
   c. Rationalization
   d. Projection

5. Karan decides to party whole week and play online games before his semester exams instead of studying. He fails his exams and tells his parents that he failed due to being sick and not getting enough sleep. Which defense mechanism is used here?
    a. Projection
    b. Displacement
    c. Denial
    d. Rationalization

6. What is an example of regression?
    a. Missing an ex-boyfriend
    b. Holding in your anger
    c. Behaving like a young child to cope with
    d. Avoiding talking about someone's death

7. Draining off the unwanted energy into socially acceptable channels is called:
    a. Substitution
    b. Sublimation
    c. Introjection
    d. Projection

8. Repression refers to:
    a. Stopping bad thoughts from coming in memory
    b. Diversion of energy into positive and socially acceptable activities
    c. Conscious exclusion of bad memories that causes anxiety
    d. Unconscious exclusion of bad memories that causes anxiety

9. A son decides to become a successful businessman just like his father. Which defense mechanism is used in this situation?
    a. Introjection
    b. Denial
    c. Compensation
    d. Identification

10. A person under heavy debt makes an excel sheet of how long would it take to repay using different payment options and interest rates. What type of defense mechanism is used here?
    a. Rationalization
    b. Intellectualization
    c. Repression
    d. Regression

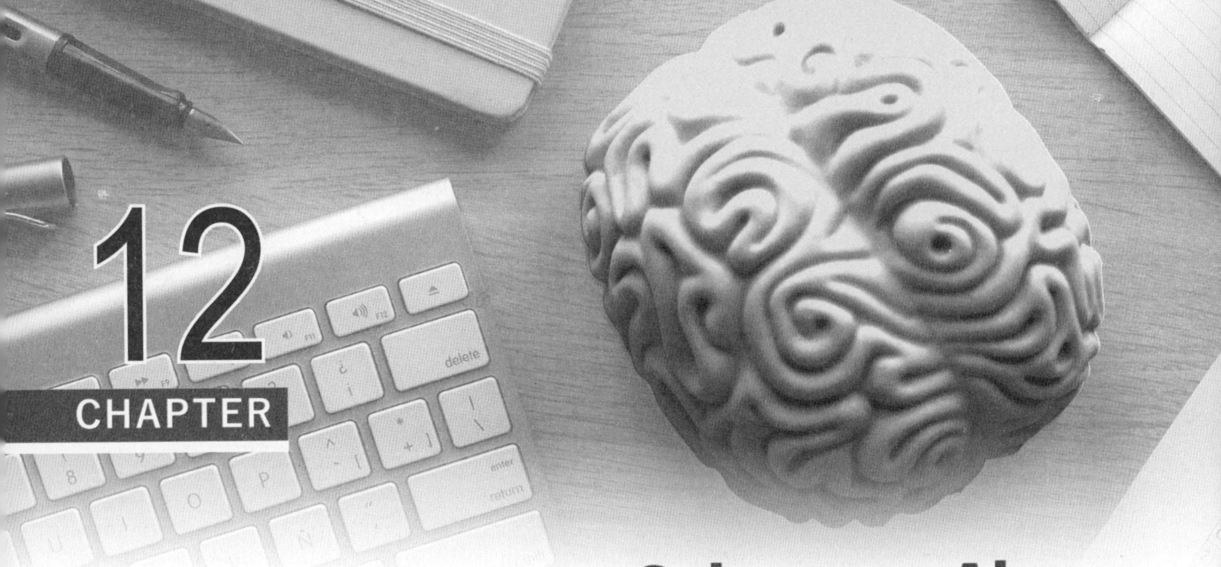

Substance Abuse

Kajal Taneja

LEARNING OBJECTIVES

After the completion of the chapter, the readers will be able to:
- Explain the meaning of "psychoactive" substances.
- Describe the scope and impact of substance use.
- Discuss the effects of various substance use disorders.
- Explain the pharmacological management of substance use disorders.
- Understand the psychosocial management of substance use disorders.

CHAPTER OUTLINE

- Introduction
- Epidemiology
- Diagnostic Criteria
- Consequences of Substance Use
- Tobacco Use Disorders
- Alcohol Use Disorders
- Opioid Use Disorders
- Cannabis Use Disorders
- Sedatives and Hypnotics
- Assessment of Substance Use Disorders
- Management

KEY TERMS

Deaddiction: It refers to the process of overcoming dependence on psychoactive substances.

Intoxication: A transient condition following administration of a psychoactive substance resulting in disturbances at the level of consciousness, cognition, perception and behavior.

Motivation: The internally generated state that stimulates us to act.

Psychoactive substance: It involves the consumption of substances that affect the mind, altering mood, perception, cognition, and behavior.

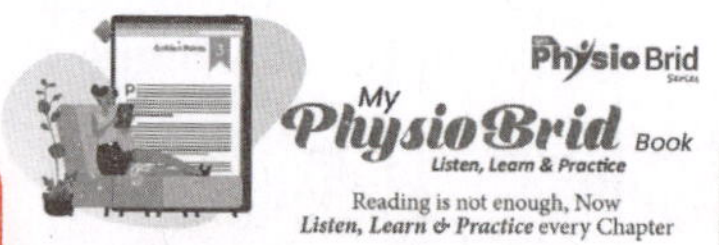

> **Relapse:** Recurrence of substance use after a period of abstinence.
>
> **Substance use:** It refers to the consumption of any psychoactive substance, which can include legal substances (such as alcohol, tobacco, and prescription medications) and illegal substances (such as cocaine, heroin, and methamphetamine).

INTRODUCTION

Since time immemorial, a person with a substance use disorder is seen as immoral and of unprincipled character and is being stigmatized in our society even today. Various ancient books like Vedas and Bible mention the historical usage of certain drugs, like opium, cannabis, marijuana for their various medicinal properties but their inappropriate use may lead to uncertain consequences which may progress to their abuse and subsequently addiction.

The World Health Organization (WHO) defines a drug as, Any substance that, when taken into the living organism, may modify one or more of its functions.[1] The definition conceptualizes 'drug' in a comprehensive way. It includes both routine medications and other pharmacologically active substances.

The words 'drug addiction' and 'drug addict' are no longer in scientific use due to their stigmatizing implication. In recent literatures, the terms, like 'substance abuse', 'substance dependence', 'harmful use', 'misuse', and 'psychoactive substance use disorders' are being used.

A psychoactive drug is the chemical compound that influences the mental functions such as the subjective perception and/or behavior.[1]

EPIDEMIOLOGY

According to a survey conducted in India in 2019, alcohol came out to be the substance consumed by the Indian population the most. Among the age group from 10 to 75 years, 14.6% of the population uses alcohol. Men were considerably surpassing women in ingesting alcohol, amounting to 27.3% compared to 1.6% only. Among alcohol consumers, the most consumed beverages were country liquor—around 30% and spirits or Indian made foreign liquor—around 30%.

The survey also revealed that about 2.8% of the population used products made of cannabis during the last year. Nearly 2.1% Indians used opioids; among which heroin (1.14%) tops the list succeeded by pharmaceutical opioids (0.96%) and opium (0.52%).[2]

Psychoactive Substances

The drugs causing major dependence are:

- **Nicotine/tobacco:** Cigarettes, chewable forms, etc.

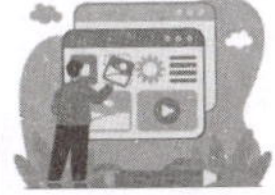

- **Alcohol:** Distilled liquors, country-made liquor, etc.
- **Opioids:** Heroin, afeem, spasmoproxyvon, etc.
- **Sedatives and hypnotics:** Barbiturates, benzodiazepines, etc.
- **Cannabinoids:** Cannabis and its various forms.
- **Stimulants:** Cocaine, amphetamine/sympathomimetics.
- **Hallucinogens:** Phencyclidine, Lysergic acid diethylamide (LSD), etc.
- Inhalants/volatile solvents.
- **Other stimulants:** Caffeine.

Etiological Factors

If we look at the substance use, from the lens of the biopsychosocial model, there are certain risk factors which interplay with each other leading to emergence of this problem. These factors are psychological factors, social and biological factors which have been shown in Table 12.1.[3,4] Biological factors constitute various genetic level problems or various physiological problems in the body. Psychological factors consist of factors related to higher mental level, and social factors involve factors related to surroundings and environment.

Table 12.1: Etiological factors in substance use disorders

Biological factors
• Genetic vulnerability (substance use disorders running in family, e.g., type II alcoholism)
• Comorbid psychiatric disorder or personality disorder
• Underlying medical disorder
• Reinforcing effects of various drug
• Withdrawal effects and craving for the substance
• Biochemical factors, e.g., dopamine and norepinephrine role in cocaine, ethanol and opioid dependence).

Psychological factors	
• To experiment: Curiosity; need for novelty seeking	• Sensation-seeking (High)
• General rebelliousness and social nonconformity	• Low self-esteem (Anomie)
• Poor impulse control	• Relief from fatigue and/or boredom
	• Poor stress management skills

Social factors	
• To fit in: Peer pressure	• Religious reasons
• Modeling: Copying behaviors of others	• Poor social/familial support
• Readily available alcohol and drugs	• Permissive social attitudes
• Intrafamilial conflicts	• Feeling distanced within the family

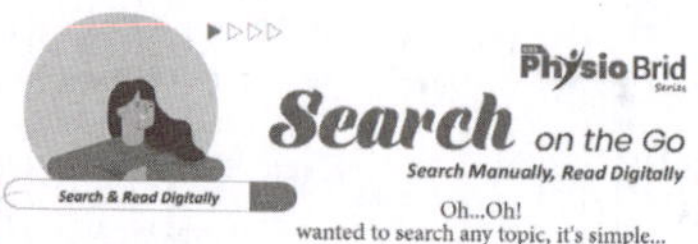

DIAGNOSTIC CRITERIA

The terminology and diagnosis of psychoactive substance use disorders is precisely described in recent guidelines prescribed by various organizations, like ICD-11 and DSM-5 in literature. ICD-11 diagnostic criteria is shown in Table 12.2.[5]

Table 12.2: ICD-11 Diagnostic criteria for disorders due to psychoactive substance use

Episode of harmful psychoactive substance use

- An episode of use of a psychoactive substance that has caused clinically significant damage to a person's physical health or mental health or has resulted in behavior leading to harm to the health of others.
- Harm to health of the individual occurs due to one or more of the following:
  - Behavior related to intoxication.
  - Direct or secondary toxic effects on body organs and systems.
  - A harmful route of administration.
- Harm to health of others includes any form of physical harm, including trauma or mental disorder that is directly attributable to behavior due to substance intoxication on the part of the person to whom the diagnosis applies.
- Harm to health is not better accounted for by another medical condition or another mental disorder, including another disorder due to substance use.

Harmful pattern of psychoactive substance use

- A pattern of continuous, recurrent or sporadic use of a psychoactive substance that has caused clinically significant damage to a person's physical health or mental health or has resulted in behavior leading to harm to the health of others.
- Harm to health of the individual occurs due to one or more of the following:
  - Behavior related to intoxication.
  - Direct or secondary toxic effects on body organs and systems.
  - A harmful route of administration.
- Harm to health of others includes any form of physical harm, including trauma or mental disorder that is directly attributable to behavior related to substance intoxication on the part of the person to whom the diagnosis applies.
- The pattern of use of the relevant substance is evident over a period of at least 12 months if substance use is episodic or at least 1 month if use is continuous.
- Harm to health is not better accounted for by another medical condition or another mental disorder, including another disorder due to substance use.

Substance dependence

- A pattern of recurrent episodic or continuous use of a psychoactive substance with evidence of impaired regulation of use of that substance that is manifested by two or more of the following:
  - Impaired control over substance use (i.e., onset, frequency, intensity, duration, termination, context);
  - Increasing precedence of substance use over other aspects of life, including maintenance of health, and daily activities and responsibilities, such that substance use continues or escalates despite the occurrence of harm or negative consequences, negative impact on health.

Contd...

- Psychological features indicative of neuroadaptation to the substance, including:
    - Tolerance to the effects of the substance or a need to use increasing amounts of the substance to achieve the same effect.
    - Withdrawal symptoms following cessation or reduction in use of that substance or
    - Repeated use of the substance or pharmacologically similar substances to prevent or alleviate withdrawal symptoms. Physiological features are only applicable for certain substances.
- The features of dependence are usually evident for a period of at least 12 months but the diagnosis may be made if use is continuous (daily or almost daily) for at least 3 months.

CONSEQUENCES OF SUBSTANCE USE

There are various consequences of using substance which are visible in various domains. Various psychiatric illnesses can be preexisting or can newly emerge with the use of substance. Disorders like anxiety, phobias, psychotic disorders, depression, posttraumatic stress disorders (PTSD), suicide attempts are linked to the use of different substances.[6]

The family members face a lot of burden in the form of shame, guilt and self-blame. Relationships become strained due to abuse happening in the form of physical, emotional or sexual abuse in the family. One parent using substance acts as a model for the children. There is unemployment leading to rise of financial burden on other earning members. It leads to disability and increased burden on society for the treatment. In order to procure substance persons might engage in stealing, robbing or selling drugs to others. There are higher chances of them coming in conflict with law. Various domains which get affected by substance use are depicted in Figure 12.1.

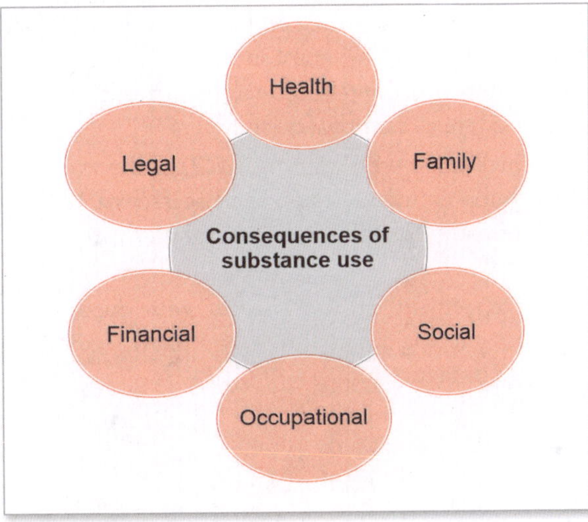

Fig. 12.1: Consequences of substance use

- **Health:** Drug use can lead to severe physical and mental health issues, including addiction, organ damage or mental disorders.
- **Family:** It often causes strain in relationships, leading to conflicts, mistrust or even estrangement.
- **Social:** Drug users may face social isolation, stigma or loss of friendships.
- **Occupational:** It affects productivity, leading to job loss or career stagnation.
- **Financial:** Substance abuse can drain savings and lead to financial instability or debt.
- **Legal:** It may result in criminal charges, imprisonment or legal complications.

TOBACCO USE DISORDERS

Among all substantial abuses, tobacco use is the most common substance abuse by Indian population. From a lower socioeconomic person to a person with higher status, tobacco use is very much prevalent in India.[2] It is readily available in various forms shown in Table 12.3.[7]

Table 12.3: Various forms of nicotine

Route of use	Preparations
Smoked	Cigarettes, Bidis, Cigars, Hookah
Oral	Guthka, Khaini, Zarda, Betel quid tobacco, Mawa
Inhaled	Snuff

Health Consequences

One of the important risk factors for chronic obstructive pulmonary disease (COPD) is cigarette smoking. There are several cancers associated with smoking. Half of all people who smoke can be expected to die from tobacco-related illnesses. Due to smoking only, there is >10% mortality, occurs due to failure of cardiovascular system.[2]

There are several tests available for the assessment of severity of nicotine dependence. One of the commonly used tests is: The Fagerstrom Test for Nicotine Dependence (FTND). It is a 6-item questionnaire. The total score can vary from 0 to 10. The higher the scoring on this test, more severe is the dependence.[8]

Management of the patient with nicotine dependence is done by various drugs and nonpharmacological methods. Nonpharmacological method constitutes **5A's approach** which is depicted in Figure 12.2.[9]

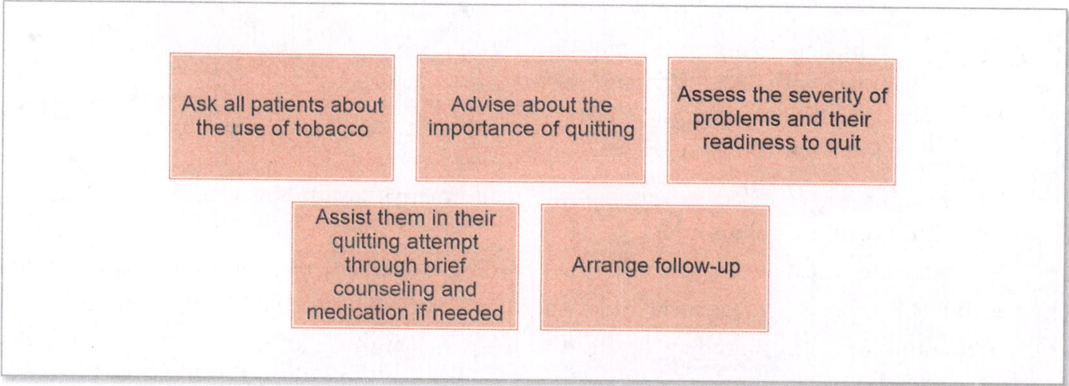

Fig. 12.2: 5A's approach to manage nicotine dependency

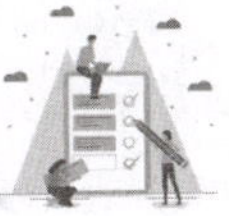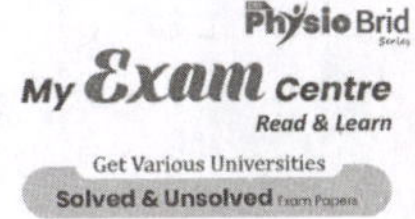

ALCOHOL USE DISORDERS

Alcoholic beverages commonly used in the society are beer, whiskey, brandy, rum, vodka, gin and wine. Different beverages have different amount of alcohol in it ranging from <1%–60%. There are locally brewed beverages like toddy, arrack and fenny popularly known as country made liquors also readily available in the markets with unknown concentrations of alcohol. Higher concentrated alcohols have various effects on the health listed in Table 12.4.[10]

Table 12.4: Acute effects of alcohol

Mental and behavioral effects	Physical effects
• Drowsiness	• Flushed face
• Attention impairment	• Rapid pulse
• Memory impairment	• Headache
• Impaired judgment	• Stomach ache
• Impulsive behavior	• Diarrhea
• Impaired occupational	• Slurred speech
• Performance	• Sweating
• Inapt social conduct	• Unsteady gait
• Inappropriate sexual behavior	• Nystagmus
• Mood lability (rapid changes)	• Respiratory depression
• Stupor/coma	

Acute Intoxication

Alcohol use leads to a short duration of excitation which is followed by generalized depression of the body's central nervous system (CNS). As the intoxication increases, the reaction time gets delayed, thinking becomes slower, motor control becomes weak and person becomes distractible. In later stages, incoordination, dysarthria and even ataxia can be seen. The person loses their self-control progressively with obvious disinhibited behavior. In acute intoxication phase sometimes, amnesia or blackouts can happen. Amount of alcohol intake and rapidity of ingestion determines the duration of intoxicated state.[10] Table 12.5 shows the effects of alcohol with respect to concentration of alcohol in blood.

Table 12.5: Effects of alcohol with respect to blood alcohol levels

Blood alcohol levels (mg%)	Effects
150–200	Signs of intoxication are obvious
300–450	Drowsiness which increases with time followed by respiratory depression; may lead to coma
400–800	Death

Pathological intoxication: In some persons even a small quantity of alcohol consumption may lead to acute intoxication.

Alcohol Withdrawal Syndrome

Hangover is the most common withdrawal syndrome seen on the very next morning. Other common symptoms with alcohol withdrawal are anxiety, insomnia, mild tremors, nausea, vomiting, irritability and weakness.[11] Due to marked morbidity with significant documented mortality, alcohol withdrawal syndrome, timely appropriate treatment is must. In some persons the severity of withdrawal symptoms is so intense that they can present as one of the following three states:

1. Alcoholic seizures
2. Delirium tremens
3. Alcoholic hallucinosis

1. Alcoholic Seizures ('Rum fits')

The very first step, if first seizure occurs during withdrawal period is to rule out organic cause or idiopathic epilepsy. **Generalized Tonic-Clonic Seizures (GTCS)** occur in nearly 10% of individuals with alcohol dependence. Usually, it manifests 12–48 hours after consumption of a large amount of alcohol. Recurrent seizures (2–6) may occur in a short span over a 24-hour period. Subsequently, patient may land up in a critical situation like **Status Epilepticus** which may succeed into **Delirium tremens** in nearly 30% of the patients.

2. Delirium Tremens

One of the presentations of severe alcohol withdrawal syndrome is delirium tremens. It is an acute organic brain syndrome. It comprises two components: Delirium and severe alcohol withdrawal. Usually, it occurs after 3–4 days of alcohol consumption. It is seen in around 5% of alcoholics. The severity of this entity is so high that if left untreated, mortality is around 10–20% of cases. Delirium tremens has a brief course and most of the patients recover within a week. Patient manifests as:

- Clouding of consciousness
- Disorientation to place and time
- Distractibility with poor attention span
- Hallucinations (auditory, visual and tactile)
- Illusions
- Autonomic disturbances—tachycardia, hypertension, pupillary dilatation, sweating and fever
- Dehydration

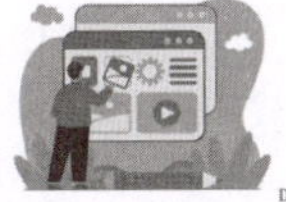
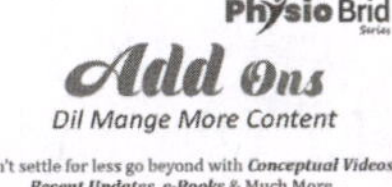

- Electrolyte imbalance
- Ataxia
- Psychomotor agitation
- Insomnia
- Reversal of sleep-wake pattern

Patient dies due to collapse of cardiovascular system, sepsis, hyperthermia or even self-inflicted injury. If the patient is having any underlying comorbid illnesses like fractures, tuberculosis, hepatic failure or renal failure, it complicates the scenario further with higher chances of having mortality.

3. Alcoholic Hallucinosis

Alcoholic hallucinosis is characterized by the presence of various hallucinations among which auditory hallucinations are the most common hallucinations. These hallucinations can be persecutory and are accompanied by fear. They may persist over a month and rarely >6 months. Usually, hallucinosis occurs when the person has clear consciousness and after the subsidence of withdrawal symptoms.

Chronic Alcohol Use

If a person consumes alcohol for a longer duration, it may lead to various complications which are listed here:

- Wernicke-Korsakoff syndrome
- Impaired memory
- Movement disorders
- Sexual dysfunction
- Alcohol related dementia
- Peripheral neuropathy
- Cerebellar degeneration

Wernicke-Korsakoff Syndrome

As the name depicts, this syndrome constitutes two components Wernicke's encephalopathy and Korsakoff's psychosis.

Wernicke's Encephalopathy (Table 12.6)

The cause for this acute manifestation is Thiamine deficiency. It is due to the hemorrhage and degeneration of the neurons seen in thalamic nuclei, hypothalamus, mammillary bodies and midbrain. Typically, the onset of encephalopathy is preceded by recurrent vomiting episodes.

Table 12.6: The important clinical signs of Wernicke's encephalopathy

Eye signs	Higher mental function disturbance	Others
• Coarse nystagmus • Ophthalmoplegia • Bilateral external rectus • Pupillary irregularities • Retinal hemorrhage • Papilledema	• Disorientation • Confusion • Recent memory disturbance • Poor attention span	• Apathy • Ataxia • Peripheral neuropathy • Serious malnutrition

Korsakoff 's Psychosis

If not treated, 80% patients with Wernicke's encephalopathy develop Korsakoff psychosis. It is chronic and irreversible.

Impaired Memory

Long-term alcohol use may result in impaired recall and the ability to form new long-term memories (anterograde amnesia).

Movement Disorders

Alcohol use alone or combined with hepatic encephalopathy can cause spectrum of movement disorders like tremor, asterixis, cerebellar dysfunction, withdrawal parkinsonism and dyskinesias.

Sexual Dysfunction

Long-term alcohol use results in problems in normal sexual functioning in the form of lack of sexual desire, premature ejaculation and erectile dysfunction. It is associated with the amount of alcohol consumed per day, severity of alcohol dependence and duration of alcohol dependence.

Alcohol Related Dementia

Alcohol use increases the risk of dementia, both directly and indirectly. It causes loss of neurons resulting in atrophy of the brain. Indirect mediation of dementia is due to liver and kidney disease, mood disorders, diabetes, arrhythmias, hypertension, heart diseases, head injuries and poisonings.

Peripheral Neuropathy

It leads to abnormalities in sensory, motor, autonomic and functions. The disease progresses gradually spanning weeks to months. It is a multifactorial process mediated by toxic effects of alcohol and modulated by genetic predisposition, malnutrition, thiamine deficiency and other systemic diseases.

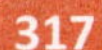

Cerebellar Degeneration

It affects up to 25% of persons with alcohol use and is the most common cause of acquired ataxia in adults. There is truncal ataxia with wide based gait, instability and variable degrees of lower limb dysmetria.

OPIOID USE DISORDERS

Opium is obtained from the unripened seeds of poppy plant. It is the prototype of opioid. An opioid is any drug that has similar action in the human body as that of opium. They are available as naturally occurring substances, semi-synthetic substances (by modifying natural substances), and pure synthetics. Different forms of opioids are given in Figure 12.3.

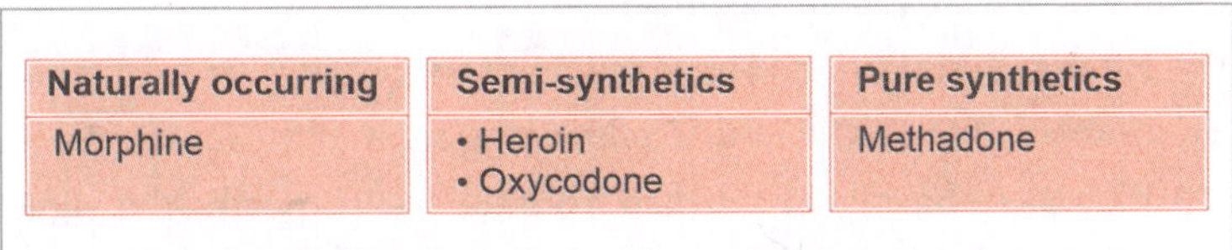

Naturally occurring	Semi-synthetics	Pure synthetics
Morphine	• Heroin • Oxycodone	Methadone

Fig. 12.3: Different forms of opioids

When someone is exposed to opioids for the first time, they may have an unpleasant feeling. But with continuous usage of morphine or heroin injection, one feels a short lived, intense experience— "rush" which remains for less than a minute. This rush state is described in literature as a state of profound happiness. Opioids are often used in history for their dramatic relief from pain, so after consuming opioid products, within minutes person gets pain relief due to inability to feel any pain. He goes in a dreamy state which is characterized by suppressed responses to the outside world.

Heroin which is popularly known to people as 'smack' or 'brown sugar', is one of the very common forms to be consumed. Different ways of consuming heroin are *via* smoking, chasing (inhaled) or injection (intramuscular or intravenous). Among these the most common mode in India is chasing. 'Chasing' is inhaling the vapors emanating from a heated metallic foil.[12]

Several other opioids which are available in the market for pain relief are also being abused. These are:

- Codeine cough syrups
- Morphine
- Buprenorphine tablets/injections
- Pentazocine injections
- Dextropropoxyphene capsules

Opioid Withdrawal Syndrome

Symptoms include:

- Nausea and vomiting
- Anxiety
- Muscle cramps
- Sweating
- Watery discharge from eyes and nose
- Diarrhea
- Yawning
- Feeling cold

To manage withdrawal syndrome, one should be given symptomatic treatment and supportive care in mild withdrawals. Otherwise, in cases of severe withdrawals, opioid substitutes can be prescribed. Opioid substitution therapy (OST) is available in the form of syrup methadone and sublingual preparation of buprenorphine.

CANNABIS USE DISORDERS

Cannabis is derived from the various parts of the plant *Cannabis sativa*, which grows wild all around the world including India.

Cannabis is available in various forms, viz.

- **Bhang:** Paste obtained by grinding of the leaves.
- **Ganja:** Obtained from dried flowering stem of the female plant.
- **Charas or hashish:** Extracted from the resin covering the plant.

Cannabis can be smoked in cigarettes, clay pipes or water pipes like the traditional hookah. In India, the most common method in religious settings and rural areas to consume cannabis is *via* clay pipes.[13] Though bhang consumption is legalized in India, consumption of charas and ganja is illegal.

If cannabis is consumed in low dose, it causes a state of wellbeing (high) and a dreamy, relaxation state. It also increases the appetite of a person. The state of enjoyment is usually followed by a period of drowsiness. Even a modest amount of cannabis intake can impair one's coordination which can be hazardous for heavy machine operators. Perceptual and sensory distortions, distortion of time sense occurs. If taken in higher doses, cannabis can lead to state of confusion and chances of developing cannabis psychosis.

SEDATIVES AND HYPNOTICS

Benzodiazepines are the most common sedative hypnotics used these days. They are commonly prescribed for sleep or to relieve anxiety and stress in addition to addiction management.[7] The commonly used and abused benzodiazepines are:

- Alprazolam
- Lorazepam
- Nitrazepam
- Diazepam
- Clonazepam
- Triazolam
- Chlordiazepoxide
- Oxazepam

These drugs are available in oral as well as injectable forms and are used in both forms by drug users.

ASSESSMENT OF SUBSTANCE USE DISORDERS

To know the severity and gravity of substance use in individuals, there are various screening tools which are discussed here. Before starting a proper and individualized treatment of substance use,

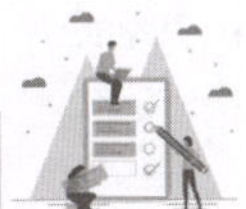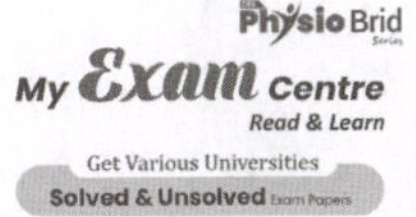

one should be aware of the comorbidities from which individual is suffering and certain facts related to substance use, which needs to get explored.

> **MUST KNOW**
> - Substance use pattern (type/quantity/frequency/current pattern/mode of use)
> - Factors associated with initiation/maintenance
> - Positive expectancy from the behavior
> - Reasons for abstinence/relapse
> - Current motivation
> - Factors that need immediate interventions

Assessment of Comorbidity:

- **Physical comorbidity:** Sexually transmitted diseases, chronic physical health issues, etc.
- **Psychiatric comorbidity:** Depression, bipolar disorder, psychosis, anxiety, attention deficit hyperactivity disorder, etc.

Screening

Usually, screening is carried out on a large group of individuals. It aids in pinpointing those individuals who have or are at risk of advancing to substance-related problems. There are numerous screening tests for analyzing the alcohol/substance consumption in individuals using a brief questionnaire or by an interview.

- **CAGE:** It is the acronym used for asking four questions. It is used in alcoholic patients.[14]

Acronym	Question
C	Have you ever felt you ought to cut down on your drinking?
A	Have people annoyed you by criticizing your drinking?
G	Have you ever felt guilty or bad about your drinking?
E	Have you ever had a drink first thing in the morning to steady your nerves or get rid of a hangover (eye-opener)?

- **MAST:** Michigan Alcoholism Screening Test
  It is a self-rated test for alcohol consumers consisting of 24 questions that are to be answered as YES or NO.[15]
- **TWEAK:** Tolerance, Worried, Eye-opener, Amnesia and K/Cut down
  It was a 5-item tool developed for pregnant women. But now it is used to identify alcohol use in general population too.[16]
- **AUDIT:** Alcohol Use Disorder Identification Test
  It is a 10-item tool developed by World Health Organization (WHO). It is available in both self-reported and clinician administered versions. Hazardous/harmful use is indicated by a score of 8 or more.[17]

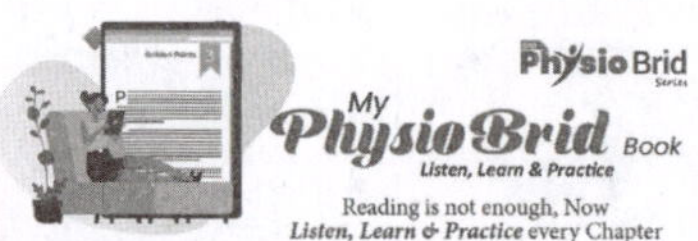

- **ASSIST:** Alcohol, Smoking and Substance Involvement Screening Test

    It is tool containing eight items, administered by healthcare professionals or can be self-rated.[18]

MANAGEMENT

Before starting the treatment, it is necessary to evaluate in which stage of motivation the individual is currently in. James Prochaska and Carlo DiClemente gave 'Stages of change model' (Trans theoretical model) which describes five stages of motivation to prevent substance use as shown in Figure 12.4. This "change" in change model is cyclical in nature and it can move bidirectionally, e.g., a person who is in contemplation stage can either succeed to the action stage or somebody who is in maintenance stage can slip back to the contemplation stage.[19]

The foremost role of the psychotherapist is to direct an individual such that he can comfortably move toward the higher stage of change.

1. **Precontemplation:** The person does not want to stop or reduce the substance.
2. **Contemplation:** There is an equivocal situation. The person wants to change but at the same time he might not know what steps to take.
3. **Preparation:** The individual has the intention of taking steps in the coming time and may start taking a few steps toward change.
4. **Action:** Active steps are being undertaken by the person to stop the use of substance.
5. **Maintenance:** Continuing the steps taken over longer periods of time.

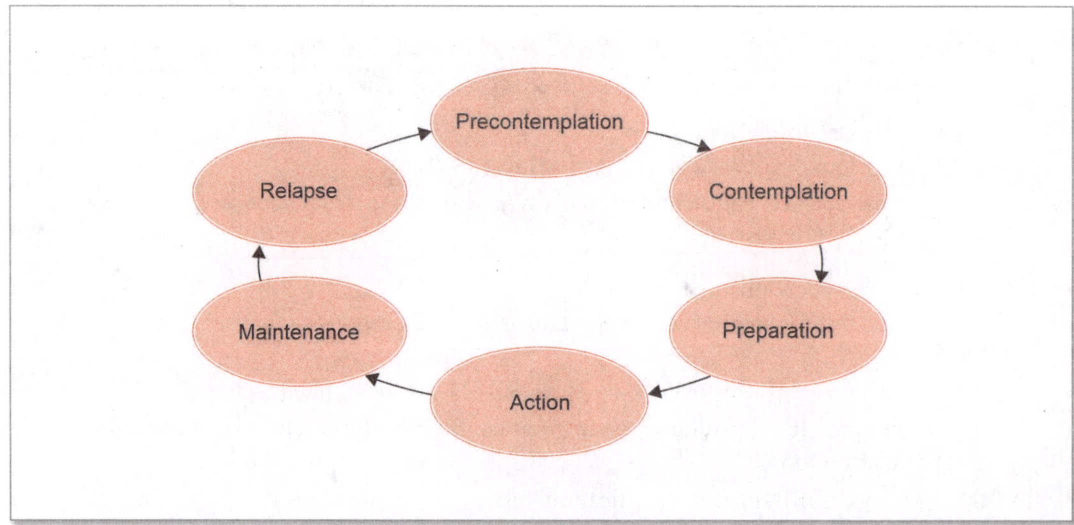

Fig. 12.4: Stages of motivation

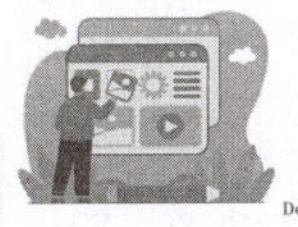

Treatment

Treatment goals not only differ for each individual but may change over the course of the treatment longitudinally. So, they need to be redefined at specific time intervals. Thus, individualizing the management and need-based plan is the key. Various treatment goals are:

- To abstain the substance
- To minimize the harm
- To improve health, occupation and social functions
- To improve quality of life.

Treatment for the substance use includes:

- Detoxification, medicines to prevent withdrawal symptoms and to maintain for longer-term (Medication maintenance)
- Psychosocial rehabilitation
- Socio-occupational rehabilitation.

Pharmacotherapy

- **Nicotine:**
  - **Nicotine replacement therapy:** It is available in the form of gum, lozenges, sublingual tablet, patch, mouth strips and topical patch.
  - **Tab. bupropion:** 150 mg once a day for one week then twice daily for next 6 weeks.
  - **Tab. varenicline:** 0.5 mg once a day for 3 days then twice daily.
- **Alcohol:**
  - **Detoxification-benzodiazepines:** First line treatment for Alcohol Withdrawal syndrome.
  - **Thiamine supplementation:** Intramuscular Thiamine 250 mg/day for 5 days followed by oral Thiamine 300–400 mg/day.
  - **Relapse prevention:**
    - **Acamprosate:** It has to be prescribed for 6 months.
    - **Disulfiram:** It inhibits the metabolism of alcohol in the liver. But accumulation of its toxic intermediate product acetaldehyde can cause alcohol-disulfiram reaction.
    - **Oral naltrexone:** To be started at 25 mg once daily and later increased to 50 mg after 3 days and then 100 mg after a week.
    - Baclofen.
- **Opioid use disorders:**
  - **Symptomatic treatment:** Nonsteroidal anti-inflammatory drugs (NSAIDs), medications for managing insomnia, anxiety, psychomotor agitation and autonomic arousal.

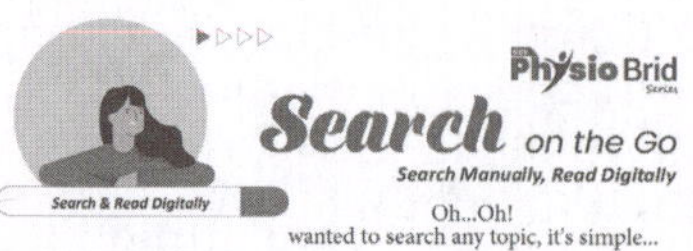

- **Agonist-assisted detoxification:** Methadone, a full opioid agonist drug and is available in liquid form. It is helpful in ensuring adherence to treatment.
- **Buprenorphine:** Partial Opioid agonist and is available in sublingual preparation. It is available either alone or in combination with Naloxone.
- **Long-term maintenance:** Can be done with agonist or antagonist (Naltrexone).

Since there is a considerable psychosocial component to the etiology of addictive illnesses, psychosocial techniques play a major role in management planning, contributing to treatment, prevention, long-term rehabilitation, and relapse prevention. Patients and their families frequently exhibit great resistance to treatment because of the many myths and misconceptions surrounding addiction diseases. Many times, the disease is thought of as a bad habit, meaning treatment is not necessary. Breaking down this barrier is crucial to including the patient and their family in their treatment.[20] Apart from medications there are many non-pharmacological psychosocial interventions which can be used as adjunct or individually.[21, 22] Some of the important psychosocial interventions are shown in Table 12.7.

Table 12.7: Important psychosocial interventions for substance use

Intervention	Basic approach	Population
Brief intervention	Feedback, responsibility Advice menu of options Empathy self-efficacy	Harmful users
Motivation Enhancement Therapy (MET)	Motivational interviewing	All type of substance users
Relapse Prevention Therapy (RPT)	Cognitive behavior approach	All substances, especially in maintenance program
Network therapy	Social networks/social support/peer support approach	Treatment nonseekers and enhancing compliance
Community reinforcement	Behavioral approach	Adolescent solvent users cannabis and cocaine users
Multi Systemic Therapy (MST)	Social cognitive approach	Adolescents (especially solvent) users
Matrix model	Combination of cognitive behavioral, empowerment education, social learning, social network approaches	Used in stimulant, alcohol and opiate users
Self-help approach	Social networks/social support	Alcohol and opiate users

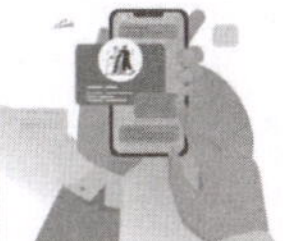
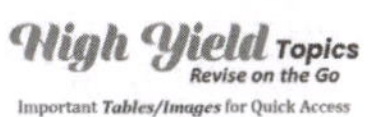

MUST KNOW

During management and rehabilitation of a patient, look out for signs of substance abuse:

- **Physical signs:** Unexplained injuries, frequent absences from treatment sessions, changes in appearance, and neglect of personal hygiene.
- **Behavioral signs:** Mood swings, irritability, poor concentration, and inconsistent attendance or performance in therapy.
- **Monitoring:** Be vigilant for signs of withdrawal, which can include anxiety, tremors, sweating, nausea, and seizures.
- **Supportive care:** Provide supportive care and refer patients to medical professionals for management of withdrawal symptoms, if necessary.

Physio CORNER

Individuals who need treatment for abstinence of various substances like nicotine, alcohol and illicit drugs, to which they are dependent, physiotherapy can act as 'adjunct' to the treatment. It aids in easing the anxiety, withdrawal symptoms and depressive symptoms during their course of treatment.

CASE STUDY

Multidisciplinary Approach for Substance Abuse Treatment

John Doe is a 32-year-old male who has been struggling with alcohol and opioid addiction for the past 10 years. He initially began drinking socially in college, but his consumption escalated following the death of his mother when he was 25. The use of opioids began after he was prescribed painkillers following a car accident at age 27.

Presenting Problem

John has been experiencing significant issues in his personal and professional life due to his substance use. He has been arrested twice for driving under the influence (DUI) and has been unable to maintain steady employment. John has recently been evicted from his apartment and is currently staying with a friend. He has sought help due to pressure from his family and after realizing he might lose the few remaining relationships he values.

Psychological Assessment

John underwent a comprehensive psychological assessment, including clinical interviews and standardized tests. Key findings include:

- **History of trauma:** The death of his mother was a significant trauma that he never fully processed. This event was a critical point in the escalation of his alcohol use.
- **Co-occurring disorders:** John was diagnosed with Major Depressive Disorder (MDD) and Generalized Anxiety Disorder (GAD). These conditions are likely to contribute to and exacerbate his substance use.
- **Family history:** There is a family history of addiction and mental illness, indicating a potential genetic predisposition to substance abuse.
- **Cognitive functioning:** Tests indicated impairments in executive functioning, particularly in decision-making and impulse control, which are common in long-term substance abuse.

Contd...

Treatment Plan

A multidisciplinary approach was recommended for John, involving the following components:

- **Detoxification:** Initially, John was admitted to a medically supervised detoxification program to safely manage withdrawal symptoms.
- **Psychotherapy:**
  - **Cognitive behavioral therapy (CBT):** To address the underlying thought patterns and behaviors associated with his substance use and co-occurring mental health disorders.
  - **Trauma-focused therapy:** To help John process the trauma of losing his mother and other significant life events.
  - **Motivational interviewing (MI):** To enhance John's motivation to change and adhere to the treatment plan.
- **Medication:**
  - **Antidepressants:** Prescribed to help manage symptoms of depression and anxiety.
  - **Medication-assisted treatment (MAT):** Such as naltrexone or buprenorphine, to reduce cravings and prevent relapse.
- **Support groups:**
  - **12-Step programs:** Such as Alcoholics Anonymous (AA) and Narcotics Anonymous (NA), to provide peer support and accountability.
  - **Family therapy:** To educate and involve John's family in his recovery process, promoting a supportive home environment.
- **Lifestyle changes:**
  - **Exercise and nutrition:** Incorporating a healthy lifestyle to improve physical well-being.
  - **Hobbies and interests:** Encouraging John to rediscover and engage in activities he once enjoyed, to provide healthy alternatives to substance use.

Progress and Prognosis

John's progress was closely monitored through regular follow-ups. After 6 months, he showed significant improvement:

- **Reduction in substance use:** John has remained abstinent from alcohol and opioids for four months.
- **Improvement in mental health:** Symptoms of depression and anxiety have decreased, and John reports feeling more hopeful about his future.
- **Social and occupational functioning:** John has re-established relationships with family members and has started part-time work.

Despite the positive progress, John is aware of the chronic nature of addiction and the potential for relapse. Ongoing support and a long-term commitment to his recovery plan are crucial.

This case study illustrates the complexity of substance abuse and the necessity for a comprehensive, individualized treatment plan addressing both the addiction and any co-occurring mental health issues.

SUMMARY

- This chapter delves into the intricate world of substance abuse, offering a comprehensive understanding of what constitutes substance use disorders, their prevalence, impact, and management strategies. It begins by laying the groundwork with definitions of key terms such as "psychoactive substances", "intoxication", "motivation", and "relapse" setting the stage for a detailed exploration of this complex issue.

Contd...

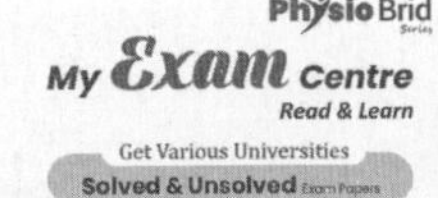

- **Historical and societal perspectives:** Substance use has been a part of human history, with ancient texts like the Vedas and the Bible mentioning the medicinal and recreational use of substances like opium and cannabis. However, the societal view of substance use has often been tinged with stigma, associating it with immorality and unprincipled behavior. The chapter highlights the evolution of terminology, moving away from stigmatizing labels like "drug addiction" to more neutral and scientifically accurate terms such as "substance dependence" and "substance use disorders".

- **Epidemiological insights:** The chapter presents data from a 2019 survey in India, revealing the extent of substance use among the population. Alcohol emerges as the most commonly consumed substance, with men showing a significantly higher consumption rate than women. The survey also sheds light on the use of cannabis products and opioids, underscoring the need for a nuanced understanding of substance use patterns.

- **Understanding psychoactive substances:** The chapter provides an extensive list of psychoactive substances, ranging from nicotine and alcohol to opioids, sedatives, hypnotics, cannabinoids, stimulants, hallucinogens, and inhalants. It discusses the various forms these substances take and the different ways they are consumed, illustrating the diversity of substance use.

- **Etiological factors:** Diving into the causes of substance use disorders, the chapter adopts a biopsychosocial model, examining the interplay of psychological, social, and biological factors. These factors, which include genetic predispositions, mental health issues, and environmental influences, are crucial in understanding the development and progression of substance use disorders.

- **Diagnostic criteria and consequences:** The chapter outlines the diagnostic criteria for substance use disorders as per the ICD-11 guidelines, providing a structured approach to identifying these conditions. It also discusses the wide-ranging consequences of substance use, including psychiatric illnesses, family dysfunction, financial strain, legal issues, and physical health complications.

- **Specific substance use disorders:** Detailed sections on tobacco, alcohol, and opioid use disorders follow, each providing an overview of the substance, its health consequences, withdrawal symptoms, and management strategies. The chapter highlights the importance of screening tools like the Fagerstrom Test for Nicotine Dependence and discusses the acute and chronic effects of alcohol, including withdrawal syndromes like delirium tremens.

- **Assessment and management:** The chapter emphasizes the importance of a thorough assessment of substance use disorders, considering not only the substance use pattern but also associated factors such as motivation, reasons for abstinence or relapse, and comorbidities. It introduces various screening tools and discusses the stages of change model, which helps in understanding an individual's readiness to change and guides the treatment approach.

- **Treatment strategies:** The management of substance use disorders is discussed in detail, with a focus on both pharmacological and psychosocial interventions. The chapter outlines specific medications used for detoxification and maintenance, as well as nonpharmacological interventions like cognitive-behavioral therapy, motivational interviewing, and support groups.

REFERENCES

1. Rudgley R. The Encyclopedia of Psychoactive Substances. New York: Macmillan Publishers, 2014.
2. Ambekar A, Agrawal A, Rao R, Mishra AK, Khandelwal SK, Chadda RK. Magnitude of Substance Use in India.2019. Ministry of Social Justice and Empowerment, Government of India.

Contd...

3. Rhodes T, Lillly R, Fernandez C, Giorgino V, Kemmesis, UE, Oseebaard HC et al. Risk Factors Associated with Drug Use: The importance of 'risk environment'. Drugs: Education Prevention and Policy.2003;10(4):303–29.

4. Stone AL, Becker LG, Huber AM, Catalano R. Review of risk and protective factors of substance use and problem use in emerging adulthood. Addict Behav.2012 Jul;37(7):747–75.

5. World Health Organization. The ICD-11 Classification of Mental and Behavioural Disorders: Clinical Descriptions and Diagnostic Guidelines. World Health Organization (WHO);2021.

6. Steinfeld MR, Torregrossa MM. Consequences of adolescent drug use. Transl Psychiatry.2023;13:313

7. Ambekar A, Lal R. Substance Use Disorders: A Manual for paramedical Personnel. National Drug Dependence Treatment Centre, AIIMS, New Delhi;Feb 2013.

8. Heatherton, Todd F, Kozlowski, Lynn T, Frecker, Richard C, et al. The Fagerstrom Test for Nicotine Dependence: A revision of the Fagerstrom Tolerance Questionnaire. British Journal of Addiction.1991; 86(9),1119–27.

9. Whitlock EP, Orleans CT, Pender N, Allan J. Evaluating primary care behavioral counseling interventions. An evidence-based approach. Am J Prev Med.2002;22(4):267–84.

10. Kranzler HR, Soyka M. Diagnosis and Pharmacotherapy of Alcohol Use Disorder: A Review. JAMA.2018;320(8):815–24.

11. Jesse S, Brathen G, Ferrara M, Kiendl M, BenMenachem E, Tanansescu R, et al. Alcohol withdrawal syndrome: Mechanisms, manifestations and management. Acta Neurol Scand.2017;135(1):4–16.

12. Rao R. The journey of opioid substitution therapy in India: Achievements and challenges. Indian J Psychiatry.2017;59(1):39–45.

13. Chopra IC ,Chopra RN. The Use of the Cannabis Drugs in India.United Nations Office on Drugs and Crime.1957;4–29.

14. Ewing JA. Detecting alcoholism: The CAGE questionnaire.JAMA.1984;252(14):1905–07.

15. Selzer M.L. The Michigan Alcoholism Screening Test. The quest for a new diagnostic instrument. Am J Psychiatry.1971; 127:1653–58.

16. Chan AW, Pristach EA, Welte JW, Russell M. Use of the TWEAK test in screening for alcoholism/ heavy drinking in three populations. Alcohol Clin Exp Res.1993;17(6):1188–92.

17. Saunders J B, Aasland OG, Babor TF, de la Fuente JR. and Grant M. Development of the Alcohol Use Disorders Identification Test (AUDIT): WHO collaborative project on early detection of persons with harmful alcohol consumption-II.Addiction.1993;88(6):791–804.

18. WHO Assist Working Group The Alcohol, Smoking and Substance Involvement Screening Test (ASSIST): development, reliability and feasibility. Addiction.2002;97(9):1183–94.

19. Prochaska JO, DiClemente CC. Stages and processes of self- change of smoking: Toward an integrative model of change. Journal of Consulting and Clinical Psychology.1983;51(3), 390.

20. Sofuoglu M, DeVito EE, Carroll KM.Pharmacological and Behavioral Treatment of Opioid Use Disorder. Psychiatr Res Clin Pract.2018;1(1):4–15.

21. Murthy P. Guidelines for psychosocial interventions in addictive disorders in India: An introduction and overview. Indian J Psychiatry.2018;60(4):S433–S439.

22. Matoo SK, Prasad S, Ghosh A. Brief intervention in substance use disorders. Indian J Psychiatry.2018; 60(4):466–472.

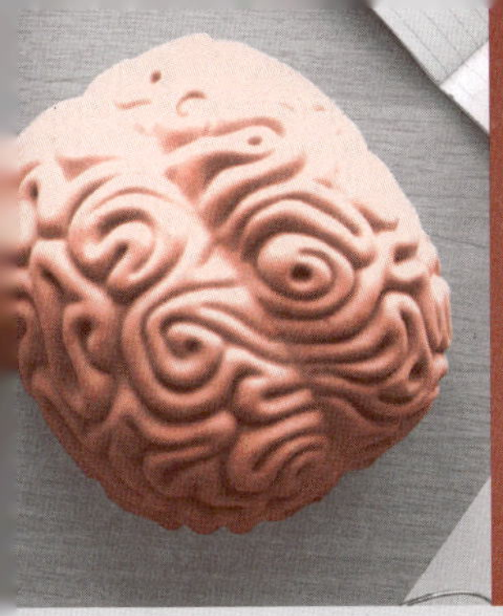

LONG ANSWER QUESTIONS

1. Explain the historical and societal perspectives on substance use, and how the terminology related to substance use disorders has evolved over time.
2. Discuss the various etiological factors that contribute to substance use disorders.
3. Explain how various factors interact to influence an individual's risk of developing a substance use disorder.
4. Outline the diagnostic criteria for substance use disorders as per the ICD-11 guidelines, and explain the importance of accurately diagnosing substance use disorders for effective treatment.
5. Describe the various treatment strategies for substance use disorders, including pharmacological, psychosocial, and nonpharmacological interventions.

SHORT ANSWER QUESTIONS

1. What is the diagnostic criteria for substance dependence?
2. Describe etiological factors for substance use disorders.
3. What are the complications of chronic alcohol use?
4. What are the symptoms of opioid withdrawal?
5. What are the psychosocial interventions for substance use disorders?

MULTIPLE CHOICE QUESTIONS

1. **What is the most commonly used substance among the Indian population according to the 2019 survey?**
   a. Cannabis
   b. Opioids
   c. Alcohol
   d. Nicotine
2. **Which of the following is NOT a psychological factor contributing to substance use disorders?**
   a. Genetic predispositions
   b. Mental health issues
   c. Cognitive impairments
   d. Social environment

3. **Which screening tool is specifically designed for use in pregnant women but is also used in the general population to identify alcohol use?**
    a. CAGE
    b. MAST
    c. TWEAK
    d. AUDIT

4. **What is the primary goal of motivational interviewing (MI) in the context of substance use disorders?**
    a. To provide immediate detoxification
    b. To enhance the individual's motivation to change and adhere to treatment
    c. To prescribe medication for withdrawal symptoms
    d. To impose strict behavioral rules

5. **Which of the following is a common symptom of opioid withdrawal syndrome?**
    a. Euphoria
    b. Muscle cramps
    c. Heightened sense of smell
    d. Visual hallucinations

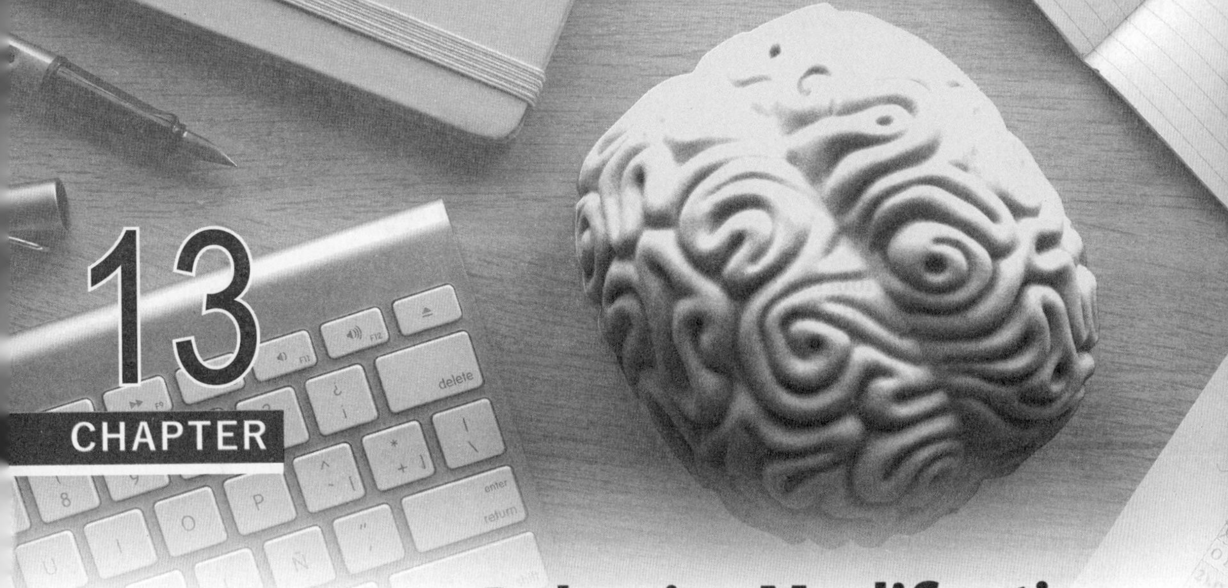

Behavior Modification

Pragya Mitra, Chandani Pandey

LEARNING OBJECTIVES

After the completion of the chapter, the readers will be able to:
- Define behavior and behavior modification as a systematic approach to changing behavior through reinforcement, punishment, shaping, and other techniques.
- Describe the fundamental principles of behavior modification and their applications in modifying patient behavior in physiotherapy settings.
- Analyze case studies and real-life examples illustrating the successful implementation of behavior modification techniques in physiotherapy practice.

CHAPTER OUTLINE

- Introduction
- Definition
- Common Labels for Behavior
- Behavior Modification
- Reinforcement and Punishment
- Other Behavioral Techniques
- Physiotherapy Application
- Recent Advancements

KEY TERMS

Backward chaining: It is a technique in which a task is broken down into steps and then taught in reverse order.

Behavioral assessment: Behavioral assessment is the process of gathering information about the frequency, duration, intensity, and antecedents/consequences of a target behavior. It is a crucial step in behavior modification, providing a foundation for designing effective intervention plans.

Behavioral contract: A behavioral contract is a written agreement between two parties outlining specific target behaviors and the consequences tied to their occurrence or nonoccurrence.

Behavioral modification: Behavioral modification is a systematic approach to changing behavior through the use of reinforcement, punishment, shaping, and other techniques. It is rooted in B F Skinner's work and aims to evaluate and enhance both overt and covert behaviors to improve daily functioning.

Chaining: It is a technique that involves breaking down a complex behavior into a sequence of smaller, manageable behaviors. Each behavior in the sequence serves as a cue for the next.

Covert behaviors: Internal activities that are not easily observable, such as thoughts or feelings.

Forward chaining: Teaching each step in the sequence from the beginning to the end is referred to as forward chaining.

Gestural prompts: Using physical gestures to guide the correct behavior.

Negative punishment: Removing a positive stimulus after a behavior to decrease its likelihood. For example, taking away a child's toy for not sharing.

Negative reinforcement: Removing an aversive stimulus after a behavior to increase its likelihood. For example, a student studying to avoid a test.

Overt behaviors: Physical actions that are observable by others, such as walking, speaking or throwing a ball.

Physical prompts: Providing physical assistance to help perform the correct behavior.

Positive punishment: Adding an aversive stimulus after a behavior to decrease its likelihood. For example, scolding a child for misbehaving.

Positive reinforcement: Adding a reward or positive stimulus after a behavior to increase its likelihood. For example, giving a child a sticker for completing homework.

Prompts and prompt fading: Prompts are tools that increase the likelihood of a correct behavior by providing cues or assistance. Prompt fading involves gradually reducing the use of prompts to transfer control to the individual.

Punishment: It involves consequences that decrease the likelihood of a behavior recurring. Like reinforcement, it also has two main types: positive and negative punishment.

Reinforcement: It involves consequences that increase the likelihood of a behavior recurring. It is a fundamental concept in behavior modification, with two main types: positive and negative reinforcement.

Shaping: Shaping is a technique used to develop a desired behavior by reinforcing successive approximations of that behavior. It involves reinforcing behaviors that gradually become closer to the target behavior.

Token economy: A token economy is a system where individuals earn tokens for exhibiting desired behaviors. These tokens can later be exchanged for rewards or privileges.

Verbal prompts: Using spoken words to guide the correct response.

INTRODUCTION

Behavior encompasses a wide spectrum of actions and reactions that shape both society's notable achievements, such as democratic governance, philanthropy, art, and scientific progress, and its pressing challenges like unhealthy lifestyles, environmental issues, racism, and terrorism. This includes the behavior of individuals in various contexts, such as a group of nursery school children playing where one child with autism prefers solitude or a nervous gymnast waiting for her turn at a championship. These scenarios highlight the complexity and diversity of human behavior, which behavior modification specialists address in their training to tackle various behavioral issues.[1,2]

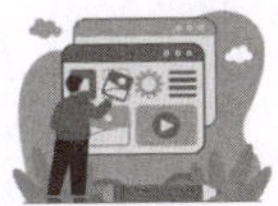

To understand such behaviors and address behavioral issues, it is necessary to understand what is behavior?

DEFINITION

Behavior refers to any physical or physiological activity of an organism, including actions, like walking, speaking aloud or throwing a ball, which are overt and observable by others. In contrast, covert behaviors are private or internal activities that cannot be easily observed by external individuals. It is important to note that in behavior, modification does not apply to the covert behaviors or those behaviors which are done in private.[1]

COMMON LABELS FOR BEHAVIOR

Summary labels are common labels used for psychological issues encompass autism spectrum disorder (ASD), attention-deficit/hyperactivity disorder (ADHD), anxiety, depression, low self-esteem, road rage, interpersonal difficulties, and sexual dysfunction. These labels offer the benefit of providing quick insights into an individual's potential performance and suggesting suitable treatment approaches. However, they can also lead to oversimplified explanations of behavior and influence negative treatment perceptions by emphasizing problem behaviors over strengths. It is crucial to recognize behaviors as either deficits (insufficient behavior of a certain type) or excesses (excessive behavior of a certain type) and instead of relying solely on labels, focusing on behavior management is essential. Techniques like behavior modification, applicable in educational, professional, and domestic settings, offer specific strategies to address behavioral concerns effectively.[1]

BEHAVIOR MODIFICATION

Behavior modification is rooted in B F Skinner's work, utilizes systematic principles of learning and techniques within the realm of behavior therapy. Its purpose is to evaluate and enhance both overt and covert behaviors to improve daily functioning. This therapeutic approach is predominantly employed to mitigate or eradicate maladaptive behaviors in individuals, especially in children or adults, with a focus on altering specific behaviors rather than addressing thoughts or emotions. The intervention's progress and effectiveness are quantifiable and assessable.[1, 2]

Behavior modification encompasses seven key characteristics:

1. It involves the measurement of behaviors in some ways.

2. Its treatment strategies and techniques focus on modifying an individual's current environment to facilitate improved functioning.

3. It relies on precise descriptions of its methods and rationales.

> **MUST KNOW**
>
> Behavior modification, evaluate and enhance both overt and covert behaviors to improve daily functioning. Modify maladaptive behavior patterns by reinforcing more adaptive behavior.

4. It commonly utilized by individuals in their daily lives.

5. It is rooted in both basic and applied research within the broader science of learning, particularly drawing from operant and Pavlovian conditioning principles.

6. It emphasizes the importance of scientifically demonstrating that a specific intervention or treatment has led to a discernible change in behavior.

7. It also places a significant emphasis on accountability among all parties involved in behavior modification programs.

Indications

Behavior modification plans are developed for various reasons, including addressing unwanted, maladaptive or aberrant behaviors, as well as teaching and reinforcing new, desired behaviors. In child psychiatry, these plans are integral to treatment for conditions, like attention-deficit hyperactivity disorder (ADHD), oppositional defiant disorder, conduct disorder, intermittent explosive disorder, and other externalizing disorders. Additionally, behavior modification plays a crucial role in Parent-Child Interaction Therapy (PCIT), where parents learn specific skills to enhance their interactions with their children both physically and verbally.[2]

Moreover, behavior modification extends beyond children and is widely applicable in treating mental illnesses in adults, such as anxiety, depression, eating disorders, and obsessive-compulsive disorder, among others.

Contraindication

Starting a behavior management plan should only happen if it can be consistently and sustainably implemented. It is normal to encounter mistakes and setbacks when aiming for behavior change, underscoring the need for caregivers and clinicians to maintain patience and consistency. Partially enforcing a behavior plan is also not recommended as it can actually worsen the targeted behavior.

Assessment

Behavior assessment is a fundamental component of behavior modification, serving as the foundation for identifying target behaviors and designing effective intervention plans.[3] In behavior modification, assessment methods such as direct observation, self-report measures, and functional analysis are commonly employed to gather information about the frequency, duration, intensity, and antecedents/consequences of the target behavior.[4]

The assessment process begins with defining the target behavior clearly and operationally, ensuring that it is observable, measurable, and specific.

- **Direct observation** methods involve systematic recording of the target behavior in its natural environment, providing valuable data for understanding its patterns and triggers.[5]

- **Self-report measures**, including questionnaires and rating scales, allow individuals to report their own behavior and experiences, offering insights into subjective aspects of behavior.[6]
- **Functional analysis**, a more complex assessment approach, involves experimental manipulation of environmental variables to identify functional relationships between antecedents, behaviors, and consequences.[7] This method is particularly useful in understanding the underlying causes and maintaining factors of challenging behaviors (Table 13.1).

Table 13.1: Examples of behavior and its consequences

Situation	Response	Consequences	Impact
Aryan had to complete his classwork.	Aryan quietly doing his classwork in the classroom.	His teacher comes and gives him chocolate for being quiet and sincere.	Later, Aryan will be more likely to complete his classwork quietly.
Mother was shopping with her baby.	Child quietly follows mother and does not show any tantrum.	Mother bought a car for the child since he showed no tantrum.	In future, child is more likely to be quiet and calm while shopping.

REINFORCEMENT AND PUNISHMENT

Skinner observed that **reinforcement** and **punishment** provide insights into how behaviors are influenced by consequences. **Reinforcers** are consequences that increase the likelihood of behavior recurring, while **punishment** decreases this likelihood. The terms "positive" and "negative" refer to whether something is added or removed.

Increasing a Behavior with Reinforcement

A positive reinforcer is something that, when given immediately after a behavior, increases the likelihood of that behavior occurring again. It is similar to a reward. **Positive reinforcement** occurs when a behavior is strengthened by the addition of a reward. For example, if a child receives a chocolate for completing the homework, the chocolate acts as a positive reinforcer because it is added when the desired behavior (completing the homework) occurs. This positive consequence makes the behavior more likely to happen again in the future. By utilizing these principles effectively, individuals can promote positive behaviors and discourage undesirable ones, contributing to behavioral change and personal growth.[1, 2, 8]

On the other hand, **negative reinforcement** involves the removal of a stimulus as a consequence, resulting in a positive outcome for the individual. An example of negative reinforcement is when a fine is waived, leading to the person avoiding jail time. Here, the removal of the negative stimulus (the fine) reinforces the desired behavior (compliance with rules or laws), making it more likely for the person to continue following those rules in the future. Positive reinforcement and negative reinforcement both play significant roles in learning and behavior modification.

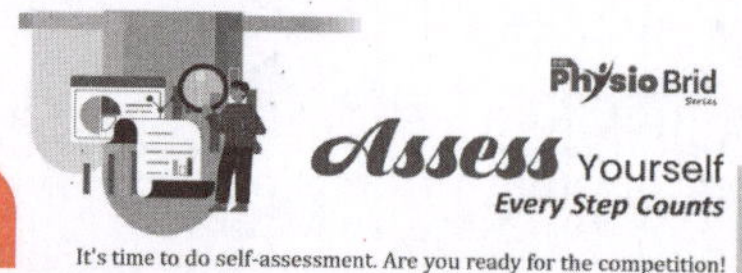

> **MUST KNOW**
>
> | | |
> |---|---|
> | **Positive reinforcement** includes situations where a behavior leads to a positive outcome (positive reinforcer) to strengthen the behavior | **Negative reinforcement** is, where a behavior leads to avoiding or stopping a negative outcome (aversive stimulus) to strengthen the behavior |

Schedules of Reinforcement

Different schedules of reinforcement can significantly impact behavior. Initially, when setting up a behavior plan, **continuous reinforcement** is often used to establish and reinforce the desired behavior consistently. As the behavior is established, continuous reinforcement can be transitioned to intermittent reinforcement, a process known as **thinning**.

There are four types of intermittent reinforcement: (1) Fixed interval, (2) Variable interval, (3) Fixed ratio and (4) Variable ratio (Table 13.2).

Table 13.2: Schedules of reinforcement

Fixed interval	Reinforcement occurs after a set number of responses. For instance, rewarding a person at the end of each day for completing the given tasks.
Variable interval	Reinforcement happens after a variable number of responses. For example, rewarding a person sometimes at the end of the day, sometimes at the end of the week or intermittently every few days.
Fixed ratio	Reinforcement is given after a certain number of responses, such as rewarding a person after completing the desired behavior a specific number of times.
Variable ratio	Reinforcement occurs after a variable number of responses, like rewarding a person after completing the desired behavior three times, then six times, then two times.

Among these schedules, variable ratio intermittent reinforcement is considered the most effective for reinforcing behavior.

Social reinforcement occurs when another person's actions produce a reinforcing consequence, like asking someone to bring you a pencil box (positive reinforcement) or asking someone to turn off a fan (negative reinforcement) while **automatic reinforcement** happens when the environment directly reinforces a behavior, such as buying something for yourself (positive reinforcement) or turning off a fan when its cold (negative reinforcement).[8]

The **Premack principle** (*David Premack* 1965) involves using a preferred activity as a reward for completing a less-preferred task, like finishing homework before getting to play, which strengthens the behavior of doing homework. Another example is when a teacher requires the student to complete his classwork before he can go for lunch. This opportunity to do lunch (a high-probability behavior) after the completion of the classwork (low probability behavior) reinforces the behavior of completing classwork.[1, 8]

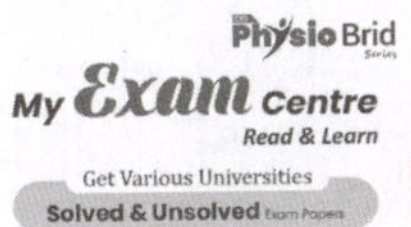

In essence, positive reinforcement involves rewarding behaviors to increase their likelihood, whether through social interactions or direct environmental consequences.

CASE STUDY

Use of Positive Reinforcement to Improve Patient Compliance

Mrs AS, a 75-year-old woman recovering from hip replacement surgery and needing physiotherapy to regain her ability to walk independently. Initially, she showed resistance to physiotherapy, specifically to walking between parallel bars with arm support. To address this, O'Neill and Gardner (1983) employed shaping techniques.

They set the initial behavior as Mrs AS going to the physiotherapy room where the bars were located. Upon her arrival in the room in a wheelchair, the therapist warmly interacted with her and provided a massage, reinforcing Mrs AS's presence in the physiotherapy room. This positive reinforcement led Mrs AS to willingly visit the physiotherapy room daily. As part of the shaping process, the therapist gradually increased expectations. Initially, Mrs AS was asked to stand between the bars for just 1 second before receiving her massage. With each successful attempt, the duration of standing was increased, reaching 15 seconds the following day. This incremental increase in the target behavior was a step-by-step process, resembling walking independently with the walker.

Once Mrs AS could stand between the bars comfortably, the therapist progressed to asking her to take a few steps initially, gradually increasing the distance until she could walk the full length of the bars independently. Ultimately, Mrs AS achieved her goal of walking independently with her walker, leading to her discharge from the hospital.

Extinction

Extinction refers to a process where a behavior, previously reinforced over time, ceases to occur because it no longer results in the expected rewards or reinforcing consequences. This lack of reinforcement leads to the gradual fading and eventual disappearance of the behavior. Skinner's experiments in 1938 with laboratory animals, such as pigeons and rats, vividly demonstrated this principle. When pigeons were no longer rewarded with food for pecking a key, their key-pecking behavior gradually diminished and eventually stopped altogether. Similarly, when laboratory rats were no longer given food pellets as a reward for pressing a lever, their lever-pressing behavior decreased over time until it ceased completely.

Extinction is a fundamental concept in behavioral psychology, highlighting how behaviors are influenced by their consequences. When the expected rewards or reinforcements are no longer present, the motivation to engage in that behavior diminishes, leading to its extinction or extinguishment. This process underscores the dynamic nature of behavior and the critical role of reinforcement in shaping and maintaining behaviors over time.

Extinction burst: During the extinction process, a notable phenomenon called an **extinction burst** often occurs. This burst refers to a temporary increase in the frequency, duration or intensity of a behavior that is no longer reinforced. For example, if Shalini tries to turn on her AC with a remote control that has dead batteries, she may push the button longer (increased duration) and harder (increased intensity) before realizing it will not work and giving up.

The extinction burst is a natural aspect of the extinction process. It is like a last effort by the individual to obtain the expected reinforcement before accepting that the behavior no longer leads to it. Another characteristic of an extinction burst is the emergence of **novel behaviors**, which are behaviors that are not typically seen in that situation. These new behaviors might only occur briefly during the extinction burst.

Additionally, during an extinction burst, individuals may exhibit **emotional responses** as part of their reaction to the lack of reinforcement. These emotions could range from frustration or anger to confusion or surprise. Overall, the extinction burst is a temporary but significant aspect of the extinction process, highlighting the dynamic nature of behavior change when reinforcement patterns shift.

When Ira's parents stopped responding to her crying at night, she initially cried longer and louder in what's known as an extinction burst. Along with this, she also displayed novel behaviors like screaming and hitting her stuffed toys and dolls.

Another aspect of extinction is **spontaneous recovery**, where a behavior that has not been observed for some time suddenly reoccurs. This natural phenomenon involves the behavior resurfacing in situations similar to those where it occurred before extinction. If extinction measures are still in place during spontaneous recovery, meaning there is no reinforcement for the behavior, it typically does not persist for long. However, if the behavior is reinforced during spontaneous recovery, the impact of extinction is negated.

Decreasing Behavior by Using Punishment

Punishment involves a behavior being followed by an immediate consequence, resulting in a reduced likelihood of that behavior occurring again in the future. This consequence, known as a punisher or aversive stimulus, weakens the behavior it follows.[1, 8]

Sumit used to tease his sister about her drawings, which initially amused his friends. However, over time, his sister became upset with his jokes. Whenever Sumit teased her about her drawings, she would yell at him. Consequently, Sumit stopped teasing his sister about her drawings.

Behavioral consequences can influence the likelihood of future behavior occurrence. Positive punishment involves an aversive stimulus following a behavior, reducing the chances of that behavior happening again. Negative punishment involves the removal of a rewarding stimulus after a behavior, leading to a decrease in the likelihood of that behavior recurring.

Two methods of negative punishment are **time-out** from positive reinforcement and **response cost.** Both entail removing a reinforcing stimulus or activity following problem behavior.

Time-out is when someone loses access to positive reinforcers for a short period due to problem behavior, resulting in a reduced likelihood of that behavior in the future. There are two types: **exclusionary time-out**, where the person is removed from the environment where the behavior occurred, and **nonexclusionary time-out**, where access to positive reinforcers is restricted while remaining in the same environment.

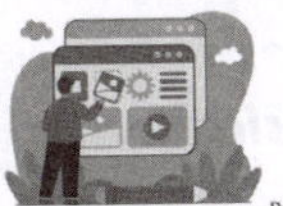

Response cost involves removing a reinforcer when problem behavior occurs, leading to a decrease in the likelihood of that behavior in the future. It is commonly used by institutions like governments and law enforcement as a form of negative punishment. For example, receiving a fine for illegal parking or speeding acts as response cost to discourage those behaviors.[8]

Issues with Punishment

There are several issues regarding the use of punishment, particularly positive punishment involving aversive stimuli. Punishment may lead to increased aggression or emotional reactions. It can also result in escape or avoidance behaviors. Ethical and acceptability issues are also associated with punishment. Additionally, its use can serve as a model for others, potentially leading to increased use of punishment by observers. People who frequently observe punishment may adopt this approach themselves, especially children who learn behavior through observation.

OTHER BEHAVIORAL TECHNIQUES

Shaping

Shaping is a technique used to encourage the development of a desired behavior that a person currently does not display. It involves reinforcing steps that progressively resemble the target behavior until the person achieves the desired behavior.

In shaping, differential reinforcement focuses on reinforcing specific behaviors while ignoring others in a given context. This reinforcement strengthens the desired behavior while other behaviors decrease due to lack of reinforcement, eventually becoming extinct. When applied to language development, shaping involves successive steps like babbling, word sounds, partial words, complete words, phrases, and sentences.

Steps to use shaping:

1. Define the target behavior clearly.
2. Assess if shaping is the appropriate method; if the person already performs the target behavior occasionally, shaping may not be necessary.
3. Identify the starting behavior, which should be something the person already does, even if infrequently.
4. Select shaping steps that gradually progress toward the target behavior, with each step being closer to the target than the previous one.
5. Choose a reinforcer to reward each step of progress in the shaping process.
6. Progress through the shaping steps systematically, ensuring mastery of each step before moving to the next one.[8]

> **MUST KNOW**
>
> Shaping entails reinforcing successive approximations of a desired behavior until the individual demonstrates the complete desired behavior.

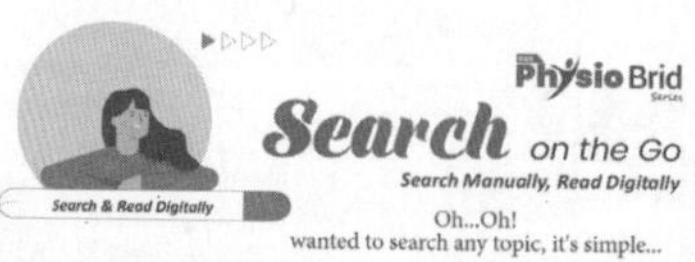

Physio CORNER

Maladaptive Syndrome refers to a collection of behaviors, thoughts, and emotional responses that are counterproductive or harmful to an individual's well-being and ability to function in daily life. These patterns are considered maladaptive because they do not effectively meet the demands of the environment or situation, often leading to distress, dysfunction or worsening of the problem.

Key Concepts of Maladaptive Syndrome

- **Maladaptive behaviors:** These are actions or habits that inhibit a person's ability to adjust to situations, solve problems or achieve goals. Examples include:
  - **Avoidance behaviors:** Avoiding situations that cause anxiety, which can lead to increased fear and withdrawal.
  - **Compulsive behaviors:** Repetitive actions that are performed to reduce anxiety but often reinforce the problem (e.g., compulsive hand-washing in OCD).
  - **Substance abuse:** Using drugs or alcohol to cope with stress, leading to addiction and further life problems.
- **Maladaptive thoughts:** These are irrational or distorted thought patterns that contribute to negative emotions and behaviors. Examples include:
  - **Catastrophizing:** Assuming the worst possible outcome in any situation.
  - **All-or-nothing thinking:** Seeing situations in black-and-white terms, with no middle ground.
  - **Overgeneralization:** Drawing broad, negative conclusions from a single event or experience.
- **Maladaptive emotional responses:** These include emotional reactions that are disproportionate or inappropriate to the situation. Examples include:
  - **Chronic anger:** Persistent anger that is not related to the current situation and leads to interpersonal conflicts.
  - **Excessive fear or anxiety:** Intense emotional responses to situations that are not inherently threatening, leading to avoidance and reduced functioning.

Examples of Maladaptive Syndromes

- **Anxiety disorders:**
  - **Generalized Anxiety Disorder (GAD):** Characterized by chronic, excessive worry about various aspects of life. The worry is often disproportionate to the actual threat, leading to avoidance behaviors and significant distress.
  - **Social Anxiety Disorder:** Involves an intense fear of social situations, leading to avoidance of social interactions, which can result in isolation and impairment in functioning.
- **Obsessive-Compulsive Disorder (OCD):** Individuals with OCD engage in compulsive behaviors (e.g., checking, cleaning) to reduce anxiety caused by intrusive, distressing thoughts (obsessions). These behaviors are maladaptive because they reinforce the anxiety and disrupt daily life.
- **Post-Traumatic Stress Disorder (PTSD):** Following a traumatic event, individuals may develop maladaptive responses such as hypervigilance, avoidance of reminders of the trauma, and emotional numbing, which interfere with their ability to recover and function normally.
- **Depression:** Depression is often characterized by maladaptive thought patterns such as hopelessness, worthlessness, and negative self-evaluation. These thoughts can lead to behaviors like withdrawal from activities, which further exacerbate the depressive symptoms.

Contd...

- **Personality Disorders:** Certain personality disorders involve pervasive maladaptive patterns of thinking, feeling, and behaving. For example:
  - **Borderline personality disorder:** Involves intense, unstable emotions and relationships, impulsive behavior, and an unstable sense of self.
  - **Narcissistic personality disorder:** Characterized by grandiosity, a need for admiration, and a lack of empathy, leading to difficulties in relationships and functioning.

Importance for Healthcare Professionals

For physiotherapists and other healthcare professionals, understanding maladaptive syndromes is essential in order to:

- Recognize when a patient's behavior may be interfering with treatment or recovery.
- Identify when a referral to a mental health professional is necessary.
- Provide a more holistic approach to care that addresses both physical and psychological factors.

Prompts and Prompts Fading

Prompts are tools that boost the chances of someone performing the right behavior at the right time. They are especially helpful during training to ensure correct behavior in specific situations. Prompting involves giving cues before or during the behavior to make it happen. This method improves teaching efficiency.[8]

There are different types of prompts used in behavior modification, including response prompts and stimulus prompts.

Response prompt refers to actions or cues from another person that encourage the desired response.

- **Verbal prompts:** These occur when someone's spoken words lead to the correct response. For example, when teaching Arjun to read, his mother showed him a flashcard with the word "CAT" and said the word aloud, prompting Arjun to respond correctly.
- **Gestural prompts:** These involve physical gestures that guide the correct behavior. If the person demonstrates the entire behavior, it is called a modeling prompt.
- **Physical prompts:** In this type, physical assistance is provided to help someone perform the correct behavior. For instance, a teacher may guide a student's hand to write the letter "B."

All these response prompts involve one person influencing another's behavior and are considered intrusive as they involve exerting control. It is important to use the least intrusive prompt first and only move to more intrusive ones if necessary to elicit the desired behavior.

On the other hand, a **stimulus prompt** alters or adds/removes a stimulus to make the correct response more likely.

Prompt fading is a widely used technique to shift control from a response prompt to the natural stimulus. This involves gradually reducing the use of a response prompt over multiple learning attempts until it is no longer needed.

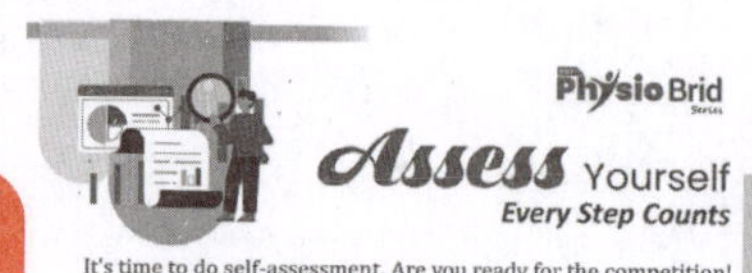

Another method, **prompt delay**, is also used for transferring stimulus control. In this, there is a delay in providing the prompt to encourage the person to respond to the natural stimulus.

When stimulus prompts are employed to elicit the correct response, changes are made to the stimulus or its environment to aid in correct discrimination. Eventually, these stimulus prompts must be phased out through stimulus fading to allow the natural stimulus to take control.

Steps to Use Prompting

If the individual has not acquired the behavior or has not learned to perform it in the right circumstances, the suitable approach involves prompting and transitioning stimulus control. Conversely, if the individual previously demonstrated the correct behavior in the right situation but now chooses not to do so, the issue is noncompliance, and prompting and transferring stimulus control would not be the most suitable method.

1. **Assess the situation:** Determine if prompting is needed based on the learner's behavior.
2. **Choose the appropriate prompting strategy:** Select the type of prompt that suits the learner and the task.
3. **Ensure attention:** Make sure the learner is focused and free from distractions.
4. **Introduce the stimulus:** Present the stimulus that should elicit the correct response.
5. **Provide prompts:** If needed, give prompts to guide the learner toward the correct response.
6. **Reinforce correct behavior:** Reward the learner immediately when they perform the correct behavior.
7. **Transfer control:** Gradually phase out prompts to shift control to the natural stimulus.
8. **Maintain reinforcement:** Continue to reinforce correct behavior even after prompts are removed.

Chaining

A behavioral chain refers to a complex behavior made up of multiple component behaviors that occur sequentially. Each chain comprises individual stimulus-response components that happen in a specific order, often referred to as a stimulus-response chain. For instance, to teach Mohan how to wear a shirt, his mother guides him through a sequence: Holding the shirt collar with his left hand, inserting his right hand into the right sleeve, adjusting the collar from the back to the left side with his left hand, holding the collar with his right hand, inserting his left hand into the left sleeve, and finally, folding the collar.[1, 8]

Task analysis involves breaking down a behavioral chain into its individual stimulus-response components. This process is essential when teaching complex tasks with multiple steps. The first step in task analysis is identifying and listing all the behaviors required to complete the task in the correct sequence.

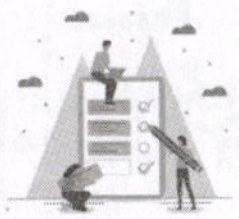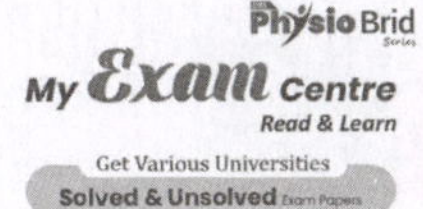

There are several methods to conduct a task analysis such as by observing someone performing the task and noting each stimulus-response component, consulting an expert who can explain all the task components. Alternatively, one can perform the task himself and record the sequence of responses.

Forward chaining teaches one component at a time and gradually chains them together. Training begins with the first component and progresses step by step, moving from the front to the end of the chain.

Backward chaining is similar to backward chaining as it an intensive training method primarily used for learners with limited abilities. It starts by teaching the last behavior in the chain first, using prompts and fading techniques.

Steps for Using Chaining

1. **Assess if chaining is suitable:** Determine if the person's inability to complete a complex task warrants a chaining approach.
2. **Create a task analysis:** Break down the task into its individual stimulus-response components.
3. **Evaluate the learner's current abilities:** Understand the learner's baseline skills related to the task.
4. **Select a chaining method:** Choose between forward or backward chaining based on the learner's abilities and the complexity of the task.
5. **Implement the chaining procedure:** Use prompting and fading techniques appropriately throughout the training.
6. **Maintain reinforcement:** Continue to provide reinforcement, even intermittently, after the learner can perform the task independently to ensure long-term retention of the behavior.

Token Economy

Token economy is a system where children receive token rewards for displaying appropriate or desired behaviors. Its aim is to reinforce positive behaviors that are uncommon and reduce negative behaviors in a structured setting. Tokens, earned for desirable actions, are exchanged later for backup reinforcers.

Steps Involved in Implementing a Token Economy

1. **Defining target behaviors:** The initial step is to clearly outline and define the positive behaviors that the token economy aims to reinforce in clients. This involves identifying specific actions or behaviors that are desirable and should be encouraged within the program.
2. **Selecting tokens:** Tokens are tangible items or symbols used as immediate rewards for demonstrating target behaviors. It is crucial to choose tokens that are practical, easy for the

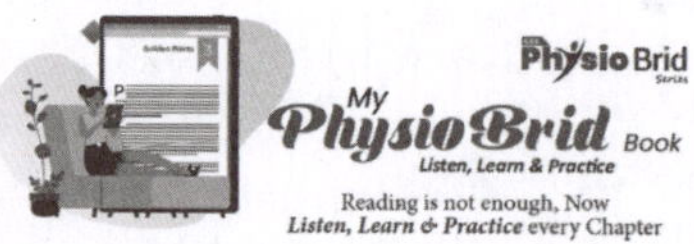

change agent to distribute, and readily available within the treatment environment whenever the desired behaviors occur.

3. **Identifying backup reinforcers:** Tokens gain their value as conditioned reinforcers through association with backup reinforcers,

> **MUST KNOW**
>
> Token economy is a behavior management system where tokens are given for desired behaviors, exchanged later for rewards, aiming to reinforce positive actions.

which are the actual rewards clients can obtain by exchanging their earned tokens. The effectiveness of the token economy hinges on the attractiveness and relevance of these backup reinforcers to the clients.

4. **Setting token exchange rates:** Each backup reinforcer in the system is assigned a specific price or exchange rate in tokens. Smaller or less valuable items require fewer tokens for exchange, while larger or more desirable items necessitate more tokens. This rate determines how tokens are exchanged for backup reinforcers.

5. **Considering response cost:** Response cost is an optional component in token economies, evaluated based on the presence of competing problem behaviors. If undesirable actions hinder desired behaviors, a response cost system may be included, deducting tokens or imposing penalties to deter these unwanted behaviors and reinforce the importance of positive actions.[8]

Behavioral Contract

A behavioral contract, also known as a contingency or performance contract, is a written agreement between two parties outlining specific target behaviors and the consequences tied to their occurrence or nonoccurrence. It is an intervention method where a client commits to behavioral changes within a set timeframe, often with stated rewards for meeting the agreed-upon goals.[8,9]

A behavioral contract comprises five crucial elements:

1. **Defining target behaviors:** The initial step involves clearly stating the specific behaviors that are the focus of the contract. These behaviors must be described objectively to ensure clarity and understanding.

> **MUST KNOW**
>
> A behavioral contract is a written agreement specifying target behaviors and consequences, facilitating behavioral changes within a timeframe, often with defined rewards.

2. **Measurement of target behaviors:** The contract must outline how the target behaviors will be measured. This is vital for the contract manager or participants to have verifiable evidence of whether the behaviors occurred as agreed upon.

3. **Timeframe for behavior performance:** Each contract should include a timeframe specifying when the behaviors must be performed or refrained from. This timeline is essential for implementing contingencies effectively.

4. **Reinforcement or punishment contingencies:** The contract manager determines the reinforcement (positive or negative) or punishment (positive or negative) contingencies that

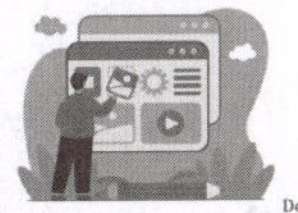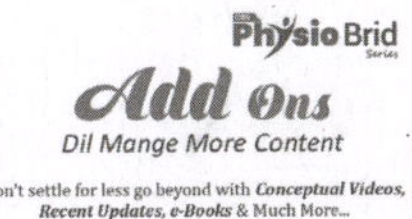

will be applied based on the performance of the target behaviors. These contingencies are clearly stated in the contract.

5. **Responsibility for contingency implementation:** The contract assigns roles to both parties involved. One party commits to the specified behaviors, while the other party is responsible for implementing the agreed-upon reinforcement or punishment contingencies.[8]

PHYSIOTHERAPY APPLICATION

Attention, rest and feedback of progress are the three main reinforcers operating in a rehabilitation setting that can be used to change behavior. Attention is often given following disruptive behavior, complaints of difficulty, complaints of pain or failing to do exercises as requested. In most cases this does not matter, but when patients are poorly motivated, they may have learned that this behavior will draw the therapist's attention. Whereas if they work quietly on their own, they will be ignored. They therefore behave in a disruptive manner. If the therapist instead gives attention while the patient is working or is quiet or cooperative, and ignores disruptive behavior and complaints, they should decrease. The amount of attention required from the therapist is the same, but it is given following different behavior.[10, 11]

In a rehabilitation environment, attention, rest, and feedback of progress serve as the primary reinforcers used to modify behavior. Attention is typically provided in response to disruptive behavior, complaints of difficulty, complaints of pain or noncompliance with exercise instructions. While this may not be problematic in most cases, patients with low motivation may have learned that such behavior gathers attention from the therapist. Consequently, they may exhibit disruptive behavior to seek attention, rather than working independently.

To address this, therapists can alter their approach by offering attention when patients are actively engaged, quiet or cooperative, while disregarding disruptive behavior and complaints. This shift in reinforcement strategy aims to reduce disruptive behaviors. Notably, the amount of attention given by the therapist remains consistent, but it is now contingent upon positive behaviors rather than disruptive ones. This approach encourages patients to exhibit desired behaviors to receive attention, fostering more productive and cooperative interactions during rehabilitation sessions.

Behavioral modification is a strategy aimed at improving well-being by reducing stress and enhancing relaxation and sleep. It's widely used in treating various disorders, including cardiovascular disease and psychiatric illnesses. One common application is boosting participation in physical activity and exercise programs. Research shows that behavioral modification helps improve exercise adherence, especially in patients with obesity, cancer, and heart failure, leading to better physiological benefits like improved aerobic performance and body composition. A recent study found that a new BM intervention led by fitness professionals was more effective than standard exercise training in improving aerobic performance, body composition, lower-body power, and heart rate variability (HRV).[12]

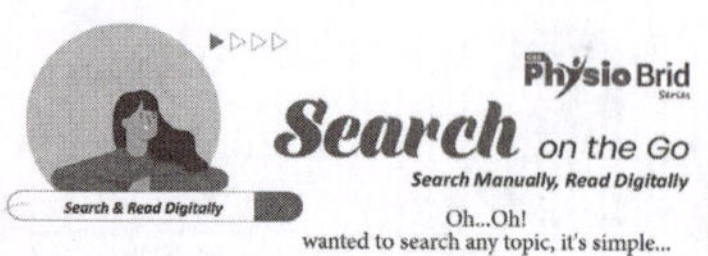

RECENT ADVANCEMENTS

Recently, physiotherapy have increasingly integrated behavioral management principles, leading to more comprehensive and effective treatment approaches. These advancements also demonstrate the evolving nature of physiotherapy, where behavioral management principles are integrated to optimize patient-centered care, improve treatment adherence or compliance, and enhance overall health outcomes.

One example of this integration is the use of cognitive-behavioral techniques in chronic pain management within physiotherapy. Research by Veehof et al. (2016) highlighted the effectiveness of combining physiotherapy with cognitive-behavioral therapy (CBT) in reducing pain intensity and improving function and quality of life for patients with chronic musculoskeletal pain. This approach addresses not only the physical aspects of pain but also the psychological factors that can contribute to its persistence.[13]

Another area of advancement is in the treatment of neurological conditions such as stroke or Parkinson's disease. Behavioral modification techniques, such as goal setting, reinforcement strategies, and mindfulness-based interventions, have been integrated into physiotherapy protocols to enhance motor learning and functional recovery. For instance, a study by Winstein et al. (2016) demonstrated the benefits of task-specific training combined with behavioral strategies in improving upper limb function poststroke.[14]

Virtual Reality (VR) and Gamification: Using VR and gamification techniques in physiotherapy has shown promise in boosting patient motivation and involvement. The focus is on developing multimodal technology-therapy programs that target specific motor activity limitations, such as posture and balance, dexterous manipulation, and functional behaviors during mobility. This includes game-based exercises for targeted strength improvement, enhancing walking function through game-based physical activities, and promoting social interaction during gaming for improved home and community participation. By combining immersive VR technology with evidence-based rehabilitation methods like muscle-specific exercises and task-specific training, the aim is to sustainably improve sensorimotor functions, alleviate cognitive load, and facilitate greater activity and social engagement in various life settings. Lange et al.'s study in 2019 illustrated how VR-based rehabilitation programs effectively enhanced motor function and mobility in patients with neurological conditions like stroke and Parkinson's disease. This recent study also suggests that this technology is beneficial and significantly effective for sensorimotor and cognitive rehabilitation, balance impairments as well as prevention of pressure ulcers.[15]

Behavioral techniques such as **goal-setting** and **motivational interviewing** are being applied in physiotherapy to enhance patient engagement and adherence to rehabilitation programs. A study suggests significantly positive changes in behavior and physical health, such as reduced weight and BMI, lower consumption of food and drinks, increased physical activity, and a greater commitment to healthy habits. These results emphasize the effectiveness of interventions that focus on setting specific goals in encouraging improvements in nutrition and exercise habits among overweight and obese people in community settings. Despite its recent introduction as a method for changing health

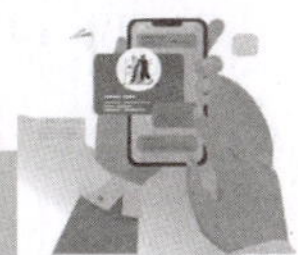

behaviors, goal setting demonstrates promise as a beneficial, affordable, and empowering strategy that can be easily incorporated into community-based weight management initiatives by healthcare professionals, researchers, and wellness practitioners.[16]

Incorporating **mindfulness-based interventions** within physiotherapy has gained attention for conditions like fibromyalgia and chronic low back pain. Moderate evidence that mindfulness-based interventions (MBIs) such as meditation, yoga, and stress reduction lower the perception of pain, increase mobility, improve functioning and wellbeing. By integrating MBIs and other therapeutic interventions in a multidisciplinary pain management plan, clinicians can improve treatment outcomes and potentially decrease pain-related medication utilization. Additional advantages of MBIs include no risk of addiction or abuse, better treatment outcomes, and improvement in comorbid conditions such as anxiety and depression. When MBIs are integrated in a comprehensive pain management plan, consumption of pain-related medications is reduced, pain interference with daily life activities decreases which leads to improvement in self-esteem, body image and activity levels.[17]

CASE STUDY

A Behavioral and Therapeutic Approach to Mobility in a Child with Left Hemiplegia

Tracy, a 6-year-old with left hemiplegia from perinatal brain damage, showed greater hypertonia in her left arm than in her leg. Her cognitive, language, and social skills were at a 2-year-old level, but her motor skills were at a 1-year-old level. She could not walk independently, had frequent toilet accidents, and displayed aggressive behaviors toward herself and others. She could stand with support, but her preferred method of movement was hitching in a sitting position using her right arm and leg. She had poor balance and difficulty crawling on all fours. Her left leg showed abnormalities in standing and walking, with an ankle that tended to collapse inward. Her aggressive behavior and resistance to certain positions made it challenging to facilitate motor patterns effectively.[18]

Behavior modification techniques, often referred to as conditioning methodology, have proven effective in teaching self-care skills to individuals with physical and mental disabilities. For instance, severely intellectually disabled children have learned to walk through a process of rewarding increasingly accurate attempts at the desired skill. Moreover, these conditioning methods have been integrated with other therapeutic approaches.

The intervention's results were visually analyzed without statistical testing. She learned the switch sequence in phase 1 but did not start moving between tables until session 12. Progress slowed after session 45, leading to frustration and temper tantrums. Video analysis revealed her balance strategy and the need for a program redesign in phase 2.

In phase 2, her aggressive behavior persisted, making it challenging to change her walking pattern. Attempts to reduce the table distance and modify arm positions did not lead to forward movement initiation. The intervention shifted to the pool, where she quickly progressed to independent walking in water.

During phase 3, she continued to improve her walking, aided by physical assistance in the gym. Verbal praise and singing were used as reinforcement, contributing to the extinction of temper tantrums when absent.

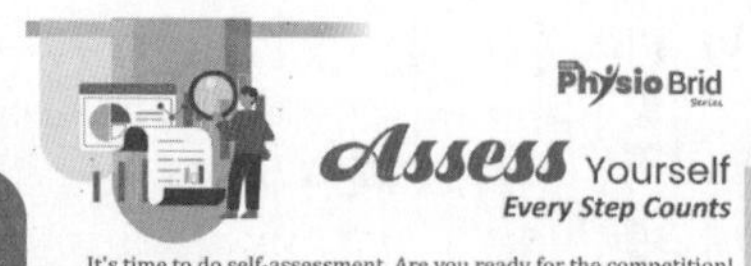

SUMMARY

- Behavior modification, rooted in B F Skinner's theories, learning principles and behavior therapy techniques to foster functional improvements through behavior changes. It emphasizes measurable alterations in behavior, employs environmental adjustments, and underscores accountability, drawing insights from learning science and operant conditioning research.
- Behavior assessment in behavior modification employs diverse methods like direct observation, self-report measures, and functional analysis. It starts with clearly defining observable behaviors and progresses to detailed analyses, such as functional assessments, for comprehensive intervention planning.
- Skinner's reinforcement and punishment concepts illustrate how consequences shape behavior.
- Positive reinforcement involves adding rewards postbehavior to boost recurrence, while negative reinforcement removes negative stimuli, reinforcing desired actions.
- Punishment reduces behavior likelihood, with positive punishment adding aversive consequences and negative punishment removing rewards, shaping future behavior in learning contexts.
- In rehabilitation settings, attention, rest, and progress feedback serve as key reinforcers molding behavior. Therapists can adjust attention strategies, rewarding positive engagement while disregarding disruptive behavior, to encourage desired patient behaviors.
- Behavioral modification within healthcare enhances exercise adherence and overall well-being, particularly benefiting individuals with obesity, cancer, and heart failure.
- Physiotherapy's evolution integrates behavioral management principles like cognitive-behavioral techniques, goal setting, and mindfulness-based interventions. These advances also include employing virtual reality and gamification to bolster motivation and integrating behavioral strategies for superior rehabilitation outcomes.

REFERENCES

1. Martin G, Pear JJ. Behavior Modification: What It Is and How To Do It. 10th ed. Psychology Press; 2014.
2. Scott HK, Jain A, Cogburn M. Behavior Modification. [Updated 2023 Jul 10]. In: StatPearls [Internet]. Treasure Island (FL): StatPearls Publishing; 2024.
3. Smith LM, Johnson TH. The role of behavior assessment in behavior modification. J Behav Ther. 2022;10(1):20–35.
4. Johnson RW, Smith A, Brown C, et al. Assessment methods in behavior modification: A comprehensive review. Behav Anal Q. 2020;25(3):78–92.
5. Wilson GH. Direct observation methods in behavior assessment. Behav Sci J. 2017;12(4):150–165.
6. Adams AB. Self-report measures in behavior assessment. J Behav Assess. 2021;15(2):45–58.
7. Miller SL, White PA. Functional analysis in behavior modification. J Appl Behav Anal. 2016;30(1):15–28.
8. Miltenberger RG. Behavior Modification: Principles and Procedures. 4th ed. Belmont, CA: Thompson Wadsworth; 2008.

Contd...

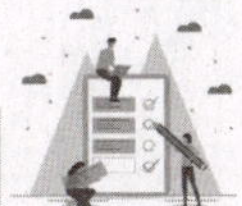
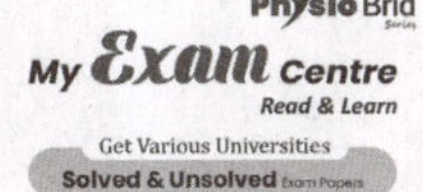

9. Neale AV. Behavioural contracting as a tool to help patients achieve better health. Fam Pract. 1991 Dec;8(4):336–42. doi: 10.1093/fampra/8.4.336. PMID: 1800

10. Lincoln N. Behavior modification in physiotherapy. Physiotherapy. 1978;64:265–267.

11. Zeidler LJ, Zimmer-Hart CL. Combining the techniques of physiotherapy and behaviour modification. Aust J Physiother. 1979 Feb;25(1):27–31

12. Dolezal BA, Boland DM, Neufeld EV, Martin JL, Cooper CB. Behavioral Modification Enhances the Benefits from Structured Aerobic and Resistance Training. Sports Med Int Open. 2019 Jul 15;3(2):E48–E57.

13. Veehof MM, Oskam MJ, Schreurs KM, Bohlmeijer ET. Acceptance-based interventions for the treatment of chronic pain: A systematic review and meta-analysis. Pain. 2016 Mar;157(3):599–611.

14. Winstein CJ, Stein J, Arena R, Bates B, Cherney LR, Cramer SC, et al. Guidelines for adult stroke rehabilitation and recovery: A guideline for healthcare professionals from the American Heart Association/American Stroke Association. Stroke. 2016 Jun;47(6):e98–e169.

15. Lange BS, Requejo P, Flynn SM, Rizzo AA, Valero-Cuevas FJ, Baker L, et al. The potential of virtual reality and gaming to assist successful aging with disability. Phys Med Rehabil Clin N Am. 2010 May;21(2):339–56.

16. Pearson ES. Goal setting as a health behavior change strategy in overweight and obese adults: A systematic literature review examining intervention components. Patient Educ Couns. 2012 Apr;87(1):32–42.

17. Majeed MH, Ali AA, Sudak DM. Mindfulness-based interventions for chronic pain: Evidence and applications. Asian J Psychiatr. 2018 Feb;32:79–83.

18. Zeidler LJ, Zimmer-Hart CL. Combining the techniques of physiotherapy and behavior modification. Aust J Physiother. 1979 Feb;25(1):27–31.

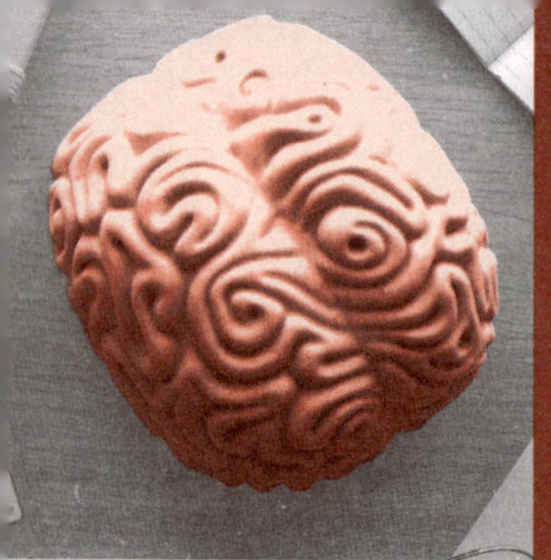

LONG ANSWER QUESTIONS

1. Discuss behavioral assessment.
2. Explain how do reinforcement and punishment affect the behavior.
3. Describe the issues associated with punishment.
4. Explain prompting.
5. Discuss how behavioral management affect the efficacy of physiotherapy.

SHORT ANSWER QUESTIONS

1. What is extinction burst?
2. Write about Premack principle with examples.
3. What are the differences between shaping and chaining?
4. Define behavioral contract.
5. Define role of time-out as a punishment.

MULTIPLE CHOICE QUESTIONS

1. If your mother tells you "You must eat your vegetables before you get ice-cream", she is using the:
   - a. Parkinson's Law
   - b. Peter Principle
   - c. Dilbert Principle
   - d. Premack Principle

2. The Principle of Reinforcement and Punishment was given by:
   - a. James Watson
   - b. Wilhelm Wundt
   - c. Edward Thorndike
   - d. B F Skinner

3. An aversive stimulus which strengthens the behavior is called:
   - a. Positive reinforcement
   - b. Positive punishment
   - c. Negative reinforcement
   - d. Negative punishment

4. A phenomenon where a temporary increase in the frequency, duration or intensity of a behavior is seen which is no longer reinforced, is called:
   - a. Punishment
   - b. Extinction burst
   - c. Reinforcer
   - d. Extinction

5. **What are the main reinforcers operating in a rehabilitation setting that is used to change behavior?**
    a. Attention
    b. Rest
    c. Feedback
    d. All of these

6. **Behavioral modification helps improve:**
    a. Exercise adherence
    b. Medicine adherence
    c. Both a and b
    d. None of these

7. **Using virtual reality and gamification techniques in physiotherapy leads to:**
    a. Enhanced motivation and engagement
    b. Fantasy life
    c. Improved sleep
    d. Improved attention

Note

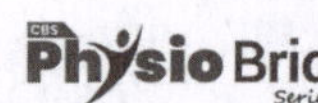

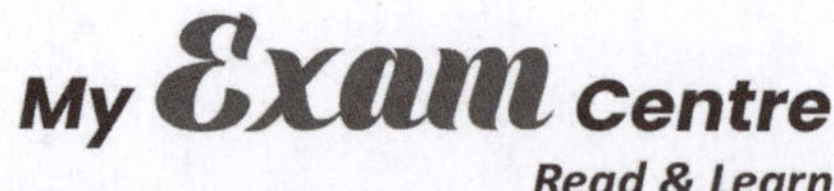

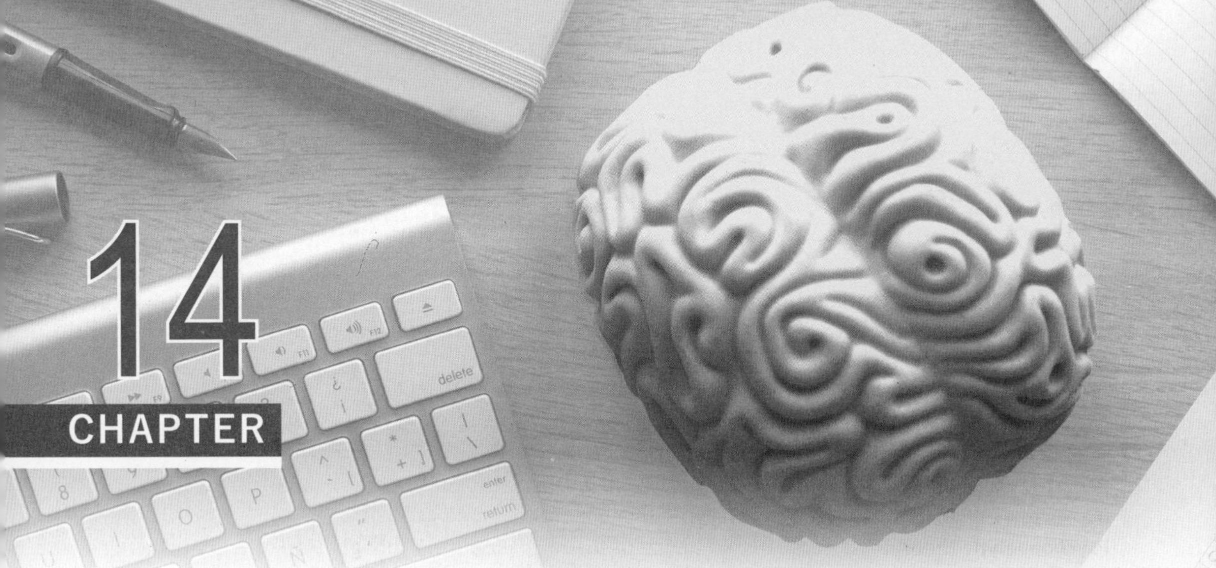

Pediatric Psychology

Riya Kalra, Kanu Goyal, Manu Goyal

LEARNING OBJECTIVES

After the completion of the chapter, the readers will be able to:
- Gain comprehensive knowledge of pediatric psychology.
- Identify various models of child development psychology.
- Articulate diverse theories that explain the process of child development.
- Enhance knowledge related to various aspects of pediatric psychology.

CHAPTER OUTLINE

- Introduction
- Origin
- Models of Development Psychology
- Child Development Theories
- Pediatric Psychologist
- Multidisciplinary Teams
- Recent Advances

KEY TERMS

Behaviorist theory: This theory focuses on observable behavior and the principles of stimulus-response associations and reinforcement.

Constructivist theory: This theory views individuals as actively creating their own knowledge from their experiences, with children possessing certain information about the world from birth.

Contextualism model: A synthesis of earlier models, emphasizing ongoing reciprocal interactions between active individuals and their environments.

Ecological theory: This theory emphasizes the impact of environmental factors on children's development, suggesting that every aspect of development is influenced by the child's environment.

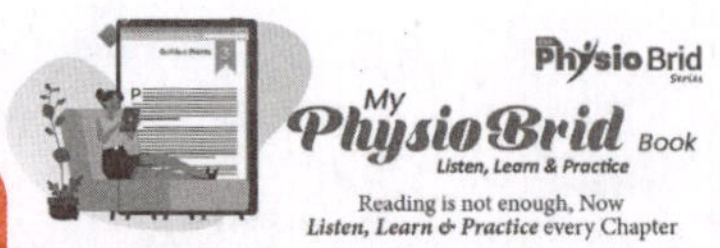

Maturation theory: This theory emphasizes the influence of genetic makeup on development, suggesting that unfavorable environmental conditions can only postpone the development of innate talents.

Mechanistic model: This model focuses on external stimuli and learning theory, suggesting that changes over time are primarily influenced by preceding and subsequent stimuli.

Organismic model: It emphasizes internal maturation processes and foundational structures and processes that evolve as individuals age.

Pediatric psychology: A specialized field that addresses the behavioral, developmental, and psychological needs of children, adolescents, and families within healthcare contexts.

Psychoanalytic theory: Examines the influence of the unconscious on thoughts, emotions, and actions, highlighting the enduring impact of early experiences on adult personality and psychological development.

Role of pediatric psychologists: Professionals who offer evidence-based assessment and therapy for children and families dealing with medical conditions, including chronic pain, unintentional injuries, genitourinary anomalies, and sexual development disorders.

Telemedicine: The use of medical data conveyed from one site to another *via* digital communication to improve a patient's clinical health status.

Virtual reality (VR): Technologies that provide controlled simulations of emotionally compelling backdrop stories, potentially enhancing learning and assessments in children with and without impairments.

INTRODUCTION

Pediatric psychology is a specialized field that addresses the behavioral, developmental, and psychological needs of children, adolescents, and families within healthcare contexts. Pediatric psychologists utilize research findings, counseling, advocacy, education, and direct patient care to prevent illnesses, encourage healthy behaviors, and manage acute and chronic medical conditions in young individuals. This discipline has emerged as a distinct area of study within clinical child psychology over the past five decades.

Logan Wright in 1967, initially described pediatric psychology as "dealing mainly with children who are in a medical setting that's nonpsychiatric in nature". Pediatric psychology focuses on the behavioral, developmental, and psychological requirements of children, adults, and families in healthcare settings. Pediatric psychologists use study findings, advice, advocacy, education, and direct patient care to prevent disease, promote healthy behaviors, and treat acute and chronic medical conditions in young people. It represents a relatively recent science, having emerged predominantly in the last 50 years as a subfield of clinical child psychology.[1, 2]

ORIGIN

Pediatricians in the 1950s and 1960s noticed a rise in behavioral and emotional issues among their patients, even as medical advancements like vaccines improved children's health. To address this, the University of Iowa established the first graduate program in pediatric psychology in 1966. Following this, there was a surge in related activities: The founding of the Society of Pediatric Psychology (SPP) in 1969, the creation of specialized training sites, and the inception of a newsletter that later became the Journal of Pediatric Psychology in 1976. Federal initiatives like the establishment of the National Institute of Child Health and Human Development in 1962 further supported developments in the field. Ultimately, SPP gained official recognition as an American Psychological Association division in 2000.[3, 4]

MODELS OF DEVELOPMENT PSYCHOLOGY

Two main models have been proposed to explain these changes as mentioned in Figure 14.1.

Organismic Model

According to the organismic model, foundational structures and processes—like Piaget's cognitive development stages, Freud's psychosexual stages, and Erickson's

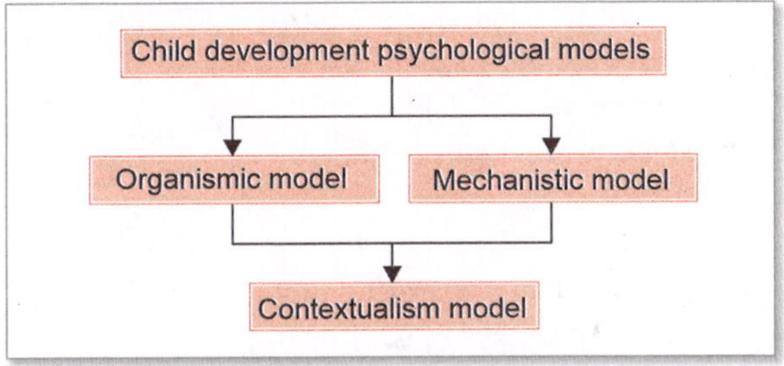

Fig. 14.1: Child development psychological models

identity development phases—evolve as individuals age, representing newly acquired, qualitatively distinct ways of engaging with the environment. In its most radical form, this view suggests that changes are primarily driven by internal maturation processes of the organism, rather than external influences. Moreover, the organism is seen as actively shaping its surroundings, rather than simply responding passively to them.[5]

Mechanistic Model

The mechanistic model of development posits that changes over time are primarily influenced by preceding and subsequent stimuli, with explanations often rooted in learning theory concepts. In its extreme form, this model suggests that individuals, regardless of age, respond relatively indifferently to complex and diverse sensory inputs compared to the organismic model. For instance, Skinner proposed that all living beings, regardless of species or age, are governed by the same law of effect and can therefore be studied similarly. This principle formed a cornerstone of behavioral psychology.

Contextualism Model

The developmental contextualism or transactional model emerged as a synthesis of earlier models, acknowledging their limitations. This paradigm emphasizes ongoing reciprocal interactions, termed transactions, between active individuals and their environments as drivers of developmental changes. Organisms are viewed as both products and shapers of their surroundings, influencing their own growth. Various mentalist perspectives generally concur that growth involves systematic, successive,

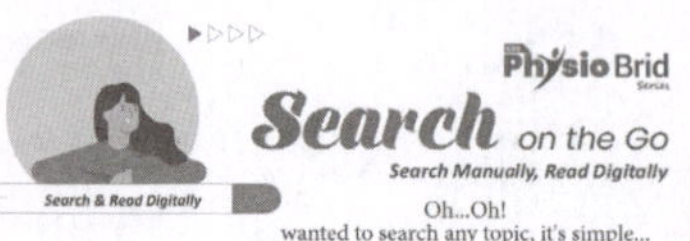

and adaptive changes in the organization, operation, and content of individuals' psychological, emotional, social, and interpersonal characteristics across life stages, although theoretical and philosophical distinctions still exist.[6, 7]

CHILD DEVELOPMENT THEORIES

A theory of child development looks at how children behave and develop, collect this information, and then analyze it (Fig. 14.2). The interpretation identifies the fundamental elements of the children's genetic make-up and the environmental circumstances that affect their growth and conduct, as well as the connections between these factors.[8–12] For more details about the theories refer to Chapter 9, Learning.

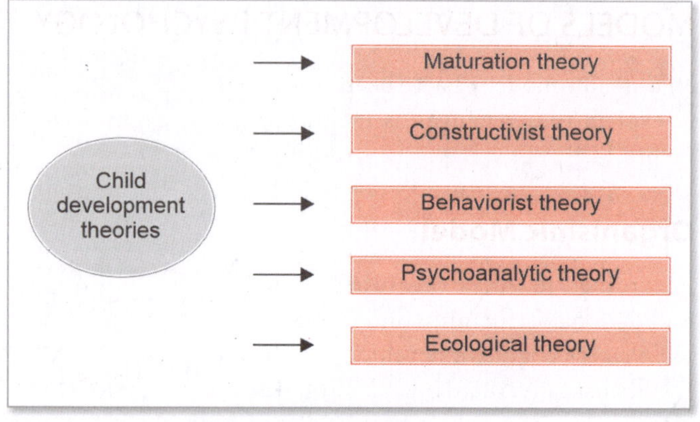

Fig. 14.2: Theories of child development

PEDIATRIC PSYCHOLOGIST

In all stages of health, illness, and accident, pediatric psychologists offer children and families evidence-based assessment and therapy. For instance, psychologists may work with children, their guardians, and their siblings to help them deal with new medical stress and problems when a child receives a new diagnosis of a persistent or severe medical condition. Psychologists collaborate closely with doctors and nurses to employ behavioral strategies that aim to improve medical outcomes for children receiving treatment, such as encouraging adherence to treatment plans. It has been increasingly involved in the shaping of new diagnostic frameworks that highlight enhanced integration of psychology[13] encompassing various aspects of pediatric psychology (Fig. 14.3).

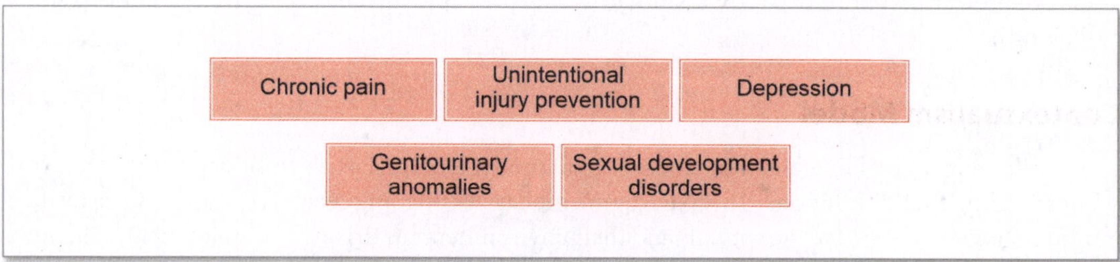

Fig. 14.3: Certain aspects of pediatric psychology

A Multidomain Approach

Considering that pediatric psychology has only been around for a short time, its clinical and scientific background is outstanding. Pediatric psychology has developed empirically validated therapies for a wide range of childhood health conditions, including cystic fibrosis, asthma, diabetes, feeding disorders, obesity, sleep disorders, encopresis, and enuresis.[13, 14]

Chronic Pain

Youth with chronic pain disorders are not uncommon; up to 25% of children and teenagers below the age of 18 report having had more than a single episode of chronic pain throughout their lives. Chronic pain disorders are linked to functional handicap and psychological comorbidities including depression and anxiety in addition to the sense of pain. Over the past 10 years, pediatric pain providers have made considerable strides toward supporting integrated, multidisciplinary therapies that involve medication, physical therapy, and psychological interventions like cognitive-behavioral therapy in order to address this intricate interaction of symptoms. Conceptually consistent with our growing comprehension of the biopsychosocial model of pain, this change is driven by studies showing that a combination of therapies may be most successful in minimizing pain and associated impairment.[15, 16]

Dealing with pain and disability is one of the psychological therapies for children having chronic pain, with the ultimate goal being the restoration of baseline functionality. Psychological therapy for chronic pain includes, among other things, the identification and management of impaired perception, relaxation techniques, psychological learning, parental training, behavioral exposure, tolerance exercises, and values education.[17, 18]

Unintentional Injury Prevention

Unintentional injuries are the biggest cause of death among children aged 1–19 in the US and other industrialized countries. Data on emergency department visits can be startling. In 2014, over 25,000 children under 20 attended emergency departments in the US for injuries. This child health concern affects families across all income levels, racial, ethnic, social, and cultural backgrounds. The majority of injuries in young children happen at home. Caregiver supervision procedures and environmental risks play a significant role in predicting injury risk. Caregiver monitoring involves paying attention, being nearby, and remaining consistent.[19, 20]

Genitourinary Anomalies

Medical professionals must have a thorough grasp of the emotional and cognitive growth of children with genitourinary (GU) diseases. Patients with complicated or long-term GU problems are more likely to experience emotional and developmental difficulties, even while individuals with relatively mild illnesses might not have any psychological aftereffects. In these populations, any deviations

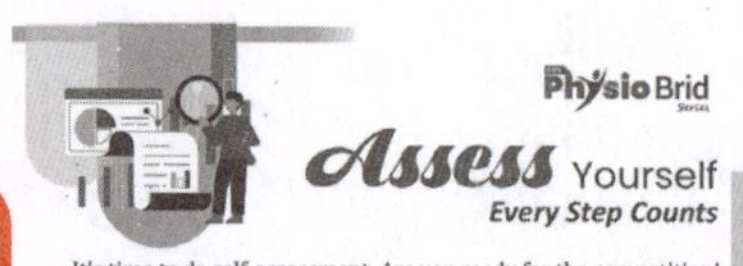

from the more conventional infant development trajectories should be closely observed. These deviations, nevertheless, might not always be obvious or understandable.[21, 22]

In the urology clinic, mental health professionals are most likely to be helpful if they can aid in preventing the emergence of chronic coping and adjustment issues. While some kids and families recover well from therapy, others require assistance. Until a crisis arises, it can be hard to predict which group families a family will belong to during routine medical appointments. Psychosocial services offered as part of the clinic's continuum of care may persuade families to seek mental health treatment at the earliest stages of a problem because interacting with a counselor or therapist who is merely another member of their healthcare team may carry less stigma. The authors advise parents of all newborns with complicated abnormalities in their clinic to schedule a meeting with the psychologist early on. Later, as part of the child's continuing treatment, the parents should have psychosocial check-ins throughout developmental or transitional periods, such as when the kid is leaving high school. These check-ins might be brief at times or they can involve discussions about emerging issues and the identification of solutions.[23, 24]

Children who have GU abnormalities may experience difficulties with several aspects of development and adjustment. Complementary mental health therapies can be advantageous for both the surgeons and their patients. Working alongside a mental health professional may give surgical teams the tools they need to handle difficult patients. Similarly, medical attention will be maximized as readily available resources will enable families and kids to get the support they need to adjust and cope to this awareness and comprehension, as well as to including the family and the kid in preventative and intervention efforts from the child's early years until maturity. For instance, the writers have assisted parents who were afraid that their toddler's GU condition would be found out and did not want them to attend preschool programs.[25, 26]

Depression

Depression causes emotions of despair, inadequacy nothingness, disappointment, and hopelessness that are unrealistic. Depression might not be a one-time occurrence. Depression is more common in children as they get older. Because fatalities of children under the age of 10 are not considered suicide, determining the association between suicide and depression in young kids is challenging.[27]

One of the techniques used to measure depression is the Children's Depression Inventory (CDI), a 27-item self-report assessment. With this tool, children choose one of three statements that best describes their current state during the last 2 weeks. The Revised Children's Manifest Anxiety Scale (RCMAS) is a self-report anxiety screening tool. With this scale, the youngster answers "yes" or "no" to 37 items.[28]

The moderate end of depression is characterized by fleeting melancholy feelings. Low to moderate depression persists and becomes ingrained in a child's attitude on life. Symptoms may include changes in eating and sleeping, poor focus, and/or depression (Sherry & Jellinek, 1996). Seasonal changes can impact energy levels, sleep, appetite, and mood in both adults and children. Phototherapy has been demonstrated to benefit people with seasonal adjustment disorder (SAD).[29]

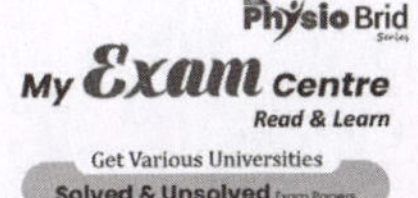

It is the responsibility of a pediatric psychiatrist with the necessary training to diagnose depression in children. When a kid is brought to a doctor or nurse practitioner due to social or behavioral issues that educators, parents or other caregivers have expressed concern about, they frequently get examined by primary care physicians first. These issues mighty be connected to education; that is, low attendance, pessimism, agitation or incapacity to complete assignments. The youngster may occasionally display changes in appetite, such as a decrease in hunger or abnormalities in sleep, such as sleeplessness.[30]

Sexual Development Disorders

"Congenital conditions in which the formation of chromosomal, gonadal or anatomical sex is atypical" are known as diseases of sex development (DSD). This diverse category of illnesses includes those that manifest as ambiguous genitalia during pregnancy or the early stages of infancy, and others that are identified later in life, usually as a result of issues with fertility or pubertal development. The possible effects of the genital exam on kids having DSD and ambiguous genitals are the main topic of this review. DSD are somewhat uncommon and typically understudied disorders, especially when it comes to how receiving medical care affects one's quality of life. Despite efforts to foster consensus, the lack of scientific direction has occasionally resulted in wildly diverse views and behaviors within and within locations. Choosing whether to perform "elective" interventions to produce genitalia that are considered "typical" for a gender-assigned kid is just one of the many complex issues at hand. Other issues include the long-term effects on fertility, sexuality and relationships, body comfort, psychological and social health, and urological function.[31, 32]

The DSD population may benefit especially from the use of "the Pediatric Psychosocial Preventative Health Model" (PPPHM), as the patients' degrees of discomfort and anxiety in the medical context are probably going to differ. The PPPHM, which uses a biopsychosocial paradigm, may be utilized to tailor treatment to the individual requirements of kids and caregivers. Three levels are proposed for treatments in this framework: Universal, focused, and resilient. At the targeted level, treatments can be tailored to acute distress and particular symptoms as needed, while universal interventions offer broad support and opportunity for risk screening. When symptoms are becoming worse and the family is at high-risk, a behavioral health professional can engage with them at the clinical/treatment level. When there's variability in reaction and suffering related to an intervention, such with the CSA health exam, this kind of model can be useful. Presumably, the genital exam may cause kids and their parents with DSD to experience widely differing degrees of discomfort, and a similar strategy could be able to provide.[33, 34]

Facilitating Child Grief

It is wise to provide youngsters with preventative care during their grieving process. Children who are grieving need security, stability, and the capacity to explore their curiosity and feelings. They also need to be given freedom to express themselves, weep, be upset, and talk about how they feel wounded and guilty. Primary preventive care entails the following: (a) Preparing kids for loss;

(b) Supporting parents or other adult caregivers during loss; (c) Explaining and discussing the experience honestly with kids; (d) Encouraging kids to participate in shared grieving rituals and the return to regular activities; and (e) Getting professional assistance as soon as possible (Black, 1996). Neglecting to assist throughout the grieving and morning process may have long-term consequences such as impeded ability to form future close connections and diminished capacity to enjoy life in general.[35, 36]

MULTIDISCIPLINARY TEAMS

In several branches of psychology, particularly rehabilitative psychology, teamwork is a prevalent practice (Table 14.1). Members of multidisciplinary teams stay firmly inside the boundaries of the designated major field while gaining knowledge from other subjects and disciplines. The boundaries between specialties are blurred and crossover occurs in multidisciplinary care. Rather than examining cognitive and speech methods independently, a psychologist and a speech pathologist could collaborate to evaluate augmentative communication device tactics. Transdisciplinary care crosses disciplinary boundaries, prioritizes the needs of the patient, and cross-fertilizes ideas to optimize problem-solving.[37, 38]

Table 14.1: Comprehensive psychological support provided for children and with physical needs

Accessibility and convenience	Psychology services are easily accessible and conveniently located, with flexible hours to accommodate families' schedules.
Integration with pediatric care	The services are closely integrated with pediatric healthcare services, ensuring a holistic approach to patient care.
Patient-centered care	The support prioritizes patient-centered care, guided by clear values and principles that focus on the well-being of both the child and their family.
Collaborative planning	Young people and families actively participate in planning their care and shaping the services they receive.
Inclusivity and stigma reduction	The services promote inclusivity and actively work to eliminate stigma associated with psychological support.
Effective communication	Emphasis is placed on effective communication between professionals, families, and relevant agencies involved in the care.
Focus on long-term well-being	In addition to addressing immediate issues, the services prioritize long-term psychological well-being, including self-esteem and relationships.
Building resilience	The services aim to build resilience and support individuals in adapting to their circumstances, focusing on strengths rather than vulnerabilities.
Transition planning	Well-defined procedures are in place for transitioning patients from pediatric services to adult services when needed.
Continuous improvement	User feedback is actively collected and used to evaluate and improve the quality of the psychological support services.

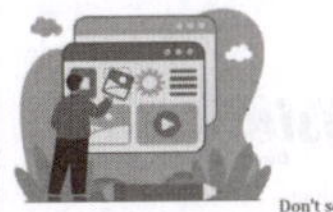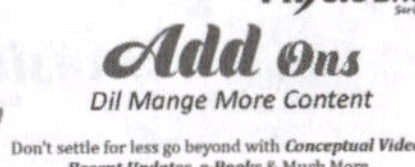

CASE STUDY

Rehabilitation with Child Psychologist

Background
A 6-year-old child, Sarah, suffered a fractured femur after falling from a playground structure. After successful surgical intervention, Sarah was referred to a physiotherapist to help her regain strength, mobility, and confidence in using her leg. However, the process of recovery was met with challenges due to Sarah's fear, anxiety, and reluctance to participate in the physiotherapy sessions.

Challenges
- **Fear of pain:** Sarah was afraid that the exercises would cause pain similar to what she experienced during the injury and subsequent surgery.
- **Separation anxiety:** Being away from her parents during sessions heightened her anxiety, making it difficult for her to cooperate with the therapist.
- **Lack of understanding:** Sarah didn't fully grasp the importance of the exercises, leading to resistance in performing them.
- **Emotional distress:** The injury had disrupted her daily activities, leading to frustration and mood swings, which further affected her engagement in the therapy.

Role of Child Psychology
Understanding and addressing Sarah's psychological state was crucial for the success of her physiotherapy. The physiotherapist collaborated with a child psychologist to develop a comprehensive treatment plan that included:
- **Building trust and rapport:** The therapist spent time getting to know Sarah, engaging in playful activities, and discussing her favorite hobbies. This helped Sarah feel more comfortable and safe during sessions.
- **Parental involvement:** Recognizing Sarah's separation anxiety, the therapist allowed her mother to stay in the room during the initial sessions. Gradually, the mother was involved less as Sarah grew more confident.
- **Pain education:** The therapist used child-friendly language and tools, like toys and storybooks, to explain the importance of the exercises and how they would help her heal. This reduced Sarah's fear of pain and made her more willing to participate.
- **Positive reinforcement:** Sarah was praised and rewarded with stickers and small treats after each session, reinforcing her positive behavior and encouraging continued participation.
- **Play therapy integration:** The therapist incorporated games and playful activities into the exercises. For example, Sarah played "Simon Says" while performing stretches or pretended to be an animal moving through an obstacle course. This made the sessions enjoyable and helped distract her from any discomfort.
- **Coping strategies:** The child psychologist taught Sarah simple breathing exercises and visualization techniques to manage her anxiety and fear during the sessions.

Outcome
With the integration of child psychology into her physiotherapy treatment, Sarah's engagement in the sessions improved significantly. She became more confident and less anxious, which allowed her to perform the necessary exercises effectively. Over time, she regained full mobility in her leg, and her emotional well-being also improved as she was able to return to her regular activities with her peers.

Contd...

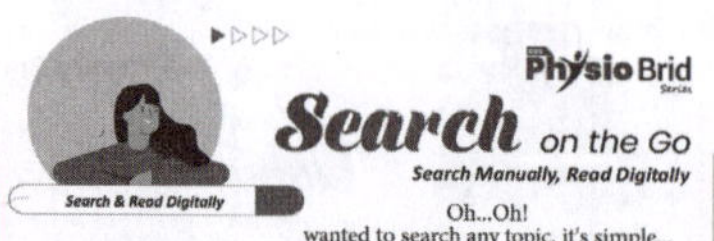

Conclusion

This case study highlights the importance of understanding and addressing the psychological needs of a child during physiotherapy treatment. By incorporating child psychology principles, therapists can create a supportive environment that fosters cooperation, reduces anxiety, and ultimately leads to better physical and emotional outcomes for young patients.

Physio CORNER

Physiotherapy and Pediatric Psychology

Rehabilitation psychology is a specialty focused on maximizing wellness as well as meaningful participation for people with disabilities in daily life. While the field primarily focuses on participation and the identification of social and environmental factors that impact participation, rehabilitation psychologists working with children also have to take a variety of pediatric-specific issues into account. When working with children, especially those who have congenital problems, rehabilitation psychologists offer therapies that are better characterized as habitation than rehabilitation services. Habitation is the term for interventions that assist people in learning new skills. It is especially crucial for children who have congenital disabilities, as many activities and skills have not yet developed to the expected level and are therefore less of a goal of rehabilitation and more of an important acquisition during the proper developmental stage. Children with severe preterm are surviving because to advancements in newborn critical care, but premature birth is associated with a high rate of problems, including motor (such as cerebral palsy) and perceptual (such as hearing, vision) impairments.[39, 40]

Although there are conventional milestones for medical and intellectual monitoring of growth for normally developing newborns, toddlers, and children, there are few standards and normed pathways for developmental and skill achievement for children with impairments. Additionally, sensory and motor limitations frequently restrict opportunities for important skill development reinforcement.[41, 42]

Psychological Factors in Pediatric Physiotherapy

In physical therapy both in research and practice, psychosocial techniques have gained more attention as a supplement to therapies that are biomedically oriented. Different definitions have been applied to offer a label that includes psychosocial techniques in the literature on physical therapy. The research's perspectives from physiotherapists demonstrated that, while thinking about using psychosocial techniques, they took into account their patients' beliefs, psychological presentation, thoughts and cognitions, capacity to manage and cope with their condition, and social and environmental aspects. Common Strategies which are used by Physiotherapist with children having psychological considerations are cognitive behavioral therapies, relaxation strategies, coping skills, imagery, visual metaphors. Physiotherapists choose certain psychosocial tactics mostly based on past experiences, approach success, perceived expertise, competence, and confidence rather than the strategies' established effectiveness.[43, 44]

RECENT ADVANCES

Telemedicine

"The utilization of medical data conveyed from one site to another *via* digital communication to improve a patient's clinical health status" is the definition of telemedicine, according to the American

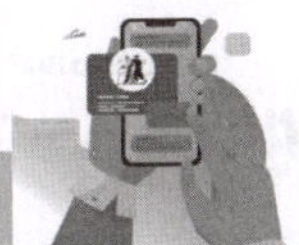

Telemedicine Association. Applications of telemedicine for children or tele-pediatrics, are utilized in medical specialties when distance is a problem. These services include diagnosis, treatment, illness prevention, education for patients and caregivers, research, and care assessment.[45, 46]

Virtual Reality

Technologies for virtual reality (VR) provide controlled simulations of emotionally compelling backdrop stories. These virtual spaces have the potential to improve social connections and experiences that are emotionally significant. In this situation, VR can help educators, therapists, neuropsychologists, and other service providers deliver safe, dependable, and adaptable treatments that can improve learning and assessments in kids with and without impairments as well as typically developing kids. Since schools are where adolescents and children spend the majority of their time, VR can offer accurate evaluations and treatments there. Despite its challenges, the potential for VR technology to be employed for distant learning in schools is exciting. VR on smartphones will become more widely available, which will increase its potential.[47]

SUMMARY

- Pediatric psychology in physiotherapy is an essential component of comprehensive care for children and adolescents with physical health conditions or disabilities.
- By integrating psychological principles and interventions into physiotherapy services, psychologists help optimize treatment outcomes, improve coping skills, and promote overall well-being in pediatric populations.
- Through collaborative efforts with physiotherapists, families, and interdisciplinary teams, pediatric psychologists ensure that children and adolescents receive holistic care that addresses both their physical and psychological needs, ultimately leading to improved health outcomes and enhanced quality of life.
- This comprehensive approach to pediatric psychology in physiotherapy underscores the importance of addressing the psychological aspects of rehabilitation to optimize outcomes and promote the well-being of young patients and their families.

REFERENCES

1. Kaufman JN, Lahey S, Slomine BS. Pediatric rehabilitation psychology: Rehabilitating a moving target. Rehabilitation Psychology. 2017 Aug;62(3):223.
2. Jehn P, Stier R, Tavassol F, Dittmann J, Zimmerer R, Gellrich NC, Krüskemper G, Spalthoff S. Physical and psychological impairments associated with mucositis after oral cancer treatment and their impact on quality of life. Oncology Research and Treatment. 2019 Jun 3;42(6):342–9.
3. Routh DK. The short history of pediatric psychology. Journal of Clinical Child & Adolescent Psychology. 1975 Sep 1;4(3):6–8.

Contd...

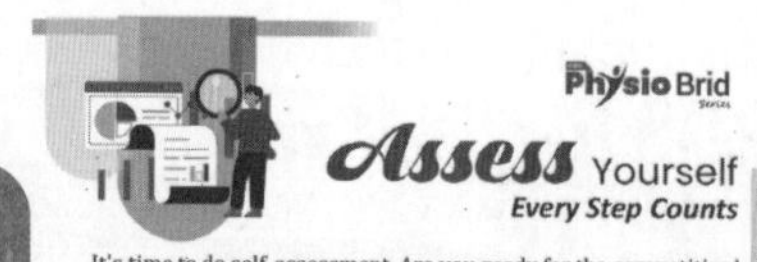

4. Drotar D. Historical analysis in pediatric psychology: From gaining access to leading. Journal of pediatric psychology. 2015 Mar 1;40(2):175–84.

5. Goodnow JJ. Parents' ideas, actions, and feelings: Models and methods from developmental and social psychology. Child development. 1988 Apr 1:286–320.

6. Evans GW, Li D, Whipple SS. Cumulative risk and child development. Psychological bulletin. 2013 Nov;139(6):1342.

7. Reese HW, Overton WF. Models of development and theories of development. InLife-span developmental psychology 1970 Jan 1 (p. 115–145). Academic Press.

8. Goodnow JJ. Parents' ideas, actions, and feelings: Models and methods from developmental and social psychology. Child development. 1988 Apr 1:286–320.

9. Saracho ON. Theories of child development and their impact on early childhood education and care. Early Childhood Education Journal. 2023 Jan;51(1):15–30.

10. Moreno JL, Moreno FB. Spontaneity theory of child development. Sociometry. 1944 May 1;7(2): 89–128.

11. Scarr S. Developmental theories for the 1990s: Development and individual differences. Child development. 1992 Feb;63(1):1–9.

12. DeRobertis EM. Deriving a humanistic theory of child development from the works of Carl R. Rogers and Karen Horney. The Humanistic Psychologist. 2006 May 1;34(2):177–99.

13. Colville G. The role of a psychologist on the paediatric intensive care unit. Child Psychology and Psychiatry Review. 2001 Sep;6(3):102–9.

14. Porritt J, Marshman Z, Rodd HD. Understanding children's dental anxiety and psychological approaches to its reduction. International journal of paediatric dentistry. 2012 Nov;22(6):397–405.

15. Deeb A, Akle M, Al Ozairi A, Cameron F. Common issues seen in paediatric diabetes clinics, psychological formulations, and related approaches to management. Journal of diabetes research. 2018 Feb 27;2018.

16. Fisher E, Heathcote L, Palermo TM, de C Williams AC, Lau J, Eccleston C. Systematic review and meta-analysis of psychological therapies for children with chronic pain. Journal of pediatric psychology. 2014 Sep 1;39(8):763–82.

17. Liossi C, Johnstone L, Lilley S, Caes L, Williams G, Schoth DE. Effectiveness of interdisciplinary interventions in paediatric chronic pain management: A systematic review and subset meta-analysis. British journal of anaesthesia. 2019 Aug 1;123(2):e359–71.

18. Dunford E, Thompson M, Gauntlett-Gilbert J. Parental behaviour in paediatric chronic pain: A qualitative observational study. Clinical child psychology and psychiatry. 2014 Oct;19(4):561–75.

19. Schwebel DC, Gaines J. Pediatric unintentional injury: Behavioral risk factors and implications for prevention. Journal of Developmental & Behavioral Pediatrics. 2007 Jun 1;28(3):245–54.

20. Kendrick D, Barlow J, Hampshire A, Stewart-Brown S, Polnay L. Parenting interventions and the prevention of unintentional injuries in childhood: Systematic review and meta-analysis. Child: Care, health and development. 2008 Sep;34(5):682–95.

21. Kramer DN, Landolt MA. Early psychological intervention in accidentally injured children ages 2–16: A randomized controlled trial. European journal of psychotraumatology. 2014 Dec 1;5(1):24402.

22. Schast AP, Reiner WG. Pediatric psychology in genitourinary anomalies. Urologic Clinics. 2010 May 1;37(2):299–305.

Contd...

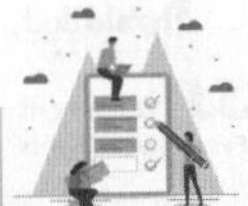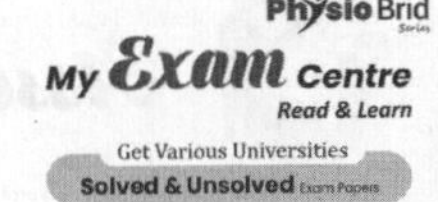

23. Rouse CM. Pediatric psychology in a urology division: Unifying complex medical and mental health treatment. Current Urology Reports. 2023 Jan;24(1):17–24.

24. Koller M. Functional Symptoms in the Genitourinary System in Children and Adolescents. InHandbook of Mind/Body Integration in Child and Adolescent Development 2023 Mar 15 (pp. 283–291). Cham: Springer International Publishing.

25. Mandal D, Maw RD, Carne CA, Opaneye A, Thirunavukarasu T. Availability of services for subjects of sexual assault in genitourinary medicine clinics. International journal of STD & AIDS. 2010 May;21(5):317–9.

26. Mandal D, Maw RD, Carne CA, Opaneye A, Thirunavukarasu T. Availability of services for subjects of sexual assault in genitourinary medicine clinics. International journal of STD & AIDS. 2010 May;21(5):317–9.

27. Loades ME, Chalder T. Same, same but different? Cognitive behavioural treatment approaches for paediatric CFS/ME and depression. Behavioral and cognitive psychotherapy. 2017 Jul;45(4): 366–81.

28. Merry SN, Hetrick SE, Cox GR, Brudevold-Iversen T, Bir JJ, McDowell H. Cochrane Review: Psychological and educational interventions for preventing depression in children and adolescents. Evidence-Based Child Health: A Cochrane Review Journal. 2012 Sep;7(5):1409–685.

29. Reynolds C, Richmond BO. Revised children's manifest anxiety scale. Psychological Assessment. 1985.

30. Pietsch K, Allgaier AK, Frühe B, Rohde S, Hosie S, Heinrich M, Schulte-Körne G. Screening for depression in adolescent paediatric patients: Validity of the new Depression Screener for Teenagers (DesTeen). Journal of affective disorders. 2011 Sep 1;133(1-2):69–75.

31. Alderson J, Hamblin RP, Crowne EC. Psychological care of children and families with variations or differences in Sex Development. Hormone Research in Paediatrics. 2023 May 30;96(2):222–7.

32. Liao L. Development of sexuality: Psychological perspectives. Paediatric and Adolescent Gynaecology. 2004 Apr 1:77–93.

33. Kleinemeier E, Jürgensen M, Lux A, Widenka PM, Thyen U, DSD Network Working Group. Psychological adjustment and sexual development of adolescents with disorders of sex development. Journal of Adolescent Health. 2010 Nov 1;47(5):463–71.

34. M Selveindran N, Syed Zakaria SZ, Jalaludin MY, Rasat R. Quality of life in children with disorders of sex development. Hormone research in paediatrics. 2017 Nov 21;88(5):324–30.

35. Mosher PJ. Everywhere and nowhere: Grief in child and adolescent psychiatry and pediatric clinical populations. Child and Adolescent Psychiatric Clinics. 2018 Jan 1;27(1):109–24.

36. Kochen EM, Jenken F, Boelen PA, Deben LM, Fahner JC, van den Hoogen A, Teunissen SC, Geleijns K, Kars MC. When a child dies: A systematic review of well-defined parent-focused bereavement interventions and their alignment with grief-and loss theories. BMC palliative care. 2020 Dec;19: 1–22.

37. Roth AD, Donnan J. Developing a competence framework for psychological interventions in a multidisciplinary paediatric context. BMJ Paediatrics Open. 2019;3(1).

38. Dovey-Pearce G, Flannery H. Integrating psychology into paediatric healthcare: A UK perspective. Clinical Child Psychology and Psychiatry. 2021 Apr;26(2):313–22.

39. Kloze AK, Buchholz A. Psychological resilience and parents' engagement in paediatric physiotherapy. Advances in Rehabilitation. 2023 Oct 1;37(4).

Contd...

40. Al Ali AA. A Critical Investigation of the Role of Psychological Pain Management on Successful Paediatric Physiotherapy and Rehabilitation. Practice. 2023; 2:06–14.

41. Sartori R, Tessitore A, Della Torca A, Barbi E. Efficacy of physiotherapy treatments in children and adolescents with somatic symptom disorder and other related disorders: Systematic review of the literature. Italian Journal of Pediatrics. 2022 Jul 27;48(1):127.

42. Ayling Campos A, Amaria K, Campbell F, McGrath PA. Clinical impact and evidence base for physiotherapy in treating childhood chronic pain. Physiotherapy Canada. 2011 Jan;63(1):21–33.

43. Bryon M, Steed E. Psychological aspects of care. Physiotherapy for Respiratory and Cardiac Problems: Adults and Paediatrics. 2008 Mar 6:252.

44. Bonduelle SL, Vanderfaeillie J, Denijs K, Lampo A, Imeraj L. Factors influencing adherence to therapeutic recommendations made after diagnostic reassessment of medically unexplained symptoms in children and adolescents. Clinical Child Psychology and Psychiatry. 2020 Jan;25(1): 62–77.

45. Van Allen J, Davis AM, Lassen S. The use of telemedicine in pediatric psychology: Research review and current applications. Child and Adolescent Psychiatric Clinics of North America. 2011 Jan;20(1):55.

46. Zabel TA, Jones E, Peterson RK, Comi-Morog N, Stephan C, Milla K, Pritchard AE, Jacobson LA. Improved parent self-efficacy following pediatric evaluation: Evidence for value of a telemedicine approach in psychological and neuropsychological assessment. The Clinical Neuropsychologist. 2023 Aug 18;37(6):1221–38.

47. Parsons TD, Riva G, Parsons S, Mantovani F, Newbutt N, Lin L, Venturini E, Hall T. Virtual reality in pediatric psychology. Pediatrics. 2017 Nov 1;140(Supplement_2):S86–91.

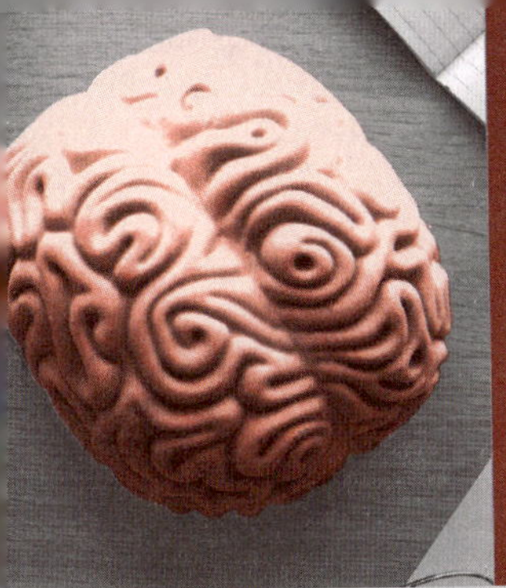

STUDENT ASSIGNMENT

LONG ANSWER QUESTIONS

1. Describe the origin and development of pediatric psychology as a specialized field within healthcare settings.
2. Differentiate between the organismic model and mechanistic model of development psychology. How do these models explain changes over time in individuals?
3. What are some empirical therapies developed by pediatric psychologists for childhood health conditions? Provide examples of such conditions.
4. How do pediatric psychologists address chronic pain disorders in children?
5. Describe the multidisciplinary approach used in treatment of a patient with various needs.

SHORT ANSWER QUESTIONS

1. Mention the importance of unintentional injury prevention and the role of pediatric psychology in reducing childhood injuries.
2. What are some psychosocial considerations for children with genitourinary anomalies?
3. How can pediatric psychologists support individuals and their families?
4. How does pediatric psychology contribute to the understanding and treatment of depression in children?
5. Write about key assessment tools used in diagnosing childhood depression.

MULTIPLE CHOICE QUESTIONS

1. **What was the focus of the first graduate program in pediatric psychology established at the University of Iowa in 1966?**
   a. Psychiatric treatment for children
   b. Behavioral and emotional issues in children within medical settings
   c. Advancements in medical technology
   d. Pediatric nutrition and wellness

2. **Which theoretical model of child development emphasizes that changes over time are primarily influenced by internal maturation processes of the organism?**
   a. Mechanistic model
   b. Psychoanalytic theory
   c. Organismic model
   d. Ecological theory

3. **According to the constructivist theory of learning, how do children create knowledge about the world?**
   a. Through passive observation
   b. By memorizing information
   c. By actively interacting with their environment
   d. By listening to adults

4. **Which theory of child development focuses on changes in behavior resulting from reinforcement and associations between stimuli in the environment and observable reactions?**
   a. Constructivist theory
   b. Ecological theory
   c. Maturation theory
   d. Behaviorist theory

5. **What is a primary focus of ecological theory in child development?**
   a. The influence of genetic makeup on development
   b. The role of unconscious desires in behavior
   c. The significance of the environment in children's lives
   d. The impact of cognitive maturation on behavior

6. **Which psychological approach emphasizes the enduring influence of early experiences on adult personality and psychological development?**
   a. Psychoanalytic theory
   b. Constructivist theory
   c. Behaviorist theory
   d. Ecological theory

7. **What is one key role of pediatric psychologists in healthcare settings according to the text?**
   a. Conducting surgeries
   b. Providing medical prescriptions
   c. Offering evidence-based assessment and therapy
   d. Training medical staff

8. **Which area of pediatric psychology focuses on interventions to address chronic pain disorders in children?**
   a. Unintentional injury prevention
   b. Genitourinary anomalies
   c. Depression
   d. Chronic pain management

9. **Which strategy is recommended for preventing unintentional injuries in children based on the text?**
   a. Increased screen time
   b. Reducing caregiver supervision
   c. Addressing environmental risks
   d. Encouraging risky behaviors

10. **What does the Children's Depression Inventory (CDI) assess?**
    a. Anxiety levels
    b. Sleep patterns
    c. Current state of depression
    d. Behavioral problems

ANSWER KEY

1. b	2. c	3. c	4. d	5. c	6. a	7. c	8. d
9. c	10. c						

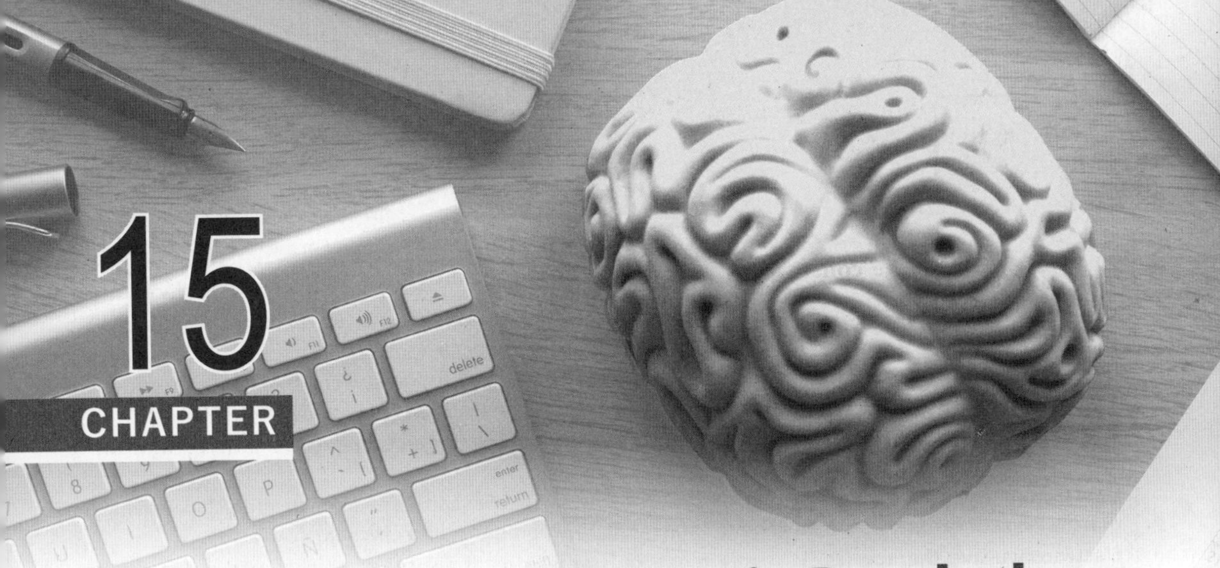

15
CHAPTER

Geriatric Psychology

Lakshay Panchal, Aditi Popli, Hem Jivani

LEARNING OBJECTIVES

After the completion of the chapter, the readers will be able to:
- Define geropsychology, its scope, and need for physiotherapist.
- Define normal aging, the process, types of aging, and its psychosocial approach.
- Common psychological challenges faced by older adults and treatment strategies.
- Recent physiotherapeutic approaches in dealing with major psychological conditions in the geriatric population.
- Psychological aspects of specific conditions: Pain, fall, and geriatric syndromes: Dementia and delirium.
- Importance of geriatric psychology in physiotherapy practice.

CHAPTER OUTLINE

- Introduction
- Geriatrics and Geropsychology
- Aging Population (Demographics and Trends)
- Challenges Faced by Older Adults and Treatment Strategies
- Recent Approaches
- Psychological Aspects of Specific Conditions

KEY TERMS

Anxiety disorders: A group of mental disorders characterized by feelings of worry, nervousness or unease. Types include generalized anxiety disorder (GAD), panic disorder, social anxiety disorder, phobias, and others.

Biological age: The age of a person as measured by biological markers, reflecting the molecular and cellular state of the body.

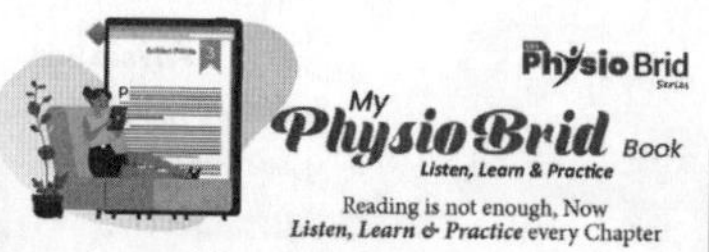

Chronological age: The actual age of a person, measured in years, months, days, minutes, and seconds.

Cranial electrical stimulation (CES): A noninvasive method of applying low-intensity current to the head to alter brain function and treat conditions like depression, anxiety, and insomnia.

Delirium: A global cerebral dysfunction that affects consciousness, attention, thinking, perception, memory, emotion, and the sleep-wake cycle, often causing changes in behavior and judgment.

Dementia: A clinical syndrome characterized by progressive cognitive decline that interferes with the ability to function independently.

Depression: A serious mental disorder characterized by persistent sadness and loss of interest in activities of daily living. It can be caused by genetic, biological, environmental, and psychological factors.

Electroconvulsive therapy (ECT): A treatment for severe mental disorders, such as major depressive disorder, involving the application of electrical stimulation to the brain under anesthetic conditions.

Functional age: An age determined by assessing an individual's biological, psychological, and social functioning, often used in clinical settings to understand a person's overall health and capabilities.

Geropsychology: A branch of psychology that focuses on the mental and physical health of older adults. It encompasses the study of the thought and behavior of older adults, including their cognitive, emotional, and behavioral aspects.

Insomnia: A sleep disorder characterized by difficulty falling asleep, staying asleep or waking up too early and being unable to go back to sleep. It can lead to daytime sleepiness and fatigue.

Normal aging: The natural process of growing older, characterized by physical, psychological, and social changes. It is categorized into primary aging (due to biological factors) and secondary aging (due to external factors).

Psychological age: A subjective measure of age, based on emotional and logical maturity, rather than physical age.

Psychosocial development: The process of personal and social growth throughout life, influenced by personality, thinking, and behavior.

Quality of life (QOL): A measure of an individual's overall well-being, including physical, mental, emotional, and social aspects.

Repetitive transcranial magnetic stimulation (rTMS): A noninvasive brain stimulation technique that uses magnetic fields to induce electrical currents in the brain, used to treat conditions like depression and PTSD.

Social age: The societal norm or expectation of behaviors associated with a certain age.

Transcranial direct current stimulation (tDCS): A noninvasive technique that modifies cortical excitability by applying a weak electrical current to the scalp.

Vagus nerve stimulation (VNS): An approach that involves applying electrical pulses to the vagus nerve to modulate brain activity, used to treat epilepsy, depression, and other conditions.

INTRODUCTION

Geriatric psychology is a branch of psychology that focuses on the mental and physical health of older adults. It explores behavioral, emotional and cognitive aspects of older adults, including memories and motivations. This chapter will provide a foundation to students for geriatric psychology.

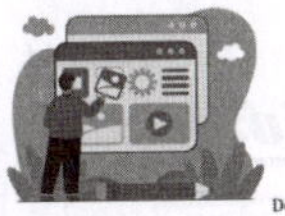
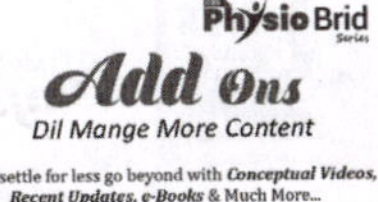

GERIATRICS AND GEROPSYCHOLOGY

Geriatrics is a branch of medicine that deals with psychological and physiological aspects of aging along with diagnosing and intervening in diseases affecting older adults.[1] Demand for psychological services among older persons is increasing constantly due to aging population, presenting a challenge to the psychology

> ### MUST KNOW
>
> "Geropsychologists are the professionals who use their knowledge of psychology and apply the methods of psychology to understand and help older persons to maintain physical and mental well-being during later life."[4]

profession to provide these services. Over the past few decades, geropsychology has evolved in response to this challenge, to meet present and future demand. Geropsychology or geriatric psychology is a branch of psychology that studies the process of aging and focuses on the physical and mental health of older individuals (Fig. 15.1). It focuses on the assessment, consultation, and intervention with older adults.[2, 3]

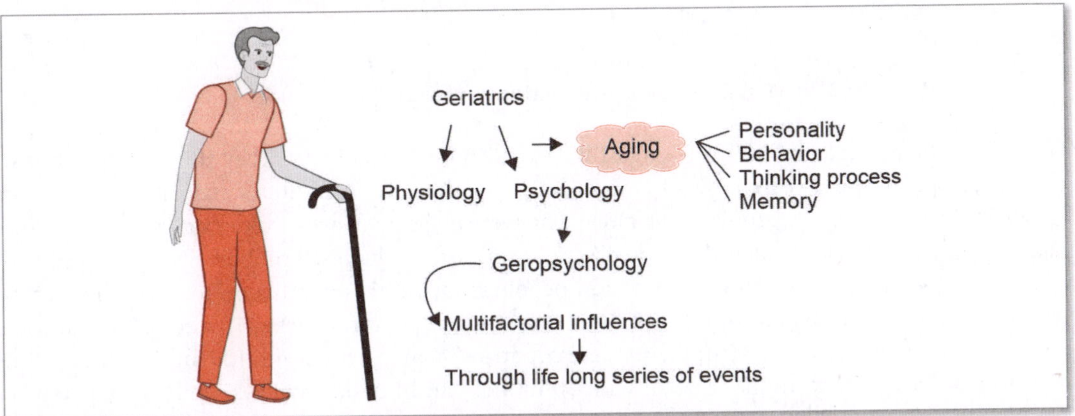

Fig. 15.1: Outline to geropsychology

AGING POPULATION (DEMOGRAPHICS AND TRENDS)

People are living longer and longer everywhere in the world. In most regions of the world, life expectancy or the average duration of life, is rising. The major global trends such as urbanization, globalization, the shift in health patterns toward noncommunicable diseases, and technological improvements. Understanding the interdependencies between these phenomena is essential to developing creative and practical aging strategies that meet the needs of the 21st century.[5, 6]

Globally, the number of elderly people is increasing with time due to improvements in healthcare. Disorders affecting individuals 60 years of age and above contribute 23% of the global disease burden. As per the World Health Organization (WHO), in 2000 people aged 60 years or

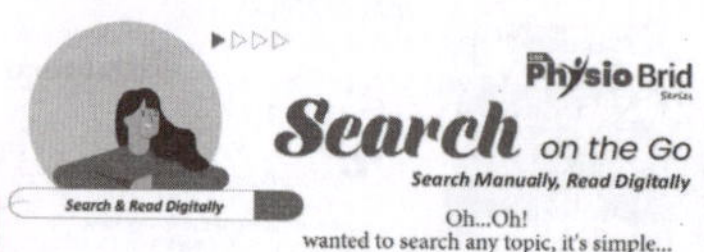

above were 600 million; and this will rise to approximately 2 billion by 2050.[7] Cardiovascular illnesses accounts for the largest portion of the disease burden in individuals 60 years of age and older (30.30%), followed by malignant neoplasms (15.10%), chronic respiratory diseases (9.50%), musculoskeletal diseases (7.50%), and neurological and mental disorders (6.60%).[8] Refer to Figure 15.2 for the distribution.

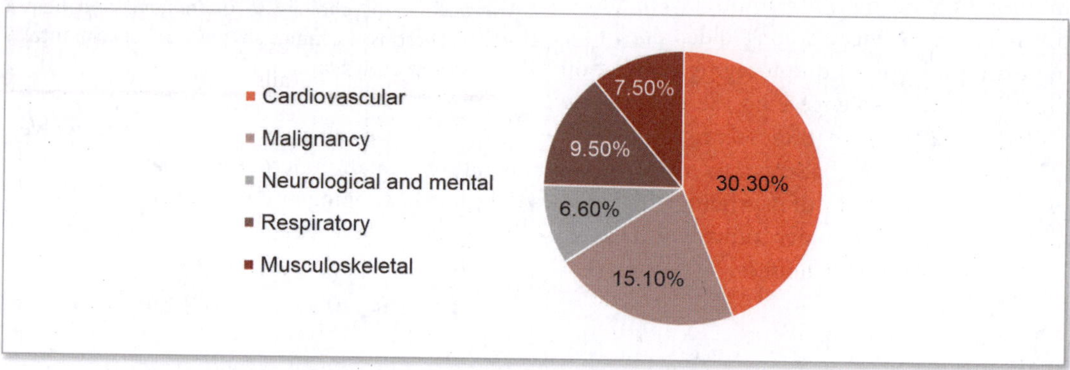

Fig. 15.2: Disease burden in geriatric population

Japanese women currently have the longest life expectancy in the world. They might anticipate an average lifespan of 86.8 years in 2014.[9] According to United Nations (2001) estimates, there were approximately 205 million people in the globe who were 60 years of age or older in 1950. Only three nations—China, India as well as the United States of America—had >10 million citizens 60 years of age or older at that time. Around 607 million people made up this population in 2000, more than tripling from the previous year. Of the 12 countries with a population of over 10 million, 5 countries had a geriatric population of >20 million: These countries include China with 129 million, India with 77 million, USA with 46 million, Japan with 30 million, and Russia having 27 million of geriatric population.[10] Refer to Figure 15.3 for the distribution.

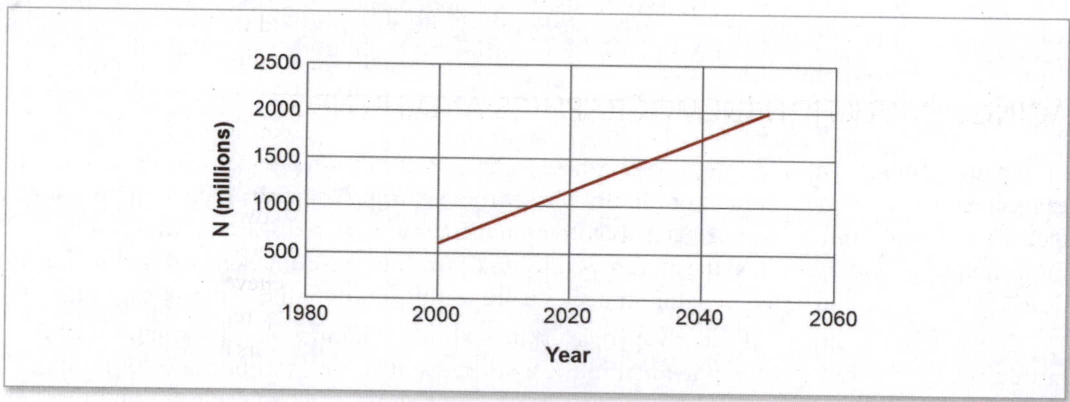

Fig. 15.3: Trends of aging (Global)

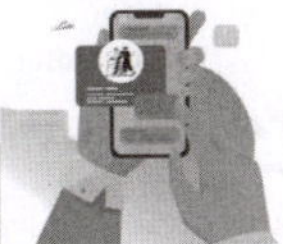
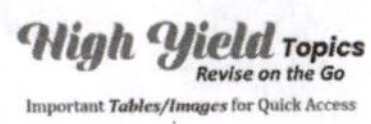

Normal Aging

Old age is subcategorized into three subgroups:

1.   Youngest-old: 65–74 years

2.   Middle-old: 75–84 years

3.   Oldest-old: 85 years and older

As a person grows older, they go through various stages of life. The process of getting aged is called aging. According to Riley, "Aging is defined as a lifelong process and entails maturation and change on physical, psychological, and social levels."[11] Every person experiences aging in their life. Aging is classified into two categories: Primary aging and secondary aging. Primary aging occurs due to cellular or molecular changes (biological factors). Secondary aging occurs due to external factors such as poor diet and lack of physical activity.[12]

Types of Age

*   **Chronological or physiological age:** This is nominal age which includes years, months, days, minutes, and seconds a person has been on the Earth.

*   **Biological age:** This is an age that can be measured *via* biomarkers on molecular and cellular levels.

*   **Psychological age:** This is a subjective age, not based on physicality, that is measured by emotional and logical maturity. Psychologists often use stage theories, which are developmental markers that most humans meet by a certain age, to determine this age.

*   **Social age:** This is the societal norm or expectation of behaviors associated with a certain age.

*   **Functional age:** With assessment materials, it is possible to quantify a person's age based on test results in the areas of biological, psychological, and social ages, in addition to chronological age. This professionally determined number is known as functional age.[13, 14]

Most humans experience changes related to aging after 50 years of age such as loosening of the skin, graying hair, and hair fall. After aging, the person's ability to perceive and memorize information declines. It's difficult for an old adult to memorize information, driving, reading, independence, and quality of life hampers after 60 years of age.

Theories of Aging

Modern biological theories of human aging can be broadly categorized into two groups: programmed and damage theories. Programmed theories suggest that aging follows a predetermined biological schedule, akin to the developmental stages of childhood. This process is believed to be influenced by changes in gene expression affecting systems responsible for maintenance, repair, and defense. On the other hand, damage theories emphasize the role of environmental stressors in causing cumulative damage to organisms at various levels, ultimately leading to aging.

Programmed theories encompass three subcategories:

1. Programmed longevity, which posits that aging results from the sequential activation and deactivation of specific genes.
2. Endocrine theory, which suggests that biological clocks regulate aging through hormonal mechanisms, particularly *via* the insulin/IGF-1 signaling pathway.
3. Immunological theory, which proposes that the immune system is genetically programmed to decline over time, rendering individuals more vulnerable to diseases and aging-related processes.

Damage theories include the wear-and-tear theory, which links aging to the gradual breakdown of vital body components due to repeated use; the rate-of-living theory, which correlates an organism's metabolic rate with its lifespan; the Cross-linking Theory, which implicates the accumulation of cross-linked proteins in cellular and tissue damage; the free radicals theory, which suggests that free radicals cause cellular damage leading to aging; and the somatic DNA damage theory, which highlights the role of accumulated DNA damage, particularly in nondividing cells, as a contributor to aging.

In summary, modern biological theories of aging in humans encompass programmed mechanisms regulated by genetic expression and environmental damage-induced processes. These theories offer insights into the complex interplay of factors contributing to the aging process, ranging from genetic regulation to cellular damage and dysfunction.[14–16]

Geriatric Consideration: Psychosocial Approach

The psychosocial development occurs at every stage of life. Personal needs fit with the needs of society through a complex relationship between the individual and society. The psychosocial development is influenced by personality, thinking, and behavior of a person.

For understanding psychosocial development there are two major theories: (1) Carl Jung theory of individualism (2) Erik Erikson psychosocial theory as shown in Table 15.1.

According to the theory of individualism, a person develops a unique personality during aging by balancing his own self and external world. When a person accepts his past, physical changes, limitation and accomplishments. While psychosocial theory states that a person needs to fulfil particular tasks at every stage of life. Erik divided life into eight stages.

1. **Infancy:** Trust versus mistrust, from birth to 18 months
2. **Toddlerhood:** Autonomy versus shame and doubt
3. **Preschool years:** Initiative versus guilt
4. **Early school years:** Industry versus inferiority
5. **Adolescence:** Identity versus role confusion
6. **Young adulthood:** Intimacy versus isolation
7. **Middle adulthood:** Generativity versus stagnation or self-absorption
8. **Late adulthood:** Ego integrity versus despair

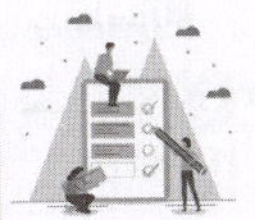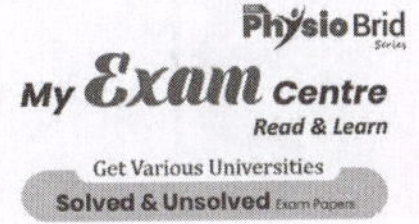

Refer to Table 15.1 to understand the different aspects of individualism and psychological theory.

Table 15.1: Different aspects of individualism and psychological theory

Aspect	Carl Jung's individualism theory	Erik Erikson's psychosocial theory
Focus	Focuses on the development of the individual's psyche and the process of individuation, striving toward self-realization and integration.	Focuses on the social and emotional development across the lifespan, emphasizing the influence of social interactions and culture.
Primary concepts	Archetypes, collective unconscious, introversion/extroversion, individuation.	Eight stages of psychosocial development, each characterized by a conflict to resolve.
Developmental stages	Doesn't propose specific stages of development but emphasizes personal growth and integration of the psyche throughout life.	Identifies eight stages of development, each associated with a psychosocial crisis or challenge.
Key contributions	Introduced the concepts of archetypes and the collective unconscious, emphasizing the importance of spiritual and symbolic dimensions of human experience.	Developed a comprehensive model of psychosocial development, highlighting the influence of social relationships and cultural context on individual growth.
Influence	Major influence in depth psychology, psychotherapy, and fields exploring the symbolic aspects of human experience.	Significant influence in developmental psychology, education, and clinical practice, particularly in understanding identity formation and lifespan development.
Application	Often applied in therapy and counseling to explore unconscious motivations, symbols, and personal growth.	Widely used in education, parenting, and clinical practice to understand and support individuals in navigating developmental challenges at various life stages.

Aging also affects Quality of Life (QOL). Health-related QOL and environment-related QOL both are influenced by aging. For example, cognitive impairment associated with dementia affects both health-related QOL (such as physical, mental, emotional, and social aspects) and environment-related QOL (such as economic dependency, capacity to form friends, etc.). Health-related QOL and environment-related QOL are correlated to each other.[17-19]

CHALLENGES FACED BY OLDER ADULTS AND TREATMENT STRATEGIES

Growing older is a normal and unavoidable process. Throughout life, a variety of changes occur that impact aging; however, not every individual experiences these changes in the same way.[20] For example, it's common for the senses to weaken, particularly vision and hearing. For some people, this weakness means wearing glasses or using a hearing aid, but for others, it might result in blindness or deafness. Numerous internal and external factors might impact the aging process.

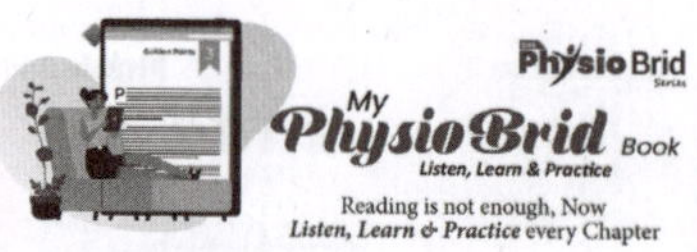

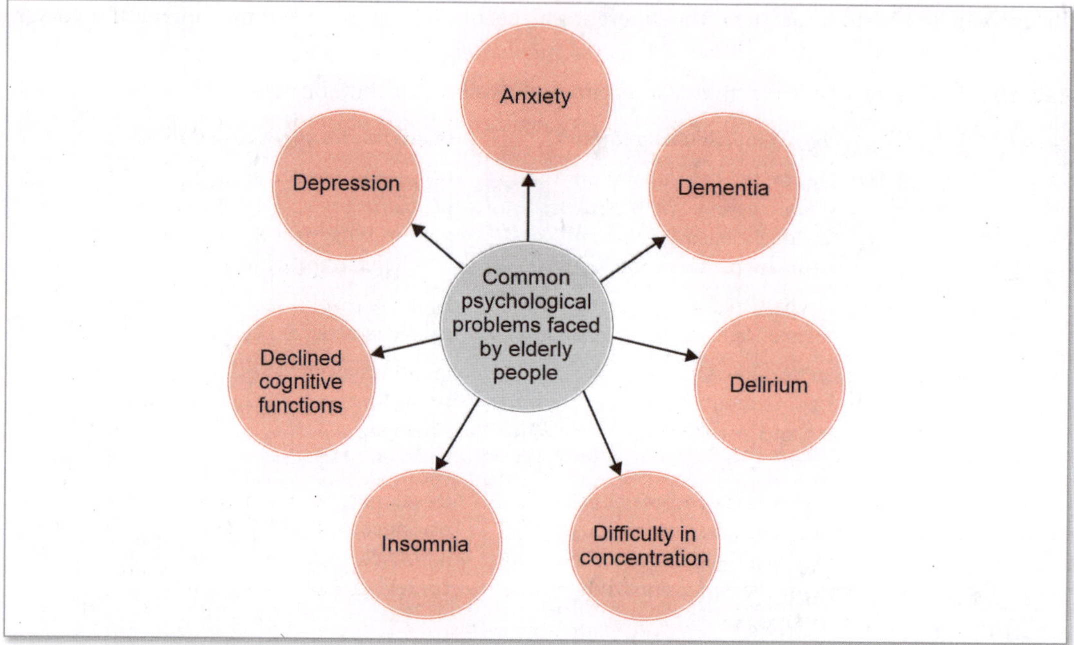

Fig. 15.4: The common psychological problems faced by elderly people

Factors such as frailty, chronic illnesses, lifestyle choices, and heredity are what ultimately determine an individual's age (Fig. 15.4). On the other hand, it is commonly known that a balanced diet and regular exercise help fend off devastating chronic illnesses like diabetes or cardiovascular disorders. Individuals frequently believe, for instance, that older individuals are losing their capacity to be mentally competent, senile, joyful, and socially engaged.[23]

Anxiety

Anxiety and fear are two normal emotions of human beings which help in protecting them from threatening situations. Our reactions to threats are: Fight, flight or freeze. Anxiety is a subjective feeling of uneasiness during stressful conditions. The overdriving of this alert while future threats or any stressful condition with an uncertain outcome is defined as an anxiety disorder. Anxiety disorder can be associated with the feeling of worry and nervousness. It can strike quickly or build up over days, weeks or even years.[21, 22]

Example: Many students feel uneasy the night before an exam. This is because an exam creates a stressful situation. You might also face this feeling. There's a lot of pressure to perform well, and the outcome (your score) is unknown. This mix of uncertainty and pressure generates fear night before

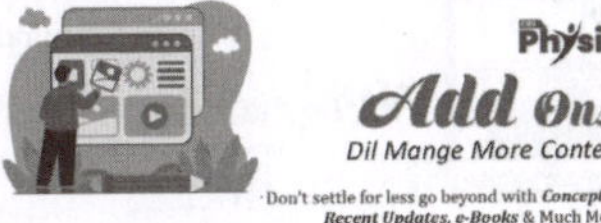

the exam. Because of a stressful condition (exam) with an uncertain outcome (your score) you are facing anxiety, but at the same time, you are facing fear due to the exam.

There are many different types of anxiety disorders, including generalized anxiety disorder (GAD), panic disorders, social anxiety, phobias, separation anxiety disorder (SAD), selective mutism, agoraphobia, Medicine-induced anxiety disorder, and anxiety disorder due to another medical condition.[23] Based on clinical features anxiety disorders can be classified into three categories:

1. Worry/distress anxiety disorder—GAD, PTSD, Acute stress disorder.

2. Fear anxiety disorder—panic disorder, phobia.

3. OCD

Anxiety disorders of the GAD kind are especially prevalent in the elderly population.[24] Clinical presentation of GAD is similar in young and older adults whereas the panic disorder in younger adults have more severe symptoms. In India, the estimated prevalence of concurrent anxiety varied from 0.3% in rural areas to 4.5% in metropolitan areas. However, in India, the estimation for very severe anxiety was only 0.2%, while the overall prevalence of severe anxiety was less than half 0.7%.[25] Anxiety in older adults is diagnosed based on the inability to control worries and the existence of three or more concomitant symptoms, such as tenseness in the muscles, restlessness, irritability, difficulties concentrating exhaustion, and insomnia.[23]

The GAD is an excessive or unreasonable anxiety. Triggers for this type of anxiety are unknown. GAD is difficult to control. Clinically GAD can be diagnosed if patient shows three symptoms out of the following six symptoms:

1. Restlessness

2. Fatigue

3. Irritability

4. Muscle tension

5. Difficulty in concentrating

6. Sleep disturbances

Assessment of anxiety includes detailed interview of the elder adult and history (medical, and family history, etc.) to diagnose anxiety disorder. There are some scales to assess the anxiety disorders shown in Table 15.2.

Table 15.2: Rating scales for assessing anxiety in geriatric population

Sl. no.	Self-reported	Multidimensional	Anxiety in depression
1.	Geriatric anxiety inventory	Hopkins symptom checklist (SCL-90 R)	Rating anxiety in dementia scale (RAID)
2.	Self-rating anxiety scale		BEHAV-AD
3.	State-trait anxiety inventory		NPI, NPI-Q

Choice of Intervention

Pharmacological approach includes drugs like SSRIs, SNRIs, buspirone, TCAs and benzodiazepines. Benzodiazepines are not a first line of drug their use is restricted in elders due to the additional adverse effect such as agitation and other neurocognitive effects. The dose in elders is lower or half than the dose in adults.[25]

Refer to Table 15.3 to know about the nonpharmacological approaches for anxiety.

Table 15.3: Nonpharmacological approaches for anxiety

Sl. no.	Recommended intervention
Behavior therapy	
1.	Relaxation therapy (such as Jacobson's technique, and Box breathing)
2.	Systemic desensitization
Cognitive therapy	
1.	Cognitive behavior therapy
Miscellaneous	
1.	Yoga, Tai Chai
2.	Music therapy
3.	Art therapy
4.	Cognitive rehabilitation
Physiotherapy and other modalities	
1.	Exercises
2.	Breathing exercises
3.	rTMS
4.	tDCS

Depression

Clinically depression or major depressive disorder or unipolar depression is a serious mental disorder characterized by persistent sadness and loss of interest in activities of daily living, for example, studying, bathing, eating, and sleeping. Factors causing depression are unknown but genetic, biological, environmental, and psychological factors can cause depression. Studies show people with family members having depression are at more risk. Depression is a leading cause of disability, for older people particularly susceptible to poor outcomes.[26] Depression in the elderly is linked with disability. Anxiety and functional and cognitive problems are more prevalent in older persons with depression than in young adults. Depression in older persons increases the risk of suicide and increases the likelihood that older adults may commit suicide.[27] Cognitive decline and a higher chance of dementia are linked to depression. Recommended intervention for depression is given in Table 15.4.[28]

Table 15.4: Recommended intervention for depression

Sl. no.	Recommended intervention
1.	Cognitive behavior therapy
2.	Problem-solving therapy
3.	Interpersonal psychotherapy
4.	Reminiscence therapy
5.	Brief dynamic therapy
6.	Exercise

MUST KNOW

In older adults, depression results in a lack of interest or lack of emotions rather than having a depressed or low mood as in younger adults. Men show anger other than sadness shown by women due to depression.

The assessment for depression includes a detailed history from the patient and the family members. The family members play a crucial role in history-taking and diagnosing the condition. Physical examination and mental status examination are important for the elimination of other conditions or finding any underlying condition.[27]

For cognitive assessment, MSME is used and DSM-5 and the Geriatric Depression Scale (GDS) are two major diagnostic tools used for the severity of the scale.[29]

CASE STUDY

Comprehensive Physiotherapy Approach for Mrs Smith: Addressing Osteoporosis, Fall-Related Anxiety, and Depression

Patient Background

Mrs Smith, a 75-year-old woman, was diagnosed with osteoporosis several years ago. Recently, she suffered a minor fall that led to a wrist fracture. Since the fall, Mrs Smith has become increasingly fearful of moving around, leading to decreased physical activity. This inactivity, combined with the stress of her condition, has contributed to the development of depression. Mrs Smith expresses feelings of hopelessness and a lack of motivation to engage in daily activities or socialize.

Physiotherapy Intervention
- **Assessment and goal setting:**
  - The physiotherapist conducts a comprehensive assessment of Mrs Smith's physical condition, including her bone density, muscle strength, and balance. They also consider her psychological state, recognizing the impact of depression on her willingness to participate in rehabilitation.
  - Together, they set realistic goals: Improving her mobility, reducing her fear of falling, and enhancing her overall quality of life.

Contd...

- **Customized exercise program:**
  - The physiotherapist designs a low-impact exercise program tailored to Mrs Smith's needs, focusing on weight-bearing activities to strengthen bones, gentle resistance training to build muscle, and balance exercises to prevent falls.
  - The exercises are introduced gradually, ensuring Mrs Smith feels comfortable and safe.
- **Addressing depression:**
  - Understanding the link between physical activity and mental health, the physiotherapist encourages Mrs Smith to engage in regular exercise, emphasizing its benefits for both her physical and emotional well-being.
  - The therapist incorporates motivational techniques, such as setting small, achievable goals and celebrating progress, to help Mrs Smith overcome her feelings of hopelessness.
- **Education and empowerment:**
  - Mrs Smith is educated about osteoporosis and the importance of staying active to manage her condition. This knowledge helps reduce her fear of movement.
  - The physiotherapist also provides guidance on safe movements and fall prevention strategies, which boosts Mrs Smith's confidence in her ability to stay independent.
- **Ongoing support and collaboration:**
  - The physiotherapist maintains regular sessions with Mrs Smith to monitor her progress, adjust the exercise plan as needed, and provide continuous encouragement.
  - Collaboration with a psychologist or counselor is suggested to address the depression more directly, ensuring a holistic approach to Mrs Smith's care.

Outcomes

Over time, Mrs Smith begins to regain her strength and mobility, which helps to reduce her fear of falling. The structured exercise routine also contributes to an improvement in her mood, as she starts to feel more in control of her health and more optimistic about her future. The combination of physical and psychological support allows Mrs Smith to lead a more active and fulfilling life, despite her osteoporosis and initial depression.

Insomnia

The most prevalent sleep disorder among elderly persons is insomnia. Insomnia is characterized by complaints of problems falling asleep, staying asleep or waking up early and not being able to go back to sleep despite having enough sleep opportunities or the perfect environment. These symptoms persist at least three times per week. Insomnia affects the quality and quantity of sleep which results in developing feelings of daytime sleepiness and fatigue. With time person's personal or professional life starts getting affected due to the development of anxiety and depression. Among older adults, the chances of either temporary or permanent cognitive damage were raised by insomnia as compared to older persons without insomnia. In older adults, persistent sleeplessness symptoms have also been linked to poor mental health or various psychological conditions. Depression was substantially correlated with symptoms of insomnia, particularly trouble falling asleep as opposed to problems staying asleep or early morning awakenings. In older men, ongoing trouble sleeping by itself predicts a decline in cognitive abilities. Insomnia can result from underlying conditions such as pulmonary disease, psychiatric conditions or the overuse of caffeine (stimulant) or alcohol (depressant).[30, 31]

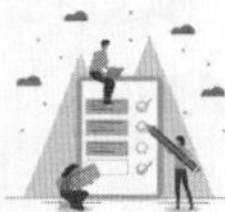
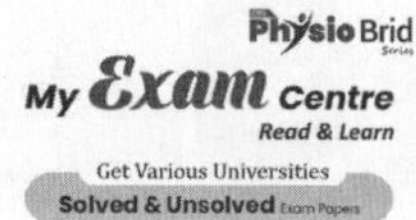

Pharmacological approach includes melatonin agonists and nonbenzodiazepine sedatives. Some drugs are low-dose doxepin, suvorexant, Z-drugs (eszopiclone, zaleplon, zolpidem), benzodiazepines, and ramelteon. Sometimes benzodiazepines are also used. Nonpharmacological interventions for insomnia include stimulus control in which the patient is asked to use his/her bed only for sleeping (Table 15.5).[32] Remove bright lights and minimize noise during sleeping if having trouble in sleep then they can use eye covers and ear plugs (Table 15.5).[31]

Table 15.5: Other nonpharmacological approaches

Sl. no.	Recommended intervention
Behavior therapy	
1.	Relaxation therapy (such as Jacobson's technique, and Box breathing)
2.	Cognitive behavior therapy
3.	Scents
4.	Sleep hygiene
5.	**Nutrition:** Avoid caffeine in the evenings, avoid alcohol consumption and heavy meals
Physiotherapy and other modalities	
1.	Breathing exercises
2.	Virtual reality
3.	Resistance and aerobic exercise
Sleep restriction therapy	

Physio CORNER

Geropsychology and physiotherapy are two fields that intersect significantly when it comes to the care of older adults. Geropsychology is the branch of psychology that focuses on the mental health and well-being of older adults, addressing issues such as cognitive decline, depression, anxiety, and the psychological impact of aging. Physiotherapy, on the other hand, involves the assessment and treatment of physical impairments, pain, and mobility issues, often prevalent in the elderly due to conditions like arthritis, osteoporosis, and general physical deconditioning.

Intersection of Geropsychology and Physiotherapy

- **Understanding the psychological impact of aging:**
  - **Cognitive decline:** As people age, they may experience cognitive decline, including memory loss and reduced problem-solving abilities. This can affect their ability to follow physiotherapy routines, remember exercises or stay motivated during rehabilitation. A physiotherapist working with older adults must consider these cognitive changes and adapt their treatment plans accordingly.
  - **Depression and anxiety:** Older adults often face significant life changes, such as retirement, loss of loved ones, and decreased independence, which can lead to depression and anxiety. These mental health issues can impact their physical health and their ability to engage in physiotherapy. Understanding and addressing these psychological factors can help improve the effectiveness of physiotherapy.

Contd...

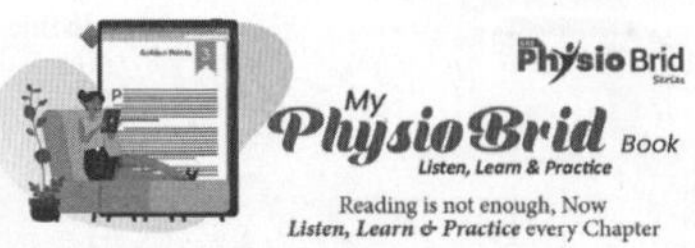

- **Motivation and compliance:**
  - **Motivation issues:** Older adults may struggle with motivation to participate in physiotherapy due to feelings of hopelessness or apathy, often related to depression or the belief that they cannot regain their previous levels of function. Geropsychology can help identify these barriers, and techniques such as motivational interviewing can be used to enhance engagement.
  - **Enhancing compliance:** Geropsychological interventions can improve adherence to physiotherapy programs by addressing mental health issues, promoting positive attitudes toward aging, and helping older adults set realistic goals for their physical health.

- **Managing chronic pain:**
  - **Psychological impact of chronic pain:** Chronic pain is common in older adults and can have a profound impact on their psychological well-being. It can lead to increased anxiety, depression, and social isolation, which in turn can reduce their participation in physiotherapy. Geropsychology provides strategies to manage the psychological effects of chronic pain, such as cognitive-behavioral therapy (CBT), which can be integrated into physiotherapy sessions.
  - **Pain management strategies:** Physiotherapists can work with geropsychologists to implement pain management strategies that include both physical exercises and psychological techniques, such as relaxation training and mindfulness, to reduce pain perception and improve overall quality of life.

- **Addressing fear of falling:**
  - **Fear of falling:** Many older adults develop a fear of falling, which can lead to reduced activity levels, loss of independence, and a decrease in physical function. This fear can be both a psychological and physical barrier to effective physiotherapy. Geropsychologists can help by providing cognitive-behavioral interventions to reduce fear and anxiety, while physiotherapists focus on balance training and strengthening exercises.
  - **Building confidence:** Both geropsychology and physiotherapy can work together to build the confidence of older adults, encouraging them to move more freely and engage in activities that they might otherwise avoid due to fear.

- **Holistic care approach:**
  - **Integrating mental and physical health:** A holistic approach to care, integrating geropsychology and physiotherapy, ensures that both the mental and physical health of older adults are addressed. This can lead to better outcomes, as physical improvements often lead to better mental health, and vice versa.
  - **Interdisciplinary collaboration:** Collaboration between geropsychologists and physiotherapists is essential for creating comprehensive care plans that address the multifaceted needs of older adults. Regular communication between these professionals ensures that the care provided is cohesive and supportive of the patient's overall well-being.

- **Promoting independence and quality of life:**
  - **Fostering independence:** The goal of both geropsychology and physiotherapy is often to promote independence in older adults. While physiotherapy focuses on maintaining or improving physical function, geropsychology addresses the psychological factors that contribute to a sense of autonomy and control over one's life.
  - **Improving quality of life:** By addressing both physical and psychological aspects of aging, the combined efforts of geropsychology and physiotherapy can significantly enhance the quality of life for older adults, helping them maintain a positive outlook and active lifestyle.

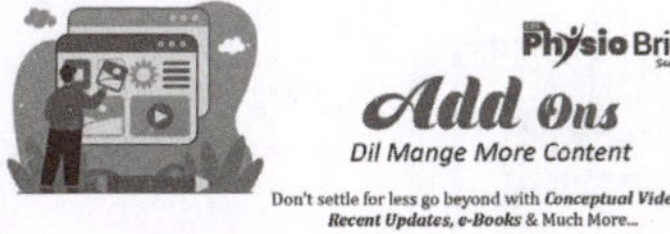

RECENT APPROACHES

Figure 15.5 shows recent modalities for mental disorders.

Electroconvulsive Therapy

Electroconvulsive therapy (ECT) is a commonly used treatment option in patients with major depressive disorder (MDD) or other psychiatric disorder that has not responded to drugs or other therapeutic options. Under anesthetic condition, ECT is applied to the patient and involves a short electrical stimulation of brain to create the generalized seizure of cerebral origin.[33] The therapeutic effects of ECT on neurotransmitters, particularly to the serotonin and dopamine systems. According to an alternative concept, depression is a proinflammatory state that can be managed using ECT by acting on cytokines, which helps in normalizing the mood. Additionally, clinical data suggests that ECT induces a brief permeability of the blood-brain barrier due to a hypertensive surge, which could potentially contribute to its therapeutic impact.[34] According to research on animals, electrically generated seizures may have epigenetic effects that increase the therapeutic efficacy of ECT. Lastly, it seems that ECT-induced modifications to structural brain plasticity are the most encouraging recent discoveries. Recent research has also shown that ECT strongly stimulates neurogenesis by encouraging stem cell multiplication and helps in depression.[35, 36]

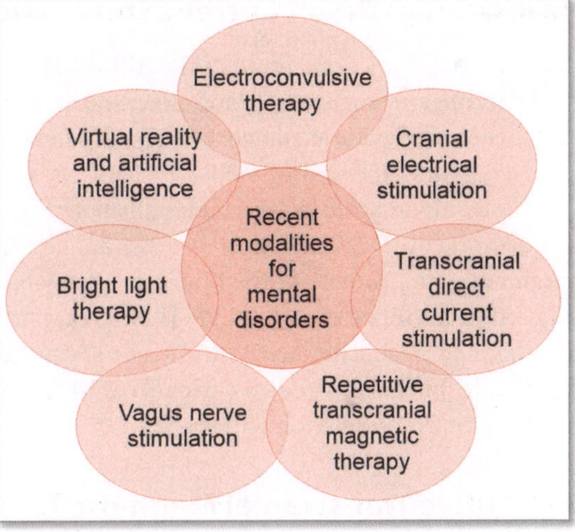

Fig. 15.5: Recent modalities for mental disorders

Cranial Electrical Stimulation

Cranial electrical stimulation (CES) is a noninvasive method of applying low-intensity current to the head of the subject. The use of CES has been increased recently to change the brain function and treat diseases like depression, anxiety, and insomnia. The CES alters the physics of the brain (electrical activities) as well as the chemistry of brain (neurotransmitters), researches have shown CES can significantly help in treating anxiety, insomnia, depression, and pain; while avoiding serious adverse effects and risks (e.g., cardiovascular complications), as compared to other interventions such as electroconvulsive therapy (ECT) and transcranial magnetic stimulation (TMS). The CES is also neurostimulation for normalizing brain activity, and in contrast, is a more cost-effective, noninvasive type of device that can be safely used by patients at home. It is being used as an adjunct to medication or psychotherapy or as a stand-alone treatment. Based on an increasing body of evidence, brain stimulation that is available now is expected to be part of the armamentarium of most psychiatrists by 2030 (George, 2019; Nasrallah, 2009).[37–40]

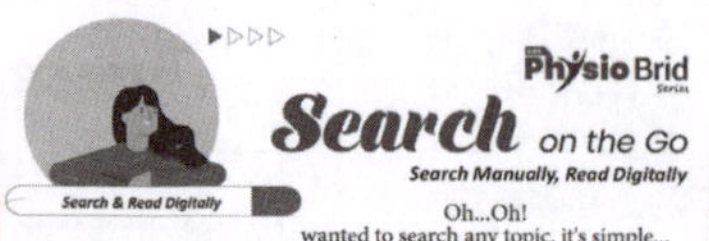

Transcranial Direct Current Stimulation

Transcranial direct current stimulation (tDCS) is a noninvasive neuromodulation technique that modifies resting membrane potential hyperpolarization or depolarization to control cortical excitability and neural network activity. There is an imbalance in dorsolateral prefrontal cortex (DLPFC) function on both sides in patients with depression due to weaker left DLPFC activity, decreased blood flow, delayed metabolism, and abnormally elevated right DLPFC activity. Therefore, the cathode of tDCS can be used to stimulate the right DLPFC to suppress its excitability, thereby modulating the activity of the brain's emotional loop and reducing depression, while the anode can be used to stimulate the left DLPFC to increase its excitability. Common side effects include burning, itching, and headaches are typically not severe enough to have a long-term impact. tDCS is more affordable, portable, safe, user-friendly, and has a significant therapeutic potential when compared to other neuromodulation techniques.[41, 42]

Repetitive Transcranial Magnetic Therapy

Repetitive transcranial magnetic therapy (rTMS) is a noninvasive brain stimulation technique that utilizes rapidly changing magnetic fields to induce electrical fields in targeted brain regions. This technique can modulate cortical excitability and is a potential approach for the treatment of neuropsychiatric disorders. The effectiveness of rTMS depends on various parameters such as cortical target, number of sessions, duration, frequency, intensity, age, disease, and medications. High-frequency rTMS (HF-rTMS) may increase cortical excitability, while low-frequency rTMS (LF-rTMS) reduces cortical excitability.[43]

Studies have shown that rTMS targeting the left dorsolateral prefrontal cortex (DLPFC) has a positive impact on posttraumatic stress disorder (PTSD) and treatment-resistant depression. The US Food and Drug Administration (FDA) approved rTMS for the treatment of MDD in 2008. Then in 2013 and 2018, rTMS received FDA approval for the treatment of chronic pain and obsessive-compulsive disorder (OCD), respectively. Additionally, rTMS can be used as the treatment of post-traumatic stress disorder (PTSD), Tourette's disorder, schizophrenia, tinnitus, and Parkinson's disease.

Generally, rTMS is considered a safe treatment, however, has some side effects such as headache, toothache, and neck pain. It is recommended that patients with certain metallic implants should not undergo rTMS treatment. rTMS targeting the left dorsolateral prefrontal cortex with a frequency of 10–20 Hz can be used for the treatment of pharmacoresistant depression and PTSD.[44, 45]

Vagus Nerve Stimulation

The vagus nerve is the longest cranial nerve and connects the brainstem with various organs throughout the body. Vagus nerve stimulation (VNS) has emerged as a therapeutic approach for the treatment of various diseases by applying electrical pulses. In 1988, the VNS was first used for the treatment-resistant epilepsy. Latterly, the FDA approved VNS in 1997 for adults and later in

2017 for children over 4 years. Studies suggest VNS may even reduce the risk of sudden unexpected death in epilepsy (SUDEP). The exact mechanism is not well known, however, it is believed that VNS interrupts the normalize electrical activity within the brain which is responsible for seizures. Animal models suggest that VNS can stop seizures and decrease their frequency. Additionally, VNS may modulate neurotransmitters such as serotonin and norepinephrine, which play an important role in seizure control. In 2005, VNS received FDA approval for treatment-resistant depression. A study had shown that VNS improved mood scores in patients who did not respond to conventional antidepressant drugs. The mechanism through which VNS treats depression is still under research.

The vagus nerve carries information about inflammatory processes throughout the body therefore VNS is a promising approach for the treatment of various conditions beyond epilepsy and depression. VNS may modulate this communication, offering potential benefits in managing inflammatory conditions. Therefore, studies are actively investigating the use of VNS for diabetes, sepsis, cardiovascular diseases, Alzheimer's, chronic pain, inflammatory bowel disease, and rheumatoid arthritis.

Transcutaneous auricular vagus nerve stimulation (taVNS) is a noninvasive approach which delivers electrical stimulation directly to the auricular branch of the vagus nerve. This method can be used in the management of pain and migraines. There are two types of taVNS, (1) Respiratory-gated Auricular Vagal Afferent Nerve Stimulation (RAVANS), and (2) Motor Activated Auricular Vagus Nerve Stimulation (MAAVNS).[46–48]

Bright Light Therapy

Bright light therapy (BLT) is a noninvasive therapy that treats a range of physiological and psychological issues by exposing patients to intense, artificial light. BLT entails sitting close to a specially made light box that simulates ambient sunlight by emitting bright light, usually 10,000 lux. Because of its ability to improve mood, regulate circadian rhythms, and lessen the symptoms of some mental health conditions, it has become more well-known in professional settings. The treatment activates the brain's suprachiasmatic nucleus, which controls circadian rhythms. It affects the synthesis of serotonin and melatonin, two chemicals essential for mood and sleep control. It is believed that BLT will have positive effects in patients with seasonal affective disorder (SAD), nonseasonal depression, sleep disorders, circadian rhythm disorders, insomnia, bipolar disorder, anxiety disorders, dementia, cognitive decline and sundowning syndrome. It is a drug-free therapy with minimal side effects and patients can be guided for self-administration at home. It provides substantial advantages for mental health and general well-being when used and monitored appropriately.[58, 59]

Virtual Reality and Artificial Intelligence

Virtual reality (VR) and artificial intelligence (AI) are integrating innovative technologies into psychology in order to improve the manner in which mental health diseases are treated. VR incorporates near-real-time computer visuals, voices and other sensory feedback to create a device created environment with which the individuals can engage. VR helps to generate therapeutically beneficial scenarios that are practically impossible to replicate in the real world. Numerous VR applications have been created to serve use in the mental well-being field including programs for the rehabilitation of specific phobias such as anxiety of flying, fear of extremes including rehabilitation of attention deficit disorder, post-traumatic stress disorder and test anxiety. To contribute in the cognitive assessment and in providing rehabilitation in cases with traumatic brain injury, dementia, stroke and schizophrenia, several VR tasks have also been developed.[60, 61] Simulating human cognitive processes is the goal of AI. Owing to the rapid advancement of methods for analytics and the growing availability of healthcare data, it is bringing about a paradigm shift in the healthcare industry. AI has several roles in healthcare profession such as various medical research and drug discovery, virtual patient healthcare, administrative applications, rehabilitation patient engagement and compliance, medical imaging and diagnostic services.[62, 63]

PSYCHOLOGICAL ASPECTS OF SPECIFIC CONDITIONS

Physiotherapist deals with the geriatric patient in clinical settings. The most common conditions where psychological approach can be used are as follows:

- **Pain management and psychological approach:** Pain management is a multidisciplinary approach to reduce the pain and help the patient by improving the QOL.[49] It includes the use of drugs combined with the alternative approach such as relaxation methods, patient education/ counseling, Cognitive behavior therapy, physiotherapy, biofeedback and social support methods.[50]

  In pain management the detailed assessment of pain is necessary it includes: Pain intensity, duration, site and onset of pain. Functionality is also an important consideration. The intensity and severity of pain can be influenced by the cognitive, behavioral, and environmental factors i.e., a person is feeling how much pain, how he is dealing with the pain and how the weather or other environmental factors are influencing the pain.[51]

- **Fall management and psychological approach:** It is one of the major incidents that cause musculoskeletal injuries. It is second leading cause of unintentional injuries and death globally. Factors responsible for fall are given in Figure 15.6. Geriatric population is high-risk population for fall. In geriatric population, the correlation between falls and fear of fall has been demonstrated in various studies. Fear of falling may cause fall and may be associated with cognitive impairments such as anxiety, depression, and balance confidence or fall efficacy. Anxiety is also correlated with balance and gait performance.[52–54]

- The most common symptom presented by the geriatric population is alteration of memory. Dementia and delirium are the most common syndrome and both terms are used interchangeably but having different symptoms, prognosis and management[55] (Table 15.6).

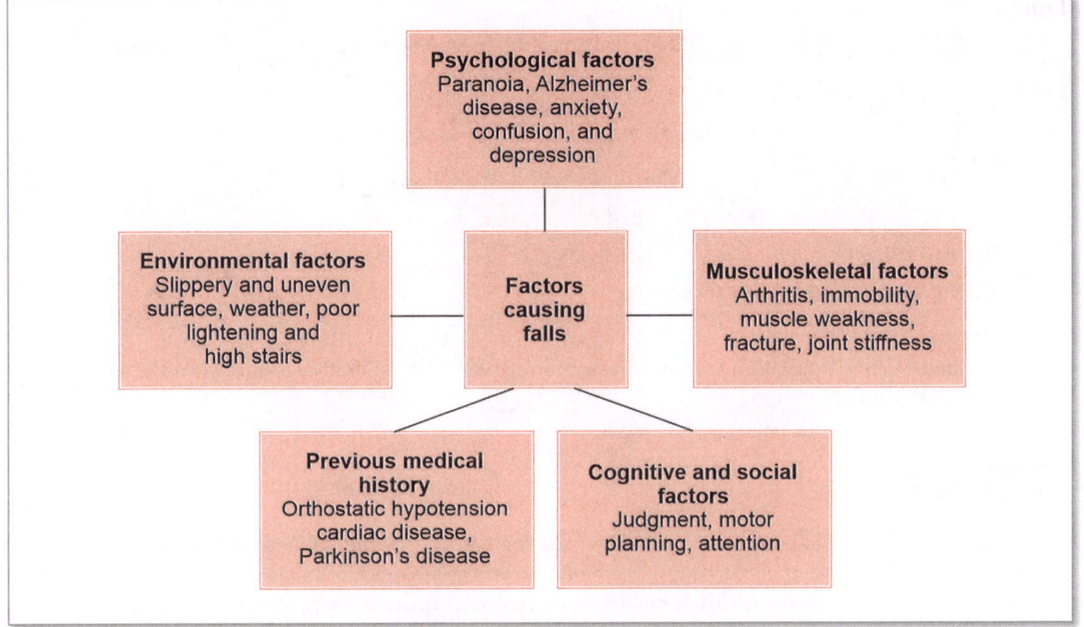

Fig. 15.6: Factors responsible for fall

Table 15.6: Comparison between delirium and dementia

Delirium	Versus	Dementia
Rapid (hours to days)	O — Onset	Insidious (months to years)
Fluctuating	C — Course	Progressive
Reversible	D — Duration	Irreversible
Altered	C — Consciousness	Often normal
Decline	A — Attention	Often normal
Immediate recall memory impaired	M — Memory	Immediate recall memory often normal
Hyperactive or hypoactive	P — Psychomotor changes	Often normal
Often reversed	S — Sleep cycle	Often normal

According to WHO, "Dementia refers to a clinical syndrome characterized by progressive cognitive decline that interferes with the ability to function independently",[56] whereas "Delirium is a global cerebral dysfunction that affects consciousness, attention, thinking, perception, memory, emotion, and the sleep-wake cycle. It can also cause changes in behavior, judgment, muscle control, and hallucinations."[57] Care considerations are given in Table 15.7.

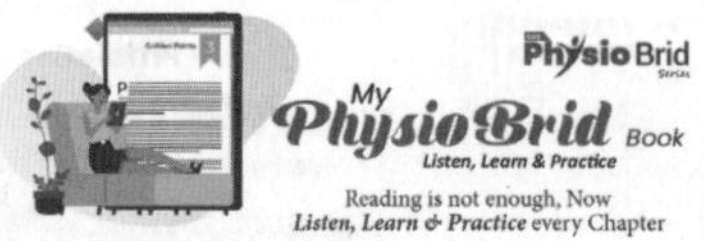

Table 15.7: The care giving considerations

Care considerations
Maintain/Provide a safe environment to the patient. Show affection.
Make patient feel safe; for example: Don't forget to knock or announce yourself before entering.
Avoid restrains
Use short, simple sentence in calm and clear voice.
Use positive commands.
Encourage family to bring familiar objects.
Give time to speak or respond.
Interventions: Such as Relaxation therapy, music therapy, validation therapy, reminiscence therapy, activity therapy, and pet therapy.

SUMMARY

- Geriatric psychology is branch of psychology that focuses on the mental and physical health of older adults. As the global population ages, the demand for psychological services among older persons is on the rise, presenting a significant challenge to the psychology profession. Geropsychology aims to address this growing need by providing specialized care that caters to the unique psychological and physiological changes associated with aging.
- The aging process is a natural part of life, characterized by a multitude of changes that affect an individual physically, mentally, and socially. These changes can have profound implications on one's quality of life, making it crucial to understand and address them effectively. The chapter begins by outlining the demographic trends of the aging population, emphasizing the increasing number of elderly individuals globally and the challenges this poses to healthcare systems.
  - **Normal aging:** The chapter discusses the various stages of old age and the different types of aging, including primary and secondary aging. It also explores the concept of aging from multiple perspectives: Chronological, biological, psychological, social, and functional.
  - **Psychosocial development:** Drawing on theories by Carl Jung and Erik Erikson, the chapter examines how aging affects an individual's personality and social interactions. It highlights the importance of psychosocial development in maintaining a healthy quality of life in older adults.
  - **Anxiety disorders:** The chapter provides an in-depth look at the prevalence, diagnosis, and treatment of anxiety disorders in older adults. It discusses various types of anxiety disorders and their impact on daily life. Treatment options for anxiety, including pharmacological and nonpharmacological approaches, are explored.
  - **Depression:** As a leading cause of disability in older adults, depression is thoroughly examined. The chapter discusses risk factors, symptoms, diagnosis, and various treatment approaches, including pharmacotherapy, cognitive behavior therapy, and interpersonal psychotherapy.
  - **Insomnia:** The most prevalent sleep disorder among the elderly, insomnia, is discussed in detail. The chapter covers its causes, impact on physical and mental health, and treatment options, including pharmacological interventions and nonpharmacological approaches such as sleep hygiene and relaxation techniques.

Contd...

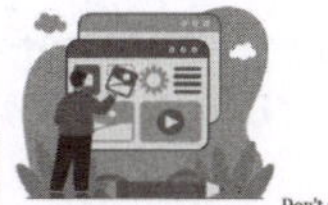
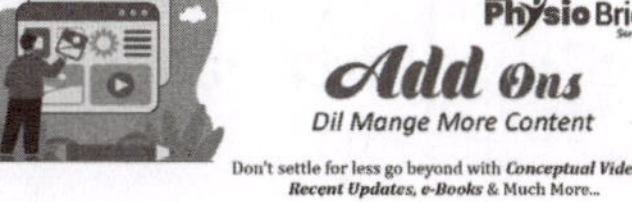

- The recent advancements in the treatment of psychological conditions in the geriatric population, focus on noninvasive brain stimulation techniques. These include:
  - **Cranial electrical stimulation (CES):** A noninvasive method that applies low-intensity current to the head to alter brain function and treat conditions like depression, anxiety, and insomnia.
  - **Transcranial direct current stimulation (tDCS):** A technique that modifies cortical excitability by applying a weak electrical current to the scalp.
  - **Repetitive transcranial magnetic stimulation (rTMS):** A noninvasive brain stimulation technique that uses magnetic fields to induce electrical currents in the brain, showing promise in treating depression and other disorders.
  - **Vagus nerve stimulation (VNS):** An approach that involves applying electrical pulses to the vagus nerve to modulate brain activity, with potential benefits for epilepsy, depression, and other conditions.
- The role of physiotherapists is managing pain, falls, and geriatric syndromes like dementia and delirium. It emphasizes the importance of a multidisciplinary approach to care, integrating physiotherapeutic and psychological interventions to improve the overall well-being of older adults.

REFERENCES

1. Stott DJ, Lowe GD, editors. Cardiovascular Disease and Health in the Older Patient: Expanded from' Pathy's Principles and Practice of Geriatric Medicine. John Wiley & Sons, Chichester, UK; 2012.
2. Makwana, G. The Growing Need of Geropsychological Intervention in Older Adults. International Journal of Indian Psychology; 2022;10(4):01–10.
3. Hinrichsen GA, et al. Guidelines for psychological practice with older adults. Am Psychol. 2014;69(1):34–65.
4. Jacobs ML, Bamonti PM. Clinical practice: A foundational geropsychology knowledge competency. Clinical Psychology: Science and Practice. 2022;29(1):28–42.
5. Magnus G. The age of aging: How demographics are changing the global economy and our world. John Wiley & Sons, Chichester, UK; 2012;27(1):10.
6. World Health Organization. World report on ageing and health. World Health Organization; 2015.
7. Montgomery R, Rowe J, Kosloski K. Family caregiving. In: Blackburn J Dulmus C Handbook of gerontology: Evidence-based approaches to theory, practice, and policy. John Wiley & Sons, New York, NY. 2007: 426–454
8. Prince MJ, Wu F, Guo Y, Robledo LM, O'Donnell M, Sullivan R, Yusuf S. The burden of disease in older people and implications for health policy and practice. The lancet. 2015;385(9967):549–62.
9. Dijkman B, Roodbol P, Aho J, Achtschin-Stieger S, Andruszkiewicz A, Coffey A et al. European Core Competences Framework for Health and Social Care Professionals Working with Older People. ELLAN, 2016. p. 43.
10. Wan Ahmad, W. I., Komang Astina, I., & Budijanto. Demographic transition and population ageing. Mediterranean Journal of Social Sciences. 2015:6(3);213–218
11. Riley, Matilda White. "Aging, Social Change, and the Power of Ideas." Daedalus 1978:107:39–52.
12. Whitbourne SK, Whitbourne SB. Adult development and aging: Biopsychosocial perspectives. John Wiley & Sons; 2010.

Contd...

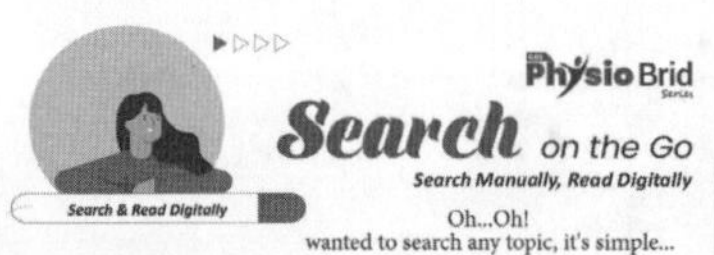

13. Séguy I, Courgeau D, Caussinus H, Buchet L. Chronological age, social age and biological age. Historical demography and paleodemography. 2019:1–7.

14. Payne W. Aging and Ableness. Human Behavior and the Social Environment II. 2020.

15. Kochman K. New elements in modern biological theories of aging. Medical Research Journal. 2015;3(3):89–99.

16. Lim K. Why did Psychologist Carl Jung have concern for Adult Development?: Educational Analysis Based on Erik Erikson. Journal of Christian Education & Information Technology. 2005;8:237–59.

17. Stein M. Individuation. The handbook of Jungian psychology 2012; 12:196–214.

18. Maree JG. The psychosocial development theory of Erik Erikson: Critical overview. The Influence of Theorists and Pioneers on Early Childhood Education. 2022:119–33.

19. Whitbourne SK. The aging body: Physiological changes and psychological consequences. Springer New York; 2012.

20. Steimer T. The biology of fear-and anxiety-related behaviors. Dialogues in clinical neuroscience. 2002;4(3):231–49.

21. LeDoux JE, Pine DS. Using neuroscience to help understand fear and anxiety: A two-system framework. American journal of psychiatry. 2016;173(11):1083–93.

22. Tuma AH, Maser JD, editors. Anxiety and the anxiety disorders. Routledge New York; 2019.

23. Guerin B, Hoorens S, Khodyakov D, Yaqub O. A growing and ageing population. Global societal trends to. 2015; 2030:1–55.

24. Elias SM. Prevalence of loneliness, anxiety, and depression among older people living in long-term care: A review. International Journal of Care Scholars. 2018;1(1):39–43.

25. Subramanyam AA, Kedare J, Singh OP, Pinto C. Clinical practice guidelines for geriatric anxiety disorders. Indian journal of psychiatry. 2018;60: S371–82.

26. Prina, A. M., Ferri, C. P., Guerra, M., Brayne, C., & Prince, M. Prevalence of anxiety and its correlates among older adults in Latin America, India and China: Cross-cultural study. British Journal of Psychiatry. 2011:199(6);485–491.

27. Arthur, A., Savva, G. M., Barnes, L. E., Borjian-Boroojeny, A., Dening, T., et al. Changing prevalence and treatment of depression among older people over two decades. British Journal of Psychiatry. 2011:343(1);49–54.

28. Rodda, J., Walker, Z., & Carter, J. Depression in older adults. BMJ. 2011:343(7825).

29. Avasthi A, Grover S. Clinical practice guidelines for management of depression in elderly. Indian journal of psychiatry. 2018;60: S341–62.

30. Patel D, Steinberg J, Patel P. Insomnia in the elderly: A review. Journal of Clinical Sleep Medicine. 2018;14(6):1017–24.

31. Milne S, Elkins MR. Exercise as an alternative treatment for chronic insomnia. British Journal of Sports Medicine. 2017;51(5):479–80.

32. Guerin B, Hoorens S, Khodyakov D, Yaqub O. A growing and ageing population. Global societal trends to. 2015;2030:1–55.

33. Abrams R. Electroconvulsive therapy. Oxford University Press; 2002; p. 328.

34. Guloksuz S, Rutten BP, Arts B, van Os J, Kenis G. The immune system and electroconvulsive therapy for depression. The journal of ECT. 2014;30(2):132–7.

35. Gazdag G, Ungvari GS. Electroconvulsive therapy: 80-year-old and still going strong. World journal of psychiatry. 2019;9(1):1.

Contd...

36. Gyger L, Regen F, Ramponi C, Marquis R, Mall JF, Swierkosz-Lenart K et al. Gradient of electro-convulsive therapy's antidepressant effects along the longitudinal hippocampal axis. Translational psychiatry. 2021;11(1):191.

37. Price L, Briley J, Haltiwanger S, Hitching R. A meta-analysis of cranial electrotherapy stimulation in the treatment of depression. Journal of psychiatric research. 2021; 135:119–34.

38. Van Rooij SJ, Riva-Posse P, McDonald WM. The efficacy and safety of neuromodulation treatments in late-life depression. Current treatment options in psychiatry. 2020; 7:337–48.

39. George MS. Whither TMS: A one-trick pony or the beginning of a neuroscientific revolution? American Journal of Psychiatry. 2019;176(11):904–10.

40. Nasrallah HA. Psychiatry's future is here. Current Psychiatry. 2009; 8:18–9.

41. Stein DJ, Fernandes Medeiros L, Caumo W, Torres IL. Transcranial direct current stimulation in patients with anxiety: Current perspectives. Neuropsychiatric Disease and Treatment. 2020:161–9.

42. Tortella G, Casati R, Aparicio LV, Mantovani A, Senço N, D'Urso G et al. Transcranial direct current stimulation in psychiatric disorders. World Journal of Psychiatry. 2015;5(1):88–102.

43. Mann SK, Malhi NK. Repetitive Transcranial Magnetic Stimulation. In: StatPearls. StatPearls Publishing, Treasure Island (FL); 2023. PMID: 33760474. Transcranial magnetic stimulation. 2021.

44. Hoogendam JM, Ramakers GM, Di Lazzaro V. Physiology of repetitive transcranial magnetic stimulation of the human brain. Brain stimulation. 2010;3(2):95–118.

45. Guse B, Falkai P, Wobrock T. Cognitive effects of high-frequency repetitive transcranial magnetic stimulation: A systematic review. Journal of neural transmission. 2010; 117(1):105–22.

46. Mandalaneni K, Rayi A. Vagus Nerve Stimulator. In: StatPearls. StatPearls Publishing, Treasure Island (FL); 2023. 32965846.

47. Ohemeng KK, Parham K. Vagal Nerve Stimulation: Indications, Implantation, and Outcomes. Otolaryngol Clin North Am. 2020;53(1):127–143.

48. Johnson RL, Wilson CG. A review of vagus nerve stimulation as a therapeutic intervention. J Inflamm Res. 2018; 11:203–213.

49. Takahashi N, Takatsuki K, Kasahara S, Yabuki S. Multidisciplinary pain management program for patients with chronic musculoskeletal pain in Japan: A cohort study. J Pain Res. 2019; 12:2563–2576.

50. Styles MH. In search of relief: Self-care strategies for clients with chronic pain Doctoral dissertation, Lethbridge, Alta.: University of Lethbridge, Faculty of Education. 2012.

51. Asmundson GJ, Gomez-Perez L, Richter AA, Carleton RN. The psychology of pain: Models and targets for comprehensive assessment. 2014.

52. Allan LM, Ballard CG, Rowan EN, Kenny RA. Incidence and prediction of falls in dementia: A prospective study in older people. PloS one. 2009;4(5): e5521.

53. Tinetti ME, Speechley M, Ginter SF. Risk factors for falls among elderly persons living in the community. New England journal of medicine. 1988;319(26):1701–7.

54. Anstey KJ, Von Sanden C, Luszcz MA. An 8-year prospective study of the relationship between cognitive performance and falling in very old adults. Journal of the American Geriatrics Society. 2006;54(8):1169–76.

55. Han JH, Suyama J. Delirium and dementia. Clinics in geriatric medicine. 2018;34(3):327–54.

56. Chertkow H, Feldman HH, Jacova C, Massoud F. Definitions of dementia and predementia states in Alzheimer's disease and vascular cognitive impairment: Consensus from the Canadian conference on diagnosis of dementia. Alzheimer's research & therapy. 2013; 5 (Suppl 1): S2.

Contd...

57. Kaplan PW. Delirium and epilepsy. Dialogues in clinical neuroscience. 2003;5(2):187–200.

58. Chen G, Chen P, Yang Z, Ma W, Yan H, Su T, Zhang Y, Qi Z, Fang W, Jiang L, Chen Z. Increased functional connectivity between the midbrain and frontal cortex following bright light therapy in subthreshold depression: A randomized clinical trial. American Psychologist. 2024 Apr;79(3):437.

59. Cheng DC, Ganner JL, Gordon CJ, Phillips CL, Grunstein RR, Comas M. The efficacy of combined bright light and melatonin therapies on sleep and circadian outcomes: A systematic review. Sleep Medicine Reviews. 2021 Aug 1; 58:101491.

60. Lynsey G, Nicholas T. Virtual reality in mental health. Social Psychiatry and Psychiatric Epidemiology. 2007 May 1;42(5):343–54.

61. Freeman D, Reeve S, Robinson A, Ehlers A, Clark D, Spanlang B, Slater M. Virtual reality in the assessment, understanding, and treatment of mental health disorders. Psychological medicine. 2017 Oct;47(14):2393–400.

62. Jiang F, Jiang Y, Zhi H, Dong Y, Li H, Ma S, Wang Y, Dong Q, Shen H, Wang Y. Artificial intelligence in healthcare: Past, present and future. Stroke and vascular neurology. 2017 Dec 1;2(4).

63. Al Kuwaiti A, Nazer K, Al-Reedy A, Al-Shehri S, Al-Muhanna A, Subbarayalu AV, Al Muhanna D, Al-Muhanna FA. A review of the role of artificial intelligence in healthcare. Journal of personalized medicine. 2023 Jun 5;13(6):951.

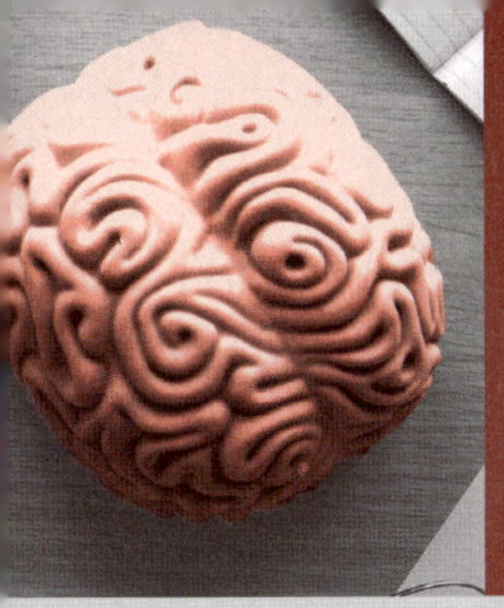

STUDENT ASSIGNMENT

LONG ANSWER QUESTIONS

1. Explain the concept of geropsychology and its growing importance in healthcare.
2. Describe the demographic trends of aging populations globally. How do these trends impact the need for geriatric healthcare services?
3. Differentiate between the various types of aging (chronological, biological, psychological, social, and functional). How do these factors interact to influence an individual's experience of aging?
4. Describe the different types of anxiety disorders and their prevalence among older adults. How are these disorders diagnosed and treated?
5. Discuss the risk factors, symptoms, diagnosis, and treatment approaches for depression in older adults.

SHORT ANSWER QUESTIONS

1. Mention how insomnia affects the physical and mental health of older adults.
2. What are the various treatment options for insomnia in this population group?
3. Compare and contrast the following noninvasive brain stimulation techniques used for treating mental health conditions in older adults:
   a. Cranial electrical stimulation (CES)
   b. Transcranial direct current stimulation (tDCS)
   c. Repetitive transcranial magnetic stimulation (rTMS)
   d. Vagus Nerve Stimulation (taVNS)
4. Write about the role of physiotherapists in managing pain, falls, and geriatric syndromes like dementia and delirium in older adults (psychological aspect).
5. How does the knowledge of psychology help a physiotherapist in treating a patient of a chronic stroke?

MULTIPLE CHOICE QUESTIONS

1. **Geriatrics is the study of:**
   a. Infants and children
   b. Adults of all ages
   c. Older adults
   d. Adolescents
2. **Geropsychology is a branch of psychology that focuses on:**
   a. The mental and physical health of children
   b. The mental and physical health of older adults
   c. The mental and physical health of adolescents
   d. The mental and physical health of people with disabilities

3. **According to the World Health Organization, which is NOT a major contributor to the disease burden in individuals 60 years of age and older?**
   a. Cardiovascular illnesses
   b. Malignant neoplasms
   c. Musculoskeletal diseases
   d. Infectious diseases

4. **Which of the following is NOT a type of aging?**
   a. Primary aging
   b. Secondary aging
   c. Accelerated aging
   d. Programmed aging

5. **Transcranial direct current stimulation (tDCS) is used to:**
   a. Modify brain activity
   b. Improve memory
   c. Treat pain
   d. All of these

6. **Vagus nerve stimulation (VNS) is used to treat:**
   a. Epilepsy
   b. Depression
   c. Pain
   d. All of these

7. **A patient with chronic low back pain reports feeling anxious and depressed due to the pain. How can a physiotherapist contribute to a multidisciplinary approach to pain management for this patient?**
   a. Prescribing pain medication
   b. Providing education on pain and relaxation techniques
   c. Referring the patient for surgery
   d. Focusing solely on manual therapy techniques

8. **Which of the following factors MOST contributes to the fear of falling in elderly patients?**
   a. Weakness in the lower limbs
   b. Lack of social interaction
   c. Presence of chronic diseases
   d. Availability of home care services

9. **When assessing pain in an elderly patient, a physiotherapist should consider which of the following factors in addition to pain intensity?**
   a. Age of the patient only
   b. Functional limitations due to pain
   c. Ability to tolerate strong medications
   d. Family history of pain

10. **Which of the following statements is MOST accurate regarding physiotherapy interventions for geriatric patients?**
   a. Physiotherapy is only necessary for patients recovering from surgery
   b. Physiotherapy can help improve mobility, function, and quality of life in older adults
   c. Physiotherapy should be avoided in patients with dementia
   d. Balance and gait training is not beneficial for fall prevention in elderly patients

---

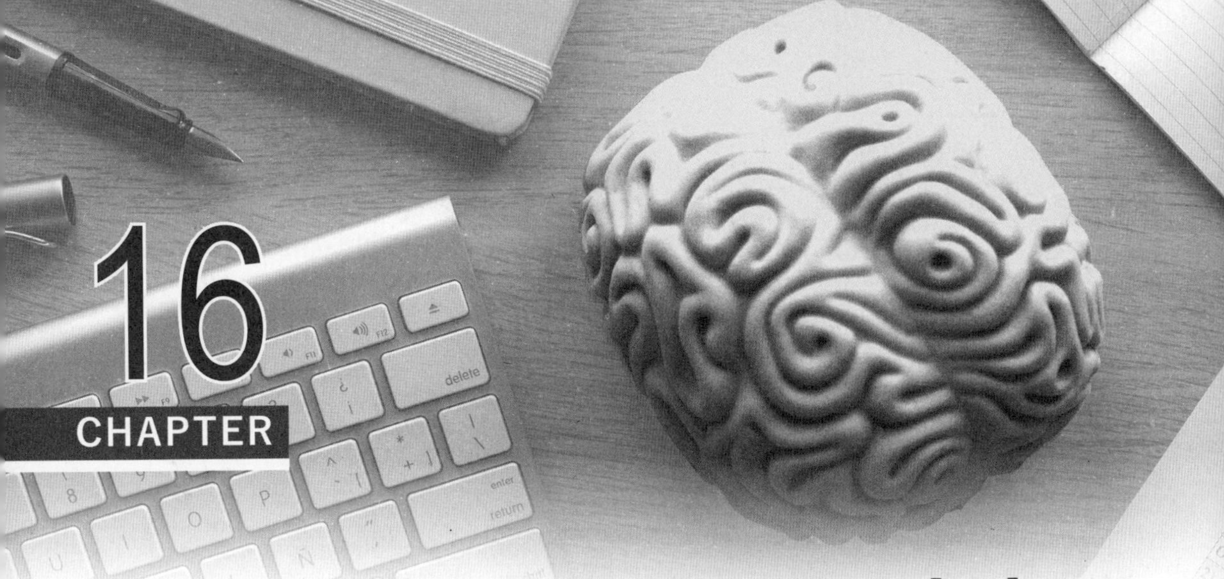

16

CHAPTER

Industrial Psychology

Divya Aggarwal, Pooja Sharma, Priyanka Sethi

LEARNING OBJECTIVES

After the completion of the chapter, the readers will be able to:
- Understand the definition and scope of industrial psychology.
- Discuss the origins of industrial psychology during the Industrial Revolution.
- Identify key milestones and influential studies in the field, such as the Hawthorne Studies and the development of psychological testing.
- Understand feedback and improvement, including constructive feedback and performance improvement plans (PIPs).
- Understand how industrial psychology enhances organizational effectiveness.

CHAPTER OUTLINE

- Introduction
- Definition and Scope
- Evolution of Industrial Psychology
- Importance
- Foundations in Theory
- Evaluation of Training Programs
- Performance Appraisal
- Practical Implications for Organizations

KEY TERMS

Diversity and inclusion: Strategies for managing diversity and promoting inclusion in the workplace, and the impact of diversity on employee interactions and organizational dynamics.

Employee performance: The study of how employees behave, think, and act in work environments, and the factors influencing their attitudes toward work, motivation, job involvement, and job satisfaction.

Ethical and legal considerations: The importance of adhering to ethical guidelines and legal standards in the practice of industrial psychology.

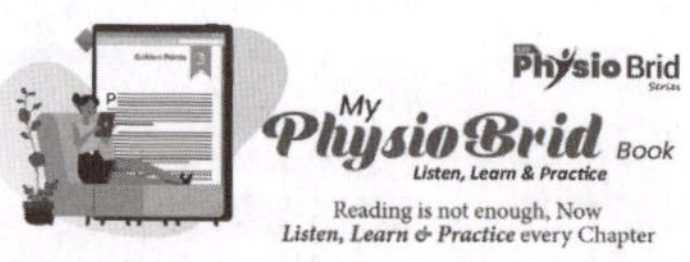

Industrial psychology: The scientific study of human behavior in the workplace, focusing on enhancing employee well-being and organizational success.

Job analysis: Systematic assessments of jobs to understand their nature and requirements, including creating job descriptions and specifications.

Job design: Organizing work to maximize efficiency and employee satisfaction, considering factors like skill variety, task identity, and autonomy.

Leadership and management: Investigating effective leadership behaviors, styles, and settings in organizations, and offering insights into efficient management practices.

Organizational culture and climate: The study of organizational culture, including norms, communication styles, and values, and how they affect work satisfaction, employee behavior, and organizational outcomes.

Performance management: Creating procedures and frameworks for managing and assessing employee performance, including performance appraisal techniques and feedback systems.

Recruitment and selection: Developing and assessing methods for attracting, choosing, and evaluating job candidates, including the use of exams, assessment centers, and interviews.

Technological advancements: The role of technology in transforming recruitment, training, performance management, and remote collaboration in the workplace.

Training and development: Identifying training needs, creating programs, and evaluating their effectiveness to improve employees' knowledge, skills, and abilities.

Work-life balance and well-being: Examining how work-related factors affect employees' quality of life and psychological health, including issues like burnout, stress, and resilience.

Workplace design and ergonomics: Focusing on creating efficient work environments that minimize health and safety risks, including the study of ergonomics to optimize human interaction with workspaces and tools.

INTRODUCTION

The applied field of industrial and organizational psychology or I/O psychology, is concerned with the study of human behavior as it relates to work, organizations, and productivity in a specific setting—that is, practically any type of organization.[1]

The goal of addressing the significant problems and challenges arising from the unique socio-economic contexts in which organizations are situated is to produce new knowledge and solutions through the theoretical and empirical study of various topics in the various subfields of I/O psychology in the academic setting.

Applied I/O psychology solves issues in the workplace by utilizing psychological concepts along with newly discovered information and research-derived solutions.[2]

The scientific study of people in their work environments, including the application of psychological theories, concepts, and research to the workplace, is known as industrial and organizational psychology.[3]

Goals of industrial psychology: The dual goals of I/O psychology are to:

1. Carry out research to broaden our knowledge and comprehension of human behavior at work; and

2. Utilize that information to enhance work behavior, the workplace, and psychological circumstances.

DEFINITION AND SCOPE

The scientific study of human behavior in the workplace and the application of psychological concepts to improve employee well-being and organizational success is known as industrial psychology (Fig. 16.1). It entails the methodical examination of organizational, group, and individual dynamics in order to maximize output, performance, and satisfaction.

The following are the scopes of the industrial psychology (Fig. 16.1).

- **Employee performance and behavior:** Industrial psychology studies how employees behave, think, and act in work environments. It aims to comprehend the variables affecting attitudes toward work, motivation, job involvement, and job satisfaction.

- **Workplace design and ergonomics:** This area of study focuses on creating work environments that are as efficient as possible while lowering health and safety hazards. It encompasses the study of ergonomics, which aims to maximize how people interact with their workspaces and other instruments.

- **Recruitment and selection:** Methods for attracting, choosing, and evaluating job candidates are developed and assessed by industrial psychologists. They create selection processes, such as exams, assessment centers, and interviews, to find people most fit for particular positions inside companies.[4]

- **Training and development:** When determining the needs for training, creating training programs, and assessing their efficacy, industrial psychology is a critical component. It entails determining where employees have skill gaps, creating training materials, and putting plans into action to improve workers' knowledge, aptitude, and skills.[2,3,5]

- **Performance management:** Industrial psychologists create procedures and frameworks for managing and assessing worker performance. This covers tactics for performance improvement, goal-setting approaches, feedback systems, and performance appraisal procedures.[4]

- **Leadership and management:** The field investigates effective leadership behaviors, styles, and settings in organizations. It offers perceptions into efficient management techniques, group dynamics, decision-making procedures, and techniques for resolving conflicts.

- **Organizational culture and climate:** The study of organizational culture and climate, encompassing conventions, communication styles, and values, is known as industrial psychology. It evaluates how organizational culture affects work satisfaction, employee behavior, and organizational results.

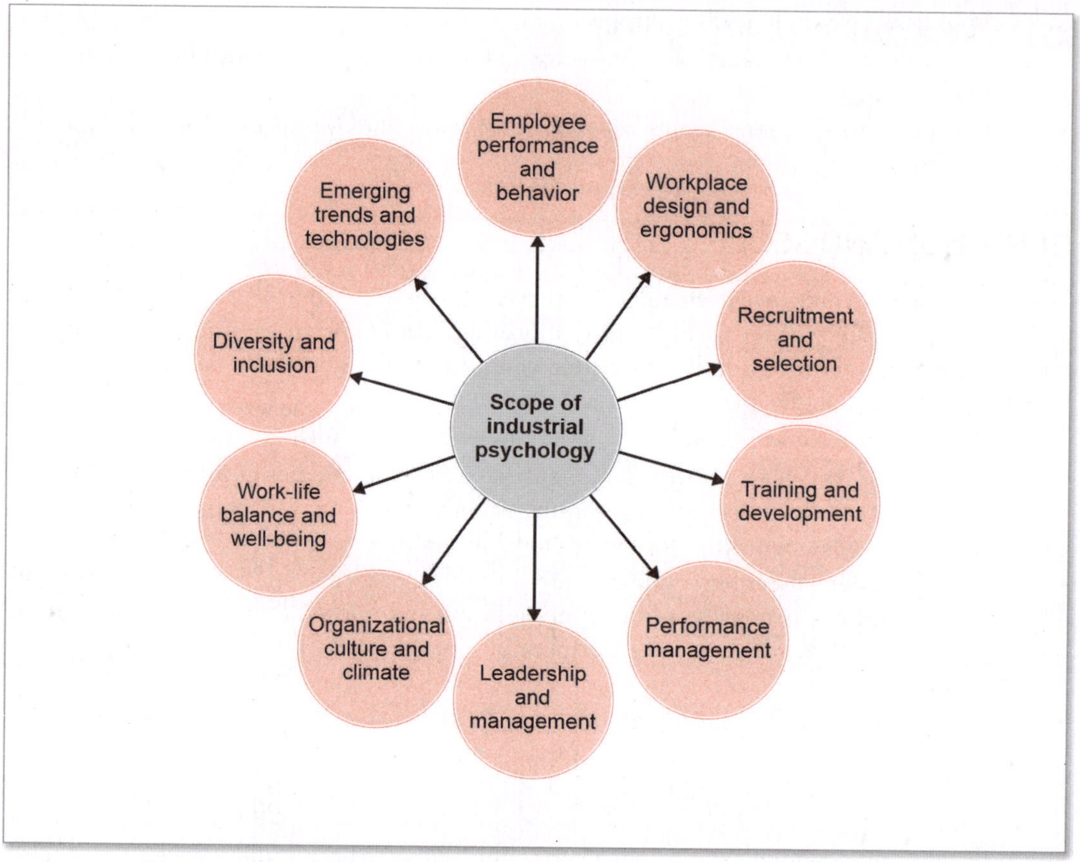

Fig. 16.1: Understanding the scope of industrial psychology

- **Work-life balance and well-being:** Industrial psychologists investigate how work-related variables affect workers' quality of life and well-being. This entails tackling problems like burnout, work-life balance, stress at work, and the development of resilience and psychological health.

- **Diversity and inclusion:** The field investigates methods for encouraging inclusion and managing diversity in the workplace. It looks at how diversity affects employee interactions, organizational performance, and organizational dynamics.[6]

- **Emerging trends and technologies:** Industrial psychology changes to keep up with new developments in technology and workplace practices. This covers the use of technology in hiring, onboarding, training, managing performance, and remote collaboration.

MUST KNOW

- A broad range of subjects pertaining to human behavior in organizational contexts are included in the field of industrial psychology.
- Understanding and enhancing human behavior in the workplace is the primary goal of industrial psychology.
- It plays an important role in increasing organizational effectiveness.

EVOLUTION OF INDUSTRIAL PSYCHOLOGY

The field of industrial psychology has a long and illustrious history, dating back to the late 1800s and early 1900s. It came into being in reaction to the industrial revolution and the increasing demand to comprehend and maximize human behavior within the framework of the workplace and business.

Early Influences

- **Scientific management:** Industrial psychology was founded on the ideas of scientific management, which Frederick Winslow Taylor introduced in the late 1800s. In order to increase production and efficiency, Taylor placed a strong emphasis on the scientific study of work processes.
- **Hawthorne studies:** The Hawthorne studies, carried out at the Western Electric Company's Hawthorne Works in the 1920s and 1930s, represented a critical turning point in the advancement of industrial psychology. Researchers who examined the impact of social and environmental elements on worker morale and productivity included Elton Mayo and Fritz Roethlisberger, underscoring the significance of interpersonal relationships in the workplace.

Early Developments

- **Psychological testing:** In order to measure individual characteristics and talents, psychological tests and evaluation instruments were developed in the early 20th century. Psychologists like Walter Dill Scott and Hugo Münsterberg used psychological concepts in hiring, training, and assigning workers.
- **Job analysis:** Systematic job assessments were initiated by industrial psychologists to comprehend the nature of labor and its prerequisites. This required creating job descriptions and specifications, breaking down jobs into discrete tasks, and determining necessary skills and competencies.[4]

Growth and Expansion

- **World Wars I and II:** The development of industrial psychology was greatly aided by these two global conflicts. During a war, psychologists were called upon to help with recruiting, training, and morale of military men. Organizational behavior and personnel psychology have advanced as a result of the application of psychological concepts to military contexts.[7]

- **Post-War era:** Industrial psychology had a boom in popularity in the post-war period, both in academic and practical contexts. The fields of organizational development, management consultancy, and human factors engineering were all influenced by industrial psychologists.[8]

- **Professionalization and institutionalization:** With the establishment of organizations like the Society for Industrial and Organizational Psychology (SIOP) and Division 14 of the American Psychological Association, industrial psychology had been acknowledged as a separate field of study.

- **Academic programs:** Universities started to provide courses in organizational and industrial psychology, preparing students to become future scholars and practitioners in the subject.

Contemporary Trends

- **Globalization and diversity:** The field of industrial psychology has evolved to meet the demands of workplace diversity and globalization. Understanding and navigating cultural differences, encouraging diversity and inclusion, and tackling difficulties related to the global workforce are becoming more and more important.

- **Technology and innovation:** When it comes to utilizing technology and innovation to improve organizational effectiveness, industrial psychologists are at the forefront. This includes applying artificial intelligence, virtual reality, big data analytics, and other cutting-edge technology to hiring, onboarding, and performance management, among other processes.

> **MUST KNOW**
>
> - Frederick Winslow Taylor introduced scientific management of workplace in 1800s which is the basis of Industrial Psychology.
> - Later psychological analysis and systematic job assessments were utilized in hiring and training.
> - Post World War era saw a phenomenal growth in the field which is now dynamic and interdisciplinary and focuses on optimizing human behavior and performance in organizational settings.

IMPORTANCE

By utilizing psychological concepts and techniques to raise employee satisfaction, increase organizational effectiveness, and maximize performance, industrial psychology plays a critical role at today's workplaces.[5] One can comprehend its significance in the workplace from a number of angles described here (Fig. 16.2):

- **Improves productivity of employees:** Organizations can better understand the variables influencing worker motivation, productivity, and job satisfaction with the aid of industrial psychologists. They can create interventions and strategies to maximize worker productivity by recognizing and addressing these variables.[9, 15]

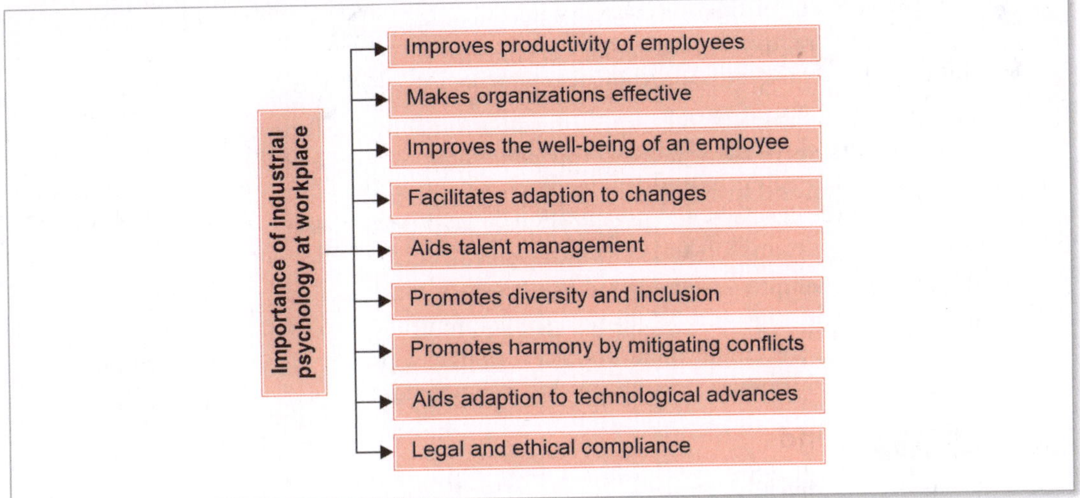

Fig. 16.2: Importance of industrial psychology at workplace

- **Makes organizations effective:** Industrial psychology helps businesses optimize hiring, training, and performance management through scientific methods. By fostering a positive work environment, enhancing leadership, and reducing workplace stress, industrial psychologists contribute to higher efficiency, lower employee turnover, and overall organizational success.[14]

- **Improves the well-being of an employee:** The goal of industrial psychology is to enhance workers' psychological health and well-being at work. Through tackling concerns like job stress, work-life equilibrium, and organizational support, industrial psychologists contribute to the establishment of a favorable work atmosphere that fosters employee contentment and involvement.

- **Facilitates adaption to changes:** Industrial psychology helps organizations adapt to change by reducing resistance and promoting a smooth transition. It uses strategies like effective communication, training, and employee engagement to foster acceptance. By supporting leadership, managing stress, and enhancing workplace flexibility, industrial psychologists ensure employees remain resilient and productive during organizational changes.

- **Aids talent management:** Effective talent management is essential to the success of any organization. Industrial psychologists help businesses find, draw in, nurture, and keep elite employees. They create and put into practice talent management plans that are in line with the aims and objectives of the company.

- **Promotes diversity and inclusion:** Workplace diversity and inclusion are topics covered by industrial psychology. Industrial psychologists assist companies in capitalizing on the advantages of a varied workforce and establishing a more equitable and respectful work environment by increasing diversity awareness, reducing prejudices, and cultivating an inclusive culture.

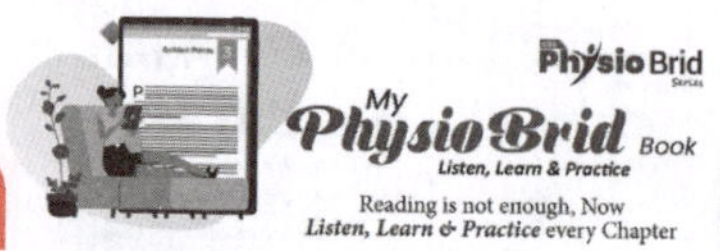

- **Promotes harmony by mitigating conflicts:** In any job, conflicts will inevitably occur. Workplace harmony and constructive management of interpersonal problems are upheld by organizations with the assistance of industrial psychologists who possess experience in mediation, negotiation, and conflict resolution.

- **Aids adaption to technological advances:** Technology is advancing so quickly that organizations must adjust to new platforms and technologies. Understanding how technology affects work processes, employee behavior, and organizational dynamics is vital for industrial psychologists to ensure a seamless transition and efficient use of technology in the workplace.

- **Legal and ethical compliance:** Industrial psychologists make sure that policies and procedures within organizations adhere to moral and legal requirements. By offering advice on matters like diversity programs, fair employment practices, employee privacy rights, and moral decision-making, they assist businesses in reducing risks and upholding moral standards.

MUST KNOW

Essential insights:

- Industrial psychology plays a critical role in today's workplaces to maximize productivity, improve organizational efficacy, support talent management and facilitate changes.
- It fosters diversity and inclusion, resolve conflicts, adjust to technological advancements, and guarantee adherence to moral and legal requirements.
- Because of its interdisciplinary approach and emphasis on human behavior, it is invaluable for tackling the intricate problems that contemporary organizations face.

FOUNDATIONS IN THEORY

The field of industrial psychology utilizes a diverse range of theoretical frameworks to comprehend and tackle the intricacies of human conduct within organizational environments.

These theoretical underpinnings offer frameworks for researching many facets of organizational dynamics, human resource management, and work behavior. The chapter examines both historical theories and modern viewpoints in industrial psychology in this part.

Early Theories

- **Taylorism (scientific management):** One of the oldest and most significant theories in industrial psychology is Taylorism, developed by Frederick Winslow Taylor in the late 19th century. In order to determine the most productive ways of producing goods, Taylor argued for the scientific examination of work processes. His scientific management philosophies placed a strong emphasis on task specialization, work process standardization, and performance-based pay. Modern methods of job design, performance management, and productivity enhancement were made possible by Taylorism.

- **Hawthorne studies:** The Hawthorne studies, carried out at the Hawthorne Works of the Western Electric Company in the 1920s and 1930s, transformed our understanding of how

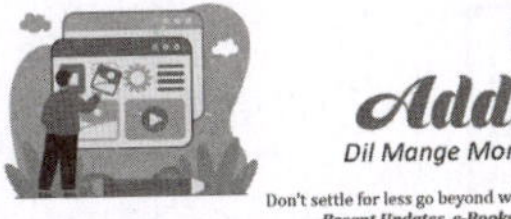

people behave at the workplace. Under the direction of scientists like Fritz Roethlisberger and Elton Mayo, the research examined how social and environmental factors affected worker morale and productivity. The results questioned conventional theories of productivity and motivation by emphasizing the role that interpersonal connections, organizational dynamics, and employee attitudes have in influencing behavior at work. The human relations approach to management emerged as a result of the Hawthorne research.

Contemporary Perspectives

Refer to Figure 16.3 to understand the contemporary perspective of industrial psychology:

- **Human relations approach:** The conclusions of Hawthorne investigation led to the development of the human relations approach. It highlights how crucial interpersonal connections, social elements, and employee wellbeing are to the success of an organization.

  Human relations proponents like Douglas McGregor and Abraham Maslow highlighted the importance of employee involvement, motivation, and job satisfaction in boosting morale and productivity. This viewpoint affected quality of work-life initiatives, participative decision-making, and employee involvement in management techniques.

- **System theory:** A comprehensive foundation for comprehending organizations as dynamic, complex systems made up of interconnected pieces is provided by systems theory. Systems theory is used by industrial psychologists to examine how people interact with groups and the broader organizational environment. The interdependence of organizational components as well as the significance of adaptation, equilibrium, and feedback loops are highlighted by systems theory. From a systemic viewpoint, it offers insights on topics including organizational structure, communication styles, change management, and performance optimization.

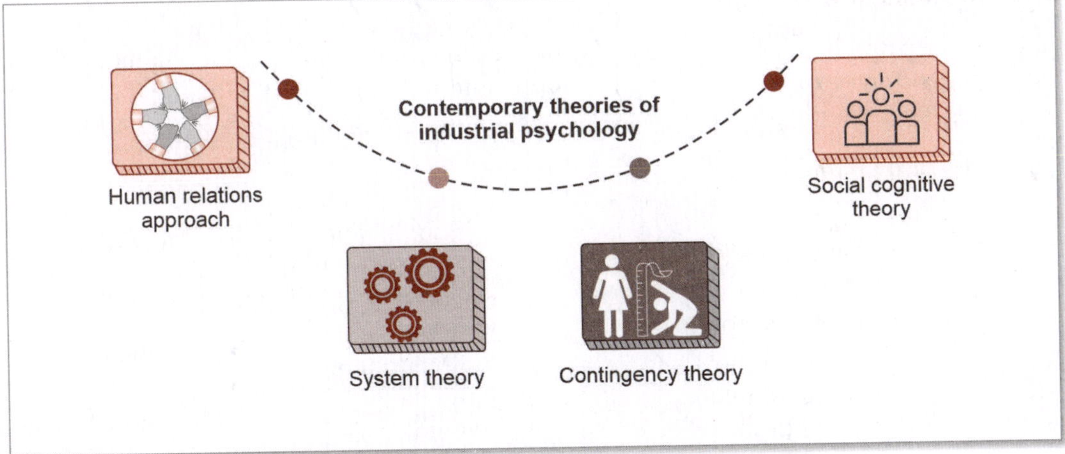

Fig. 16.3: Contemporary theories of industrial psychology

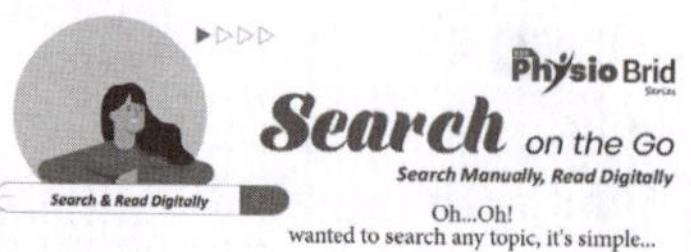

- **Contingency theory:** According to contingency theory, there is no one-size-fits-all method of managing an organization; rather, the success of a management strategy is contingent upon the particular circumstances and context. Contingency theory is used by industrial psychologists to help them understand how HR procedures, organizational structures, and leadership philosophies should be customized for each organization's particular needs. According to contingency theory, there is no one-size-fits-all method of managing an organization; rather, the success of a management strategy is contingent upon the particular circumstances and context. This viewpoint emphasizes that effective management of people and organizations requires flexibility, adaptation, and response to environmental contingencies.

- **Social cognitive theory:** Albert Bandura's Social Cognitive Theory places a strong emphasis on the roles that cognitive functions, observational learning, and self-regulation play in behavior. Social cognitive theory is used by industrial psychologists to study how people pick up knowledge, abilities, and attitudes through modeling, reinforcement, and observation.

  This viewpoint is especially pertinent to fields where learning and behavior modification are major goals, such performance management, leadership development, and training and development.

MUST KNOW

- The theoretical underpinnings of industrial psychology span a wide spectrum of viewpoints, from early theories like the Hawthorne experiments and Taylorism to more modern theories like human relations, systems theory, contingency theory, and social cognitive theory.
- The development of workable interventions and tactics for improving organizational success and employee well-being is influenced by these theoretical frameworks
- They offer insightful information about the nuances of human behavior in organizational settings.

Job Analysis and Design

In industrial psychology, job analysis and design are essential procedures that entail methodically examining and organizing the elements of occupations inside companies (Fig. 16.4).

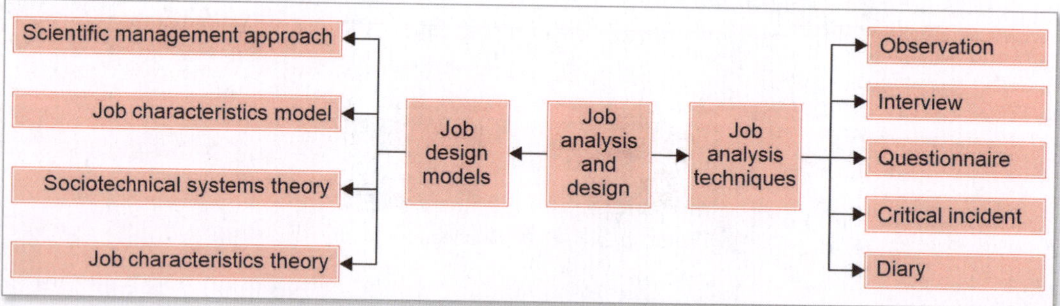

Fig. 16.4: Techniques in job analysis and models of job design

These procedures are necessary to maximize worker performance, comprehend job requirements, and improve organizational efficacy. (Wilson M A, 2014)

Job Analysis Techniques

- **Observation method:** Directly seeing workers as they carry out their duties is part of the observation method. The tasks completed, the order in which they were completed, the tools and equipment utilized, and the surrounding circumstances are all recorded by observers. With this approach, you can gain firsthand knowledge of the demands and expectations of the work.[10, 20]

- **Interview method:** In order to obtain information regarding job activities, responsibilities, and requirements, the interview approach entails conducting organized interviews with subject matter experts, supervisors, and job incumbents. Individual or group interviews can yield comprehensive qualitative information about the nature of the work.

- **Questionnaire method:** The questionnaire approach gathers data on job-related elements like tasks, knowledge, skills, abilities, and work environment by giving supervisors and job occupants standardized questionnaires. Utilizing questionnaires can help with quantitative analysis and collect data from a large number of employees.

- **Diary method:** Under the diary technique, employees are expected to keep a journal or track of all the things they do during the workday or week. Diaries offer a thorough documentation of the quantity, duration, and kind of work assignments, along with any disruptions or departures from regular schedules.

- **Critical incident technique:** The critical incident technique is locating pivotal moments or significant occurrences that represent successful or unsuccessful work performance. These occurrences are recorded and examined in order to determine the fundamental duties, attitudes, and proficiencies needed for effective work performance.[11, 15]

Job Design Models

- **Scientific management approach (Taylorism):** Frederick Winslow Taylor invented the scientific management approach, which places a strong emphasis on methodically analyzing and improving work processes in order to increase production and efficiency. According to this concept, job design entails standardizing work procedures and segmenting activities into smaller, more focused parts in order to produce the most effective results.

- **Job characteristics model (Hackman & Oldham):** Five essential job features—skill variety, task identity, task importance, autonomy, and feedback—are identified by the job characteristics model as having a positive impact on meaningful work and intrinsic motivation. Higher levels of these traits in a job increase the likelihood of favorable employee outcomes including motivation, job satisfaction, and performance.

- **Sociotechnical systems theory:** The interplay between the social and technological dimensions of work design is highlighted by socio-technical systems theory. This method acknowledges that the technical demands of the work as well as the social needs and preferences of the employees should be taken into account when designing a job. Jobs are made to maximize worker pleasure as well as job efficiency.[6]

- **Job characteristics theory:** The job characteristics theory is a well-known theoretical framework for comprehending the connection between employee motivation and job design, which was established by Hackman and Oldham. This idea states that professions with high levels of autonomy, feedback, task relevance, task identity, and skill variation are more likely to provide good results including increased motivation, job satisfaction, and performance.

> **MUST KNOW**
>
> - Job analysis and design are essential procedures in industrial psychology that entail methodically dissecting and organising the elements of occupations inside businesses.
> - Through the utilisation of work design models like the work characteristics model and the application of diverse job analysis tools, organizations can optimise job roles to maximize employee motivation, job satisfaction, and performance.
> - A balance between the social and technological dimensions help to maximize the job efficiency.
> - For training and development of personnel, a thorough analysis of organization, task and individual should be done.
> - Adequate training should be provided according to the diverse needs of learners. On site and Simulation trainings can help in skill enhancement.
> - A post-training evaluation should be carried out to assess the efficacy of training program and understand the scope of improvement.

EVALUATION OF TRAINING PROGRAMS

A key component of industrial psychology is program evaluation, which measures the influence and efficacy of training interventions on worker performance and organizational results. The function of industrial psychology in the planning, execution, and assessment of training initiatives is examined.

Theoretical Frameworks in Training Evaluation

- **Kirkpatrick's four levels of evaluation:** Describe the four levels of training evaluation included in Kirkpatrick's model, which are reaction, learning, behavior, and results (Fig. 16.5). Talk about the framework that industrial psychologists use to evaluate the efficacy of training at every stage.[18, 22]

- **Systems theory in training evaluation:** Examine how systems theory can be used to evaluate training, with a focus on how training programs interact with organizational systems and procedures. Talk about the ways that training evaluation design and analysis are influenced by systems thinking.

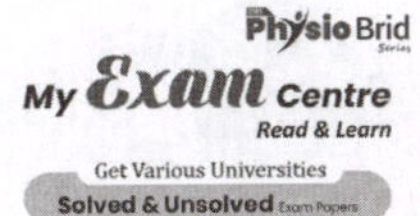

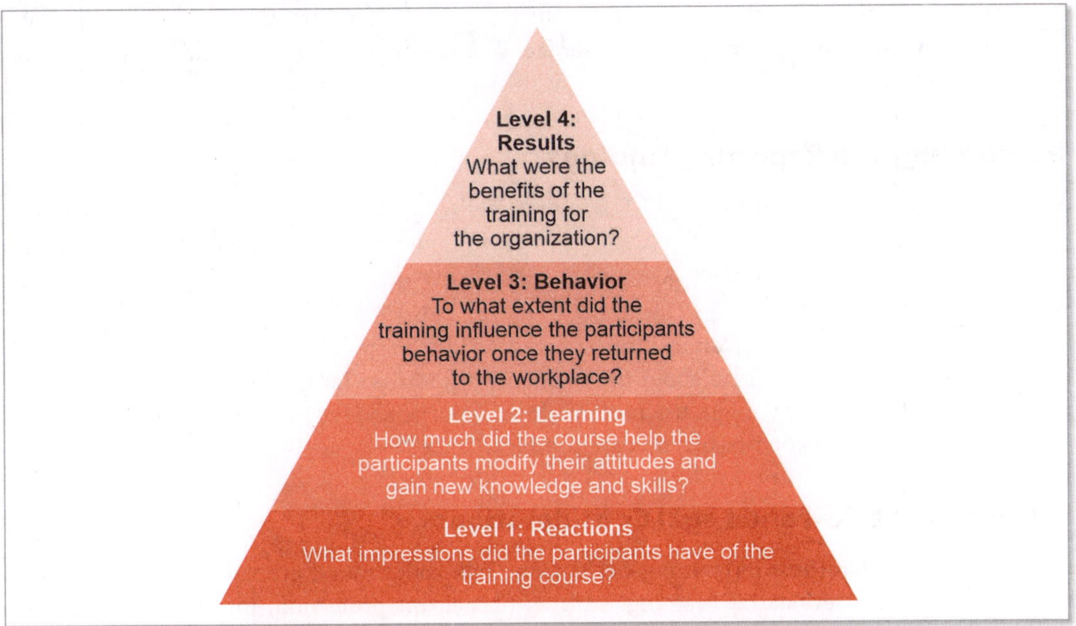

Fig. 16.5: Kirkpatrick's four levels of evaluation

Designing Evaluation Studies

- **Research design and methodology:** Talk about the several research designs and techniques—such as mixed-method approaches, experimental designs, and quasi-experimental designs—that are employed in training evaluation studies. Stress how crucial it is to choose the right designs in order to evaluate training outcomes and answer research questions.

- **Data collection methods:** Examine the many approaches to gathering data for training evaluation, including observations, interviews, surveys, and performance evaluations. Talk about the benefits and drawbacks of each technique as well as factors to take into account while gathering data in actual organizational contexts.

Analyzing Training Evaluation Data

- **Quantitative analysis techniques:** Introduce quantitative analysis methods like regression analysis, inferential statistics, and descriptive statistics that are frequently used in training evaluation. Talk about the methods industrial psychologists use to examine training data and find correlations between the variables being trained and the results.[12, 23]

- **Qualitative analysis techniques:** Examine qualitative analysis methods for open-ended questions, interview transcripts, and qualitative data gathered from training assessments.

These methods include theme analysis, content analysis, and narrative analysis. Talk about the importance of qualitative insights in comprehending training program participants' experiences and views.[12, 23]

Interpreting and Reporting Findings

- **Interpreting evaluation findings:** Talk about methods for analyzing assessment results and making judgments regarding the efficacy of training initiatives. Stress how crucial it is to take into account contextual elements, competing theories, and ramifications for upcoming training programs.[13, 24]

- **Communicating results:** Examine the best ways to inform sponsors, organizational executives, and front-line staff members about the evaluation's findings. Talk about the various ways that industrial psychologists might use presentations, reports, and data visualization approaches to clearly convey evaluation results that are complex.

Addressing Ethical and Legal Considerations

- **Ethical considerations in training evaluation:** Talk about moral precepts and directives that are pertinent to evaluating training, such as participant protection, informed consent, and confidentiality. Examine moral conundrums that could occur in training assessment studies and ethical solutions for them.

- **Legal considerations in training evaluation:** Analyze the legal aspects of training evaluation, such as intellectual property rights, data protection laws, and privacy laws. Talk about the ways that industrial psychologists can make sure that training assessment studies are conducted in accordance with the law.

> **MUST KNOW**
> - Industrial psychology emphasizes on assessment of training programs, from planning evaluation studies and data analysis to evaluating results and presenting conclusions.
> - Industrial psychologists utilise ethical principles, research methodologies, and theoretical frameworks to help create a trained and productive workforce and continuously enhance training initiatives.

PERFORMANCE APPRAISAL

The foundation of organizational management is performance appraisal, which offers a methodical way to assess worker performance and encourages criticism and development. This section examines the goals, procedures, and tactics related to performance appraisal, emphasizing the role it plays in promoting both individual and organizational effectiveness.[14, 25]

Objectives

- Providing performance comments to staff members.

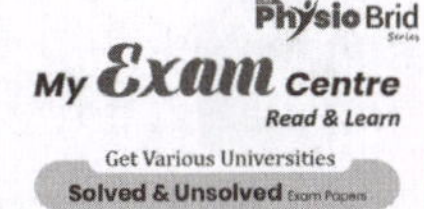

- Recognizing one's advantages and shortcomings.
- Assisting with succession planning and career development.
- Providing information to support decisions on awards, promotions, and training opportunities.
- Coordinating individual performance with the aims and objectives of the company.

Importance

- Increases worker enthusiasm and engagement by offering praise and helpful criticism.
- Encourages an environment of openness and transparency by facilitating communication between managers and staff.
- Contributes to the growth and development of employees by identifying areas for skill development and training activities.
- Supports the decision-making procedures for performance management, compensation adjustments, and promotions.
- Increases the effectiveness of the organization as a whole by strengthening the alignment between individual and organizational goals.

Feedback and Performance Improvement

- **Giving sufficient recommendations:**
  - Responses ought to be precise, timely, and useful. Highlight your advantages and room for development.
  - Promote candid discussion and two-way communication.
- **Plans for performance improvement (PIPs):**
  - Determine the areas where performance is lacking and set specific objectives for improvement.
  - Establish deadlines and concrete actions for progress.
  - Offer assistance and resources to enable the improvement of performance.
- **Mentoring and training:**
  - To assist in the development of your employees, provide coaching and mentorship.
  - Provide them the chance to advance their careers and enhance their skills.
  - Keep an eye on developments and offer constant assistance and criticism.

> **MUST KNOW**
> - The multidimensional process of performance appraisal is essential to improving both organizational success and personnel performance.
> - Organizations can cultivate a culture of perpetual learning, expansion, and excellence by putting into practice efficient performance appraisal techniques and offering constructive criticism and assistance for better performance.

Motivation at the Workplace

Workplace engagement and employee performance are significantly influenced by motivation. Chapter 4 Motivation examines a number of motivational theories, incentive programs, and techniques, along with the idea of employee engagement, emphasizing the importance of each in creating a positive and effective work atmosphere.[10, 15]

Applications of Industrial Psychology: Enhancing Organizational Effectiveness

A wide range of applications in industrial psychology are available to maximize organizational effectiveness and improve employee well-being. Through case studies, real-world examples, and the identification of possibilities and obstacles faced by organizations in integrating psychological concepts, investigates the practical applications of industrial psychology.[16, 17]

CASE STUDY

Effectiveness of Industrial Psychology

XYZ Corporation, a mid-sized tech company, noticed a decline in employee motivation and performance. Despite competitive salaries and benefits, productivity had stagnated, and employee turnover had increased. The company's leadership team decided to bring in an organizational psychologist to address these issues and improve overall workplace dynamics.

Challenges

- **Lack of engagement:** Employees felt disconnected from the company's goals and their roles, leading to decreased engagement and enthusiasm.
- **Stress and burnout:** High workloads and unrealistic deadlines had led to increased stress levels and burnout among employees.
- **Poor communication:** There was a significant breakdown in communication between management and employees, resulting in misunderstandings and unmet expectations.
- **Lack of recognition:** Employees felt their hard work and achievements were not adequately recognized, leading to dissatisfaction and decreased motivation.

Psychological Interventions

The organizational psychologist conducted a thorough assessment through surveys, interviews, and observation. Based on the findings, the following interventions were implemented:

- **Goal setting and clarity:** The psychologist introduced specific, measurable, achievable, relevant, time-bound (SMART) goal-setting framework. Managers worked with employees to set clear, achievable goals that aligned with the company's objectives. This provided employees with a sense of direction and purpose, increasing their engagement and motivation.
- **Stress management and well-being programs:** Workshops on stress management techniques, such as mindfulness, time management, and relaxation exercises, were introduced. The company also

Contd...

implemented flexible working hours and remote work options to help employees balance their work and personal lives better. These initiatives reduced burnout and improved overall well-being.

- **Improved communication channels:** The psychologist recommended regular town hall meetings, open-door policies, and anonymous feedback systems to enhance communication between management and employees. This fostered a more transparent and open work environment where employees felt heard and valued.
- **Recognition and reward systems:** A formal recognition program was established to celebrate employees' achievements, both big and small. This included monthly awards, public acknowledgment in meetings, and personalized thank-you notes from management. Recognizing employees' hard work boosted their morale and motivation to perform well.
- **Team building and collaboration:** The psychologist facilitated team-building activities and workshops to improve collaboration and teamwork. These activities helped build stronger interpersonal relationships, improving communication, trust, and overall team performance.
- **Career development and growth opportunities:** The company introduced mentorship programs, skill development workshops, and clear career progression paths. This made employees feel invested in and provided them with opportunities for growth, which increased their commitment to the organization.

Outcome

Within 6 months of implementing these psychological interventions, XYZ Corporation saw significant improvements in employee motivation and performance:

- **Increased engagement:** Employees reported feeling more connected to their work and the company's mission, leading to higher levels of engagement.
- **Improved productivity**: Productivity increased by 25%, as employees were more motivated and focused on achieving their goals.
- **Reduced turnover:** Employee turnover decreased by 15%, as job satisfaction improved, and employees felt more valued and supported.
- **Enhanced communication:** The open communication channels led to fewer misunderstandings and a more cohesive work environment.
- **Higher morale:** The recognition and reward systems significantly boosted employee morale, leading to a more positive and motivated workforce.

Conclusion

This case study demonstrates the importance of psychological principles in enhancing workplace motivation and performance. By addressing key psychological factors such as goal clarity, stress management, communication, recognition, and career development, organizations can create a more motivated, productive, and satisfied workforce. The success at XYZ Corporation highlights the value of integrating psychology into organizational strategies to achieve better outcomes for both employees and the business.

PRACTICAL IMPLICATIONS FOR ORGANIZATIONS

- **Implementing selection and recruitment practices:** Using concepts from industrial-organizational psychology, talk about doable tactics for creating and executing hiring and selection procedures that support company objectives and values.

- **Training and development initiatives:** Examine the real-world effects of utilizing learning and developmental psychology findings to create training and development plans that are customized to the preferences and learning styles of staff members.[12, 17]
- **Performance management systems:** Examine how businesses may use performance psychology concepts to create and execute performance management systems that offer insightful feedback, acknowledge accomplishments, and foster staff development.

Challenges and Opportunities

- **Addressing diversity and inclusion challenges:** Talk about the difficulties businesses have in encouraging inclusion and diversity in the workplace. Then, using knowledge from organizational behavior and social psychology, investigate methods for building an inclusive and diverse culture.[18, 21]

- **Leveraging technology for talent management:** Discuss best practices for integrating technology into human resource management, based on concepts from organizational psychology and human-computer interaction.

   Examine the benefits and drawbacks of using technology for talent management processes, such as hiring, performance reviews, and training.

- **Adapting to changing workforce dynamics:** Discuss strategies for effectively managing and engaging a diverse workforce, drawing on insights from organizational behavior and industrial-organizational psychology.

   Examine the opportunities and challenges presented by changing workplace dynamics, such as remote work, gig economy trends, and multigenerational workplaces.[13, 19]

SUMMARY

- Industrial Psychology is a branch of psychology that focuses on the study of human behavior in the workplace and has evolved significantly over the years. Its origins can be traced back to the Industrial Revolution when it became imperative to understand and optimize human performance in rapidly changing work environments.
- The early influences on industrial psychology, include the contributions of pioneers like Frederick Winslow Taylor and Hugo Münsterberg. Hawthorne Studies revolutionized our understanding of workplace dynamics, and the development of psychological testing, which laid the foundation for modern recruitment and selection processes.
- The case studies illustrate the practical applications of industrial psychology and discuss how the field has been instrumental in addressing workplace issues, enhancing organizational effectiveness, and promoting employee well-being.

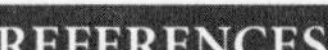

REFERENCES

1. Cascio WF, Aguinis H. Research in industrial and organizational psychology from 1963 to 2007: Changes, choices, and trends. Journal of applied psychology. 2008 Sep;93(5):1062.

2. Schreuder D, Coetzee M. An overview of industrial and organizational psychology research in South Africa: A preliminary study. SA Journal of Industrial Psychology. 2010 Jan;36(1):1–1.

3. Riggio RE. Introduction to industrial and organizational psychology. Routledge; 2015 Jul 17.

4. Gërxhani K, Koster F. Making the right move. Investigating employers' recruitment strategies. Personnel Review. 2015 Aug 3;44(5):781–800.

5. Russo G, Rietveld P, Nijkamp P, Gorter C. Issues in recruitment strategies: An economic perspective. International Journal of Career Management. 1995 Jun 1;7(3):3–13.

6. Wilson MA. A history of job analysis. InHistorical perspectives in industrial and organizational psychology 2014 Feb 4 (p. 249–272). Psychology Press.

7. Bagraim JJ. Organizational Psychology and Workplace Control: The Instrumentality of Corporate Culture. South African Journal of Psychology. 2001;31(3):43–49. doi:10.1177/008124630103100306

8. Hodgkinson G, Ford JK. International Review of Industrial and Organizational Psychology 2006 Volume 21. John Wiley & Sons; 2006.

9. Hodgkinson GP. The interface of cognitive and industrial, work and organizational psychology. Journal of Occupational and Organizational Psychology. 2003 Mar;76(1):1–25

10. O'Neil HF, Allred K, Baker EL. Review of workforce readiness theoretical frameworks. In Workforce readiness 2014 Mar 5 (p. 3–25). Psychology

11. Gelfand MJ, Aycan Z, Erez M, Leung K. Cross-cultural industrial organizational psychology and organizational behavior: A hundred-year journey. Journal of Applied Psychology. 2017 Mar;102(3):514.

12. Koppes LL. The Expanding Role of Workplace Training: Themes and Trends Influencing Training Research and Practice. InHistorical Perspectives in Industrial and Organizational Psychology 2014 Feb 4 (p. 311–340). Psychology Press.

13. Fitzpatrick ME, Cotter EW, Bernfeld SJ, Carter LM, Kies A, Fouad NA. The importance of workplace bullying to vocational psychology: Implications for research and practice. Journal of Career Development. 2011 Dec;38(6):479–99.

14. Moralo TS, Graupner LI. An industrial psychology perspective of workplace counselling in the changing world of work. SA Journal of Industrial Psychology. 2022 May 27;48:1988.

15. Donaldson-Feilder EJ, Bond FW. The relative importance of psychological acceptance and emotional intelligence to workplace well-being. British Journal of guidance and counselling. 2004 May 1;32(2):187–203.

16. Van Vuuren LJ. Industrial psychology: Goodness of fit? Fit for goodness?. SA Journal of Industrial Psychology. 2010 Jan;36(2):1–6.

17. Luthans F, Frey R. Positive psychology in the workplace: The important role of psychological capital (PsyCap). InPositive Psychology 2017 Sep 1 (p. 169–196). Routledge.

18. Ones DS, Sinangil HK, Viswesvaran C, Anderson N. The SAGE Handbook of Industrial, Work & Organizational Psychology: Personnel Psychology and Employee Performance.

19. Kanfer R. Motivation theory and industrial and organizational psychology. Handbook of industrial and organizational psychology. 1990 Sep;1(2):75–130.

Contd...

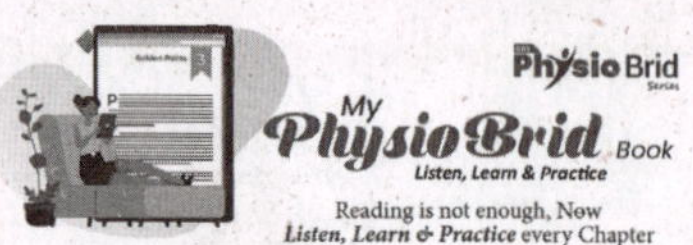

20. Cronshaw SF. Job analysis: Changing nature of work. Canadian Psychology/Psychologie canadienne. 1998 Feb;39(1–2):5.

21. Anderson N, Born M, Cunningham-Snell N. Recruitment and selection: Applicant perspectives and outcomes. Kornhauser A. Industrial psychology as management technique and as social science. American Psychologist. 1947 Jul;2(7):224.

22. Kraiger K, Ford JK, Salas E. Application of cognitive, skill-based, and affective theories of learning outcomes to new methods of training evaluation. Journal of applied psychology. 1993 Apr;78(2):311.

23. Barnard G, Fourie L. A conceptual framework to explore the roles and contributions of industrial psychologists in South Africa (Part 1). SA Journal of Industrial Psychology. 2007 Jan 1;33(2):34–44.

24. Passmore J, Velez MJ. Training evaluation. The Wiley Blackwell handbook of the psychology of training, development, and performance improvement. 2014 Oct 1:136–53.

25. Farr JL, Levy PE. Performance appraisal. InHistorical perspectives in industrial and organizational psychology 2014 Feb 4 (p. 341–358). Psychology Press.

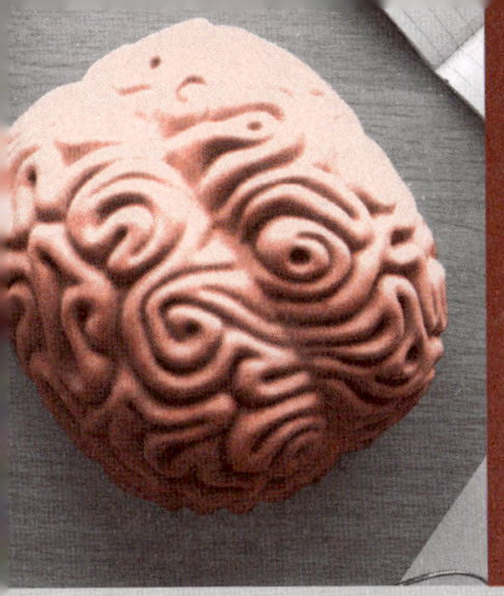

LONG ANSWER QUESTIONS

1. Discuss the evolution of industrial psychology from its early beginnings to contemporary trends. Include key milestones and influential studies that have shaped the field.
2. Evaluate the role of industrial psychology in enhancing employee performance and organizational effectiveness. Provide examples of how industrial psychologists can address workplace issues.
3. Analyze the impact of technology on industrial psychology. How have advancements in technology changed recruitment, training, and performance management practices?
4. Critically examine the ethical and legal considerations in industrial psychology. How do industrial psychologists ensure fairness and equity in their practices?
5. Explore the relationship between leadership and employee motivation. How can industrial psychologists contribute to developing effective leadership within organizations?

SHORT ANSWER QUESTIONS

1. Define industrial psychology and explain its primary objectives.
2. Briefly describe the significance of the Hawthorne Studies in the field of industrial psychology.
3. What are the core components of a job analysis?
4. What do you understand by the concept of work-life balance and its importance in industrial psychology?
5. Mention two modern methods of performance appraisal.

MULTIPLE CHOICE QUESTIONS

1. **Which of the following is a primary goal of industrial psychology?**
   a. To conduct clinical therapy sessions
   b. To improve workplace productivity and employee well-being
   c. To develop new psychological theories without application
   d. To provide medical treatments for physical injuries

2. **The Hawthorne Studies highlighted the importance of which factor in the workplace?**
   a. Financial incentives
   b. Employee training programs
   c. Social and environmental factors
   d. Technological advancements

3. **Which of the following is NOT a method used in job analysis?**
   a. Observation method
   b. Interview method
   c. Diary method
   d. Statistical method

4. **Frederick Winslow Taylor is associated with which theory?**
   a. Human relations approach
   b. Scientific management
   c. Contingency theory
   d. Systems theory

5. **What is the main focus of ergonomics within industrial psychology?**
   a. Employee recruitment
   b. Workplace design and efficiency
   c. Leadership training
   d. Performance appraisal

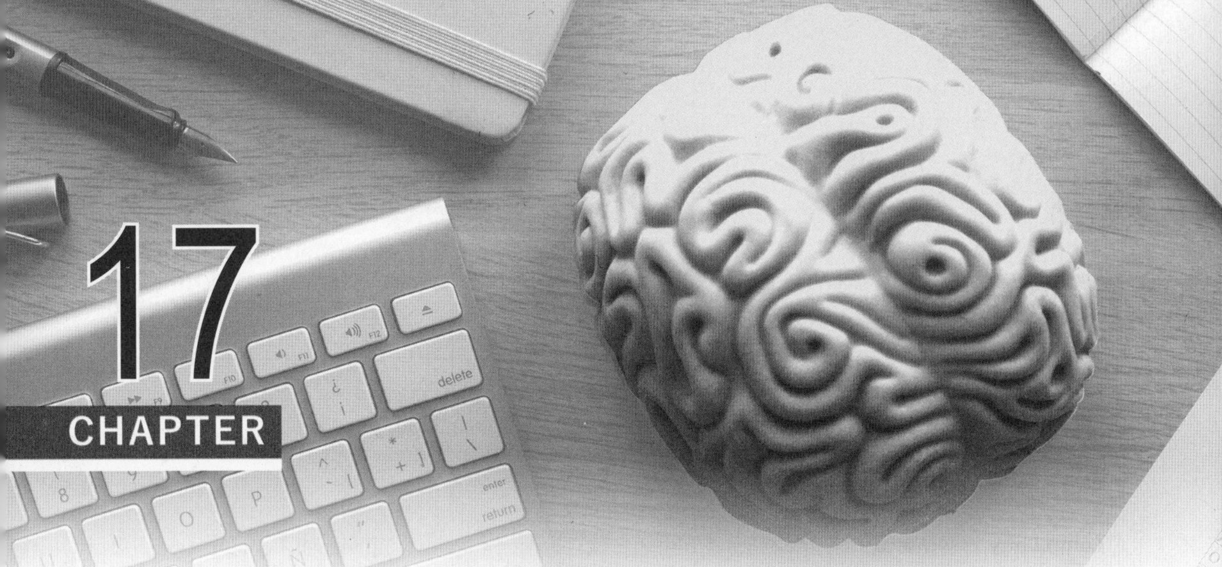

17

Social and Clinical Psychology

Shweta Sharma, Urvi, Parul Sharma

LEARNING OBJECTIVES

After the completion of the chapter, the readers will be able to:

- Understand the foundations of social and clinical psychology.
- Discuss the importance of combining insights from social and clinical psychology to understand human behavior and mental health.
- Analyze how the integration can lead to more effective therapeutic interventions.
- Define and explain concepts such as social perception, attitudes, persuasion, group dynamics, and interpersonal relationships.
- Describe the assessment and diagnosis of mental health disorders.
- Explain various therapeutic approaches, including cognitive behavioral therapy, psychodynamic therapy, and humanistic therapy.
- Discuss the role of pharmacotherapy in managing mental health symptoms.
- Discuss mental health promotion interventions and community psychology principles.
- Explain how cultural factors influence social behavior and mental health.
- Discuss advances in research methods, technology, and interdisciplinary collaboration in social and clinical psychology.

CHAPTER OUTLINE

- Introduction
- Overview of Social Psychology
- Overview of Clinical Psychology
- Intersection of Social and Clinical Psychology
- Historical Foundations
- Theoretical Frameworks
- Integration of Theories
- Social Psychological Processes
- Clinical Psychology Processes
- Applications
- Chronic and Terminal Illness
- Cross-Cultural Perspectives
- Current Trends and Future Directions
- Implications for Practice and Research
- Challenges and Opportunities in Social and Clinical Psychology

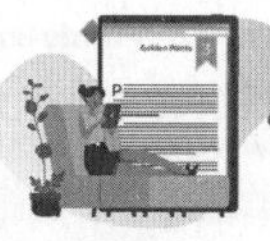
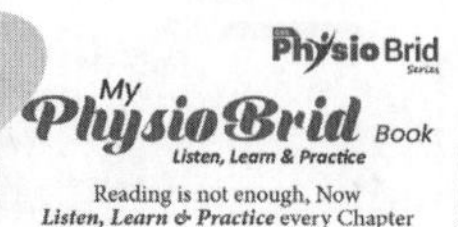

KEY TERMS

Attitudes: Evaluations of objects, people or concepts that influence behavior and decision-making.

Behavioral genetics: The study of how genetics influence behavior and mental health.

Clinical psychology: The field of psychology that focuses on the assessment, diagnosis, and treatment of mental, emotional, and behavioral problems.

Cognitive behavioral therapy (CBT): A therapeutic approach that focuses on identifying and changing unhealthy thought patterns and behaviors.

Community psychology: A field that emphasizes understanding individuals within their social environments and addressing social issues through interventions.

Cross-cultural psychology: The study of how cultural factors influence behavior and mental health.

Cultural competence: The ability of healthcare professionals to understand, communicate with, and engage with patients from diverse cultural backgrounds.

Digital technology in psychology: The use of technology, such as telepsychology and online therapy platforms, to provide mental healthcare.

Global mental health: The occurrence, management, and prevention of mental illnesses on a global scale.

Group dynamics: The behavioral and mental processes that occur within social groups.

Humanistic therapy: A therapeutic approach that emphasizes the individual's experience and self-actualization.

Interdisciplinary collaboration: The integration of different disciplines, such as psychology, social work, medicine, and education, to address complex mental health issues.

Interpersonal relationships: The interactions and behaviors between individuals.

Mental health promotion: Interventions aimed at enhancing psychological well-being and preventing the onset of mental health disorders.

Persuasion: The process of changing attitudes through communication.

Pharmacotherapy: The use of medications to manage and reduce symptoms of mental health disorders.

Psychodynamic therapy: A therapeutic approach based on Freudian theories, exploring how past events and unconscious processes influence current behavior.

Social influence: The process by which individuals adapt their ideas, emotions, and actions in response to their social environment.

Social perception: The process by which individuals form impressions and make judgments about the traits and actions of others.

Social psychology: The study of how social situations and interactions shape our thoughts, feelings, and behaviors.

INTRODUCTION

Social and clinical psychology are two dynamic yet complementary fields of medical science that illuminate the world of human behavior and mental health. Social psychology explores how the connections and social situations around us shape our ideas, feelings, and behaviors, revealing the potent powers of social perception, persuasion, and conformity.[1] Clinical psychology, on the other hand, is concerned with the identification and management of mental health issues. It does this by utilizing therapeutic procedures that are supported by research to reduce psychological suffering

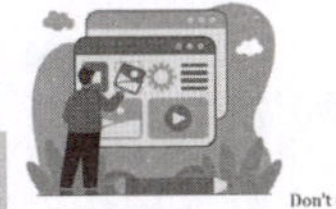

and improve overall health.[2] The confluence of these domains provides significant understanding of the ways in which social environments affect mental health and psychological disorders affect social relationships. Through their ability to connect the dots between personal dysfunction and the social milieu, these fields offer a comprehensive understanding of the human mind. An introduction of clinical psychology and social psychology will be given in this chapter, along with an examination of the junction of these two disciplines and their contributions to theoretical understanding and real-world applications. Gaining insight into how society and the individual mind interact can provide us with effective strategies for promoting mental health and navigating the difficulties of interpersonal interactions.

OVERVIEW OF SOCIAL PSYCHOLOGY

Social psychology examines how humans are impacted by the social situations in which they live, with a particular emphasis on how people interact, perceive, and influence one another.[3] Social perception, social impact, interpersonal dynamics, and intergroup connections are important subjects in this study. Social psychologists investigate a broad range of topics, including prosocial behavior, prejudice, aggressiveness, and conformity.[1]

To thoroughly examine ideas and hypotheses, social psychology makes use of a range of methodological techniques, such as surveys, observational studies, experiments, and meta-analyses.[4] Social psychology research yields valuable insights that may be applied in a variety of contexts, including the workplace, education, health, and law. For example, knowing group dynamics may improve leadership and collaboration in corporate settings, while knowing the mechanics of social influence can aid in the design of successful public health initiatives.[5, 6]

OVERVIEW OF CLINICAL PSYCHOLOGY

The examination, evaluation, and management of mental diseases are the main areas of concentration for clinical psychology. It combines clinical practice and academic study to comprehend and treat psychological disorder and discomfort.[7] To address each patient's unique requirements, clinical psychologists use a variety of therapeutic modalities such as Cognitive Behavioral Therapy (CBT), Psychodynamic Therapy, Humanistic Therapy, and others.

Two essential elements of clinical psychology are assessment and diagnosis.[7] To recognize and comprehend mental health disorders, practitioners employ a variety of instruments, including behavioral evaluations, structured interviews, and standardized psychological testing. The American Psychiatric Association's Diagnostic and Statistical Manual of Mental diseases (DSM-5) offers a thorough categorization system for mental diseases that aids in diagnosis and treatment planning for medical professionals.[8] In addition, clinical psychology deals with professional and ethical concerns, making sure that procedures follow guidelines that safeguard the well-being of patients and encourage efficient care. The practice of clinical psychology is based on core ethical principles, which emphasize the importance of client-centered treatment and include confidentiality, informed consent, and competence.[9]

INTERSECTION OF SOCIAL AND CLINICAL PSYCHOLOGY

The intersection of social and clinical psychology reveals how social circumstances and interactions have a major influence on mental health, while psychological problems have an impact on social conduct. By incorporating knowledge from both disciplines, this interdisciplinary approach offers a more comprehensive understanding of human behavior and improves the way complicated psychological challenges are addressed.

Social psychology plays a crucial role in informing therapeutic treatment in relation to social determinants of mental health, including cultural influences, socioeconomic position, and social support.[10-12] Strong networks of social support, for example, have been demonstrated to improve recovery and resilience in people with mental health concerns, whereas social exclusion and prejudice are known risk factors for mental illness.[13] Comprehending these social variables enables medical professionals to create treatment regimens that are more thorough and appropriate for the given environment.[14]

Furthermore, the inclusion of social psychology theories on bias and discrimination is beneficial for the research of stigma and mental health. Improving the accessibility of mental health services and guaranteeing that people receive the assistance they require depend on lowering the stigma attached to mental illness. The study of attitudes, preconceived notions, and social impact in social psychology offers insightful tactics for eradicating stigma and raising mental health awareness.[15]

Social psychology ideas can also be applied to therapeutic therapies. For instance, group dynamics are used in group therapy to assist and encourage participant transformation.[16] Social psychology research is directly applied to methods like role-playing and social skills training, which help clients feel less symptomatic and function better in interpersonal situations.

Researchers and practitioners may create more effective therapies and promote a greater knowledge of the intricate interactions between social circumstances and psychological well-being by combining the concepts and methodology of both social and clinical psychology.[17] This multidisciplinary approach promotes practical outcomes in social functioning and mental health treatment in addition to theoretical understanding.

HISTORICAL FOUNDATIONS

Development of Social Psychology

Historical developments, theoretical breakthroughs, and methodological improvements have all played a dynamic interplay in the evolution of social psychology as a science. Social psychology, a vibrant scientific subject devoted to comprehending how people's ideas, feelings, and behaviors are impacted by the social environments in which they are enmeshed, sprang from philosophical studies into human nature and social behavior. We will now embark on this historical journey to witness the progression of key concepts and how research perspectives have evolved throughout time.

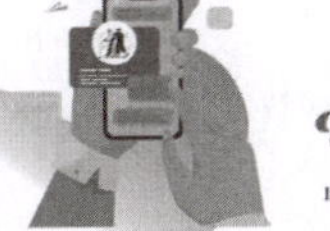
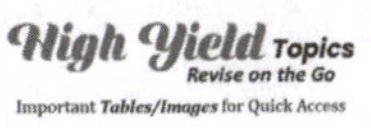

Figure 17.1 lists some of the pioneers who played a crucial role in the development of social psychology.

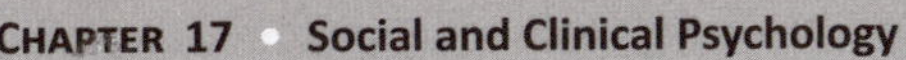

Leon Festinger	Kurt Lewin	Henri Tajfel	Albert Bandura	Stanley Milgram
Developed cognitive dissonance theory	Father of modern psychology	Developed social identity theory	Introduced social learning theory and the concept of self-efficacy	Conducted groundbreaking research on obedience

Fig. 17.1: Pioneers and their contributions to social psychology

The progression of social psychology from its philosophical roots through to its contemporary breadth and methodological sophistication (Each period highlights key theoretical advances, methodological improvements, and ethical considerations) has been listed in Table 17.1.

Table 17.1: Progression of social psychology

Period	Key developments
Early foundations	• Influenced by Aristotle, Plato, Comte, Spencer.[18] • Wilhelm Wundt and William James lay foundation for psychology as a scientific field.[19]
Formalization and experimental roots	Quantitative measurements begin • Norman Triplett's study on social facilitation (1898).[20, 21] • Floyd Allport distinguishes social psychology from sociology (1924).[22–24] • Kurt Lewin and Leon Festinger pioneered experimental methods (1940s–50s).[25, 26]
Expansion and theoretical development	• World War II influences studies on attitudes, persuasion and group dynamics.[27, 28] • Stanley Milgram's obedience experiments (1963).[29] • Solomon Asch's conformity studies (1952).[29] • Philip Zimbardo's Stanford Prison Experiment (1971).[30] • Theoretical frameworks emerge: Cognitive Dissonance Theory (1957), Social Learning Theory (1963) and Attribution Theory (1968).[31–33]
Methodological and ethical refinements	• Advances in experimental design and statistical methods.[34] • Development of social cognition.[34] • Ethical concerns lead to IRBs and ethical regulations (e.g., APA standards).[35]
Contemporary social psychology	• Expands into technology, social identity, intergroup relations.[36] • Applied to environmental conservation, health promotion and organizational behavior.[36] • Emphasis on cultural context and cross-cultural studies.[37]

Development of Clinical Psychology

With a long history that has integrated scientific research, theoretical developments, and real-world applications, clinical psychology is the area of psychology that focuses on the identification and management of mental, emotional, and behavioral problems.

Early Foundation, Formalization and Growth

The early 1900s saw the emergence of clinical psychology, which was impacted by the wider advancement of psychology as an academic discipline. Wilhelm Wundt, who is frequently seen as the founder of contemporary psychology, founded the very first laboratory for psychology in 1879 and placed a strong emphasis on the use of experimental techniques.[38] The foundation for therapeutic approaches was laid by the research of Sigmund Freud on psychoanalysis in the late 19th and early 20th centuries, which popularized the notion that mental illnesses could be cured by discussion and understanding.[39]

Clinical psychology officially began in the early 20th century when Lightner Witmer, a student of Wundt, established the first psychological clinic at the University of Pennsylvania in 1896. Witmer's strategy laid the groundwork for further advancements in the discipline by fusing scientific methodology with useful therapy.[40]

The Boulder Model and Beyond

A pivotal moment in the history of clinical psychology occurred in the middle of the 20th century with the development of the scientist-practitioner paradigm or Boulder paradigm. The integration of therapeutic practice and empirical studies was stressed in this approach, which was created during the 1949-Boulder Conference on Graduate Education in Clinical Psychology. Even in modern clinical psychology training programs, the Boulder Model is still a mainstay.[41]

Carl Rogers developed client-centered therapy at this time, highlighting the value of unity, compassion, and unconditional positive regard in the therapeutic alliance. This humanistic perspective offered a substitute for behaviorist and psychoanalytic techniques.[42]

Cognitive Revolution and Evidence-Based Therapy

The development of cognitive psychology in the latter half of the 20th century had a huge impact on therapeutic practice. The emphasis moved to comprehending and changing problematic thought processes with the advent of cognitive therapy developed by Aaron Beck and rational emotive behavior therapy developed by Albert Ellis.[43, 44]

The shift to evidence-based practice, which prioritizes the use of therapies backed by scientific studies, gained pace in the 1980s and 1990s. This strategy was formalized *via* the creation of organizations like the Society of Clinical Psychology (Division 12 of the American Psychological Association).[45]

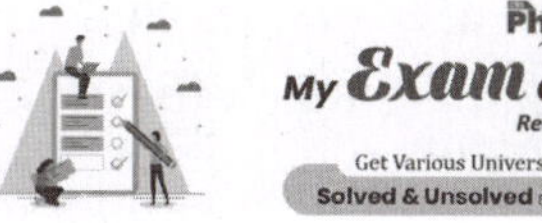

Contemporary Clinical Psychology–Integration and Diversity

Clinical psychology is still in developing stage, using a variety of theoretical stances and methods. The biopsychosocial paradigm has gained widespread acceptance as a means of diagnosing and treating mental diseases.[46] It takes into account biological, psychological, and social variables. Furthermore, the significance of cultural competency in clinical practice—which addresses the necessity of comprehending and respecting a variety of cultural backgrounds—is becoming more widely acknowledged.[47] Refer to Figure 17.2 to know about some of the noteworthy academicians who contributed immensely to clinical psychology.

The key developments in clinical psychology from its early foundations to contemporary practices, highlighting significant milestones, theoretical shifts, and methodological advancements are shown in Table 17.2.

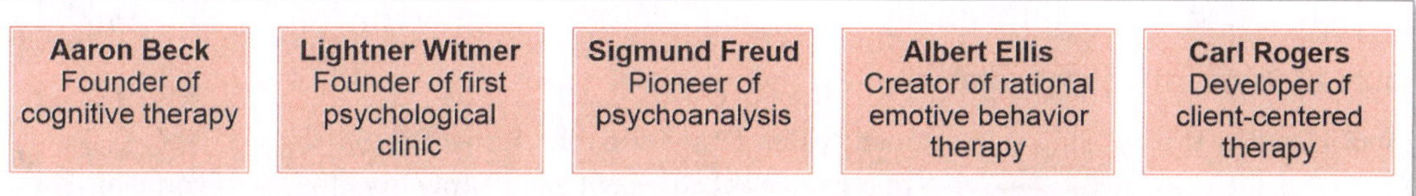

Fig. 17.2: Pioneers and their contributions to clinical psychology

Table 17.2: Clinical psychology and its development process

Period	Development of clinical psychology
Early 1900s	• Emergence influenced by advances in psychology as an academic discipline. • Wilhelm Wundt established first psychology laboratory in 1879, emphasizing experimental techniques. • Sigmund Freud's psychoanalysis (late 19th– early 20th centuries) popularized therapy through discussion and understanding. • Lightner Witmer founded the first psychological clinic in 1896 at the University of Pennsylvania, merging scientific methodology with practical therapy.
Mid-20th century	• Boulder Model (1949) established the scientist-practitioner paradigm, integrating therapy and empirical research. • Carl Rogers developed client-centered therapy, emphasizing empathy and unconditional positive regard.
Late 20th century	• Cognitive psychology (latter 20th century) shifted focus to understanding and altering problematic thought processes. • Aaron Beck developed cognitive therapy, focusing on changing maladaptive thoughts. • Albert Ellis developed rational emotive behavior therapy (REBT), emphasizing challenging irrational beliefs. • Rise of evidence-based practice in the 1980s–1990s, promoting therapies validated by scientific research.

Contd...

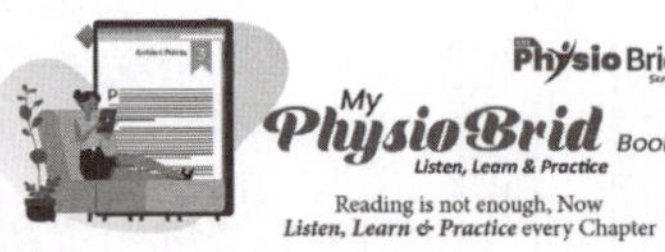

Period	Development of clinical psychology
Contemporary	• Biopsychosocial paradigm gains acceptance, incorporating biological, psychological, and social factors in diagnosis and treatment. • Emphasis on cultural competency in clinical practice, recognizing the importance of understanding and respecting diverse cultural backgrounds. • Continued evolution with diverse theoretical approaches and methodologies.

THEORETICAL FRAMEWORKS

Refer to Tables 17.3 and 17.4 to know about various social psychological theories and clinical psychological theories and the academician who conceived them.

Table 17.3: Social psychological theories

Social identity theory	• Developed by Henri Tajfel and John Turner (1979). • Posits that people get some of their identity from the social groupings they are a part of. • Understanding concepts like bias, discrimination, and group dynamics has been made possible thanks in large part to Social Identity Theory (SIT).[29]
Social learning theory	• Developed by Albert Bandura (1977). • Essential for comprehending how people pick up attitudes, behaviors, and emotional responses by watching other people. • Incorporates cognitive processes that take place in social environments, going beyond the conventional ideas of behavioral learning theories.[34]
Attribution theory	• Introduced by Fritz Heider (1958). • Further developed by Harold Kelley and Bernard Weiner. • Addresses how people understand and attribute causes to actions and occurrences. • Examines how attributions affect emotions and actions by differentiating between inner (dispositional) and outer (situational) attributions.[48]

Table 17.4: Clinical psychological theories

Cognitive behavioral therapy	• Developed by Aaron Beck and Albert Ellis (1960s). • Popular therapeutic method focusing on the interaction of ideas, feelings, and actions. • Asserts that emotional and behavioral issues are caused by dysfunctional thought patterns. Through recognition and adjustment of these tendencies, people can attain improved mental health results.[43]

Contd...

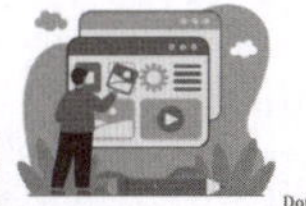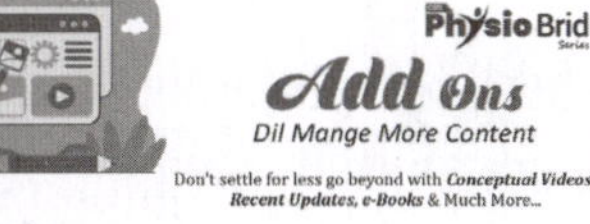

Psychoanalytic/ psychodynamic theory	• Developed by Sigmund Freud (1926). • Investigates how early events, defensive systems, and internal disputes affect mental health. • Modern psychodynamic techniques frequently use understandings from interpersonal interactions and attachment theory.[49]
Humanistic theory	• Associated with Carl Rogers and Abraham Maslow (1950s). • Emphasizes each person's unique experience and potential for self-actualization and places a strong emphasis on the role that the therapeutic connection, compassion, and positive reinforcement have in promoting psychological health and personal development.[50]

INTEGRATION OF THEORIES

Our comprehension of human conduct and mental health may be greatly improved by examining the junction of social and clinical psychology. Both social psychology and clinical psychology theories—which stress the diagnosis and treatment of mental disorders—offer important insights into how social circumstances and group dynamics impact individual behavior. A more comprehensive strategy that addresses the internal psychological processes as well as the exterior social variables that contribute to mental health difficulties is made possible by integrating various points of view. Better therapy results, more successful treatments, and a greater understanding of the intricate interactions between a person's social setting and psychological health can all result from this synthesis.[51]

There are several advantages of combining social and clinical psychology theories:

- **Integrated understanding:** By taking into account both individual cognitive processes and societal effects, integration offers a more thorough understanding of behavior.[49]

- **Improved interventions:** By integrating theories, more efficient therapy strategies that take into account both internal psychological processes and exterior social aspects may be developed.[45]

- **Better assessment and therapy:** Accurate diagnosis and successful treatment results can be achieved by comprehending the interaction among social and clinical aspects.[47]

- **Applications of integration (Fig. 17.3):** Recognition and management of mental health problems including depression and social anxiety disorder (SAD) can be significantly improved through the integration of social and clinical psychology ideas. For example, a thorough method of treating SAD is offered by the combination of Social Identity Theory and Cognitive Behavioral Therapy (CBT).[51] Social Identity Theory describes how people's self-image and impressions of social status are influenced by society norms and group dynamics, which in turn causes social anxiety. By addressing the cognitive illusions and avoidance actions that sustain social anxiety, cognitive behavioral therapy offers techniques for changing these tendencies. Combining these viewpoints allows therapists to create therapies that take into account the social environment as well as the cognitive processes of the patient, leading to more successful SAD therapy.[52]

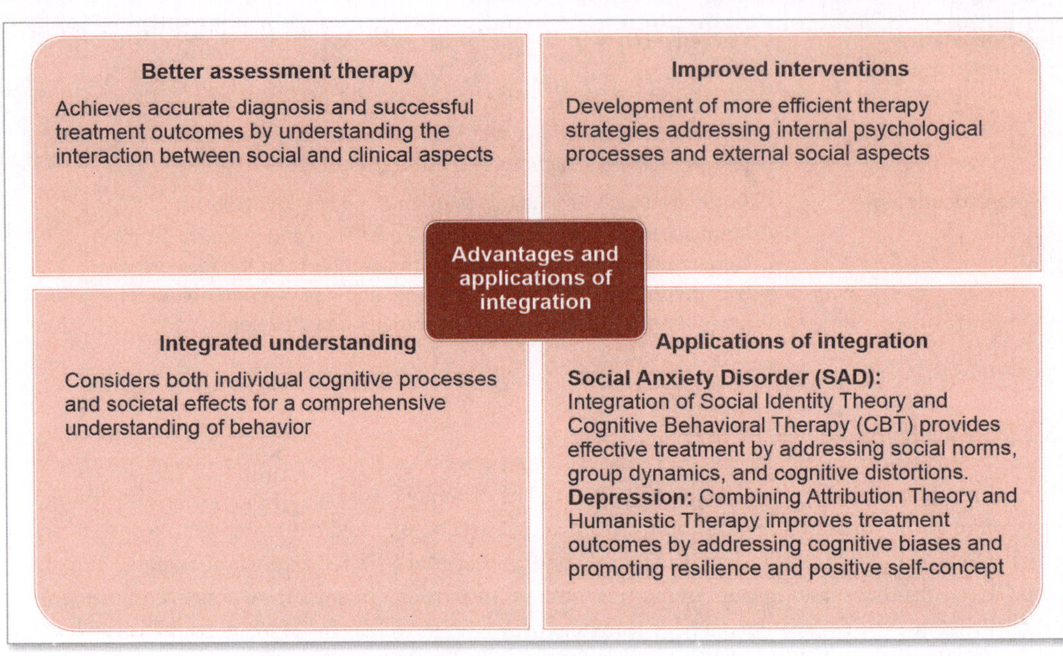

Fig. 17.3: The advantages and applications of integrating social and clinical psychology theories in the context of mental health treatment

In a similar vein, combining Attribution Theory with Humanistic Therapy improves depression treatment. The application of Attribution Theory to the study of how people assign reasons to occurrences in life might shed light on the cognitive tendencies that underlie depression.[53] Depressive attributional styles, for instance, might lead people to persistently link unfavorable experiences to internal, stable, and external sources, which exacerbates feelings of hopelessness and powerlessness. People can build resilience and a more positive self-concept by utilizing humanistic therapy, which emphasizes compassion, positive reinforcement, and self-realization.[54] By using these beliefs, therapists can better assist patients with depression by addressing cognitive errors and creating a nurturing, a growth-focused therapy environment.[53]

SOCIAL PSYCHOLOGICAL PROCESSES

Studying social psychological processes is essential to comprehending how people interact with their social environment. These processes cover an extensive variety of phenomena, such as how individuals form and modify attitudes (attitudes and persuasion), how they think about and understand others (social perception and cognition), and how they act in interactions and in groups (group dynamics and interpersonal relationships). Psychologists can learn more about the fundamental principles guiding social interactions, cultural standards, and human conduct by examining these processes.

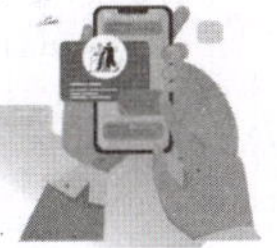

Social Perception and Cognition

The core concepts of social psychology are social perception and cognition, which deal with how people see, comprehend, and react to social cues. The mechanism by individuals create judgments and views about the traits and actions of others is known as social perception. Contextual knowledge, social roles, and nonverbal cues are some of the variables that affect this process.[35] The formation of these impressions is greatly influenced by cognitive functions like inference, memory, and attention.[55]

The attribution theory is a crucial idea in social cognition that examines how people rationalize the reasons behind their actions. The concept that people attribute activities to either inherent inclinations or outside circumstances was first put out by Fritz Heider in 1958. This phenomenon was further explained by Harold Kelley's (1967) covariation model, which takes consensus knowledge, uniqueness, and consistency into account when assigning blame.[56] These mental algorithms or cognitive shortcuts, frequently result in fallacies like the basic attribution mistake, which occurs when people overstate personality qualities and understate environmental elements when attempting to explain the conduct of others.[57]

Attitudes and Persuasion

Attitudes are judgments about things, people or concepts that affect how one behaves and makes decisions. Affective (sentimental reaction), cognitive (opinions and concepts), and behavioral (actions or visible behavior) are their three constituent parts.[58] In social psychology, attitudes and how they develop and evolve are major subjects.

Altering viewpoints *via* dialogue is the process of persuasion, which is informed by a number of theoretical frameworks. There are two paths to persuasion, according to Petty and Cacioppo's (1986) Elaboration Likelihood Model (ELM): (1) The center/primary route and (2) the Periphery way. The primary path entails a thorough and deliberate analysis of the arguments put forth, resulting in a permanent shift in perspective.In contrast, the peripheral route depends on surface-level indicators, such the source's beauty or legitimacy, which might cause a transient shift in attitude.[59]

Leon Festinger's 1957 Cognitive Dissonance hypothesis is another well-known hypothesis. It suggests that people feel uncomfortable (dissonance) when their conduct contradicts their views or when they have competing beliefs. People are driven to alter their actions or attitudes in order to lessen the discomfort, which ultimately results in attitude modification.[60]

Group Dynamics and Interpersonal Relationships

The behavioral and mental processes that take place inside social groupings are referred to as group dynamics. Comprehending these dynamics is essential to grasping how belonging to a group affects one's actions and how groups operate collectively. Group decision-making, conformity, and social influence are important ideas in this field.

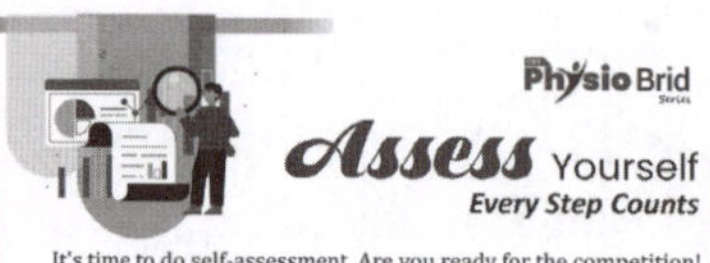

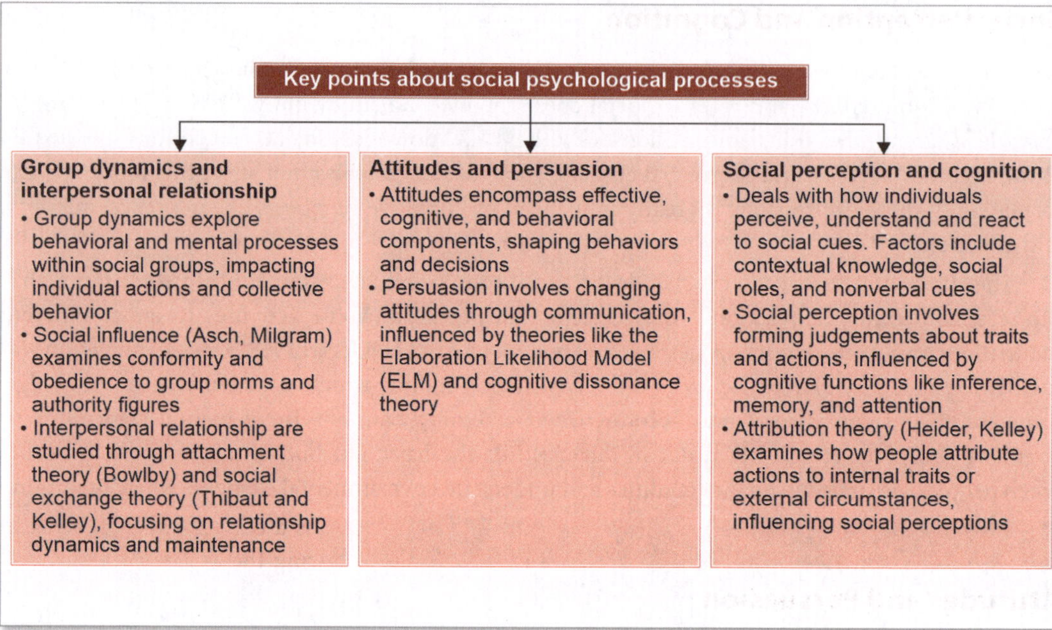

Fig. 17.4: The key points about social psychological processes

The process by which people adapt their conduct to fit the expectations of a social setting is known as social influence. According to Solomon Asch's (1951) conformity tests, individuals frequently follow group standards even when they go against their personal opinions. In the same spirit, Stanley Milgram's (1963) research on obedience demonstrated the degree to which people are prepared to submit to authoritative figures, even if it means doing damage to others.[61]

Another important area of social psychology that focuses on the connections and behaviors between people is interpersonal relationships (Fig. 17.4). John Bowlby (1969) established attachment theory, which examines how early ties with providers affect the nature of connections in the future. According to Thibaut and Kelley's (1959) social exchange theory, interpersonal connections are sustained by the benefits and costs that come with them. According to this hypothesis, people try to reduce expenses and maximize benefits in their relationships.[62]

CLINICAL PSYCHOLOGY PROCESSES

Clinical psychology uses both empirical study and real-world application to better understand, diagnose, and treat mental health conditions. This discipline covers a wide range of procedures, including as diagnosis and evaluation, treatment of different mental health issues, and treatment methods like medication and psychotherapy.

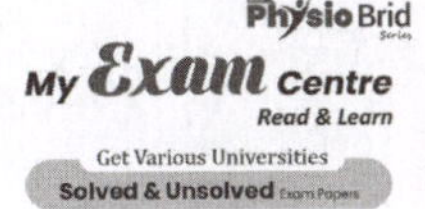

Assessment and Diagnosis

Clinical psychology relies heavily on assessment and diagnosis as they lay the groundwork for efficient treatment and intervention planning. When someone presents with psychological difficulties, clinical assessment entails the methodical examination and measurement of psychological, biological, and social components. Clinical interviews, behavioral analyses, psychological examinations, and neuropsychological tests are examples of common techniques.[63]

The Diagnosis and Statistical Manual of Mental Disorders (DSM-5), which is published by the American Psychiatric Association, provides guidelines that are generally followed during the diagnosis process.[64] These guidelines guarantee uniformity and dependability in diagnosis. It contains thorough explanations of the signs, characteristics, and diagnostic standards for a variety of mental health issues, ranging from personality disorders and psychotic disorders to mood disorders and anxiety disorders.

Therapeutic Approaches

- **Psychotherapy:** Psychotherapy, also referred to as talk therapy, is a collection of therapeutic modalities designed to assist people in comprehending and altering their feelings, ideas, and actions. There are several forms of psychotherapy, such as:

  - **Cognitive behavioral therapy (CBT):** A popular and scientifically validated psychotherapy modality. It was created by Aaron Beck and focuses on recognizing and changing unhealthy thought patterns and behavior patterns. A variety of problems, such as anxiety, PTSD, and depression, can be effectively treated with CBT.[65]

  - **Psychodynamic therapy:** Based on the theories of Freud, psychodynamic therapy investigates how past events and unconscious processes shaped a person's behavior in the present. This method assists people in understanding their internal problems and creating more positive behavioral patterns.[66]

  - **Humanistic therapy:** Person-centered therapy and other humanistic therapies emphasize the individual's experience and self-actualization. They also place a strong emphasis on establishing a therapeutic atmosphere that is both nonjudgmental and helpful. This method works especially well for problems pertaining to growth and self-worth.[67]

- **Pharmacotherapy:** Pharmacotherapy is the process of managing and reducing mental health diseases' symptoms *via* the use of pharmaceuticals. This method is frequently used with psychotherapy to offer all-encompassing care. Typical categories of psychiatric drugs consist of:

  - **Antidepressants:** These drugs, which treat anxiety and depression, include serotonin-norepinephrine reuptake inhibitors (SNRIs) and selective serotonin reuptake inhibitors (SSRIs).[68]

  - **Antipsychotics:** The main purpose of these drugs is to treat the hallmarks of psychotic conditions like schizophrenia. They include antipsychotics, both conventional and atypical, that lessen delusions and hallucinations.[69]

- **Mood stabilizers:** Anticonvulsants and lithium are examples of drugs that are used to treat mood disorders like bipolar disorder.[70]
- **Anxiolytics:** These drugs, which include β-blockers and benzodiazepines, are used to treat panic attacks and anxiety symptoms.[71]

Therapeutic approaches and treatments for mental health disorders are given in Table 17.5.

Table 17.5: Therapeutic approaches and treatments for mental health disorders

Therapeutic approaches	Description
Psychotherapy	
Cognitive behavioral therapy (CBT)	Focuses on identifying and changing unhealthy thought patterns and behaviors. Effective for anxiety, PTSD, depression, and other issues.[65]
Psychodynamic therapy	Based on Freudian theories, explores how past events and unconscious processes influence current behavior. Helps in understanding internal conflicts.[67]
Humanistic therapy	Emphasizes individual experience, self-actualization, and creating a supportive therapeutic environment. Effective for issues related to growth and self-worth.[67]
Pharmacotherapy	
Antidepressants	Includes SSRIs and SNRIs, used to treat depression and anxiety disorders by affecting serotonin levels in the brain.[68]
Antipsychotics	Treats psychotic symptoms like hallucinations and delusions in conditions such as schizophrenia. Includes both conventional and atypical antipsychotics.[69]
Mood stabilizers	Examples include lithium and anticonvulsants, used to manage mood swings in bipolar disorder.[70]
Anxiolytics	Includes benzodiazepines and β-blockers, used to alleviate symptoms of anxiety disorders such as panic attacks and generalized anxiety disorder (GAD).[71]
Common mental health disorders and treatment	
Depression	Characterized by persistent sadness and loss of interest, treated with CBT to address negative thinking patterns and SSRIs for symptom management.[68]
Anxiety disorders	Includes social anxiety disorder, panic disorder, and GAD. Treated with CBT for cognitive restructuring and exposure therapy, along with medications like benzodiazepines.[65, 71]
Schizophrenia	Involves hallucinations, delusions, and disordered thinking. Treated primarily with antipsychotic medications and complemented by psychosocial therapies like CBT.[72]
Bipolar disorder	Alternating episodes of mania and depression. Managed with mood stabilizers (e.g., lithium, anticonvulsants) and supported by psychoeducation and CBT.[73]

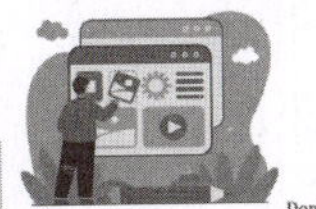

Mental Health Disorders and Treatment

Clinicians primarily focus on studying the causes, manifestations, and therapies of mental health illnesses. Examples of common mental health conditions and how they are treated are provided here:

- **Depression:** Depression is a common mental illness marked by enduring melancholy, interest loss, and a range of cognitive and physical manifestations. Usually, medication and psychotherapy are used for treatment. When it comes to treating the negative thinking tendencies linked to depression, cognitive behavioral therapy or CBT, is very helpful. The SSRIs and other antidepressants are frequently recommended to treat symptoms.[68]

- **Anxiety disorders:** Excessive and ongoing concern and dread are symptoms of anxiety disorders, which include social anxiety disorder, panic disorder, and generalized anxiety disorder (GAD). Cognitive behavioral therapy (CBT) is a common treatment method that uses exposure tactics and cognitive restructuring to help patients control their anxiety.[65] Benzodiazepines and SSRIs are two examples of medications that can be used to treat symptoms.[71]

- **Schizophrenia:** Hallucinations, delusions, disordered thinking, and poor functioning are hallmarks of schizophrenia, a severe psychotic illness. Antipsychotic drugs are commonly used as a kind of treatment to lessen psychotic symptoms. In order to assist people, manage their disease and enhance their quality of life, psychosocial therapies including cognitive behavioral therapy and social skills training are also crucial.[72]

- **Bipolar disorder:** Mania and sadness bouts alternate in bipolar illness, a mood disease. The main pharmaceutical therapies for mood swings are mood stabilizers, such as anticonvulsants and lithium.[73] Psychoeducation and CBT in particular are essential for helping people comprehend and control their symptoms.

APPLICATIONS

Social Influence and Behavior Change

The term "social influence" describes how people adapt their ideas, emotions, and actions in reaction to their social surroundings. Promoting behavior change in a variety of practical contexts, including health, education, and environmental protection, requires an understanding of these mechanisms.

- **Theories and mechanisms of social influence:** The workings of social influence are explained by several ideas. There are several principles of influence, such as scarcity, likeability, authority, social proof, reciprocity, and commitment and consistency. It is possible to create treatments that support desired behaviors by applying these ideas. For example, ads advocating healthy habits can take use of social proof, which is the concept that individuals look to others to decide proper conduct, by emphasizing how widely certain activities are adopted throughout the society.[74]

- **Applications in behavior change:** One prominent usage is in the field of public health, where social influence techniques are employed to encourage lifestyle modifications including giving up smoking, getting more exercise, and maintaining a balanced diet. For instance, programs that make use of social norms and peer pressure have been successful in lowering teenage smoking rates. In environmental psychology, social influence tactics are also used to promote energy-saving and recycling habits. According to studies, giving neighbor's input into how much energy they use can drastically cut down on home energy use.[75]

CHRONIC AND TERMINAL ILLNESS

The psychology of chronic and terminal illness involves understanding the emotional, cognitive, and behavioral responses that individuals and their families experience when dealing with long-term, often life-altering conditions. Here's an overview of the key psychological aspects related to chronic and terminal illness:

- **Emotional responses:**
  - **Shock and denial:** Upon diagnosis, individuals often experience shock, disbelief, and denial. These initial reactions can serve as a defense mechanism, allowing them to gradually come to terms with their condition.
  - **Anxiety and fear:** Chronic and terminal illnesses can trigger significant anxiety and fear related to the progression of the disease, loss of autonomy, and fear of death or worsening symptoms.
  - **Depression:** Feelings of sadness, hopelessness, and despair are common, especially as individuals grapple with the reality of living with a long-term illness or facing the end of life. Depression can be a significant barrier to quality of life and adherence to treatment.
  - **Anger and frustration:** Individuals may feel anger toward their situation, the healthcare system or even loved ones. This can stem from a sense of injustice, loss of control or frustration with the limitations imposed by their illness.
  - **Grief and loss:** Chronic and terminal illnesses often involve a process of grieving, not just for the potential loss of life, but also for the loss of one's previous health, independence, and future plans.

- **Cognitive responses:**
  - **Adjustment and adaptation:** Over time, individuals work through the psychological process of adjusting to their illness. This involves rethinking personal goals, life expectations, and daily routines.
  - **Cognitive distortions:** People with chronic or terminal illnesses may experience negative thought patterns, such as catastrophizing (expecting the worst) or overgeneralizing (believing that their illness will negatively affect all areas of life).
  - **Meaning-making:** Many individuals engage in a process of finding meaning in their illness, which can lead to personal growth, a re-evaluation of life priorities or spiritual development. This can be a crucial factor in coping with the illness.

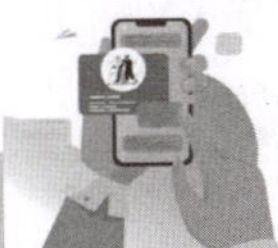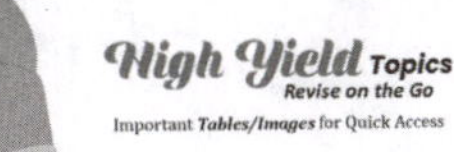

- **Behavioral responses:**
  - **Treatment adherence:** Psychological factors greatly influence whether individuals adhere to prescribed treatments. Depression, hopelessness, and cognitive distortions can lead to non-adherence, while positive coping strategies and support can improve adherence.
  - **Lifestyle changes:** Chronic illnesses often require significant lifestyle changes, such as diet modification, exercise, and stress management. How individuals adapt to these changes is influenced by their psychological state.
  - **Social withdrawal or engagement:** Some individuals may withdraw socially due to feelings of shame, embarrassment or a desire to conserve energy. Others may seek out social support and become more engaged with loved ones and support groups.

- **Coping mechanisms:**
  - **Active coping:** This involves taking direct action to manage the illness, such as seeking information, following treatment plans, and making lifestyle adjustments. It is associated with better psychological outcomes.
  - **Avoidant coping:** This involves denial, avoidance or distraction to cope with the stress of the illness. While it may provide short-term relief, avoidant coping is generally associated with poorer long-term psychological outcomes.
  - **Spiritual and religious coping:** Many individuals turn to spirituality or religion to find comfort, meaning, and hope. This can provide significant emotional support, though it may also lead to conflict if the illness challenges previously held beliefs.

- **Social and interpersonal dynamics:**
  - **Family dynamics:** Chronic and terminal illnesses impact not just the individual, but also his family. Families may experience role changes, increased stress, and emotional strain, which can affect relationships.
  - **Support systems:** The presence of a strong support system, including family, friends, and healthcare providers, is crucial for the psychological well-being of individuals with chronic or terminal illnesses. Support systems provide emotional support, practical help, and a sense of belonging.
  - **Communication:** Open and honest communication about the illness, prognosis, and emotional needs is essential in maintaining healthy relationships and ensuring that the patient's needs and wishes are met.

- **Quality of life:**
  - **Maintaining dignity:** For individuals with terminal illness, maintaining a sense of dignity and autonomy is a critical aspect of their psychological well-being. This includes having control over treatment decisions, end-of-life care, and how they spend their remaining time.
  - **Pain and symptom management:** Effective management of pain and other distressing symptoms is closely linked to psychological well-being. Uncontrolled pain can lead to increased anxiety, depression, and a decreased quality of life.

- **Life review and legacy:** Many individuals engage in a process of life review, reflecting on their life experiences and accomplishments. This can be a source of comfort and help them find peace. Some may also focus on creating a legacy, such as writing memoirs or creating lasting memories with loved ones.
- **End-of-life issues (for terminal illness):**
    - **Acceptance of mortality:** Coming to terms with the reality of impending death is a profound psychological process. Some individuals achieve a sense of peace and acceptance, while others may struggle with this.
    - **Advance care planning:** Engaging in discussions about end-of-life wishes, such as advance directives, palliative care, and hospice, can help individuals feel more in control and reduce anxiety about the unknown.
    - **Grief and bereavement:** As the end of life approaches, both the individual and their loved ones begin to experience anticipatory grief. Counseling and support can help in processing these emotions and preparing for the eventual loss.
- **Psychological interventions:**
    - **Counseling and psychotherapy:** Counseling can provide a space for individuals to express their emotions, work through difficult thoughts, and develop coping strategies. Cognitive behavioral therapy (CBT), acceptance and commitment therapy (ACT), and mindfulness-based therapies are particularly useful.
    - **Support groups:** Group therapy and peer support groups offer individuals the chance to connect with others facing similar challenges, which can reduce feelings of isolation and provide practical and emotional support.
    - **Palliative care:** Palliative care focuses on improving quality of life by addressing physical, emotional, and spiritual needs, and providing support to both patients and their families.

The Five Stages of Grief

Elisabeth Kübler-Ross was a Swiss-American psychiatrist who is best known for her work on death, dying, and grief. She introduced the "Five Stages of Grief" model, which describes a series of emotional stages that people often go through when faced with death or significant loss. These stages were first outlined in her groundbreaking 1969 book, *On Death and Dying*.

Kübler-Ross's model includes the following stages:

1. **Denial:**
    - **Reaction:** In this initial stage, individuals may struggle to accept the reality of the situation. They may think, "This cannot be happening" or "This is not real". Denial serves as a defense mechanism, providing a temporary emotional buffer against the overwhelming shock and pain of loss.
    - **Example:** A person might refuse to acknowledge the seriousness of a terminal diagnosis or might continue to act as if a deceased loved one is still alive.

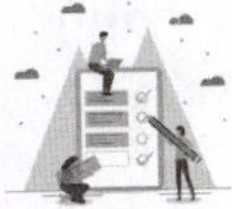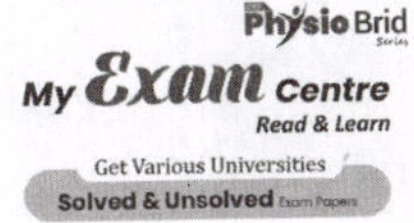

2. **Anger:**
   - **Reaction:** As denial begins to fade, the reality of the situation sets in, often leading to feelings of anger and frustration. This anger can be directed at oneself, others or even at the deceased person. Some may question, "Why me?" or "Why did this happen?"
   - **Example:** A person may express anger toward healthcare providers, family members or even God, feeling that the situation is unfair or unjust.

3. **Bargaining:**
   - **Reaction:** In this stage, individuals may attempt to negotiate or make deals with a higher power, themselves or others in an effort to reverse or minimize the loss. It often involves "what if" or "if only" statements.
   - **Example:** A person might say, "If only I had taken them to the doctor sooner" or "I will do anything to have more time".

4. **Depression:**
   - **Reaction:** As the reality of the loss fully sinks in, individuals may experience deep sadness, despair, and hopelessness. This stage involves mourning the loss of what was and what could have been. Depression in this context is a natural and necessary response to significant loss.
   - **Example:** Individuals may withdraw from others, lose interest in activities they once enjoyed, and feel overwhelmed by the weight of the loss.

5. **Acceptance:**
   - **Reaction:** In this final stage, individuals come to terms with the reality of the loss. Acceptance does not mean being "okay" with the loss, but rather reaching a point of peace and understanding. It involves acknowledging the permanence of the loss and beginning to move forward with life.
   - **Example:** Individuals may start to reorganize their life around the loss, finding ways to adjust and continue living without the person or situation that was lost.

Important Considerations

- **Nonlinear process:** It is important to note that the stages are not necessarily experienced in a linear fashion. People may move back and forth between stages, experience multiple stages at once or skip some stages altogether.
- **Individual variability:** The model was intended as a framework to help understand common reactions to loss, but individual experiences of grief are highly personal and can vary widely. Some may not experience all the stages or they may experience them in a different order.
- **Broader application:** While originally developed in the context of terminal illness and death, the stages of grief have been widely applied to various forms of loss, including the end of relationships, job loss or significant life changes.

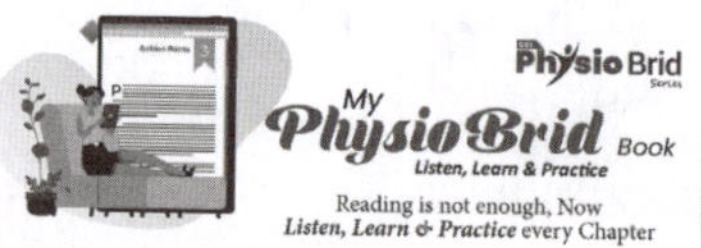

Impact

Kübler-Ross's work had a profound impact on the way society understands and approaches death and dying. She brought attention to the emotional and psychological needs of the dying and their families, advocating for more compassionate care at the end of life. Her model of grief remains one of the most influential frameworks in understanding the human response to loss, though it is now recognized as one of many ways to conceptualize the grieving process.

CASE STUDY

Coping with Limb Loss Through the Five Stages of Grief

Patient Background

John, a 45-year-old male, was involved in a severe car accident that resulted in the amputation of his right leg above the knee. Prior to the accident, John was an active individual who enjoyed running, hiking, and participating in sports. The amputation was a life-changing event that not only affected his physical abilities but also his psychological well-being.

The five stages of grief and John's experience:

1. **Denial:**
   - **John's reaction:** Initially, John struggles to accept that he has lost his leg. He frequently expresses disbelief, saying things like, "This cannot be real. I will wake up tomorrow, and my leg will be there". John avoids looking at his amputated limb and refuses to discuss prosthetic options with the medical team.
   - **Physiotherapist's role:** The physiotherapist approaches John with empathy, allowing him the space to express his feelings while gently introducing the reality of his situation. Physiotherapist started with non-threatening activities, like basic upper body exercises, to slowly build trust and help John stay engaged in his care without forcing him to confront the loss directly until he is ready.

2. **Anger:**
   - **John's reaction:** As reality sets in, John becomes increasingly angry. He directs his anger toward the medical staff, his family, and himself. He often questions, "Why did this happen to me?" and expresses frustration with the limitations imposed by his new condition.
   - **Physiotherapist's role:** The physiotherapist listens to John's frustrations without judgment, validating his feelings of anger. They help John channel this anger into his rehabilitation, using it as motivation to regain as much independence as possible. The physiotherapist also educates John on the benefits of physical activity in managing emotional stress, thereby helping to redirect his energy positively.

3. **Bargaining:**
   - **John's reaction:** John begins to engage in bargaining, both mentally and verbally. He might say things like, "If I work hard enough, maybe I can get back to the way I was before" or "If only I had taken a different route that day, I would not have lost my leg". He starts to set unrealistic goals for his recovery, hoping that by achieving them, he can somehow undo the loss.
   - **Physiotherapist's role:** The physiotherapist helps John set realistic, achievable goals, guiding him through the rehabilitation process step by step. The physiotherapist emphasizes the importance of small victories and incremental progress, helping John understand that while he may not regain his previous physical condition, he can still achieve a high quality of life. This helps John reframe his thinking from "what if" to "what's next".

Contd...

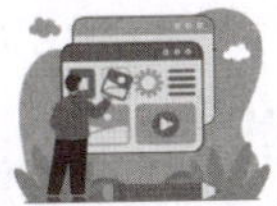
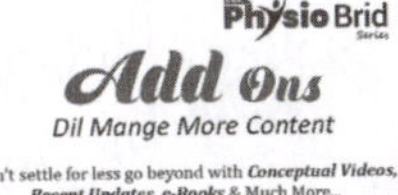

4. Depression:

- **John's reaction:** As John realizes the permanence of his loss, he falls into a deep depression. He becomes withdrawn, loses interest in physical therapy sessions, and expresses feelings of hopelessness, saying things like, "What is the point? I will never be the same again".
- **Physiotherapist's role:** Recognizing the signs of depression, the physiotherapist works closely with John, offering a compassionate and supportive presence. They may involve a psychologist or counselor to provide additional support. During sessions, the physiotherapist focuses on activities that John used to enjoy or new activities that might spark his interest, gently encouraging him to engage. They remind John of the progress he has made, however small, to foster a sense of achievement and hope.

5. Acceptance:

- **John's reaction:** Over time, John begins to accept his new reality. He starts to engage more actively in his rehabilitation, discusses prosthetic options with interest, and begins to plan for his future. He no longer focuses solely on what he has lost but starts to think about what he can achieve moving forward.
- **Physiotherapist's role:** The physiotherapist supports John in this stage by helping him set long-term goals, such as learning to walk with a prosthetic leg or participating in adaptive sports. The physiotherapist works on strengthening exercises, balance training, and mobility exercises tailored to John's needs. The physiotherapist also encourages John to connect with peer support groups where he can share experiences and gain inspiration from others who have gone through similar situations.

How the physiotherapist can help throughout the process?

- **Building trust and rapport:** The physiotherapist plays a crucial role in building a trusting relationship with John. This relationship provides a foundation of support throughout the different stages of grief, ensuring that John feels understood and supported.
- **Individualized care:** The physiotherapist tailors John's rehabilitation plan to his emotional state and physical needs at each stage of grief. He adjusts the intensity and focus of therapy based on how John is coping, ensuring that the treatment aligns with his current capabilities and mental readiness.
- **Interdisciplinary collaboration:** Recognizing that John's needs extend beyond physical rehabilitation, the physiotherapist collaborates with psychologists, social workers, and other healthcare providers to address the emotional and psychological aspects of his recovery. This holistic approach ensures that John receives comprehensive care.
- **Education and empowerment:** Throughout the process, the physiotherapist educates John about his condition, potential outcomes, and the rehabilitation process. This knowledge helps John feel more in control and empowered to take an active role in his recovery.
- **Promoting resilience and hope:** The physiotherapist encourages John to focus on his strengths and the progress he has made. By highlighting small successes and fostering a positive outlook, the physiotherapist helped John develop resilience and a hopeful attitude toward his future.

Interventions for Mental Health Promotion

The goals of programs for the promotion of mental health are to enhance psychological well-being and delay the emergence of mental illnesses. These treatments, which combine ideas from social and clinical psychology, can be provided at the individual, group, and society levels.

- **Preventive interventions:** The goal of preventive treatments is to delay the onset of mental health problems by decreasing risk factors and increasing protective variables. Research has demonstrated that school-based initiatives that foster emotional control, problem-solving abilities, and perseverance can lower the prevalence of anxiety and depression in kids and teenagers.[76] Social-emotional learning (SEL) concepts and cognitive-behavioral methods are frequently included in these programs.

- **Community-based interventions:** Community-based interventions leverage social networks and community resources to promote mental health. For example, the Mental Health First Aid program trains individuals to recognize the signs of mental health crises and provide initial support until professional help is available. This program has been effective in improving mental health literacy and reducing stigma associated with mental illness.[77]

Community Psychology and Social Interventions

Community psychology places a strong emphasis on helping people understand themselves within their social environments and on putting social concerns and community wellness into practice through treatments (Fig. 17.5).

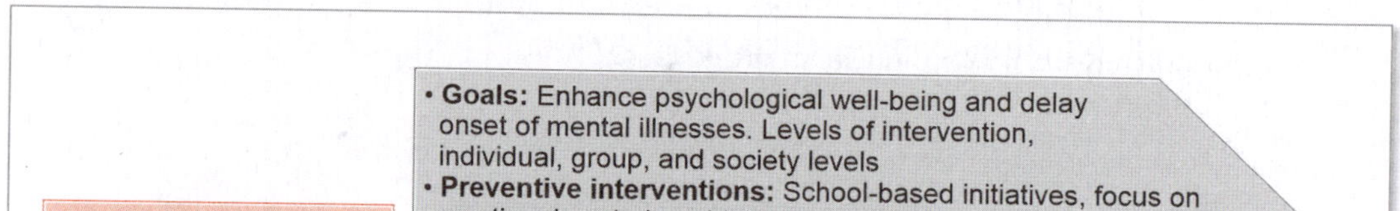

Fig. 17.5: The key interventions and principles related to mental health promotion, community psychology, and social interventions

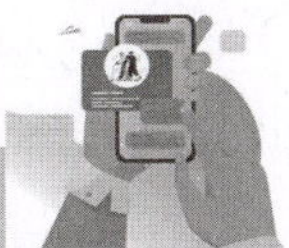
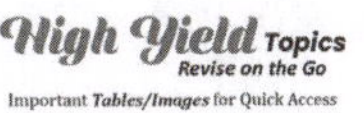

- **Principles:** The three main tenets of community psychology are ecological viewpoints, social justice, and empowerment. This method acknowledges the close relationships between social, economic, and environmental variables and an individual's well-being; as a result, treatments must target these larger factors that influence health.[78]

- **Social interventions:** In community psychology, social interventions work to enhance quality of life by targeting systemic problems including prejudice, poverty, and resource availability. The Housing First strategy, which offers immediate, long-term housing without requiring sobriety or treatment compliance, is one example of how to combat homelessness. This strategy has been demonstrated to lessen psychiatric symptoms and increase housing stability for homeless people with mental illnesses.[79] Community development programs that include locals in the design and execution of projects targeted at enhancing neighborhood circumstances are another example. These initiatives can strengthen community cohesiveness, expand access to resources, and encourage a feeling of empowerment and ownership among participants.

CROSS-CULTURAL PERSPECTIVES

In a society growing more interconnected by the day, comprehending the ways in which psychology and culture interact is essential to solving the complex problems of mental illness and behavior. Following key subfields in social and clinical psychology provides insights into how cultural environments affect mental health outcomes, clinical procedures, and individual and group behavior.

Cultural Influences on Social Behavior

The various ways in which cultural norms, values, and beliefs impact people's relationships and behaviors within a society are collectively referred to as cultural effects on social behavior. Studies reveal notable differences in social behavior between cultures, impacted by things like power distance, uncertainty avoidance, and individualism versus collectivism.[80]

People who live in individualistic cultures—where freedom and personal aspirations are valued—tend to act in ways that encourage self-expression and accomplishment. As a result of their emphasis on interdependence and group harmony, collectivist societies, on the other hand, encourage actions that promote social cohesiveness and the wellbeing of the whole.[81] According to research, individuals in collectivist cultures, for example, are more inclined to act prosocially and comply to social norms in order to preserve peace within the group.[82]

Additionally, social relationships are impacted by power gap or the degree to which society's weaker members tolerate an uneven allocation of power. People in high power distance cultures are more inclined to respect authoritative figures and hierarchical systems, which can have an impact on family relations and workplace conduct.[80] Low power distance cultures, on the other hand, typically encourage equality and candid communication between members of different social classes.

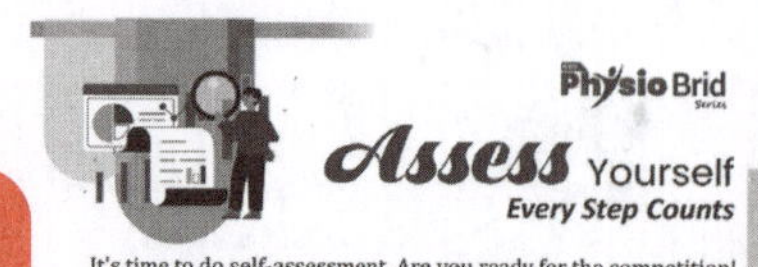

Cultural Competence in Clinical Practice

In the context of clinical medicine, cultural competence pertains to the capacity of medical professionals to comprehend, communicate, and engage with patients from a variety of cultural backgrounds. This proficiency is necessary to guarantee that every patient receives considerate and pertinent care, which is especially crucial in communities that are becoming more and more multicultural.

In addition to addressing any biases and preconceptions held by healthcare practitioners, achieving cultural competency entails acknowledging the cultural elements that impact health attitudes and practices.[83] Comprehending cultural perspectives on mental health, for example, can enhance evaluation and therapy compliance. Certain cultures stigmatize mental illness, which makes people postpone getting treatment or display their symptoms in ways that are unique to their culture.[84]

Healthcare workers must participate in educational courses in order to become culturally competent. Cultural sensitivity, effective communication, and culturally aware caregiving techniques are frequently covered in these programs. Studies indicate that providing treatment that is culturally sensitive can result in higher levels of satisfaction among patients, improved wellness, and a decrease in healthcare inequalities.[85]

Global Mental Health Issues

The occurrence, management, and avoidance of mental illnesses in various parts of the world are all included under the umbrella of global mental health. Cultural, economic, and social variables impact the prevalence of mental illnesses and the efficacy of therapies, making mental health concerns a major worldwide public health concern.

According to the World Health Organization (WHO), depression is the primary cause of disability globally and mental health problems account for a significant amount of the global illness burden.[86] Access to and the quality of mental healthcare vary significantly between wealthy and low- and middle-income nations. There is a serious lack of mental health specialists and restricted access to necessary mental health treatments in many communities with limited resources.[87]

Cultural influences are also very important in determining the course of mental health. For instance, people may find it difficult to seek care and receive treatment in a timely manner if they are stigmatized by society about mental illness. Furthermore, conventional methods of healing and social networks for support may work in tandem or against biological approaches to mental health treatment.[88] Implementing culturally relevant therapies, encouraging community-based care, and integrating mental health services into primary healthcare are some of the steps being taken to address global mental health challenges. To enhance mental health outcomes globally, international partnerships and collaborations are crucial for exchanging best practices, resources, and information.[89]

 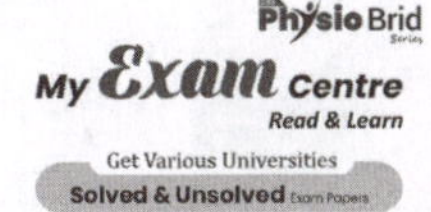

CURRENT TRENDS AND FUTURE DIRECTIONS

Advances in Social Psychology Research

Thanks to methodological advancements and the growing use of technology in research, social psychology has made tremendous strides in recent years. The extensive study of human behavior *via* the use of big data and social media analytics is one noteworthy development.[90] By using this method, researchers may examine patterns and trends in social interactions and gain understanding of phenomena including interpersonal dynamics, social influence, and the dissemination of false information.[90]

The use of neuroscience methods in social psychology represents a significant further breakthrough. Researchers are learning more about the brain foundations of social functions including empathy, bias, and decision-making by utilizing functional magnetic resonance imaging (fMRI) and other neuroimaging techniques.[91] This multidisciplinary method, which connects psychological theory with biological mechanisms, is sometimes called social neuroscience. Clarity and repeatability have also received increased attention in social psychology studies. Researchers are embracing open scientific approaches in response to the replication issue, such as preregistering papers, sharing data, and working together on large-scale replication efforts. The goal of these initiatives is to increase the validity and reliability of study findings.[92]

Innovations in Clinical Psychology Practice

Significant advancements have also been made in clinical psychology, namely in the fields of evaluation, intervention, and care delivery. The use of digital technology in clinical practice is one significant trend. Access to mental health treatments has increased because of telepsychology and online therapy platforms, especially for those living in underprivileged or distant places. These platforms assess patient progress and provide evidence-based therapies through the use of digital monitoring tools, smartphone applications, and video conferencing.[93]

In addition, clinical psychology is changing as a result of advances in artificial intelligence (AI). AI-powered instruments are being created to support treatment planning, diagnostics, and individualized care. Machine learning algorithms have the capability to examine extensive datasets and detect patterns linked to certain mental health disorders. This can lead to improved diagnostic precision and customized treatment strategies.[94] The application of virtual reality (VR) in therapeutic contexts is another noteworthy discovery. The VR is being used in conjunction with immersive simulations and exposure therapy to treat problems including post-traumatic stress disorder (PTSD), anxiety disorders, and phobias. With the use of this technology, patients may face and control their anxieties in a secure and regulated setting.[95]

Emerging Areas of Integration and Collaboration

Progressive integration and collaboration across domains is what will shape the future of clinical and social psychology. Behavioral genetics—the nexus of psychology and genetics—is one developing field. This area of study investigates how genetics influence behavior and mental health, providing information on the inheritance of psychological characteristics and illnesses.[96]

Furthermore, the value of diversity and cultural competency in psychological research and practice is becoming increasingly apparent. More diverse and culturally sensitive methods are being used in both research and therapeutic settings as a result of cross-cultural psychology's growing awareness of the ways in which cultural environments affect behavior and mental health.[97]

Treatment improvements for complicated illnesses are also being fostered *via* interdisciplinary cooperation. For instance, the incorporation of psychology into social work, medicine, and education is encouraging all-encompassing care models that attend to the many needs of patients. Since mental and physical health are intimately related to chronic illnesses, a holistic approach is especially pertinent for addressing these conditions.[98]

Global mental health issues, summarizing key points such as the impact of cultural influences, disparities in access to care and strategies for improvement are listed in Table 17.6.

Table 17.6: Global mental health issues

Section	Global mental health issues
Global mental health	
Scope	Occurrence, management, and prevention of mental illnesses globally.
Impact factors	Cultural, economic, and social variables influence prevalence and treatment efficacy.
Challenges	Disparities in mental healthcare access and quality between different income nations. Stigma associated with mental illness affects timely care seeking.
Interventions	• Culturally relevant therapies • Community-based care integration • Mental health services in primary healthcare.
Collaboration	International partnerships crucial for sharing best practices and resources.
Emerging areas of integration and collaboration	
Areas of integration	• **Behavioral genetics:** Study of genetics' impact on behavior and mental health. • **Cross-cultural psychology:** Increasing cultural competency in research and practice.
Interdisciplinary cooperation	Psychology integrated with social work, medicine, and education for comprehensive patient care models.
Focus	Holistic approaches to address mental and physical health connections, especially in chronic illness contexts.

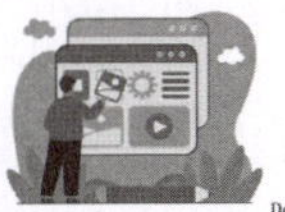

IMPLICATIONS FOR PRACTICE AND RESEARCH

The amalgamation of social and clinical psychology has noteworthy consequences for pragmatic implementations in mental health environments and forthcoming investigations. New research areas and improved treatment methods can result from an awareness of and ability to use the interaction between an individual's mental health and larger societal dynamics.

In order to improve treatment effectiveness and patient outcomes, practitioners might take a holistic approach that takes into account social environment in addition to individual psychological states. Therapeutic procedures can be enhanced by incorporating concepts like social support, social identity, and group dynamics.[99] Strong social support networks are essential parts of treatment regimens since research links them to better mental health outcomes.[100] Supportive settings that facilitate rehabilitation can be fostered by clinicians.

It's critical to comprehend how prejudice and social stigma affect mental health. By addressing stigmas associated with mental illness, race, gender, and sexual orientation, therapy relationships can be strengthened and more people can be motivated to seek assistance. Research has demonstrated that interventions targeted at lowering stigma against oneself in mental health patients enhance treatment adherence and self-esteem.[101]

In therapy, cultural competency is crucial. Interventions that are culturally sensitive can improve participation and results in a variety of populations.[84] It is recommended that clinicians include culturally appropriate methods into their treatment approaches. The convergence of clinical and social psychology creates a wealth of opportunities for further research. Examining the effects of socioeconomic determinants on the development, progression, and management of mental health illnesses is one important topic. Subsequent studies ought to explore the ways in which social circumstances influence psychological well-being and how these effects might be utilized in therapeutic contexts.

The long-term impacts of social networks and support systems on mental health are shown by longitudinal research. For instance, studies can clarify the ways in which social integration and isolation affect the course of anxiety and depression over time.[102] Analyzing social interactions in digital and online spaces is another interesting avenue. Given the widespread use of digital communication, it is essential to comprehend how technology affects mental health. Research has examined the effects of social media use and online social support on psychological well-being, showing both beneficial and detrimental effects.[103] These dynamics should be further investigated in future studies in order to guide digital treatments for mental health.

To understand the similarities and differences between social and clinical psychological processes across cultures, cross-cultural study is crucial. Deeper understanding of how cultural settings influence mental health experiences and the efficacy of interventions may be gained through comparative research conducted in various cultural contexts. Global mental health solutions that take cultural variances into account can benefit from this research. Finally, combining social and clinical psychology has important ramifications for both research and practice. By taking into account social and cultural circumstances, practitioners can improve therapy outcomes.

Meanwhile, researchers can investigate the relationship between social surroundings and mental health to create more potent therapies. Collaboration across these fields will continue to expand our knowledge and enhance mental health services globally.

CHALLENGES AND OPPORTUNITIES IN SOCIAL AND CLINICAL PSYCHOLOGY

The unification of social and clinical psychology poses notable obstacles as well as encouraging prospects for improving knowledge and procedures in the field of mental health. Bridging the historical divide between these disciplines—which have historically placed an emphasis on distinct approaches and focus points—is one of the most important difficulties. Fostering multidisciplinary communication and dismantling institutional silos that obstruct the integration of social and clinical views are necessary to overcome these obstacles.[104] Another major obstacle in the industry is cultural sensitivity. Therapists must traverse and respect a variety of cultural ideas, values, and customs in order to provide successful mental healthcare.[105] In order to guarantee that treatment techniques are effective and connect with a variety of groups, culturally competent procedures are crucial.

In addition, the emergence of social media and digital communication has brought up new dynamics that affect mental health. These platforms can improve social support and connectedness, but they also carry concerns, such the possibility of cyberbullying and prolonged screen time, which can have a negative impact on psychological health.[103] Therapists must adjust and create plans that maximize the advantages of digital contacts while minimizing their drawbacks in order to strike a balance between the risks and rewards.

The combination of social and clinical psychology presents a number of potentials for improving mental health treatment, in contrast to these obstacles. Practitioners can create more thorough treatment plans by using an integrated approach that takes into account both specific psychological processes and larger societal circumstances.[100] With this integrated approach, therapists may treat the underlying social factors of psychological suffering in addition to the symptoms of mental disease.

Novel approaches based on social psychology concepts offer an additional pathway for advancement. For example, the idea of social support emphasizes the significance of creating supportive situations that promote resilience and healing.[102] Through the integration of these concepts into therapeutic procedures, physicians can improve treatment outcomes and foster patients' long-term well-being.

By offering insights into elements of mental health that are both universal and culturally particular, cross-cultural research contributes to the field's enrichment. Studies that compare various populations aid in the identification of successful tactics that take cultural variances into account.[47] This global viewpoint influences the creation of inclusive mental health policy globally as well as culturally appropriate interventions.

There are many opportunities for improving mental healthcare through holistic approaches, creative interventions, and culturally aware practices when integrating social and clinical psychology. However, there are also challenges, like disciplinary integration, cultural sensitivity, and navigating the digital age. Sustained investigation and interdisciplinary cooperation will be essential in capitalizing on these prospects to enhance mental health results globally.[106, 107]

SUMMARY

- To sum up, the investigation of social and clinical psychology uncovers the complex relationship between a person's mental health and larger societal dynamics. Throughout history, these areas have developed along separate but connected trajectories, shaped by key concepts and revolutionary procedures.
- Diverse viewpoints that emphasize the complexity of human behavior and mental processes have affected the field of psychological study, from Freud's psychoanalysis to Bandura's social learning theory.
- The merging of social and clinical psychology emphasizes how important it is to approach psychological difficulties holistically in order to comprehend and treat them.
- A more thorough treatment plan that takes into account the patient's internal psychological states as well as the exterior social factors that have an impact on mental health is made possible by this integration. Thus, social psychology provides valuable insights into therapeutic techniques, enabling more effective interventions that support general well-being.
- Cross-cultural approaches shed light on how cultural circumstances influence psychological processes, which advances our understanding even further. By promoting culturally competent behaviors in social and therapeutic contexts, this understanding guarantees that treatments are pertinent and considerate of a range of backgrounds.
- Cross-cultural insights are becoming more and more important to incorporate into psychological practice as globalization continues to erase cultural barriers.
- All things considered, the integration of theoretical frameworks, integrative methods, historical advancements, and cross-cultural viewpoints in social and clinical psychology offers a strong basis for next studies and methods.
- Psychologists can address the complex issues of mental health in our varied and interconnected environment by continuing to build bridges between various disciplines and developing more nuanced and effective techniques.

REFERENCES

1. Merhad A., Veiga J.D., Kasparian J., Cardoso M., Hernandez I. Understanding and Exploring Social Psychology in Context of Human Behavior. *Open Science Journal.* 2023; 8(2).
2. Wahass SH. The role of psychologists in healthcare delivery. J Family Community Med. 2005;12(2):63–70.
3. Allport G. W. The historical background integration of social psychology. In: G. Lindzey & E. Aronson (Eds.), The Handbook of Social Psychology, *Oxford: Oxford University Press*, 1998.
4. Figgou Lia & Pavlopoulos Vassilis. Social Psychology: Research Methods. *International Encyclopedia of the Social & Behavioral Sciences.* 2015;10,1016

Contd...

5. Forsyth, D. R. *Group Dynamics*, 6th ed., Wadsworth Cengage Learning. 2014.

6. Robert B. Cialdini, Influence: Science and Practice, 5th ed, Pearson 2005

7. Roccella M, Vetri L. Adventures of Clinical Psychology. *J. Clin. Med.* 2021; 10, 4848.

8. van Heugten-van der Kloet D, van Heugten T. The classification of psychiatric disorders according to DSM-5 deserves an internationally standardized psychological test battery on symptom level. Front Psychol. 2015 Aug 4; 6, 1108.

9. American Psychological Association. Ethical Principles of Psychologists and Code of Conduct. 2017

10. Sue, Derald Wing. and David Sue. Counseling the Culturally Diverse: Theory and Practice. 7th edition. Hoboken, New Jersey, John Wiley & Sons, Inc, 2016.

11. Adler NE, Stewart J. Health disparities across the lifespan: Meaning, methods, and mechanisms. Ann N Y Acad Sci. 2010 ;1186:5–23.

12. Cohen, S. Social Relationships and Health. *American Psychologist, 2004; 59*(8), 676–684.

13. Santini Z. I., Koyanagi A., Tyrovolas S., Mason C., & Haro J. M. The association between social relationships and depression: A systematic review. *Journal of Affective Disorders*, 2015, 175, 53–65.

14. Braveman P., & Gottlieb L. The social determinants of health: It's time to consider the causes of the causes. *Public Health Reports*, 2014, 129(2), 19–31.

15. Corrigan P. W., Druss B. G., & Perlick D. A. The impact of mental illness stigma on seeking and participating in mental healthcare. *Psychological Science in the Public Interest*, 2014, 15(2), 37–70.

16. Malhotra A., Baker J. Group Therapy. In: StatPearls. Treasure Island (FL): StatPearls Publishing; 2024 Jan

17. Swierc, Susan & Routh, Donald. Introduction to the Special Issue on International Clinical Psychology. Journal of Clinical Psychology. 2003, 59. 631–4.

18. Hergenhahn B. R., & Henley, T. B. *An Introduction to the History of Psychology* (7th ed.). Wadsworth, Cengage Learning. 2013.

19. Schultz D. P. & Schultz S. E. A History of Modern Psychology (10th ed.). Cengage Learning. 2015.

20. Kruglanski. A., & Stroebe. W. *Handbook of the History of Social Psychology.* Philadelphia, PA: Psychology Press. 2011.

21. Stroebe, Wolfgang. The Truth About Triplett (1898), But Nobody Seems to Care. Perspectives on Psychological Science. 2012; 7. 54–57.

22. Greenwood J. D. A conceptual history of psychology: Exploring the tangled web. *Cambridge University Press*. 2014.

23. Joas H. The Creativity of Action. *University of Chicago Press*. 1996.

24. Shalin, D. N. Pragmatism and Social Interactionism. American Sociological Review, 1986; 51(1), 9–29.

25. BurnesB., &Bargal D. Kurt Lewin: 70 years on. *Journal of Change Management*. 2017,17(2), 91–100.

26. Jost J. T. Resistance to change: A social psychological perspective. *Social Research: An International Quarterly*. 2015, 82(3), 607–636.

27. Moscovici S. *The Age of the Crowd: A Historical Treatise on Mass Psychology*. Cambridge University Press. 1985.

28. S. McKeown, R. Haji, & N. Ferguson (Eds.), *Understanding peace and conflict through social identity theory: Contemporary global perspectives*. Springer International Publishing. 2016; 3–17.

Contd...

29. Haslam S. A., Reicher, S. D., & Birney, M. E. Nothing by mere authority: Evidence that in an experimental analogue of the Milgram paradigm participants are motivated not by orders but by appeals to science. *Journal of Social Issues*. 2014, 70(3), 473–488.

30. Zimbardo P. G. *The Lucifer Effect: Understanding How Good People Turn Evil*. Random House. 2008.

31. Burnes B., & Cooke B. Kurt Lewin's field theory: A review and re-evaluation. *International Journal of Management Reviews*. 2013, 15(4), 408–425.

32. Cooper J. Cognitive dissonance: Where we've been and where we're going. *International Review of Social Psychology*. 2019, 32(1), 1–11.

33. Bandura A. Toward a psychology of human agency: Pathways and reflections. *Perspectives on Psychological Science*. 2018, 13(2), 130–136.

34. Fiske S. T., & Taylor S. *Social Cognition: From Brains to Culture*. SAGE Publications. 2013.

35. Van Bavel, J. J., Mende-Siedlecki, P., Brady, W. J., &Reinero, D. A. Contextual sensitivity in scientific reproducibility. *Proceedings of the National Academy of Sciences*. 2016, 113(23), 6454–6459.

36. Kassin S., Fein S., & Markus, H. R. *Social Psychology*. 10th ed. Cengage Learning. 2017.

37. Chiu C.-Y., & Hong Y.-Y. Social psychology of culture. *Psychological Inquiry*. 2013, 24(1), 1–5.

38. Nicolas, Serge & Ferrand, Ludovic. Wundt's Laboratory at Leipzig in 1891. History of psychology. 1999, 2, 194–203.

39. McLeod, S. Sigmund Freud: Theories. *Simply Psychology*. 2013.

40. Benjamin LT Jr. A history of clinical psychology as a profession in America (and a glimpse at its future). Annu Rev Clin Psychol. 2005; 1, 1–30.

41. Baker DB, Benjamin LT Jr. The affirmation of the scientist-practitioner. A look back at Boulder. *Am Psychol*. 2000; 55(2):241–7.

42. Kirschenbaum, Howard & Jourdan, April. The Current Status of Carl Rogers and the Person-Centered Approach. Psychotherapy: Theory, Research, Practice, Training. 2005, 42, 37–51.

43. Beck, J. S. *Cognitive Behavior Therapy: Basics and Beyond* (3rd ed.). Guilford Press. 2019.

44. Turner MJ. Rational Emotive Behavior Therapy (REBT), Irrational and Rational Beliefs, and the Mental Health of Athletes. Front Psychol. 2016; 20;7:1423.

45. Kazdin Alan. Evidence-based psychotherapies II: Changes in models of treatment and treatment delivery. South African Journal of Psychology. 2015; 45, 3–21.

46. Engel GL. The need for a new medical model: A challenge for biomedicine. Science. 1977; 196(4286):129–36.

47. Sue, D. W., Rasheed, M. N., & Rasheed, J. M. *Multicultural Social Work Practice: A Competency-Based Approach to Diversity and Social Justice* (2nd ed.). Wiley. 2015.

48. Weiner, B. The legacy of an attribution to motivation and emotion: A no-crisis zone. *Motivation Science,* 2018; 4(1), 4–14.

49. Westen D. The scientific status of unconscious processes: Is Freud really dead? J Am Psychoanal Assoc.1999; 47(4):1061–106.

50. Maslow, A. H. *A Theory of Human Motivation*. Start Publishing LLC. 2013.

51. Daniels, Jo. An Introduction to Cognitive Behavioral Therapy: Skills and Applications David Westbrook, Helen Kennerley and Joan Kirk, London: Sage Publications, 2007; 296.

52. Turner, R. N., & Crisp, R. J. Imagining intergroup contact reduces implicit prejudice. *British Journal of Social Psychology,* 2010, 49(1), 129–142.

Contd...

53. L. B. Alloy & J. H. Riskind. Cognitive vulnerability to emotional disorders. 2nd ed. Psychology Press. 2005; 121–134.

54. Elliott, R., Watson, J., Goldman, R. N., & Greenberg, L. S. Learning Emotion-Focused Therapy: The Process-Experiential Approach to Change. American Psychological Association. 2013.

55. Rogers, C. R. *On Becoming a Person: A Therapist's View of Psychotherapy*. Houghton Mifflin Harcourt. 1961.

56. Malle, B. F. Attribution theories: How people make sense of behavior. In D. Chadee (Ed.), Theories in social psychology. Wiley Blackwell. 2011; 72–95.

57. Baron, R. A., & Branscombe, N. R. *Social Psychology*. 13th ed. Pearson.2013.

58. Kruglanski, Arie&Jasko, Katarzyna &Milyavsky, Maxim & Chernikova, Marina & Webber, David & Pierro, Antonio & Di Santo, Daniela. Cognitive Consistency Theory in Social Psychology: A Paradigm Reconsidered. Psychological Inquiry. 2018; 29. 45–59.

59. Petty, R. E., &Briñol, P. The elaboration likelihood and metacognitive models of attitudes: Implications for prejudice, the self, and beyond. In M. Mikulincer, P. R. Shaver, E. Borgida, & J. A. Bargh (Eds.), *APA Handbook of Personality and Social Psychology, Volume 1: Attitudes and Social Cognition*.2015, 69–112.

60. Harmon-Jones, E., & Mills, J. An introduction to cognitive dissonance theory and an overview of current perspectives on the theory. In E. Harmon-Jones (Ed.), *Cognitive Dissonance: Re-examining a Pivotal Theory in Psychology*. 2019; (2),3–24.

61. Burger, J. M. Replicating Milgram: Would people still obey today? *American Psychologist*. 2009; 64(1).

62. Reis, H. T., & Clark, M. S. Responsiveness. In J. A. Simpson & L. Campbell (Eds.), *The Oxford handbook of close relationships*. 2013; 400–423.

63. Groth-Marnat, G., & Wright, A. J. *Handbook of Psychological Assessment*, 6th ed.Wiley. 2016.

64. Hofmann SG, Asnaani A, Vonk IJ, Sawyer AT, Fang A. The Efficacy of Cognitive Behavioral Therapy: A Review of Meta-analyses. Cognit Ther Res. 2012; 36(5):427–440.

65. Shedler, J. The Efficacy of Psychodynamic Psychotherapy. *American Psychologist*. 2010, 65(2), 98-109. Therapy?

66. Cain, D. J. *Person-Centered Psychotherapies*. American Psychological Association. 2010.

67. Stahl, S. M. *Stahl's Essential Psychopharmacology: Neuroscientific Basis and Practical Applications*. 4th ed. Cambridge University Press. 2013.

68. Muench, J., & Hamer, A. M. Adverse effects of antipsychotic medications. *American Family Physician.* 2010; *81*(5), 617–622.

69. Malhi GS, Bassett D, Boyce P, Bryant R, Fitzgerald PB, Fritz K, Hopwood M, Lyndon B, Mulder R, Murray G, Porter R, Singh AB. Royal Australian and New Zealand College of Psychiatrists. Aust N Z J Psychiatry. 2015; 49(12)

70. Baldwin DS, Anderson IM, Nutt DJ, Allgulander C, Bandelow B, den Boer JA, Christmas DM, Davies S, Fineberg N, Lidbetter N, Malizia A, McCrone P, Nabarro D, O'Neill C, Scott J, van der Wee N, Wittchen HU. Evidence-based pharmacological treatment of anxiety disorders, post-traumatic stress disorder and obsessive-compulsive disorder: A revision of the 2005 guidelines from the British Association for Psychopharmacology. J Psychopharmacol. 2014; 28(5):403–39.

71. Leucht S, Arbter D, Engel RR, Kissling W, Davis JM. How effective are second-generation antipsychotic drugs? A meta-analysis of placebo-controlled trials. Mol Psychiatry. 2009; 14(4):429–47.

Contd...

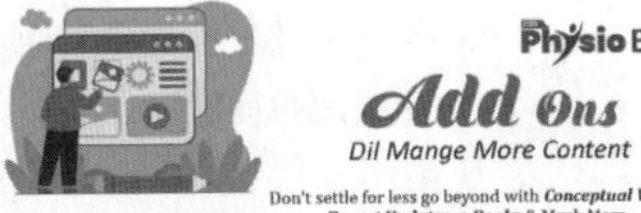

72. Geddes JR, Miklowitz DJ. Treatment of bipolar disorder. Lancet. 2013; 381(9878):1672–82.

73. Van Lange, P. A. M., Kruglanski, A. W., & Higgins, E. T. (Eds.). (2012). Handbook of theories of social psychology. SAGE.2012.

74. Allcott, H. Social norms and energy conservation. Journal of Public Economics, 2011, 95(9-10), 1082–1095.

75. Durlak, J. A., Weissberg, R. P., Dymnicki, A. B., Taylor, R. D., & Schellinger, K. B. The impact of enhancing students' social and emotional learning: A meta-analysis of school-based universal interventions. Child Development, 2011, 82(1), 405–432.

76. Jorm, A. F., Kitchener, B. A., Sawyer, M. G., Scales, H., & Cvetkovski, S. Mental health first aid training for high school teachers: A cluster randomized trial. BMC Psychiatry. 2010, 10(1), 1–12.

77. Nelson, Geoffrey &Prilleltensky, Isaac. Community Psychology: In Pursuit of Liberation and Well-being. 2005

78. Tsemberis S, Gulcur L, Nakae M. Housing First, consumer choice, and harm reduction for homeless individuals with a dual diagnosis. Am J Public Health. 2004;94(4):651–6.

79. Hofstede, G., Culture's Consequences: Comparing Values, Behaviors, Institutions, and Organizations Across Nations, 2nd ed. Sage, Thousand Oaks, CA. 2001.

80. Triandis, H. C. *Individualism and Collectivism*. Routledge. 2018.

81. Markus, H. R., & Kitayama, S. Culture and the self: Implications for cognition, emotion, and motivation. *Psychological Review.* 1991; *98*(2), 224–253.

82. Betancourt JR, Green AR, Carrillo JE, Ananeh-Firempong O 2nd. Defining cultural competence: A practical framework for addressing racial/ethnic disparities in health and healthcare. Public Health Rep. 2003 Jul-Aug; 118(4).

83. Sue S, Yan Cheng JK, Saad CS, Chu JP. Asian American mental health: A call to action. Am Psychol. 2012 Oct; 67(7):532–44.

84. Saha S, Beach MC, Cooper LA. Patient centeredness, cultural competence and healthcare quality. J Natl Med Assoc. 2008 Nov; 100(11):1275–85.

85. World Health Organization. Depression and Other Common Mental Disorders: Global Health Estimates. World Health Organization. 2017.

86. Patel V, Chisholm D, Parikh R, Charlson FJ, Degenhardt L, Dua T, Ferrari AJ, Hyman S, Laxminarayan R, Levin C, Lund C, Medina Mora ME, Petersen I, Scott J, Shidhaye R, Vijayakumar L, Thornicroft G, Whiteford H; DCP MNS Author Group. Addressing the burden of mental, neurological, and substance use disorders: key messages from Disease Control Priorities, 3rd edition. Lancet. 2016 Apr 16; 387(10028):1672–85.

87. Kohrt, B.A., & Mendenhall, E. (Eds.). Global Mental Health: Anthropological Perspectives (1st ed.). Routledge. 2015.

88. Kleinman A. Global mental health: A failure of humanity. Lancet. 2009 Aug 22;374(9690):603-4.

89. Kosinski M, Matz SC, Gosling SD, Popov V, Stillwell D. Facebook as a research tool for the social sciences: Opportunities, challenges, ethical considerations, and practical guidelines. Am Psychol. 2015 Sep; 70(6):543–56.

90. Cacioppo JT, Cacioppo S, Dulawa S, Palmer AA. Social neuroscience and its potential contribution to psychiatry. World Psychiatry. 2014 Jun; 13(2):131–9.

91. Nosek BA, Ebersole CR, DeHaven AC, Mellor DT. The preregistration revolution. Proc Natl Acad Sci U S A. 2018 Mar 13; 115(11):2600–2606.

Contd...

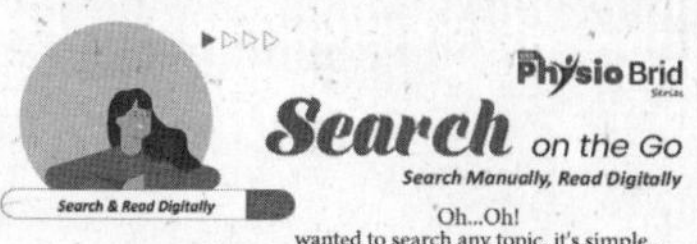

92. Godine, N., & Barnett, J.E. The Use of Telepsychology in Clinical Practice: Benefits, Effectiveness, and Issues to Consider. *Int. J. Cyber Behav. Psychol. Learn.,* 2013; *3,* 70–83.

93. Shatte ABR, Hutchinson DM, Teague SJ. Machine learning in mental health: A scoping review of methods and applications. Psychol Med. 2019; 49(9):1426–1448.

94. Maples-Keller JL, Bunnell BE, Kim SJ, Rothbaum BO. The Use of Virtual Reality Technology in the Treatment of Anxiety and Other Psychiatric Disorders. Harv Rev Psychiatry. 2017; 25(3):103–113.

95. Plomin, R. Blueprint: How DNA Makes Us Who We Are. *MIT Press.* 2018.

96. Henrich J, Heine SJ, Norenzayan A. The weirdest people in the world? Behav Brain Sci. 2010;33(2-3):61–83.

97. Kazdin AE, Blase SL. Rebooting Psychotherapy Research and Practice to Reduce the Burden of Mental Illness. PerspectPsychol Sci. 2011; 6(1):21–37.

98. Haslam, S.A., Reicher, S.D., &Platow, M.J. The New Psychology of Leadership: Identity, Influence and Power. 2nd ed. Routledge. 2020

99. Taylor, Shelley. Social Support: A Review. See Friedman 2011. 2012; 189–214.

100. Corrigan PW, Morris SB, Michaels PJ, Rafacz JD, Rüsch N. Challenging the public stigma of mental illness: A meta-analysis of outcome studies. Psychiatr Serv. 2012; 63(10):963–73.

101. Haslam, Catherine, Steffens, Niklas K., Branscombe, Nyla R., Haslam, S. Alexander, Cruwys, Tegan, Lam, Ben C. P., Pachana, Nancy A., and Yang, Jie. *The importance of social groups for retirement adjustment: evidence, application, and policy implications of the social identity model of identity change. Social Issues and Policy Review 2019; 13* (1) 93–124.

102. Seabrook EM, Kern ML, Rickard NS. Social Networking Sites, Depression, and Anxiety: A Systematic Review. JMIR Ment Health. 2016; 3(4).

103. Kazdin, Alan E., *Innovations in Psychosocial Interventions and Their Delivery: Leveraging Cutting-Edge Science to Improve the World's Mental Health.* Oxford Academic. 2018.

104. Ryder, Andrew & Ban, Lauren & Chentsova-Dutton, Yulia. (2011). Towards a Cultural–Clinical Psychology. Social and Personality Psychology Compass. 2011; 5. 960–975.

105. Patel V, Saxena S, Lund C, Thornicroft G, Baingana F, Bolton P, Chisholm D, Collins PY, Cooper JL, Eaton J, Herrman H, Herzallah MM, Huang Y, Jordans MJD, Kleinman A, Medina-Mora ME, Morgan E, Niaz U, Omigbodun O, Prince M, Rahman A, Saraceno B, Sarkar BK, De Silva M, Singh I, Stein DJ, Sunkel C, UnÜtzer J. The Lancet Commission on global mental health and sustainable development. Lancet. 2018; 392(10157)

106. Kirmayer LJ, Pedersen D. Toward a new architecture for global mental health. Transcult Psychiatry. 2014; 51(6):759–76.

107. Haslam, S. & Reicher, Stephen. Rethinking the Psychology of Leadership: From Personal Identity to Social Identity. Daedalus. 2016; 145. 21–34.

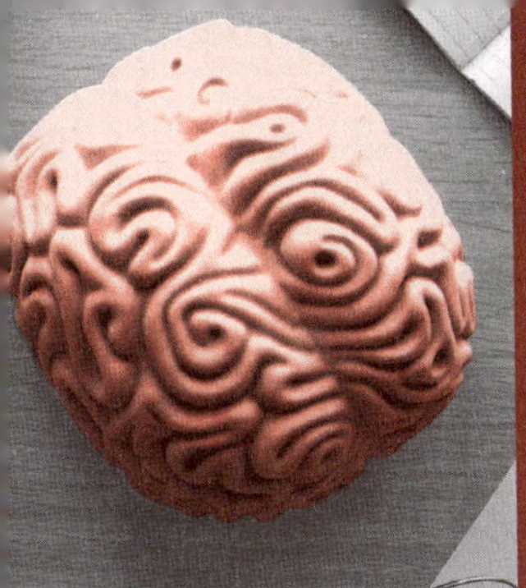

STUDENT ASSIGNMENT

LONG ANSWER QUESTIONS

1. How has clinical psychology improved our understanding and treatment of mental health issues?
2. What are the main contributions of social psychology to our understanding of human behavior?
3. How does clinical psychology approach the assessment and diagnosis of mental health disorders?
4. What are the main therapeutic approaches in clinical psychology, and how do they differ?
5. How do cultural factors influence social behavior and mental health?

SHORT ANSWER QUESTIONS

1. What is the role of the diagnostic and statistical manual of mental disorders (DSM-5) in clinical psychology?
2. How does cognitive behavioral therapy (CBT) differ from psychodynamic psychotherapy?
3. What is meant by cultural competence in clinical practice?
4. What are some of the challenges faced by global mental health initiatives?
5. How can digital technology improve access to mental healthcare?

MULTIPLE CHOICE QUESTIONS

1. **Which of the following is NOT a core concept in social psychology?**
   a. Social perception
   b. Conformity
   c. Neuropsychological testing
   d. Group dynamics

2. **Who is often referred to as the "Father of Social Psychology"?**
   a. Sigmund Freud
   b. Wilhelm Wundt
   c. Kurt Lewin
   d. Albert Bandura

3. **Which therapeutic approach is based on the theories of Sigmund Freud?**
   a. Cognitive behavioral therapy
   b. Psychodynamic therapy
   c. Humanistic Therapy
   d. Behavioral therapy

4. **What is the primary purpose of the diagnostic and statistical manual of mental disorders (DSM-5)?**
    a. To provide guidelines for mood psychological testing
    b. To offer a classification system for mental disorders
    c. To outline therapeutic techniques for various disorders
    d. To document historical developments in psychology

5. **Which of the following is NOT a principle of social influence?**
    a. Scarcity
    b. Likeability
    c. Authority
    d. Isolation

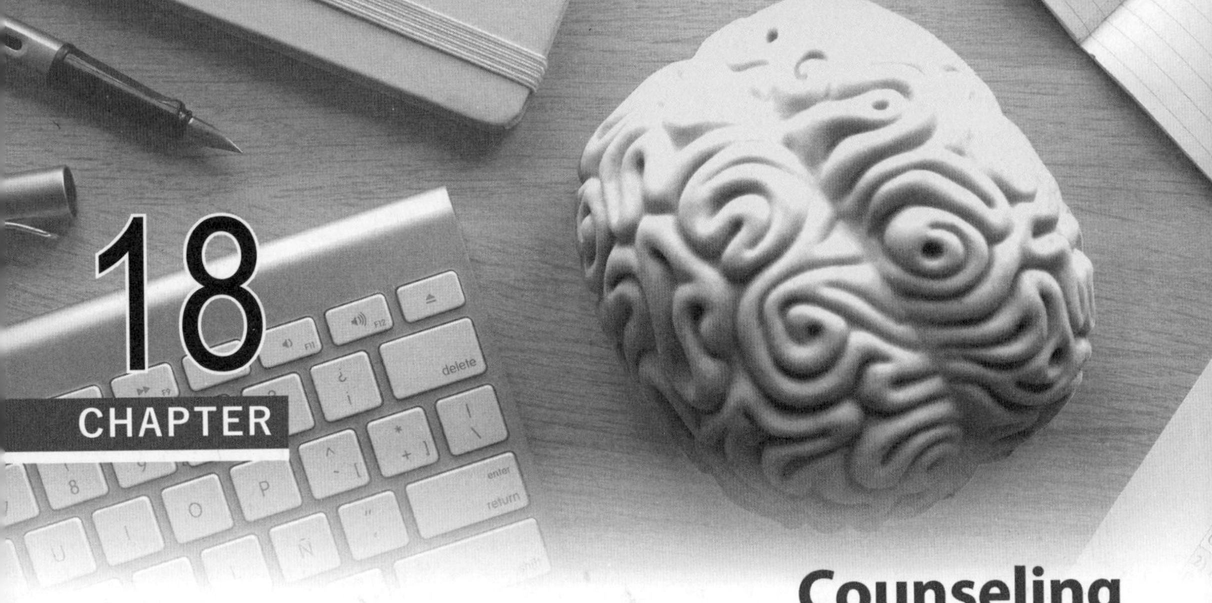

Counseling

Chandani Pandey, Pragya Mitra

LEARNING OBJECTIVES

After the completion of the chapter, the readers will be able to:
- Understand the basic principles of counseling, its process, historical background and various approaches.
- Develop practical skills in applying various counseling techniques such as active listening, empathy, and effective communication skills.
- Gain awareness of cultural, social, and personal factors that influence the counseling process.
- Discuss the ethical standards and legal considerations in counseling practice.
- Develop the competencies necessary to support and guide the clients effectively, fostering positive change and promoting physical and mental health and well-being.

CHAPTER OUTLINE

- Introduction
- Scope of Counseling
- Definitions of Counseling
- Aims of Counseling
- History
- Process
- Approaches
- Skills and Techniques
- Ethical and Legal Considerations
- Physiotherapy and Mental-Health

KEY TERMS

Active listening: A technique where the counselor fully engages with the client, demonstrating attentiveness and understanding.

Body awareness and dissociation: Techniques to improve body awareness and manage dissociative symptoms.

Confidentiality and privacy: The protection of a client's personal information and the right to keep their details private.

Counseling: The process of assisting individuals in exploring, understanding, and resolving personal, social or psychological issues.

Empathy: The ability to understand and share the feelings of another person.

Ethical and legal considerations: Guidelines and frameworks that govern the practice of counseling to ensure ethical standards and legal compliance.

Ethical guidelines: Formal frameworks that outline recommended behaviors for counselors to ensure safe and ethical practice.

Falls and mobility issues: Addressing physical issues that affect mobility and independence.

Identifying patterns and behaviors: Recognizing and addressing maladaptive thought and behavior patterns that cause distress.

Informed consent: The process of obtaining a client's agreement to participate in therapy, ensuring they understand the purpose and potential outcomes.

Interdisciplinary collaboration: Working together with other healthcare professionals to provide comprehensive care.

Lifestyle and weight management: Developing programs to improve lifestyle choices and manage weight for better health.

Mental health integration: Combining mental healthcare with physiotherapy to provide holistic treatment.

Motivation and self-management: Encouraging patients to take an active role in their recovery and self-care.

Nonpharmacological pain management: Using nondrug methods to alleviate pain and improve mental well-being.

Note-taking: The practice of documenting sessions to aid memory, maintain confidentiality, and support legal requirements.

Psychoeducation: Offering information and education about illnesses, symptoms, and management techniques.

Questioning: Asking open-ended and closed-ended questions to fully understand the client's experiences and emotions.

Relaxation exercises: Techniques such as progressive muscle relaxation, deep breathing, and guided imagery to reduce anxiety and stress.

Self-disclosure: The process of revealing personal information to another person to foster intimacy and trust.

Summarizing: Providing a concise overview of the session's key points to ensure clarity and understanding.

Supportive therapy: Providing support to individuals facing serious physical health issues, emphasizing acceptance and coping strategies.

Tailored exercise programs: Individualized exercise regimens to enhance mood and overall well-being.

Therapeutic relationship: The bond between the counselor and client, essential for effective therapy.

INTRODUCTION

Counseling is a wonderful invention of the 20th century. In today's intricate, fast-paced world, we encounter various challenges that can be overwhelming. While we often manage to navigate through life smoothly, there are moments when we confront situations beyond our immediate capacity to handle. Typically, we seek solace and guidance from loved ones, community members, spiritual

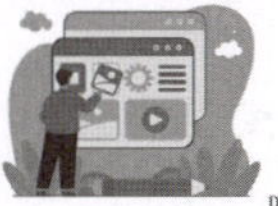

leaders or healthcare professionals to address these issues. However, there are instances when their support may not suffice or we feel hesitant to confide in them due to embarrassment or a lack of suitable solutions.[1]

Counseling serves as a valuable resource during such moments. It's often readily accessible and affordable now. Rather than diagnosing or labelling the patients, counselors focus on listening and collaborating with their clients to understand and resolve the issues. For most individuals, just one to six counseling sessions can significantly alleviate their concerns. These sessions offer a chance in our society to be genuinely heard, respected, and understood without any expectations of reciprocity. Counselors are trained mental health professionals that are equipped with various qualities that help them connect with fellow human beings more deeply.[2]

SCOPE OF COUNSELING

The scope of counseling is not only limited to psychological issues, it is well implicated in various physical diseases as well such as hypertension, neurological disorders, cardiac issues, etc. (Fig. 18.1).[2]

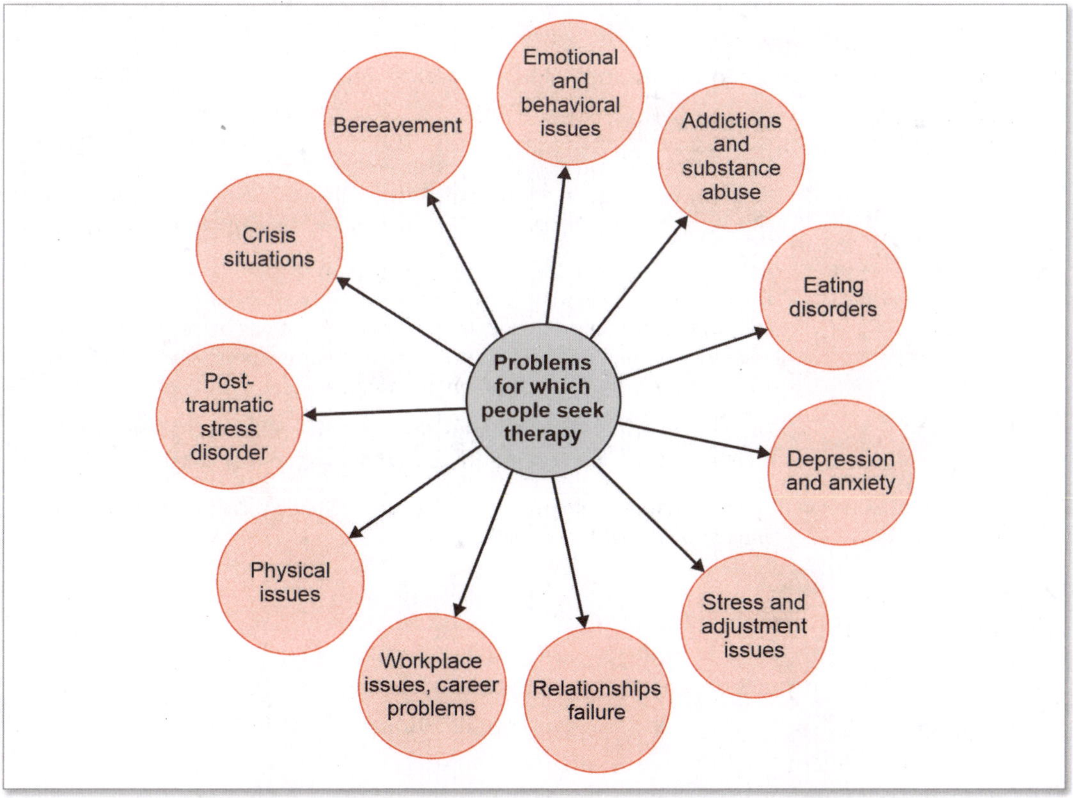

Fig. 18.1: Various problems due to which clients seek counseling

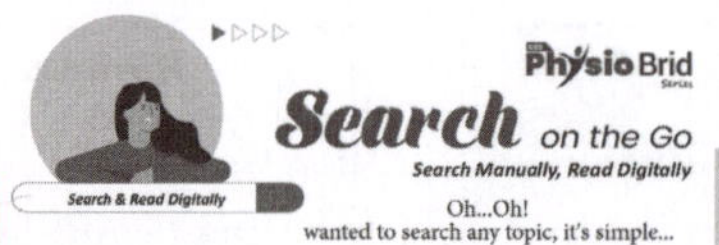

DEFINITIONS OF COUNSELING

Counseling has been defined by many professional bodies which are as follows:

The definition of counseling includes work with individuals and with relationships which may be developmental, crisis support, psychotherapeutic, guiding or problem-solving. The task of counseling is to allow the 'client' to explore, discover and clarify ways of living more satisfyingly and resourcefully.[3] **(BAC, 1984).**

Counseling refers to a professional and therapeutic relationship between therapist and client. This includes one-to-one interaction with clients, sometimes more than two. It is designed to help clients to understand and clarify their views of their life space, and to learn to reach their self-determined goals through meaningful, well-informed choices and resolution of problems of an emotional or interpersonal nature.[4] **(Burks and Stefflre, 1979).** Refer to Table 18.1 to understand the differences between the functions of various health professionals.

> **MUST KNOW**
>
> The various professionals work together to provide holistic mental health services to individuals by collaborating and making referrals to interdisciplinary professionals.

Table 18.1: Differences between various mental health professionals

Professional group	Specialization
Counselors/psychologists	Counselors/psychologists work with clients who can function and fulfil their day-to-day activities but experience mild difficulties due to stress, adjustment issues, family issues, marital issues, self-confidence issues, sleep issues, etc.
Clinical psychologists	They are involved in understanding the symptomatology of various severe mental health issues that are causing difficulties in day-to-day life and that need immediate treatment such as bipolar disorder, personality disorders, schizophrenia, neurodevelopmental disorders, etc.
Psychiatrists	They are involved in prescribing medications to clients suffering from significant mental health issues that are also affecting their normal functioning.
Psychiatric-social workers	They work at the community level and provide healthcare facilities to state and national healthcare centers.

AIMS OF COUNSELING

These are the various outcomes or goals that can be achieved through counseling.

- **Gaining insight:** To understand the root causes of emotional difficulties and gain control over feelings and actions.[5]

- **Improving relationships:** Developing the ability to form and maintain meaningful connections with others in family or work settings.

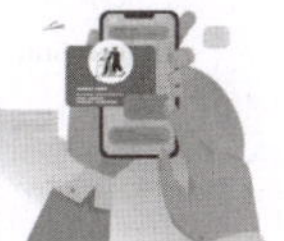
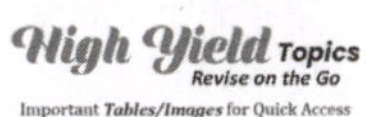

- **Enhancing self-awareness:** Becoming more conscious of suppressed thoughts and feelings and gaining a clearer understanding of how others perceive oneself.
- **Embracing self-acceptance:** Cultivating a positive attitude toward oneself involves acknowledging and accepting previously criticized aspects of one's identity.
- **Pursuing self-actualization:** Progressing toward fulfilling one's potential and integrating conflicting aspects of oneself.
- **Attaining enlightenment:** Aiding the client in reaching a higher spiritual awakening or understanding.
- **Solving problems:** Finding solutions to specific issues that the client has been unable to resolve independently, and gaining general problem-solving skills.
- **Educating on psychology:** Providing clients with concepts and techniques to comprehend and manage behavior.
- **Developing skills related to social situations:** Initiating and maintaining conversations, and assertiveness skills.
- **Changing thought patterns:** Altering or replacing irrational beliefs or harmful thought patterns linked to self-destructive behavior.
- **Modifying behavior:** Changing or replacing maladaptive behavioral patterns.
- **Instituting systemic change:** Introducing alterations to the functioning of social systems, like families.
- **Empowerment:** Equipping the client with skills, awareness, and responsibility to be the master of their own decisions.
- **Quality of life:** Focusing on the quality of life and leading a more purposeful and meaningful life.

HISTORY

Development Before 1900

The field of counseling was evolved over a period when counseling was not done by professionals but teachers, advocates and reformers were the main ambassadors who did counseling mainly to provide information and to make people aware of various issues. It started with the start of the social welfare movement.

Development During 1900–1909

This era was all about these three persons who were addressed as pioneers in the field of counseling: *Frank Parsons, Clifford Beers and Jesse B. Davis.*[5]

- **Frank Parsons,** father of counseling psychology, is well known for his multidisciplinary career and his selfless energy in helping others. He also established Boston's Vocational Bureau in 1908

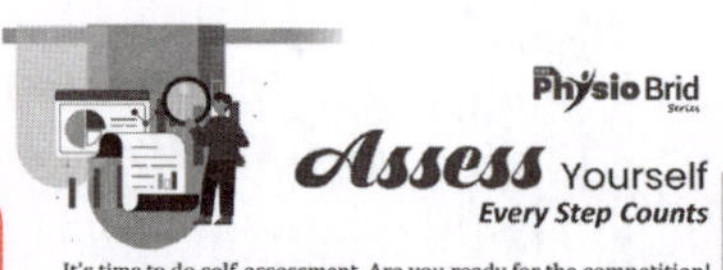

which was aimed to help youngsters to choose their career as per their aptitude and interest areas. He also constructed several questionnaires that could help people in choosing careers as per their "experiences", "preferences" and "morals".

- **Clifford Beers** was struggling with depression and found insufferable mental health facilities during his multiple admissions to the hospital and penned down his feelings in his book, named "A Mind That Found Itself". He addressed counseling "as a means of helping people adjust to themselves and society".

Development in 1910

Three major episodes that clearly define the growth of counseling during 1910:

1. **National Vocational Guidance Association (1913):** Print writing about vocational counseling and guidance.
2. **Smith-Hughes Act (1917):** Financial contribution to support the vocational guidance in the educational institutes.
3. **World War-I (1914–1918):** Establishment of Army Alpha and Army Beta and other psychometric tests.

Development in 1920

Commencement of educational courses: In 1920, the counseling field got authenticity by commencing certificates and professional courses in counseling. Education courses were developed to become a counselor and it was first started at Harvard University in 1911. Also, certification of the counselors was initiated in Boston and New York during the mid-1920s.

Development During 1930

- E G Williamson's work became prominent in the 1930s and 1940s, particularly with the publication of his book "How to Counsel Students" in 1939. His development is also known as "trait-factor theory" or the "Minnesota Point of View" which focused on a counselor-centered approach. The main aim of this approach was to figure out the deficits of the client and suggest solutions to fulfill the deficits so that the client could make decisions independently. The subjects with whom Williamson majorly worked were the unemployed ones.

- **Counseling as a part of school curriculum:** John Brewer in his book Education as Guidance (1932) emphasized the role of teachers as counselors so that they could prepare students for the outer world in which they have to survive after the completion of their studies.

- **Dictionary of occupational tiles (DOT):** US employment service was also developed by the government and it further launched the DOT in 1938 and it became the main platform that provide knowledge of the guidance specialists.

Development in 1940

- **Carl Roger's theory:** Carl Roger proposed a client-centered theory in which solution was planned and thought by the client only. He emphasized few qualities such as listening and being empathetic and unconditional positive regard as a counselor to achieve common goal.

- **World War II:** Military recruiters were looking for men and women who possessed the aptitude to serve in the army irrespective of gender. In simple words, the war crises compelled the government to recruit men and women according to their aptitude not based on their gender. Thus, during World War II, the US government was looking for trained professionals and psychologists who could perform psychometric assessments to recruit men and women in the army.

Development During 1950–1960

Refer to Figure 18.2 to understand the major developments that took place during 1950–1960.

Development in 1970

- **Development of new concepts of counseling:** Counseling was not limited to the fields of vocation and education. The counseling psychology became popular almost in every area and the recruitment process of hiring counselors began even for hospitals, clinics, rehabilitation centers, community mental health clinics, and even for assistance programs as well.

- **American Mental Health Counseling (1976):** AMHC was established to define the goals and roles of the counselors as per the standards of the code of ethics.

- **State Licensure:** As counseling became a profession and law became restricted and it became a law that one had to pass an exam to become a professional counselor. Virginia was the first state to acquire a state license in 1976.

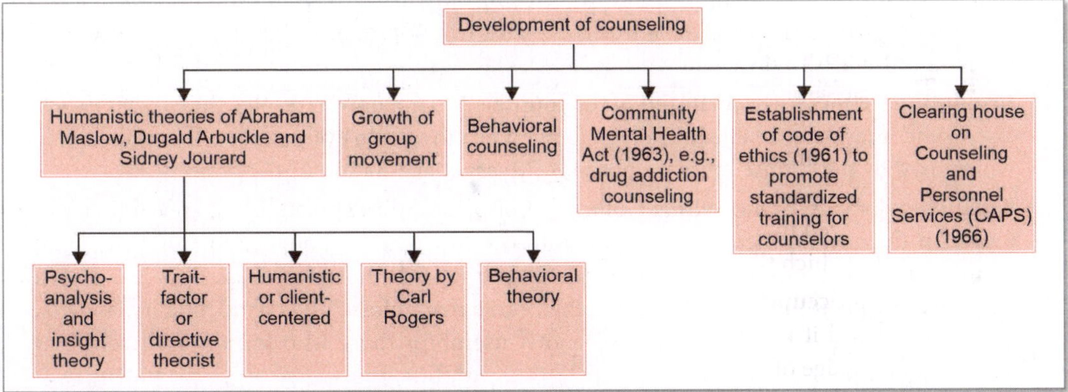

Fig. 18.2: Development during 1950–1960

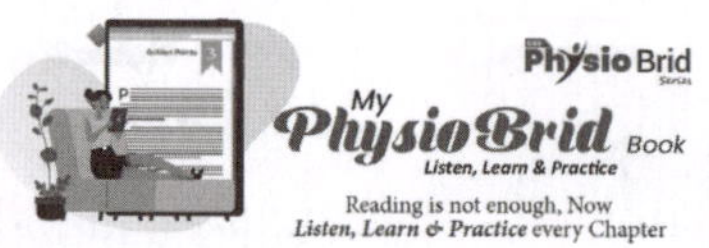

- **Guidelines for higher qualifications in counseling:** Guidelines and outlines had prepared and issued by the Association of Counselor and Supervisors in 1973 to pursue master's and doctoral in counseling.

Development During 1980–1990

- **Council for Accreditation of Counseling and Related Educational Programs:** It was established in 1981 and in 1987, it got the membership of Council of Postsecondary Accreditation. The main of this body is to systematize the educational programs at school, graduation, master and doctoral level of counseling psychology.
- **National Academy of Certified Clinical Mental Health Counselors:** The academy started training professionals and supervisors of mental health counselors in 1988.
- **American Association of Counseling Association:** After 1984, American Personnel and Guidance Association (APGA) changed its name from APGA to the American Association of Counseling Association to define the changing goals and roles of the counselor.
- **Publishing Journals:** Journal of Counseling and Development, March 1987, Journal of Counseling and Development, May 1986, Journal of Mental Health Counseling, January 1985, Elementary School Guidance and Counseling, October 1989.

Current Trends

- **Crisis plan management for critical issues:** Terrifying incidents such as terrorist attacks, sudden loss of dear ones, and road accidents usually make persons more vulnerable to experiencing post traumatic stress disorder (PTSD) and acute stress disorder (ASD). The symptoms of PTSD were observed among people of the US after a terrorist attack on September 9, 2001 in New York. Crisis counseling plays a crucial role in helping individuals to overcome the trauma and healthily lead their lives.
- **Managed care:** It can be understood in terms of third-party (e.g., Maybe the hospital or the organization where the counselor works) system which promotes the quality of services that counselor provides to the client.
- **Promoting wellness:** The main aim of the counselors is not only to resolve the current issues but also to encourage and enable the person to live a healthy life in every aspect. The wellness model which used by the counselors is proposed by Myers et al. (2000).
- **Technology or cyber-counseling:** Counselors also use different platforms to reach their clients and with the advancement of technology it becomes easy for both (counselor and client) to connect. Earlier the technology was used to keep records, however, these days it is also used to communicate, to interact with each other while maintaining the confidentiality, and also to preserve the client's responses. This is majorly useful for those who are physically challenged, and living in remote areas.

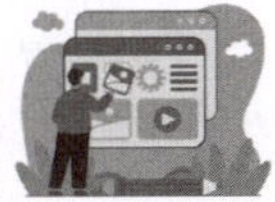

Conclusion

The field of counseling has progressed from the root and works almost in every aspect of life to promote a healthy and fruitful lifestyle of individuals. It uses the holistic or eclectic approach to deal effectively with the stressors of life.

PROCESS

Counseling relies on a structured framework for guidance, benefiting both the counselor and the client. While not always strictly adhered to, this framework acts as a map or reference point in counseling practice. In 1994, Egan[6] presented a three-stage framework for the counseling process, as detailed in Figure 18.3. In his book "The Skilled Helper" (1994), Egan elaborates on these three stages with additional subsections. However, an alternative model might examine the preliminary steps before clients begin working with counselors.

- **Precontemplation:** The client starts considering seeking help.
- **Establishing the contact:** A referral is usually made to the client or they can approach the counseling.
- **Envisioning the relationship:** The client envisions the counselor and the relationship they will form.
- **Initial meeting:** The client and counselor discuss pressing issues, leading to emotional expression and potential catharsis.
- **Clarity and focus:** The client gains clarity on problem situations, experiences reduced tension, and feels understood.
- **Addressing other issues:** Past-related problems may emerge and require attention.

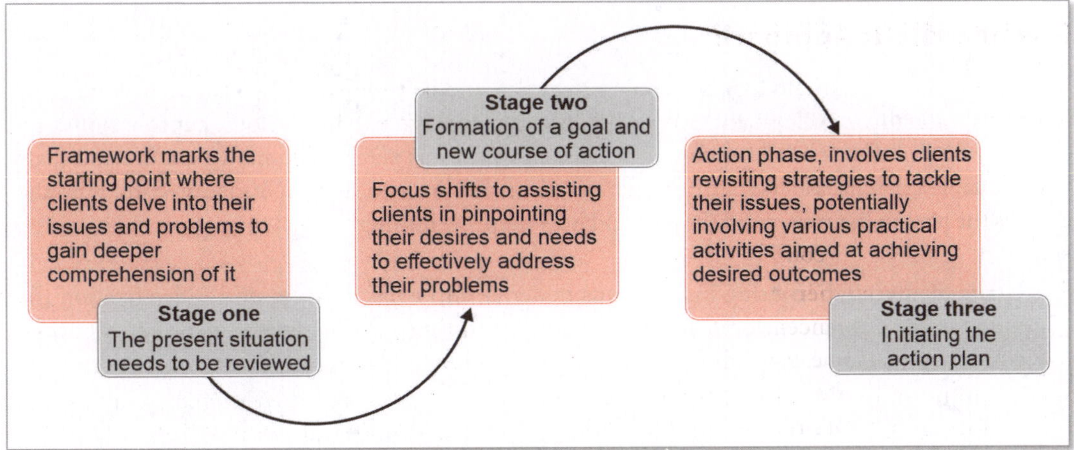

Fig. 18.3: Stages of counseling

- **Fears/worries about change:** The client expresses worry regarding the process of change and how it will impact their life and that needs to be freely discussed with the therapist.
- **Attainment of goals:** The goals can be achieved by targeting them with significant actions and seeing the changes in their actions.
- **Termination:** The counseling relationship concludes, and the client feels more self-reliant and capable of coping independently.

Factors Affecting the Counseling Process

Refer to Table 18.2 to know about the factors affecting counseling.

Table 18.2: Factors affecting counseling

Client's variables	Counselor's variables	Environmental variables
Sociodemographic factors	Sociodemographic factors	Traveling and distance
Motivation	Educational qualification, skills and training	Infrastructure
Insight level	Personality factors	Ventilated counseling rooms
Personality factors	Belief system and flexibility	Noise proof rooms
Intelligence	Emotional intelligence	Cost and affordability of counseling sessions
Coping styles	Experience and expertise	Availability of test materials like manuals and stationery

APPROACHES

Psychoanalytic Approach

Sigmund Freud concentrated on personality structure and considered Id, Ego, and Superego as the basis of personality development. Also, take into consideration the conscious, subconscious, and unconscious mind to resolve the conflicts. This approach was also an attempt to understand many unreasonable current behaviors of the person. It is also known as insight-oriented therapy that enables the person to understand the past and how these events might affect the person in his current situation.[7]

- **Goals of therapy:** To bring unconscious material into consciousness, to resolve fixation that might occur during developmental stages, and to resolve the repressed traumatic experiences of childhood that are causing difficulties in the client's life.[8]
- **Techniques of therapy:** Analysis of dreams, free association technique, analysis and interpretation of resistance, analysis of transference and countertransference.

Behavioral Approach

B F Skinner's approach emphasizes the modification of undesirable behavior by using different behavioral modification techniques such as reinforcements, rewards, and desensitization. This approach is based on the notion that behavior can be learned and unlearned, clearly explained by Pavlov and Skinner in their experiments.

- **Goals of therapy:** Reducing undesirable behaviors and focusing on increasing desirable behaviors.[9]
- **Techniques of therapy:** Systematic desensitization, relaxation exercises, flooding, token economy, contingency management, differential reinforcement, etc.

Cognitive Behavior Therapy

Dr Aaron Temkin Beck focuses on the negative core beliefs and encourages them to challenge these negative thoughts with evidence. This theory believes that thoughts lead to feelings and feeling further leads to behavior. Thus, undesirable action or behavior can be modified by molding the thoughts. This therapy also figures out the cognitive distortions and makes the client aware of the pattern of their thoughts by charting it down in a thought recording chart.[8,9]

- **Goals of therapy:** It aims to improve emotional regulation and develop effective coping strategies for various psychological issues.
- **Techniques of therapy:** Socratic questioning, daily thought record, relaxation techniques, grounding techniques, responsibility chat, activity scheduling, etc.

Rational Emotive Behavior Therapy

Dr Albert Ellis states that Rational Emotive Behavior Therapy (REBT) deals with the task of modifying irrational beliefs into rational beliefs. The therapist will be helping the patients understand their irrational beliefs and see through the more logical thoughts and explanations through confrontation and by analyzing the event.[9]

- **Goals of the therapy:** REBT helps people to understand thoughts that are not rational. It is the emotional and personal reaction to the events or situations that cause the problems, not the situations themselves. The therapy helps to identify the thoughts that are leading to negative emotions and then modify it with logical ones to decrease the stress and difficulties associated with it.
- **Techniques of therapy:** It include disputing irrational beliefs (DIBs), where irrational thoughts are challenged and replaced with logical ones, and the ABC Model, which helps individuals analyze the link between Activating events, Beliefs, and emotional or behavioral Consequences to promote healthier responses.

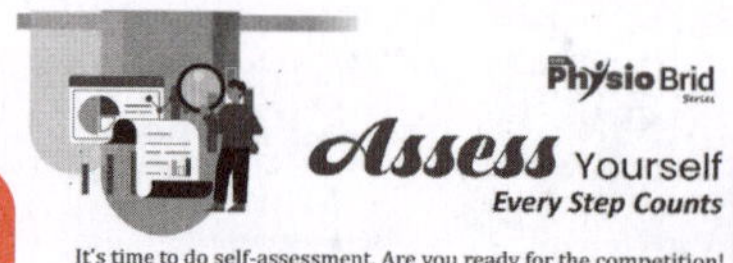

Humanistic Approach/Person-Centered Therapy

- Dr Carl Rogers came up with six main factors responsible for the development of a person:
    i. Therapist client psychological contact
    ii. Client incongruence or vulnerability
    iii. Therapist congruence or genuineness
    iv. Therapist unconditional positive regard (UPR)
    v. Therapist empathy
    vi. Client perception.[10]
- Rogers formulated his hypothesis of the 'necessary and sufficient conditions'. The strength of the change lies like relationship between the therapist-client.[11]
    - The client is having incongruence between their real and ideal self.
    - The therapist should have unconditional positive regard toward the clients.
    - The therapist should be more accepting, empathetic and genuine toward the clients.[10, 11]
- **Techniques of therapy:** Active listening, empathy, unconditional positive regard, reflecting and genuineness.

Existential Therapy

- Existential therapy, shaped by the contributions of Rollo Reece May and Viktor Emil Frankl, centers on the individual's pursuit of meaning, freedom, and responsibility. It addresses existential concerns such as isolation, mortality, and decision-making, encouraging individuals to live with authenticity and purpose.
    - Existentialists think that the person writes his own life story by the choices that they make.
    - Problems and symptoms start when the client is not able to make meaningful choices, has an existential crisis in their life, and thus not utilize their full potential.
    - Anxiety acts like a motivating force to achieve the full potential while sometimes it also acts as the hindrance or limiting factor that is stopping a client from achieving his full capacities.[12]
    - Frankl states that every person looks for the meaning of life, and although this meaning may be different, it never stops to be.[12, 13]
    - The fundamental dimensions of the human condition are the following: The ability to be self-aware, freely exercising their will, developing their own identity and forging significant connections as the only important part of their lives, to find the meaning, the purpose of life, finding their own beliefs, values, the meaning of life and the inevitable truth of death.[12]
- **Techniques of therapy:** The technique employed in existential counseling is the relationship with the client. On the other hand, the clients realized that they need to take responsibility of their own choices, decisions and hence their own life and destiny.[13]

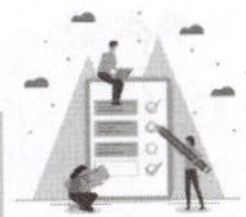 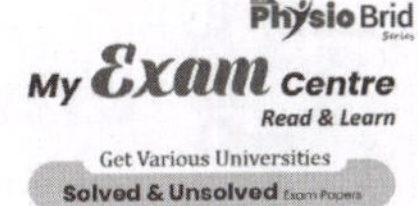

SKILLS AND TECHNIQUES

Counseling Interview

- Interview is an important tool for data collection. An interview is a very important method for collecting detailed information related to a client's life that could help us in understanding the problems and thus making a better case formulation and treatment part. It has specific goals and a defined way of achieving those goals in a standardized way.

- The assessment includes the discussion of painful, traumatic and distressing experiences between the therapist and the client.

- The objective is to obtain reliable and adequate information through one-to-one interaction and to understand the perception of the client and how he/she sees his/her problem. The events themselves are not the issue, but how we are perceiving is rather more important.

- The interview can be of three types:

    i. **Structured interview:** It has a predefined set of questions for all the clients. It follows a strict set of frameworks that does not provide much scope of flexibility and opportunity in gathering information. This type of interview provides very little flexibility and follows a rigid and strict process.[8, 13]

    ii. **Semi-structured interview:** It usually starts with a predefined question and later the conversation continues according to the responses given by the clients. It gives more flexibility as compared to the structured interview.

    iii. **Unstructured interview:** This interview has no predefined questions and usually takes the form of free-flowing questions that could take any path depending on the answers given by the client. It lacks structure. This type of interview sometimes deviates from the goals of the interview, thus important data cannot be collected or might get lost in the steam of other topics.

Therapeutic Relationship

The relationship of counselor and client plays a vital role in the therapeutic process and also determines the outcome of therapy. The therapist shall be nonjudgmental, empathetic, warm, open to sensitive issues and a good listener.[9, 14]

- **Observation of behaviors:** Observation of verbal and nonverbal behaviors to understand the problems of the client.[14]

- **Carl Rogers** (1951) defined various principles that are an important part of a therapy process and these are discussed here:

    - **Real versus ideal self-congruency:** Carl Rogers believes that there should be congruency between the real and ideal self, i.e., the internal feelings and the external feelings. The capacity of the client and what they aspire to achieve.[11, 14]

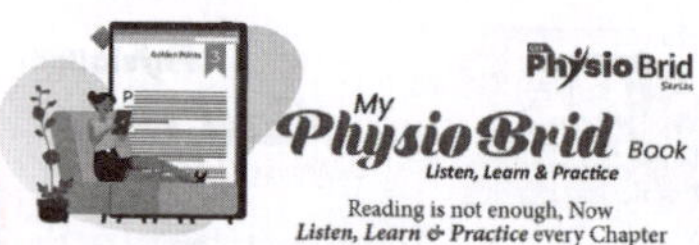

- **Positive regard:** The therapist shouldn't judge or evaluate the clients based on their feelings and behaviors rather than accepting them as they are. They should see their clients in a very natural way.[10, 11]

- **Empathy:** Empathy involves understanding people's situation from their perspective, feeling what they feel, and communicating that understanding back to them to enhance their own experience and meaning. It goes beyond sympathy, which is simply recognizing and caring about someone else's suffering. While often used interchangeably, empathy involves feeling the other person's pain, whereas sympathy is more about acknowledging it. While both are sincere, empathy can create a deeper connection and facilitate more meaningful communication between individuals or between a leader and his followers.[6, 15]

  Various skills are associated with empathy such as verbal and nonverbal skills, skills paraphrasing, Reflecting client's feeling, then meaning of messages shared by the client.

- **Attending or active listening** in counseling encompasses the counselor's presence, both physically and emotionally, with their clients. Being fully present communicates to clients that they are being heard and that their experiences are valued. Effective attending enables counselors to listen attentively to their clients.

  The acronym SOLER as shown in Table 18.3 serves as a tool to demonstrate respect and authenticity throughout the counseling session, especially crucial in building rapport during the initial stages of interaction.

Table 18.3: The acronym of SOLER

S	Straightly facing the client.
O	Posture should be open and accepting.
L	Appropriately leaning toward the client to show curiosity and interest.
E	Eye contact with the client shows that the therapist is paying attention and also showing empathy.
R	Making the client feel relaxed so they can express themselves freely.

Skills of Paraphrasing

Involve focusing on understanding the thoughts and feelings of the messages conveyed by the clients, where their keywords and concepts are reflected to them in a condensed and rephrased manner. This technique reassures the client of your attentive listening and helps them gain clarity on their situation.[14, 15]

The various steps of an effective paraphrasing include:

1. **Active listening:** The message conveyed by the client should be attending actively without forgetting or missing the important parts of it and later remembering it.

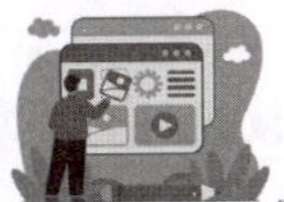

2. Determine important issues related to specific people, situations, settings, etc.

3. Concisely rephrase important words and concepts presented by the client and presenting them from a very different perspective.[14]

4. Assessing the understanding of the client's problems by using brief questions like "It sounds like..." or "Let me see if I understand this", allowing the client to confirm or correct your paraphrasing.

Effective paraphrasing can provide clearer, more focused reflections than the original statements, often resulting in client responses like "That's right" to show agreement.

Tips for paraphrasing is to begin responses with "you" to reflect the client's internal viewpoint, slow your speech rate to allow more time for thinking, and develop a strong vocabulary, and memory by practicing paraphrasing regularly.

Reflecting Client's Feeling

This involves respectfully and openly reflecting the clients' verbal and nonverbal communication, capturing both their words and body language, as well as making reasonable inferences about their emotional state. It is crucial for the helper to carefully select words that accurately convey these emotions back to the client.[14]

Ways to Show Empathy

1. **Step 1:** Establish a supportive and secure atmosphere between the therapist and client, ensuring physical and emotional comfort. This involves maintaining a tidy, private space and projecting a calming presence as the counselor.[8, 9]

2. **Step 2:** Employ encouraging behaviors to elicit further disclosure from the client regarding their life circumstances. These can include nonverbal signals like gestures, body posture, facial expressions, etc., and verbal prompts like "Okay", "I see", "I understand" and "Please elaborate".[8, 14]

3. **Step 3:** Engaging in active listening, paying close attention to the verbal and nonverbal expressions of the client. The attention should be directed toward understanding the perspective of the client and empathizing with their experiences.

Self-Disclosure

Self-disclosure involves the communication process where an individual reveals personal information to another person. This information can encompass descriptions or evaluations, including thoughts, emotions, aspirations, successes, failures, fears, dreams, preferences, and dislikes. It is regarded as a valuable strategy for fostering intimacy and strengthening interpersonal connections through the sharing of information.

Through self-disclosure, individuals allow themselves to be perceived authentically, making it easier for others to relate to them as genuine human beings, complete with both flaws and strengths, thoughts, and emotions. When viewed as human, communication and relationships can flourish more readily.

Sharing one's experiences and maintaining therapy boundaries at the same time is one of the crucial components of self-disclosure that can create a feeling of similarity with the client's own experiences. It is important to note that empathy is not about sharing similar experiences, but rather about expressing understanding and care toward the client's feelings and thoughts. Self-disclosure goes beyond merely imparting information; scholars define it as revealing details to others that they wouldn't typically learn or uncover. This process entails a degree of risk and vulnerability for the individual expressing their feelings.

Johari Window

A different way of viewing oneself can be assessed through the Johari Window (Fig. 18.4). It is a method to understand how much one knows about oneself and how much other people know about him.

Information about ourselves and others, categorized by what is known or unknown, comprises several concepts:

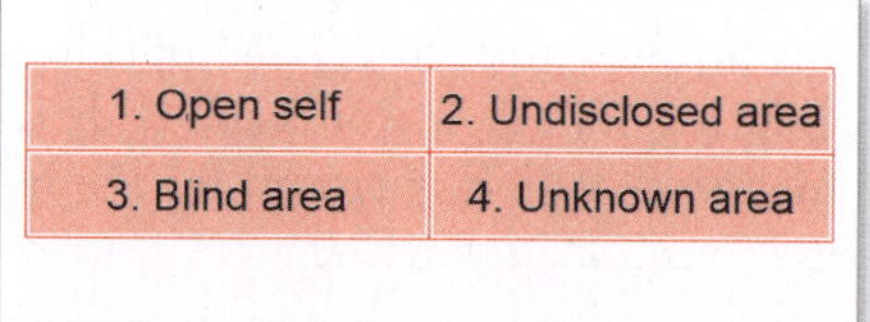

Fig. 18.4: Johari Window

1. **Open self:** This encompasses aspects of ourselves that are readily apparent and acknowledged by both ourselves and others, such as physical attributes like hair color, occupation, and general appearance.

2. **Undisclosed area:** This pertains to aspects of ourselves that we are aware of but choose not to disclose to others, such as personal dreams or ambitions, creating a hidden dimension of our identity.

3. **Blind area:** This refers to aspects of ourselves that others perceive but of which we remain unaware. An example could be when others view us as displaying strong leadership skills, while we may not recognize this trait in ourselves.[14]

4. **Unknown area:** This includes aspects of ourselves that neither we nor others are aware of. These could be hidden talents or potential qualities that have yet to be discovered or explored.

Self-disclosure, while often beneficial, carries certain risks:

- It may shift the focus from the other person to yourself, potentially leading to an unfavorable response or failing to elicit the desired impression. Self-disclosure doesn't guarantee positive outcomes.

- There's a risk of creating an imbalance in the relationship, where the other person gains power or feels pressured to support or protect you due to the information shared.

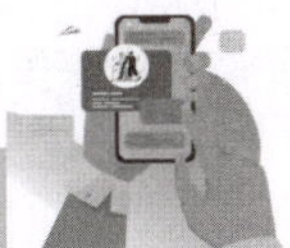

- Self-disclosure can be misinterpreted as advice, potentially leading to misunderstandings or conflicts.
- Excessive or premature self-disclosure in a relationship can undermine its foundation and damage trust and intimacy.

Acceptance

Acceptance is fundamentally recognizing and acknowledging "What is" without passing judgment on a situation. It involves embracing a mindset that enables you to release feelings of frustration, disappointment, stress, anxiety, regret, and unfulfilled expectations. Acceptance fosters inner peace by acknowledging the inherent limits of your control. While a simple concept, it's a challenging practice. Fortunately, life offers numerous opportunities to cultivate acceptance. The reality is that life presents countless moments where one might wish for different outcomes.

Acceptance should not be equated with giving up or condoning others' behavior to persist. It doesn't entail surrendering to circumstances that are unhealthy or uncomfortable. The primary obstacle to acceptance often lies in the desire for control, yet control itself is illusory. Life's certainty is its unpredictability; you cannot dictate events, others' actions or the past and future. What you can control are your thoughts, beliefs, attitudes, interpretations, and expectations. Investing energy in trying to control things that are not controllable will only lead to anger and frustration. Accepting what one can and cannot control is the key to solving many problems.

Engaging in acceptance involves practicing simple matters. For instance, when faced with rain, acknowledge its presence without judgment. Should your mind veer toward negative thoughts, return to the simple acknowledgment of the rain's existence. Employ mindfulness techniques, such as tuning into your senses, to fully experience and embrace the moment. By accepting what is, you can cultivate a sense of calm and inner peace amidst life's uncertainties.

Counselors must cultivate self-acceptance regarding their attitudes, values, and beliefs, recognizing how these aspects may influence both personal lives and professional practice. They should reflect on how their perspectives might impact their interactions with clients, particularly when faced with differing opinions. In the counseling profession, practitioners engage with individuals from diverse backgrounds, encompassing various races, cultures, and religions. Counselors need to acknowledge and respect these differences, understanding that clients may hold beliefs and values divergent from their own.

Genuineness

Genuineness, also known as congruence, is a fundamental aspect of effective counseling characterized by authentic attitudes and behaviors. Being genuine entails being truthful and authentic, presenting oneself exactly as one truly is without imitation. Genuine individuals are transparent, with no hidden agendas or personas. They are comfortable in their interactions and do not feel the need to alter themselves to gain acceptance.

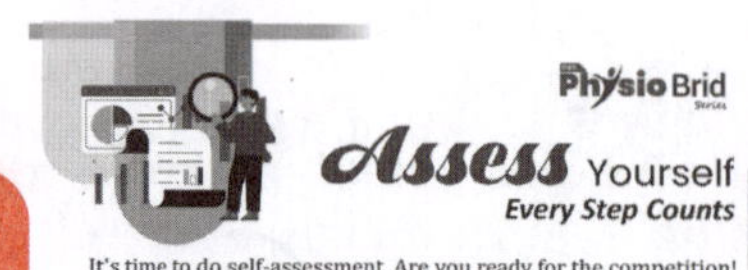

In the context of counseling, genuineness is considered paramount, particularly according to Rogers. It involves therapists being authentic to themselves during client interactions. While being genuine doesn't necessitate therapists disclosing their problems, it does involve sharing their emotional reactions to clients' experiences. Genuineness fosters a direct and sincere connection between counselor and client, where the therapist engages on a person-to-person level without a facade.

Ultimately, the development of a sound therapeutic relationship between the client and the therapist laid the foundation of the therapeutic process, facilitating trust, openness, and effective communication.

- **Informed consent:** In this, the client has been informed regarding the purpose of the test, how the results will be used to answer the referral question, and who will have access to the findings of the assessment. The psychologists will proceed only after the client agrees to begin with the assessments.[15]

- **Privacy and confidentiality:** The right to confidentiality means that the test results are only accessible to appropriate parties and will not be shared otherwise. The appropriate parties usually include the client, therapist, and referral professionals. So, any transmission of results to other parties will warrant the informed consent of the client.

  The right to privacy essentially pertains to an individual's willingness to share personal information with others, whether that information is factual or related to feelings and attitudes.

- **Note taking:** Aid for the memory-previous session, confidentiality, court orders, diagnosis, prognosis. Date, name, age/sex, session no, session participants, therapy method, session objective, therapist reflection, next session, plan.

- **Summarizing:** Counselor's feedback, summarizing the salient points mentioned by the client so that it couldn't be missed by the therapist. It includes a concise summary of the whole session. The client should know that the therapist heard, and understood him and can clarify any thoughts and emotions, if not clear enough for both the client and therapist.

- **Questioning:** Asking questions to fully understand, the depth of the client's emotions. Not too many questions, language is important.

  - **Open-ended questions:** Begin, elaborate, rich, How- feelings, what- emergence of facts, when- timing of problems, where- environment, why- reasons.
  - **Closed-ended questions:** Keeping from wandering off, fill in specific information gaps.

Identifying Patterns and Behaviors

Identifying the maladaptive patterns of thoughts, behaviors and emotions that is causing distress to the individual and helping them through various approaches of counseling for alleviating their distress and promotes well-being and quality of life.[15]

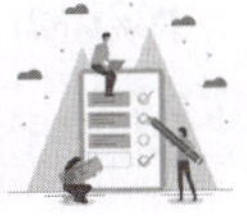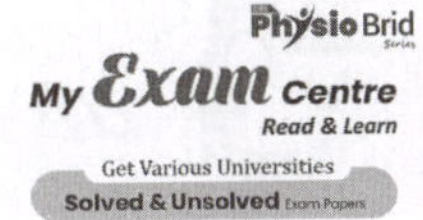

ETHICAL AND LEGAL CONSIDERATIONS

Ethics are recommended behavioral norms derived from a shared set of values. Typically, a code of ethics serves as a formal framework for ethical norms. A code of ethics must be developed as the group moves closer to professionalism to ensure safe professional practice. Counselors can access ethical guidelines that have been produced by professional bodies of counseling.[15, 16]

The following are professional associations for counselors and psychotherapists:

- American Psychological Association (APA)
- American Counseling Association (ACA)
- British Association for Counseling (BAC)

Since 1953, APA has published and updated ethical guidelines, with the latest version being the ethical principles of psychologists and code of conduct, released in the year 1992.

General Principles

- **Beneficence and nonmaleficence:** Psychologists aim to help their clients, avoid causing harm to them and work to protect the rights and well-being of both themselves and other impacted parties, as well as the welfare of study subjects who are animals, in the course of their work.

- **Fidelity and responsibility:** A trustworthy and genuine relationship with their clients should be made by psychologists. Psychologist should understand their obligations to society, to maintain ethical and professional standards at the community level by being truthful to their responsibilities toward society.[16, 17]

- **Integrity:** The aim is to promote transparency and accuracy related to research, assessments, training, education, and practice in psychology. Psychologists should never indulge themselves in behaviors that hide the truth, mislead, misinterpret, confound the assessments or reports, and make rash or ambiguous decisions. They have the responsibility to maximize the benefits of the clients and minimize any harm. If they think, they are not the expert in any particular area of assessment and therapy, then referrals should be made to another expert.

- **Justice:** They should provide equal access and opportunity to people from all areas of life irrespective of gender, race, caste, religion, background, socioeconomic status (SES), etc. They shouldn't indulge in any unfair means of practice and safeguard the rights of people in society.

- **Respecting rights and dignity of people:** They should safeguard the confidentiality, privacy and self-determination as well as the worth and dignity of the individuals irrespective of their vulnerability whether they are capable of making a decision or not. They should connect the individuals to many levels of services available at the community level.[17]

Ethical Issues and Dilemmas

- **Honoring the individuality and diversity of the client:** If a client's right to freedom is not upheld, the following issues may arise such as building client dependence, difficulty concluding

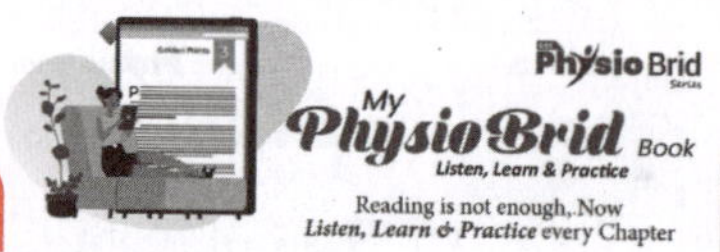

a case, pushing clients to take on tasks they are unable to perform on their own, keeping the assistance process opaque and discrimination.[15, 16]

- **Transparency and clear boundaries in dual professional relationships**: A dual connection is when a professional takes on two or more roles with the person seeking assistance, either concurrently or sequentially, such as friendship and business dealings. Because of the unequal power and status relationships between counselors and their clients, judgment is likely to be impacted and weakened, which increases the risk of exploitation.[18, 19]

PHYSIOTHERAPY AND MENTAL-HEALTH

Physiotherapy (PT) is a healthcare profession that deals with restoring and managing various physical conditions that could occur due to any injury thus affecting the day-to-day functioning of the individuals. It helps in the management of mobility, chronic pain, stiffness and many other conditions through physical rehabilitation.[20]

These healthcare professionals work at a general hospital, private clinics, community health centers, and sports clubs, and organize various camps, workshops, charities research work, etc. Physiotherapy offers valuable assistance to individuals of all age groups dealing with various health issues, including:

- **Bones, joints, and soft tissue:** This includes conditions like pain in the back, neck shoulder, and injuries related to sports where physical interventions could aid in pain management and rehabilitation.

- **Brain or nervous system:** Physiotherapy addresses movement difficulties stemming from conditions such as multiple sclerosis (MS), and dementia such as Alzheimer's, Parkinson's, and stroke helping individuals regain mobility and functionality.[20, 21]

- **Heart and circulation:** Following a heart attack, physiotherapy plays a crucial role in cardiac rehabilitation, promoting cardiovascular health and aiding in the recovery process.[22, 23]

- **Lungs and breathing:** Physiotherapy interventions are beneficial for managing conditions like chronic obstructive pulmonary disease (COPD) and cystic fibrosis, improving lung function and enhancing breathing efficiency.[24, 25]

By focusing on physical activity enhancement and injury prevention, physiotherapy empowers individuals to lead healthier lives and minimize the risk of future injuries.[26, 27]

There are various reasons why individuals seek the assistance of a physiotherapist.[28]

Here are some common scenarios:

- **Illness:** Following a prolonged illness or during/after an illness affecting mobility, balance or motor skills, physiotherapy can aid in recovery and rehabilitation.

- **Chronic health conditions:** Certain chronic health conditions, such as diabetes, may impair mobility and balance, necessitating physiotherapy intervention to manage symptoms and improve function.

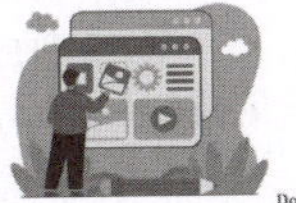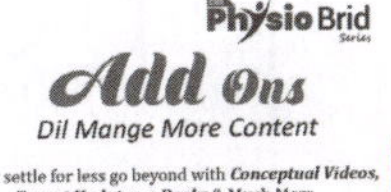

- **Postsurgery:** After undergoing surgery, engaging in physical therapy is crucial for the healing process. Physiotherapy helps individuals regain mobility and function in affected body parts, such as hands, feet or the back, facilitating recovery and rehabilitation.[28]

- **Injury management:** Physiotherapy is effective in managing injuries that cause significant pain or limit mobility, facilitating recovery and restoring function.

- **Aging:** As individuals age, they may encounter changes in their bodies that affect movement and function. Physiotherapy can assist in mitigating these effects, helping individuals regain function or adapt to changes.

- **Major health crisis:** Following major health crises such as heart attacks, strokes or traumatic brain injuries, physiotherapy plays a crucial role in aiding patients' recovery and restoring everyday function.[28, 29]

- **Comorbid psychological problems:** Many psychological issues such as stress, depressive symptoms, panic attacks, generalized anxiety disorder, somatoform, substance abuse, insomnia, obsessive-compulsive disorder (OCD), cognitive deficits, etc.

- **Enhanced physical performance:** Athletes and individuals aiming to improve their physical performance often turn to physiotherapy to learn techniques for optimizing their body's capabilities, thereby enhancing performance in fitness pursuits.

- **General wellness:** Physiotherapy is utilized by individuals seeking to maintain overall health and mobility, counteracting the effects of aging, and acquiring strategies for staying active and healthy.

Physiotherapy also plays a significant role in enhancing mental health, a fact often overlooked by some practitioners. The saying "no health without mental health" underscores the integral relationship between physical and mental well-being. Physiotherapists, renowned for their expertise in physical healthcare, offer a range of interventions that positively impact mental health.[29, 30]

- **Nonpharmacological pain management:** Physiotherapists provide nondrug approaches to pain management, which can alleviate discomfort and enhance mental well-being.[31, 32]

- **Tailored exercise programs:** Individualized exercise regimens prescribed by physiotherapists can boost mood, promote overall well-being, and address comorbidities associated with mental health conditions.

- **Addressing physical barriers:** Physiotherapy interventions target physical issues hindering social participation and recovery in individuals with mental health diagnoses, such as side effects of psychotropic medications.

- **Motivation and self-management:** Physiotherapists play a crucial role in motivating patients and promoting self-management strategies for both mental and physical health issues.

- **Falls and mobility issues:** Physiotherapists manage falls and mobility issues in older adults and address developmental challenges in children and young people.

- **Body awareness and dissociation:** Expert advice and interventions aim to improve the awareness of the body like any sensation, pain, stiffness or numbing.

- **Lifestyle and weight management:** Physiotherapists develop tailored lifestyle and weight management programs to enhance overall health and well-being.
- **Relaxation exercises:** Progressive muscle relaxation, deep breathing, and guided imagery could help with anxiety and physiological symptoms related to mental health issues.
- **Supportive therapy:** Supporting people suffering from serious physical health issues where one could not alter the debilitating consequences and acceptance is one of the major components.
- **Psychoeducation:** Providing important information regarding the illness, symptomatology, and management techniques can help alleviate the distress of the individuals.
- **Counseling:** Counseling can provide help with the numerous factors that are interfering with the recovery process of the individual.

Research highlights the profound impact of physical activity on psychological well-being, with physical exercises proven to lessen the symptoms of many mental health issues such as stress, depression, anxiety, etc. Recognizing the substantial burden of mental health disorders and their correlation with musculoskeletal conditions, physiotherapists advocate for a holistic multidisciplinary approach to management.[32, 33]

Implications

Apart from helping individuals with physical issues and comorbid psychological issues that can affect the recovery from their illness and also the symptoms could worsen if mental health issues weren't targeted, the same challenges could affect those working in the healthcare field including the mental health of physiotherapists themselves.[33, 34]

Physiotherapists can also suffer from various mental health issues due to burnout, fatigability, lack of resources, infrastructure, human resources, etc. Mental health issues in these professionals could affect their work productivity and in turn, could impact the delivery of healthcare services to the people at large. Mental health issues like depression, anxiety, stress, generalized anxiety disorder, panic disorder, substance abuse, obsessive and compulsive disorder, etc., could affect any healthcare worker.[35]

The timely interventions in these conditions that include, supportive therapy, behavior therapy, cognitive behavior therapy, mindfulness, relaxation, etc., could alleviate the distress of the physiotherapists and can improve their quality of life which in turn could improve the delivery of healthcare services at large.

> **MUST KNOW**
>
> Physiotherapists can help by providing basic counseling skills to their patients but it is also very important to remember that they need to refer the patient to a psychologist/clinical psychologist or psychiatrist for serious mental health concerns or if their counseling skills are not able to alleviate their distress. Timely referral is very important, so the Multidisciplinary Team (MDT) works well for the overall management of patients in clinics).

Physio CORNER

Guidance and counseling are essential components of a physiotherapist's practice, as they contribute significantly to the overall well-being and recovery of patients. Here are the primary purposes of guidance and counseling in the context of physiotherapy:

- Enhancing patient compliance and engagement
- Addressing psychological barriers to recovery
- Improving communication and understanding
- Supporting behavioral change
- Managing chronic pain and coping strategies
- Enhancing patient empowerment and independence
- Facilitating emotional and psychological support
- Improving social and interpersonal relationships
- Preventing relapse and long-term maintenance
- Integrating multidisciplinary care

CASE STUDY

Integrating Counseling and Physiotherapy for Chronic Pain Recovery

Patient Background

John, a 45-year-old man, suffered a severe lower back injury from a car accident. After initial medical treatment, he was referred to physiotherapy to aid in his recovery. Despite attending regular physiotherapy sessions, John's progress was slow, and he reported ongoing pain, frustration, and a lack of motivation to continue the exercises. His physiotherapist noticed that John's psychological state might be hindering his physical recovery and recommended integrating counseling into his treatment plan.

Challenges

- **Chronic pain and fear-avoidance behavior:** John experienced persistent pain, which led to fear-avoidance behavior. He was afraid that movement would exacerbate his pain, causing him to limit his activity levels and resist certain physiotherapy exercises.
- **Emotional distress:** The accident and its aftermath caused significant emotional distress, including anxiety, depression, and feelings of helplessness, which further impeded his recovery.
- **Lack of motivation:** John struggled with staying motivated during his rehabilitation, often feeling that the exercises were too difficult or that his condition would never improve.
- **Negative coping mechanisms:** John began using unhealthy coping mechanisms, such as excessive alcohol consumption, to manage his pain and emotional distress, which further negatively impacted his physical and mental health.

Counseling Interventions

Recognizing the need for psychological support, John's physiotherapist referred him to a counselor specializing in pain management and rehabilitation. The following interventions were implemented:

- **Cognitive behavioral therapy (CBT):** The counselor used CBT to address John's fear-avoidance behavior and negative thought patterns. By helping him reframe his thoughts about pain and movement, John

Contd...

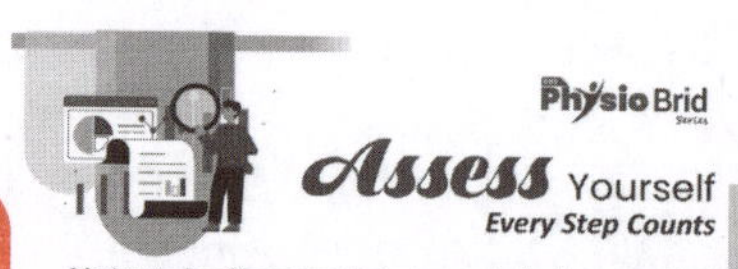

began to see his exercises as a pathway to recovery rather than a source of increased pain. This shift in mindset encouraged him to engage more actively in his physiotherapy sessions.

- **Pain management techniques:** The counselor introduced John to relaxation techniques, such as deep breathing exercises and guided imagery, to help him manage his pain more effectively. These techniques were also incorporated into his physiotherapy sessions, allowing John to feel more in control during exercises.

- **Motivational interviewing:** The counselor used motivational interviewing to help John explore his own reasons for wanting to recover and regain his previous level of functioning. This intervention increased his intrinsic motivation and commitment to the rehabilitation process.

- **Addressing emotional distress:** Through regular counseling sessions, John was able to process the emotional trauma related to the accident. The counselor provided a supportive environment where John could express his fears and frustrations, which helped reduce his anxiety and depression.

- **Developing healthy coping mechanisms:** The counselor worked with John to identify healthier coping mechanisms to replace his alcohol use. This included developing a daily routine that incorporated activities he enjoyed, setting achievable goals, and building a support network with friends and family.

- **Collaborative approach with the physiotherapist:** The counselor maintained regular communication with John's physiotherapist to ensure that the psychological and physical aspects of his recovery were aligned. This collaborative approach helped tailor John's physiotherapy exercises to his evolving psychological state.

Outcome

With the integration of counseling into his treatment plan, John experienced significant improvements in both his physical and psychological well-being:

- **Improved pain management:** John learned to manage his pain more effectively, which reduced his fear of movement and allowed him to participate more fully in his physiotherapy exercises.

- **Increased motivation and engagement:** His motivation to engage in physiotherapy increased as he began to see progress and believed in his ability to recover.

- **Enhanced emotional well-being:** John's anxiety and depression symptoms decreased, leading to a more positive outlook on his recovery process.

- **Healthier coping strategies:** John reduced his reliance on alcohol and developed healthier ways to cope with stress and pain, contributing to his overall well-being.

- **Accelerated physical recovery:** As a result of his improved psychological state, John's physical recovery accelerated. He regained strength, mobility, and confidence, eventually returning to his daily activities and work.

Conclusion

This case study illustrates the critical role that counseling can play in enhancing physiotherapy outcomes. By addressing the psychological barriers to recovery, counseling helped John overcome his fear of movement, manage his pain, and stay motivated throughout his rehabilitation. The collaborative approach between the counselor and physiotherapist ensured a holistic treatment plan that supported both John's physical and emotional recovery, leading to a successful outcome.

SUMMARY

- Counseling for mental health issues has significant implications in the field of physiotherapy, enhancing both the physical and psychological well-being of patients. Integrating mental health with physiotherapy promotes a holistic approach to patient care. Patients receiving mental health support alongside physiotherapy tend to have better treatment outcomes. Addressing issues such as anxiety, depression, and stress can improve patient engagement, adherence to physiotherapy regimes, and overall recovery rates. This leads to the development of individualized care plan can lead to more effective and tailored treatments.[30, 35]
- Counseling equips patients with coping strategies to manage chronic pain, disability or recovery from injury. Techniques such as cognitive behavioral therapy (CBT) can help patients change negative thought patterns and improve their pain management and rehabilitation efforts. Many physical symptoms can be exacerbated by psychological factors. Addressing mental health issues can reduce psychosomatic symptoms, thereby enhancing the effectiveness of physiotherapy.
- Mental health counseling can provide techniques for stress and pain management, such as mindfulness, relaxation exercises, and stress reduction strategies, which can complement physical therapy exercises. Effective counseling can strengthen the therapist-patient relationship, building trust and open communication. This rapport is crucial for patients to feel comfortable sharing their concerns and for therapists to provide comprehensive care.[33, 35]
- Incorporating counseling within physiotherapy encourages interdisciplinary collaboration. Physiotherapists may work closely with psychologists, psychiatrists, and other mental health professionals to provide integrated care.
- Overall, the integration of mental health counseling within physiotherapy is essential for comprehensive patient care, leading to improved physical and mental health outcomes, enhanced treatment adherence, and overall patient well-being.[34, 35]

REFERENCES

1. McLeod J. An Introduction to Counseling. 3rd ed. Open University Press; 2003.
2. Hough M. Counseling Skills and Theory. 3rd ed. Hodder Education; 2010.
3. British Association for Counseling. Code of Ethics and Practice for Counselors. Rugby: BAC; 1984.
4. Burks HM, Stefflre B. Theories of Counseling. 3rd ed. New York: McGraw-Hill; 1979.
5. Gladding S. T. Counseling: A Comprehensive Profession. 3rd ed. Englewood Cliffs, New Jersey: Prentice-Hall; 1996.
6. Egan G. The Skilled Helper: A Systematic Approach to Effective Helping. 5th ed. Belmont, CA: Brooks Cole; 1994.
7. Freud S. Five Lectures on Psychoanalysis. London: Penguin Books; 1909.
8. Kabir SMS. Essentials of Counseling (Banglabazar, Dhaka): Abosar Prokashana Sangstha; 2017.
9. Bloch S, Crouch E, Reibstein J. Therapeutic factors in group psychotherapy. Archives of General Psychiatry. 1981;38(5):519–526.
10. Rogers C. R. Counseling and Psychotherapy. Boston: Houghton Mifflin; 1942.

Contd...

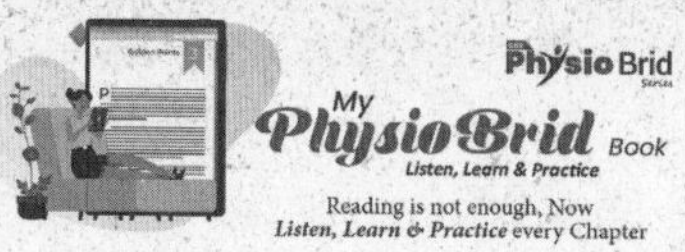

11. Rogers, C. R. The necessary and sufficient conditions of therapeutic personality change. Journal of Consulting Psychology.1957; 21(2):95–103.

12. Yalom I. D. Existential Psychotherapy. New York: Basic Books; 1980.

13. Yontef G. M. Gestalt therapy. In A. S. Gurman and S. B. Messer (eds) Essential Psychotherapies: Theory and Practice. New York: Guilford Press; 1995.

14. Kabir, S.M.S. Basic Guidelines for Research: An Introductory Approach for All Disciplines. Book Zone Publication, Chittagong, Bangladesh; 2016.

15. Avasthi A, Grover S, Nischal A. Ethical and legal issues in psychotherapy. Indian J Psychiatry. 2022; 64(1): S47–S61.

16. American Psychological Association. Ethical Principles of Psychologists and Code of Conduct. 1992; 47(12):1597–1611.

17. Oliver P. The Student's Guide to Research Ethics. Maidenhead: OU Press; 2003.

18. Kottler J. A. Counselors finding their way. Alexandria, VA: American Counseling Association; 2002.

19. Marshall S. Difference and Discrimination in Psychotherapy and Counseling. London: Sage Publications; 2004.

20. Hawkins P, Shohet R. Supervision in the Helping Professions. UK: Open University Press; 2004.

21. Rowan J. Future of Training in Psychotherapy and Counseling: Instrumental, Relational and Transpersonal Perspectives. UK: Brunner Routledge; 2005.

22. Culley S. Integrative Counseling Skills in Action. 2nd ed. London: Sage Publications; 2004.

23. British Association for Counseling and Psychotherapy Online Learning: CPD and Regulation. London: BACP; 2009.

24. Marshall S. Difference and Discrimination in Psychotherapy and Counseling. London: Sage Publications; 2004.

25. Bond T. Standards and Ethics for Counseling in Action. 3rd ed. London: Sage Publications; 2009.

26. Cooper M. Ethical Research Findings in Counseling and Psychotherapy. London: Sage Publications; 2008.

27. Davies M. B. Doing a Successful Research Project. London: Palgrave Macmillan; 2007.

28. Hart C. Doing a Literature Review: Releasing the Social Science Research Imagination. London: Sage Publications; 1998.

29. Hawkins P, Shohet R. Supervision in the Helping Professions UK: Open University Press; 2004.

30. McLeod J. Doing Counseling Research. 2nd ed. London: Sage Publications; 2003.

31. Walker S. Culturally Competent Therapy: Working with Children and Young People. UK: Palgrave Macmillan; 2005.

32. Starker S. Do-it-yourself therapy: The prescription of self-help books by psychologists. Psychotherapy. 1998; 25(1):142–146.

33. Steenberger B. N. Toward science–practice integration in brief counseling and therapy. Counseling Psychologist. 1992; 20(3):403–50.

34. Whiteley J M, Sprinthall N A, Mosher R L, Donaghy R T. Selection and evaluation of counselor effectiveness. Journal of Counseling Psychology.1967;14(3): 226–34.

35. Tatar M. Counseling immigrants: School contexts and emerging strategies. British Journal of Guidance and Counseling. 1998; 26(3):337–52.

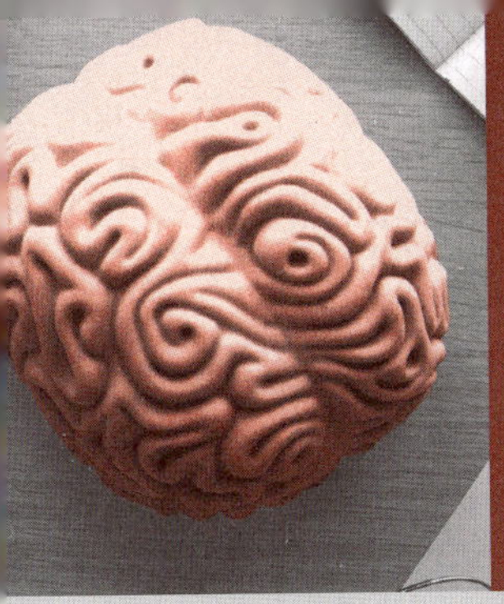

LONG ANSWER QUESTIONS

1. What is counseling? What are the most common approaches to counseling, and how do they differ?
2. Elaborate on the various skills and techniques of counseling.
3. How do cognitive-behavioral techniques integrate into counseling sessions?
4. What are some common barriers to effective counseling, and how can they be overcome?
5. What are the key ethical issues counselors face, and how can they be addressed?
6. In what ways can physiotherapists integrate mental health screenings into their practice?
7. How can physiotherapists and mental health professionals collaborate to provide holistic care for patients?

SHORT ANSWER QUESTIONS

1. Define active listening technique with relevant example.
2. Write about confidentiality and privacy of a counseling process.
3. What do you understand by the client-centered approach of counseling?
4. What is Johari Window?
5. What are the common mental disorders that are prevalent in a physiotherapy clinic?
6. Define self-disclosure.

MULTIPLE CHOICE QUESTIONS

1. **What is a primary goal of counseling in mental health?**
   a. Prescribing medication
   b. Providing physical therapy
   c. Facilitating self-understanding and change
   d. Conducting medical procedures

2. **How can physiotherapists support mental health during physical rehabilitation?**
   a. By prescribing antidepressants
   b. By integrating mindfulness and relaxation techniques
   c. By referring all patients to psychiatrists
   d. By focusing solely on physical recovery

3. **Which strategy is most effective for building a strong therapeutic alliance in counseling?**
   a. Being authoritative and directive
   b. Using technical jargon
   c. Demonstrating empathy and active listening
   d. Minimizing personal interaction

4. **When should a physiotherapist refer a patient to a mental health professional?**
   a. When the patient requests a referral
   b. When mental health issues are beyond the physiotherapist's scope of practice
   c. When physical therapy goals are met
   d. When the patient shows no physical improvement

5. **What is an indicator of a successful physiotherapy and mental health intervention?**
   a. Increased dependence on therapy
   b. Enhanced physical function and improved mood
   c. Solely physical recovery
   d. Reduced need for social interactions

6. **In physiotherapy, which technique is often used to help reduce anxiety and improve mental well-being?**
   a. High-intensity interval training
   b. Progressive muscle relaxation
   c. Deep tissue massage
   d. Cryotherapy

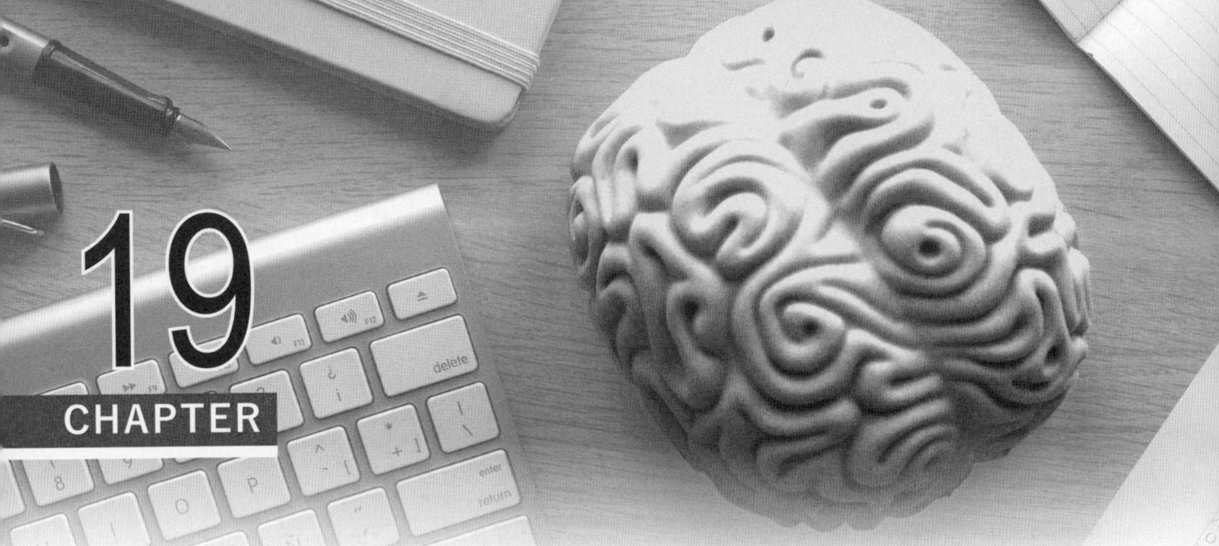

19

CHAPTER

Psychology and Physiotherapy

Muskan Gupta, Shweta Sharma, Parul Sharma

LEARNING OBJECTIVES

After the completion of the chapter, the readers will be able to:
- Know the relation between psychology and physiotherapy.
- Understand the psychological factors in pain perception.
- Understand the integration of behavioral modification techniques and mind-body techniques into physiotherapy interventions.
- Assess the psychosomatic symptoms in a patient.
- Analyze the effectiveness of integrating psychological strategies with physiotherapy interventions.

CHAPTER OUTLINE

- Introduction
- Psychophysiotherapy
- Biopsychosocial Model
- Neurological Basis of Behavior and Movement
- Pain Perception and its Management
- Stress
- Strategies for Improving Adherence in Rehabilitation
- Communication and Therapeutic Relationship
- Mind-Body Interventions
- Cognitive Behavioral Therapy
- Principles of Professional Ethics in Psychophysiotherapy
- Psychological Primitives for a Physiotherapist
- Clinical Application

KEY TERMS

Behavioral modification techniques: Methods used to change or modify behavior patterns. They are crucial for addressing various health issues, including chronic pain and stress.

Biopsychosocial model: An interdisciplinary approach to healthcare that considers the interactions between biological, psychological, and social factors in understanding health and illness.

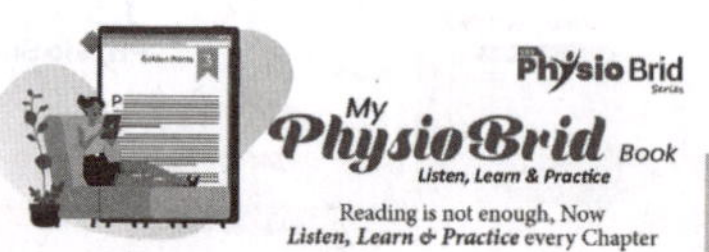

Cognitive behavioral therapy (CBT): A form of psychotherapy that focuses on identifying and changing dysfunctional thoughts and behaviors.

Holistic care: An approach to healthcare that considers the whole person, including their physical, mental, and social well-being.

Interdisciplinary approach: An approach that involves collaboration among various healthcare professionals to provide comprehensive care.

Mind-body interventions: Techniques that focus on the connection between the mind and body to improve health and well-being.

Motivational strategies: Techniques used to encourage patients to adhere to treatment plans and engage in self-care.

Multidisciplinary: Involving professionals from multiple disciplines working together to provide comprehensive care.

Neuroplasticity: The brain's ability to change and adapt in response to new experiences or injury.

Pain perception: The process by which the brain interprets and experiences pain.

Psychophysiotherapy: An interdisciplinary field that combines principles from physiotherapy and psychology to address the mental and physical aspects of health and well-being.

Stress management: Techniques and strategies used to reduce and manage stress. Effective stress management is crucial for maintaining physical and mental health.

Therapeutic relationship: The connection between a healthcare provider and a patient, characterized by mutual trust and respect.

Triangle model: A model that highlights the interconnectedness of brain and body functions and the importance of interdisciplinary teamwork in patient care.

Well-being: A state of being comfortable, healthy or happy. It is a key goal of healthcare, aiming to improve patients' overall quality of life.

INTRODUCTION

A thorough examination of integrated healthcare practices that put mental and physical health first is given in this chapter on psychophysiotherapy and the biopsychosocial model. It draws attention to the triangle model, highlighting the relationship between brain and body functions and the value of interdisciplinary teamwork in patient care. By empowering patients to actively manage their own health, this model lowers reliance on medication and improves patients' quality of life in general. The biopsychosocial model, which takes into account the intricate interactions between social, psychological, and biological factors that influence health outcomes, is crucial. It provides individualized treatment programs that combine psychological and social support to lessen social isolation and stress. Using a variety of healthcare specialties, the model is used to show how comprehensively addressing medical, psychological, and other healthcare needs can improve patient well-being.

PSYCHOPHYSIOTHERAPY

Psychophysiotherapy is an interdisciplinary field that addresses the mental and physical elements of health and well-being by blending principles from physiotherapy and psychology.[1–4]

Triangle Model

- **Brain-body association:** Studies have found that your thoughts directly impact your physical health. Furthermore, this concept does not require much validation; otherwise, no one suffering from anxiety would have voiced physical discomfort.[5–8]

- **Comprehensive approach:** Healthcare was never intended to be limited to the physical. Health has always meant having a healthy body, mind, and soul. The concept emphasizes treating a patient as a whole rather than just his or her symptoms.[9–11]

- **Interdisciplinary approach:** The health system works together, whether it is a medical practitioner, nurse, allied health professional, physiotherapist or psychologist. A patient or case does not require a single person, but rather the entire team for comprehensive care.[12–15]

Figure 19.1 shows the triangle model.

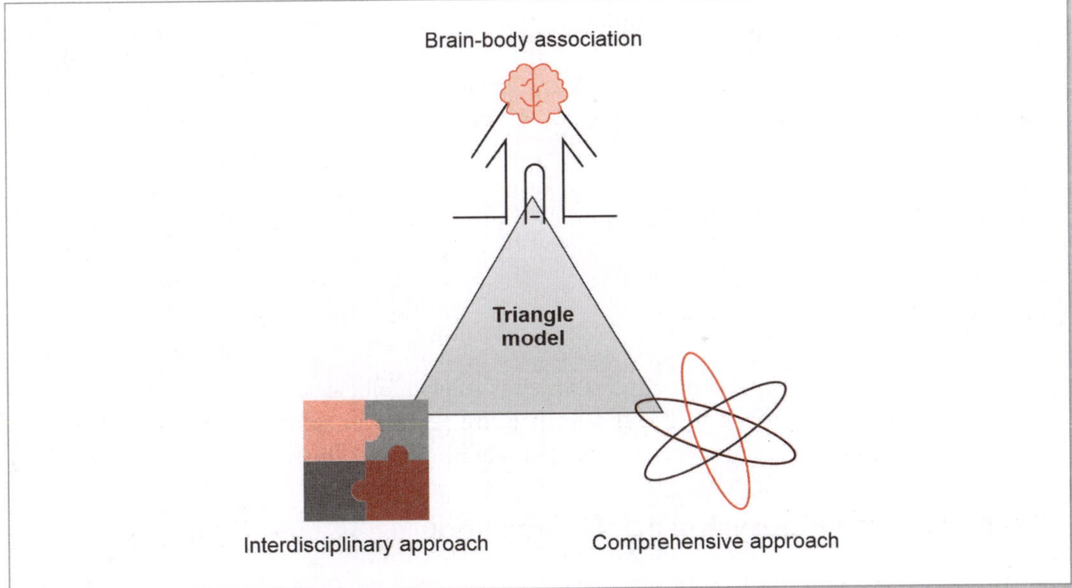

Fig. 19.1: Triangle model

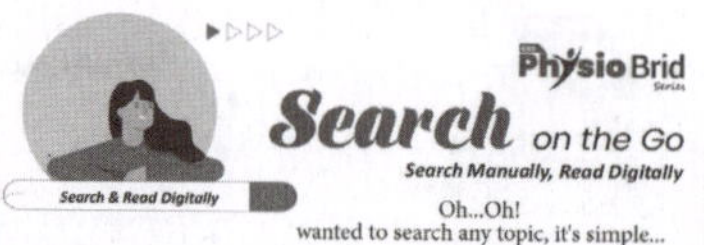

Importance of Integrating Psychology and Physiotherapy

- The dependency of patients on medications and assistance reduces when one is treated as a whole. Combining physical and psychological therapies can minimize side effects, drastically reduce the need for medication, and save costs associated with healthcare.[16–19]

- A holistic approach helps patients develop the knowledge and abilities to take charge of their own health, which boosts their autonomy, confidence, and sense of self-efficacy.[20]

  Physiotherapy and psychology are integral components of comprehensive medical care that aim to promote holistic well-being by addressing both physical and mental health aspects of patients. This personalized treatment, which addresses both emotional and physical issues, ensures better outcomes.[21]

- All facets of a patient's health are addressed holistically in comprehensive treatment, which can greatly enhance overall quality of life and produce more effective and long-lasting results.[21, 22]

Implications of Psychophysiotherapy

To lessen pain and enhance function, physical therapy and psychosocial approaches are used in chronic pain treatment. Prolonged stress can have an impact on the autonomic nervous system, which raises cortisol levels. Autonomic reactions can be modulated by methods such as biofeedback, relaxation training, and cognitive behavioral therapy.[42] Enhancing neuroplasticity and adhering to rehabilitation programs are important for motor recovery and rehabilitation. Restoring mental health requires treating brain circuits and abnormalities in neurotransmitter systems.[43] Both psychological counseling and physical exercise can enhance neurotransmitter function. Facilitating behavioral change through psychological strategies and physical treatment is the essence of behavioral change and lifestyle modification. Neural circuits are linked to cognitive function, and exercise can improve it.[44]

BIOPSYCHOSOCIAL MODEL

Unlike the traditional biomedical paradigm, which is solely biological, the biopsychosocial model is an interdisciplinary approach to healthcare that stresses the interconnectedness of biological, psychological, and social components in understanding health and illness.[23, 24]

Vital Parts of the Biopsychosocial Framework

- **Biological factors:**
  - Pathology refers to the presence of diseases, infections, and physical injuries.
  - Genetics is the study of inherited traits and predispositions.
  - Physiology is the study of how body systems work.

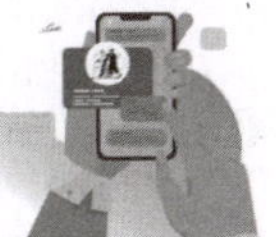
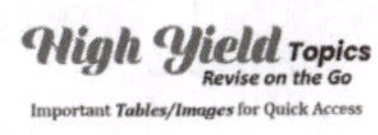

- **Psychological factors:**[25–29]
  - Emotions include stress, anxiety, depression, and general well-being.
  - Behavior includes lifestyle decisions such as nutrition and exercise.
  - Cognition refers to thoughts, beliefs, attitudes, and perceptions of health and illness.
- **Social factors:**[25–29]
  - Socioeconomic impacts on healthcare access
  - Wealth, schooling, and job all influence healthcare access.
  - Cultural beliefs, behaviors, and conventions influence health and wellness.
  - Sources of support include family, friends, community networks, and social interactions.

The biopsychosocial model is a great paradigm for giving patients comprehensive care since it addresses all facets of health.[29, 30]

To improve patient-centered care, personalized healthcare requires developing tailored treatment plans that take into consideration each patient's unique social, biological, and psychological background.[27, 30]

It improves patient outcomes by integrating social and psychological support, as well as reducing social isolation and stress, both of which can be detrimental to physical health.[27, 28, 30]

Preventative treatment prioritizes early intervention and lifestyle changes while identifying social and psychological variables that contribute to health problems.

Systemic illness treatment successfully addresses social and psychological difficulties as well as physical symptoms, enabling continuing, comprehensive care that aids in long-term disease management.[25–30] Figure 19.2 shows the biopsychosocial model.

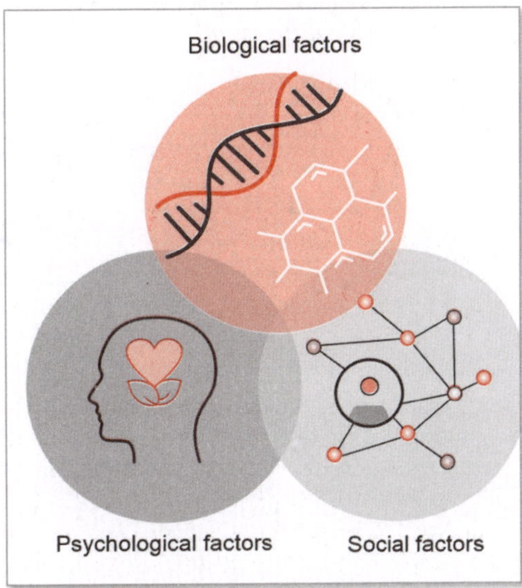

Fig. 19.2: The biopsychosocial model

Applications

Primary care physicians use the biopsychosocial model to better understand their patients' overall health and provide exceptional treatment. Nowadays, family physicians encourage routine to conduct assessments to identify physical indicators related to social factors influencing health and mental well-being.[26, 31]

Counselors, psychologists, and psychiatrists utilize this framework to enhance their comprehension of the interplay between mental and physical health. They promote all-encompassing treatment strategies, including medication, counseling, and social services.[27, 30, 31]

Physiotherapists, occupational therapists, and other rehabilitation specialists employ this approach to treat injury or illness by incorporating support and social reintegration into the healing process, resulting in both physical recovery and psychological adaption for patients.

To treat chronic pain, experts use the biopsychosocial approach, which addresses not only physical pain but also emotional and social factors that influence pain perception and treatment.

CASE STUDY

Examining the Biopsychosocial Model in Physiotherapy: Case Studies on Chronic Pain Management and Rehabilitation Challenges

According to the biopsychosocial model of health, social circumstances, behavioral aspects, and biological traits all have an impact on health and illness. Mrs. Chatsworth had a total hip replacement due to osteoarthritis in her knees, hips, and shoulders; this has resulted in pain and restricted range of motion. She needs to do strengthening exercises because she can only bear a portion of the weight. Her healthcare provider will recommend these activities and make sure the treatment plan is both successful and manageable in terms of physical demands. Her rehabilitation may also be impacted by social and psychological issues, such as stress or despair following her husband's passing. It is important to acknowledge her concern of bearing weight on her right leg and her desire to adhere to a recovery plan.[32]

The biopsychosocial approach is examined in this study with a focus on barriers and facilitators among physiotherapy students. Using purposive and snowball sampling together with in-depth interviews, the study employed a case study methodology. Students found it difficult to put the biopsychosocial approach into practice, despite their awareness of it, according to the findings. Proactive views toward individuals with chronic pain, robust social skills, emotional intelligence, skilled professional oversight, supervisor support, and personal pain experience were among the facilitators. Obstacles included clinical supervision, a lack of interaction with interdisciplinary team members, and unfavorable views toward people with chronic pain. According to the study, there is a gap between the theoretical understanding of the biopsychosocial paradigm and its actual implementation in the treatment of chronic pain.[33, 34]

This study employs the biopsychosocial (BPS) model to examine the impacts of physiotherapist-guided therapy on spinal disorders. The study has a particular emphasis on patients with spinal disorders who were treated with BPS-based therapies. The study is helpful in consolidating data for BPS therapies and directing the development of future physical therapy treatments, despite its limitations.[35]

NEUROLOGICAL BASIS OF BEHAVIOR AND MOVEMENT

The neurological foundation of behavior and movement studies the intricate relationships between neurons, neurotransmitters, and brain circuits, governing voluntary and involuntary movements.

It also investigates how the brain controls motor output, interprets sensory information, and adjusts to changes through neuroplasticity. This knowledge provides insights into mobility issues, behavior, and rehabilitation techniques.

Anatomical Basis

- **Brain:** The cerebrum is an important brain region that regulates movement and perception, conscious and unconscious behavior, emotions, memory, and intellect. It is divided into two hemispheres: The right, which is responsible for spatial thinking, and the left, which is responsible for speech and abstract reasoning. The cerebrum is made up of four lobes: Frontal, parietal, temporal, and occipital.[37] The frontal lobe controls all aspects of language, cognition, and motor function. The parietal lobe interprets all visual, auditory, motor, sensory, and memory activity. The temporal lobe is responsible for processing sensory data as well as understanding written and spoken words. The occipital lobe processes visual information. The cerebellum receives sensory information from the brain and spinal cord to permit precise motor action and govern voluntary movement.[38]

- **Spinal cord:** An indispensable organ, the spinal cord transmits motor orders, sensory data, and reflexes from the brain to the body.[37] It acts as a conduit, sending sensory data to the cortex and motor signals to the muscles. Reflex arcs are used by the spinal cord to coordinate reflexes in instances where brain signals are not present. Moreover, interneurons or central pattern generators, are present to regulate rhythmic movements. Without step-specific sensory feedback or volitional motor control, the lumbar spinal cord produces rhythmic muscle activation, suggesting a role in human locomotion.[39]

- **Nervous system:**[36]
  - **Autonomic nervous system:** The peripheral nervous system's autonomic nervous system controls involuntary physiological functions like blood pressure, respiration, digestion, sexual arousal, and heart rate.
  - **Somatic nervous system:** The somatic nervous system, which is mainly made up of sensory fibers and motoneurons, is in charge of triggering both muscular contraction and relaxation as well as voluntary bodily motions.

- **Hormones:** Dopamine is associated to happiness. It produces oxytocin, a hormone that improves emotional bonding and lessens the feeling of pain. Crush, however, can result from dissociation of the amygdala, which is active against negative emotions like fear. The hormone cortisol helps the body become ready for stressful situations.[40]

Concept of Neuroplasticity

The process by which the nervous system modifies its structure and function in response to stimuli, such as a stroke or traumatic brain damage, is referred to as neuroplasticity, also known as neural or brain plasticity. It entails realigning the connections, functions or structure following an injury. The interprofessional team's contribution to better patient care is discussed in this process, along with evaluation and management.[41]

PAIN PERCEPTION AND ITS MANAGEMENT

Pain perception is a multifaceted interaction of sensory, emotional, and cognitive processes shaped by biological, psychological, and social influences.

Impact

Many elements, such as attention, interpretation, attitudes, expectations, and anxiety, affect how people perceive pain. Pain perception can be influenced by management techniques including attention divertissement and different interpretations. Beliefs and feelings regarding pain are also influenced by cultural variables.[45] By concentrating on the worst-case scenario, catastrophic thinking can make suffering worse. Another element is a feeling of agency because patients are able to self-administer painkillers. Anticipations have a big impact on how individuals perceive pain, and the placebo effect suggests that therapies function better when patients think they will.[46] Positive emotional states, such as listening to music, might lessen pain, but anxiety can exacerbate it. Hands-holding reduces pain, according to research. Since emotions, attitudes, and behaviors play a crucial role in the human pain experience, psychological factors have a considerable impact on how pain is perceived.[47]

Management

A group of medical specialists with differing degrees of specialization collaborate and often consult with one another while treating pain using a multidisciplinary approach. There is mounting evidence that this method, which addresses the physical, psychological, medical, occupational, and social components of chronic pain, is successful. Anesthesiologists, psychologists, nurses, physical and occupational therapists, surgeons, neurologists, internists, physiatrists, psychiatrists, social workers, nutritionists, and pharmacists should all be part of the core team.[48] Individualized treatment plans should combine medical and physical therapies, as well as cognitive behavioral therapy (CBT)-based psychological interventions. The CBT techniques help patients reduce the impact of their pain and return to their regular daily activities by addressing several contributing factors.[49]

Integrative care requires interdisciplinary teamwork, which combines expertise, experience, and knowledge to produce the best results. Every member of the ICU team has a distinct duty depending on the demands of the patient. Physiotherapists are vital because they should be able to communicate and comprehend others well to deliver high-quality, coordinated therapy.[50]

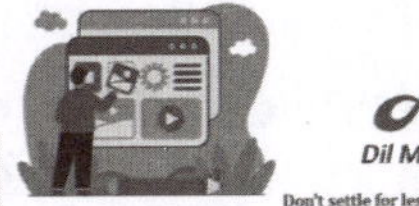

STRESS

Stress is a natural physiological and psychological response to the demands or challenges faced in daily life, which can vary in intensity and impact depending on individual perceptions and coping mechanisms.

Types of Stress Responses

- **Physiological responses:** Numerous physiological systems, including the neurological, muscular, reproductive, endocrine, digestive, respiratory, and cardiovascular systems are impacted by physical stress.[51] While chronic stress activates the sympathetic nervous system and results in higher stress hormones, inflammation, atherosclerosis, and problems with vascular function, acute stress causes an increase in heart rate and muscular contractions. Dyslipidemia is a result of changes in lipid metabolism brought on by stress, which raises the risk of cardiovascular disease. For the removal of carbon dioxide and the delivery of oxygen, the respiratory and cardiovascular systems are essential. Stress, whether acute or chronic, can impair immunological function, breathing patterns, inflammation, and bronchial hyperresponsiveness. Stress releases catecholamines, which have an impact on the gastrointestinal tract and lead to slowed intestinal transit and delayed stomach emptying. Increased stress hormones and physiological reactions are also a result of chronic stress.[51, 52]

- **Psychological responses:** Early mortality, medical morbidity, mood disorders, aggressive dyscontrol, hypoimmune dysfunction, anxiety, and structural abnormalities in the central nervous system are all increased by prolonged exposure to stress during the formative years.[51] Stress affects the whole body, including neural pathways and mind frameworks, which are essential for memory and cognition.[53] Psychological stress can increase the risk of cardiovascular diseases, as anxiety affects heart function, blood pressure, and there is a weak association between symptoms of indigestion and heartburn.[54] Up to 64% of people with anxiety and gastroesophageal ebb disorder experience irritation from their side effects.

To manage stress and improve mental health, individuals can engage in mindfulness workouts, physical activity, and regular exercise.[55] Examples of such workouts include swimming, muscle preparation, kayaking, climbing, and roll classes.

In conclusion, managing stress through mindfulness, physical activity, and regular exercise is crucial for overall health.

Coping Mechanisms

Stress is a widespread social ailment that most people experience during times of change, trauma, difficulties, and bereavement. It has a major effect on productivity and efficiency, but how much of an impact depends on how intense the pressure is and how much coping is required. Even though they are well-adjusted, most people go through brief episodes of distress throughout these times.[56, 57]

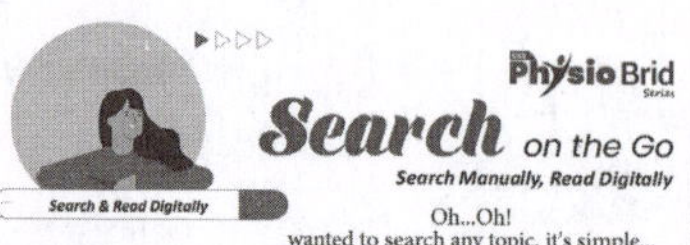

In contrast to automatic or subconscious adaptive reactions that try to minimize or accept stress, coping is the deliberate and purposeful mobilization of ideas and behaviors to manage stress.

Comparing female university students to their male counterparts, a study found that the former employ four coping strategies: Self-amusement, encouragement, practical assistance, and sharing. Although it is seen to be a useful coping strategy, self-distraction cannot remove stress. Higher coping mechanisms include emotional support, with instrumental help being more common in women. Although it is a passive tactic, venting might make stress worse. Men tend to rely more on strategies that directly address the problem they're facing, while women often prefer strategies that focus on managing their emotional responses to the situation.[58]

Peer connections, social status, academic expectations, and family problems are among the things that cause stress in adolescents. They use self-comfort, spirituality, diversion, and reasoning as coping mechanisms. They do, however, require assistance from society and family, especially constructive dialogue with adults.[56, 57]

Additionally, the previous levels of both positive and negative impact at different times were examined in available literature. The content analysis showed that adults reported different forms of stressors at different ages. It was discovered that there are three different kinds of coping strategies: problem-focused, positive emotion-focused, and negative emotion-focused. Older adults tend to use problem-focused coping strategies less often than younger adults. Additionally, they report experiencing lower levels of positive emotions compared to younger adults.[59]

Stress Management Techniques in Rehabilitation

- **Aerobic exercises:** It has been demonstrated that aerobic exercise (AE) lowers stress and enhances neurocognitive function. After a 20–30 minutes workout, individuals report feeling more at ease.[60] Nevertheless, little is known about the molecular mechanisms by which AE impacts brain function, particularly in stress-related circuits. As indicated by the biomarkers cortisol (CORT) and salivary α-amylase (sAA), AE is thought to enhance neurocognitive health by altering the amounts of stress-related hormones and signaling components linked to the HPA axis and autonomic nervous system (ANS) in the bloodstream. This theory suggests that the positive benefits of AE on neurocognitive health may be mediated by changes in stress biomarkers, such as CORT and sAA. Higher levels of aerobic fitness may help lower HR, perceived work stress, and tense muscles.[61]

- **Breathing exercises:** Stress can be decreased by using breathing techniques including alternate nostril breathing (ANB), timed slow breathing, diaphragmatic breathing, and breathing with biofeedback.[62] These techniques, which have their roots in both ancient yogic pranayama beliefs and contemporary scientific research, can be used to treat clinical anxiety and reduce stress in collegiate athletes.[63] They are scalable, cost-free, and widely available, allowing people to use them without the need for medical assistance or experiencing any negative side effects. Breathing exercises have a profound effect on the brain and autonomic nervous system, promoting increased parasympathetic tone and affecting mood, thought processes, and neural circuit dynamics. By enhancing heart rate variability, respiratory sinus arrhythmia, and altering central nervous system activity, slow breathing techniques stimulate autonomic alterations.[64] Increased comfort, relaxation, pleasantness, energy, and alertness are the outcomes of these modifications, which also lessen arousal, anxiety, depressive, angry, and confused feelings.

- **Stretching:** Depression symptoms are brought on by the release of cytokines such as TNF-α, IL-1β, and IL-6 during stress reactions. These inflammatory markers have an impact on the central nervous system, which can result in decreased monoamine levels, sleep disturbances, and cognitive loss.[65, 66] Since high cortisol levels impede cortisol activity, they can be detrimental.

- Yoga can improve general health and promote physiological changes including lower blood pressure, blood glucose, and cortisol levels, which can help manage stress-related mental diseases like anxiety and depression.[65] Yoga influences the hypothalamus, which in turn impacts the adrenal gland and lowers cortisol synthesis by suppressing the anterior pituitary gland's activity and lowering ACTH production.[67]

Stress management techniques in rehabilitation are given in Table 19.1.

Table 19.1: Stress management techniques in rehabilitation

Exercise	Benefits
Aerobic exercise	• Reduces stress levels • Improves neurocognitive function • Modulates stress-related hormones and signaling pathways • Decreases heart rate (HR), perceived work-related stress, and muscle tension[60, 61]
Breathing exercise	• Mitigates stress • Treats clinical anxiety • Enhances parasympathetic tone • Improves mood and cognitive processes • Increases heart rate variability • Facilitates autonomic adjustments • Enhances comfort, relaxation, pleasantness, energy, and alertness • Reduces arousal, anxiety, depression, anger, and confusion[62–64]
Stretching	• Alleviates symptoms of depression • Enhances overall health and well-being • Reduces blood pressure, blood glucose levels, and cortisol levels • Manages stress-related mental disorders such as anxiety and depression • Modulates hypothalamic activity • Decreases cortisol production by diminishing anterior pituitary activity and ACTH secretion[65–67]

STRATEGIES FOR IMPROVING ADHERENCE IN REHABILITATION

To encourage patients to adhere to rehabilitation regimens, medical experts employ a variety of techniques. These include forming therapeutic relationships, raising health literacy, establishing realistic objectives, tailoring the curriculum, controlling the feelings associated with exercise, applying positive reinforcement, avoiding distracting stimuli, and asking for help. These techniques increase patient empowerment and enhance healing results.

Researchers look at several approaches adopted by medical practitioners to encourage patients who have fractured lower limbs to follow their rehabilitation regimens. According to Bandura's self-efficacy model, a person's behavior, thoughts, and emotions can be influenced by their confidence in their capacity to complete a task or reach a goal. Adherence to rehabilitation may be impacted by self-efficacy. Four primary domains have been the focus of research: verbal persuasion, vicarious experience, psychological monitoring, and mastery experiences.[68]

Creating a therapeutic relationship that encourages mutual respect and collaboration is crucial for achieving positive outcomes in rehabilitation. This connection facilitates mastery experiences, where patients feel empowered and motivated to actively engage in their recovery process. It encourages the patient to participate actively in their own recovery by building a rapport and understanding between the patient and the healthcare provider. Strong therapeutic alliances have been linked to improved long-term outcomes, reduced symptoms, and higher levels of satisfaction with one's health, according to numerous studies.[69]

Based on the information they have learned about the patient, medical experts can customize the rehabilitation program to fit each patient's needs, objectives, and capabilities. This involves designing an exercise program that takes the patient's medical problems into account and is tailored to their needs, abilities, and goals. Nonetheless, there is a chance that exercising will cause unpleasant side effects like pain.[70] Healthcare providers may choose to modify the exercise regimen, take prescription drugs or apply heat or cold to alleviate unpleasant sensations.

Sharing examples of people who have gone through comparable things and effectively reduced their discomfort through self-management techniques is known as vicarious experiences. This strategy can be especially useful for people who find it difficult to learn through conventional techniques like oral instruction or practical experience.

Patient motivation can also be achieved through visual persuasion. It entails complimenting the patient's effort, praising past and current accomplishments, and motivating and recognizing the participants' ability to complete a particular activity.[71]

Finally, patients recovering from injury need to engage in physical exercise and functional training. The review is a useful tool to support healthcare providers in their day-to-day work and provides them with practical motivational strategies to incorporate into their patient care regimens.

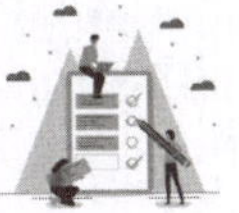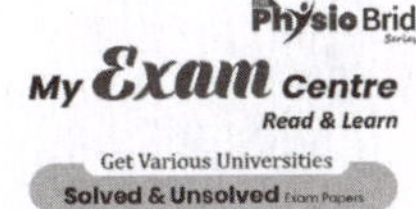

Psychological Impact of Injury

Athletes who sustain injuries may experience both healthy and unhealthy psychological reactions. An athlete's susceptibility to injury and challenges during recovery can be influenced by various preinjury factors such as biological, physical, psychological, social, and stress-related factors. Postinjury, there are interconnected elements involving cognition, emotions, and behavior that mutually impact each other, both in the short and long term.[72] Stress, for instance, can disrupt focus, divert attention, and heighten self-awareness, all of which can impair performance and increase injury risk. Additionally, persistent stress has been shown to elevate hair cortisol levels across different contexts, including pain management, endurance sports, and in individuals experiencing severe depression.[74]

It is crucial for athletic trainers, team physicians, athletes, coaches, and administrators to acknowledge that while emotional reactions to injuries are normal, concerning responses are those that endure, worsen over time or seem disproportionate. Adolescents with high mental toughness exhibit fewer symptoms of depression and demonstrate greater resilience to stress. A physical injury can trigger additional negative responses, including feelings of despair. Emotional and mental health challenges often impact athletic performance, with athletes experiencing depression or stress being more susceptible to injury.[73, 74]

Several substances are used to manage emotions, and substance use and addiction are common problematic reactions. Student athletes also exhibit undesirable responses such as fighting, gambling, and legal issues. About 21% of collegiate athletes who had their depression examined also had excessive alcohol use and alcohol-related disorders.[75]

Athletes may experience psychological and physical suffering as well as a decline in quality of life metrics following a long period recovery injury. Student-athletes may find it extremely difficult to cope emotionally with concussions, especially if they have had major damage to their knees. It is critical to be aware of treatment options and keep an eye out for any unfavorable reactions to injuries.[76]

While the goal of traditional rehabilitation programs is to return an athlete to physical condition, research is starting to show how important it is to address psychological responses in the context of rehabilitation. The integrated approach to addressing sports injuries—according to rehabilitation, situational and personal factors might affect an athlete's emotional state, cognitive assessment, and behavioral reactions.[77] It has been shown that athletes can manage their pain, stress, anxiety, and self-efficacy with the use of psychosocial techniques such as goal-setting, visualization, positive self-talk, and relaxation. Athletic trainers (ATs), among other experts in sports medicine, feel that in order to be efficient in their work, they need to treat psychological elements of injuries.[78] Unfortunately, there are no clear, standardized procedures for imparting this knowledge, which makes ATs unconfident and unprepared to handle the psychological components.

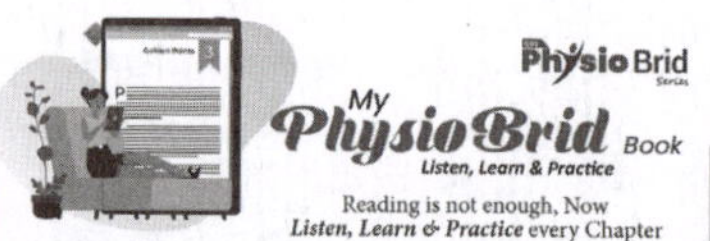

COMMUNICATION AND THERAPEUTIC RELATIONSHIP

Doctor-patient relationship is based on effective communication between the two parties.[79, 80]

Let's explore the elements of therapist communication that patients find most valuable.

- **Speaking confidently:** I am confident because the doctor is confident.

- **Empathetic:** The doctor pays great attention to me, listens to what I am going through emotionally and physically, and then translates that understanding to me.

- **Humane:** The doctor is compassionate, sensitive, and thoughtful.

- **Personal:** The doctor talks with me, acknowledges me as an individual, and takes an interest in me as a person rather than just a patient.

- **Frank:** When explaining things to me, the doctor is straightforward and uses basic language.

- **Respectful:** The doctor interacts with me and listens to my recommendations.

- **Extensive:** The doctor is conscientious and tenacious (Fig. 19.3).

- **Behavior and attitude:** It was observed that occupations require highly developed communication skills in addition to a firm basis in specific specialty knowledge.

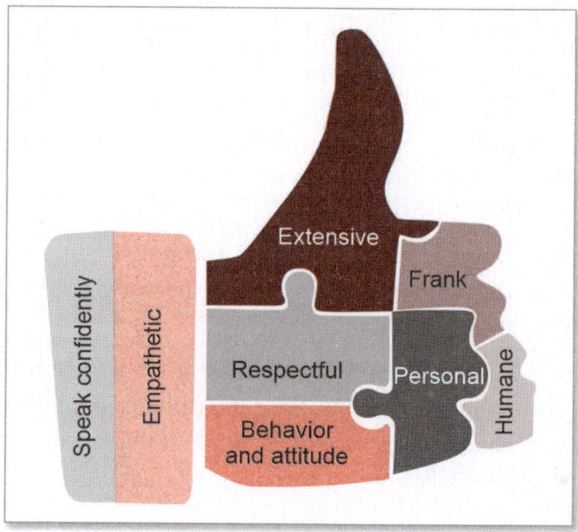

Fig. 19.3: Elements of therapist communication[79, 80]

MIND-BODY INTERVENTIONS

- **Yoga:** Through pranayama and asanas, yoga facilitates controlled breathing processes, hence promoting harmony between man and nature. FVC, FEV_1, and PEFR of the participants of a study significantly changed as a result of enhanced respiratory muscle tone and decreased sympathetic activity.[81] Yogic breathing techniques, such as diaphragmatic, thoracic, and abdominal breathing, enhance lung function and vital capacity. After a year of practice, the study also discovered a significant rise in pulmonary function markers, such as VO_2 max, which was determined using the Bruce treadmill test.[82] Yoga poses strengthen the skeletal muscles, which benefits the cellular machinery and the lungs.

- **Meditation:** Mindfulness, meditation, and reflection are essential for daily life, promoting brain changes, improved cognitive and executive functions, and improved mental and physical health. They also impact immune health, genes, and cell longevity. The complexity of our brain remains a mystery, but our thoughts can become reality. A crucial component of our everyday lives is mindfulness, which is often referred to as meditation and introspection. It deals with the

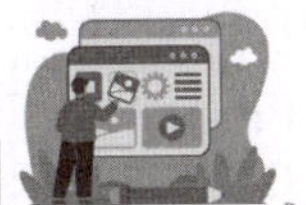

interaction between our internal and external consciousness.[83] It has been demonstrated to cause profound alterations in the brain, such as the activation of the cognitive and emotional centers. Research has demonstrated that meditation enhances cognitive and executive functioning, lowers IL-6 levels, and modifies genes to postpone aging and lengthen cell life. Although the diversity and complexity of our brains are yet unknown, our ideas have the power to manifest into reality.[84] The Buddhist practice of meditation has been shown to improve mental health in clinical settings, especially when treating PTSD and related conditions. It promotes social relationships, elevates happiness and good emotional reactions, and ameliorates cancer patients' mood disorders.[85]

- **Biofeedback:** Biofeedback techniques can help patients with chronic pain, exhaustion, and insomnia by relieving their symptoms and improving their quality of life.[86, 87] By empowering patients to take charge of their illness, these strategies preserve their sense of self-efficacy and general well-being. Patients are capable of making long-lasting adjustments without the use of these devices with sufficient training sessions. Moreover, biofeedback can lower drug usage, preventing polypharmacy and adverse drug reactions. Results, however, differ from person to person and are more likely to be observed in conjunction with physical therapy, cognitive behavioral therapy, and relaxation methods. The advantages of biofeedback techniques can be maximized by an interdisciplinary team of primary care physicians, pain specialists, neurologists, physical therapists, and behavioral health nurses with specialized training.[88]

- **Mental imagery:** This is a strategy for improving performance by imagining movement in the mind rather than physically moving. Working memory can resurrect particular motor movements because of its self-generation *via* visual and sensory mechanisms. The process of imagination is based on central processing systems rather than the capacity to perform a movement. As a result, the ability to construct mental representations of locomotor motions is required.[89] These representations can be created from two points of view:

  i. The third-person viewpoint (also known as external imaging) when seeing someone else walking.

  ii. The first-person perspective (also known as internal imagery) when imagining oneself walking.

- **Visual and auditory cues:** Although they did so in various ways, visual and auditory cues help patients perform better throughout their gaits. While visual cueing increases stride length, auditory cueing considerably enhances cadence. Patients are instructed to place their feet on the stripes provided on the walking surface, attention may be drawn to the stepping procedure.[90]

  Auditory cues are another form of cueing that has been demonstrated to be helpful for patients' improved gait. Cueing techniques like metronomes, rhythmic clapping, and musical beats have been utilized to assist patients in walking more freely.[90, 91]

- **Massage:** Studies that have only included those who are willing to get massage treatment have demonstrated that massage therapy has no negative effects and can even increase the likelihood of getting pregnant and maintaining pregnancies. The scientists hypothesize that greater blood flow, relaxation, less tension, and less uterine contractions may all contribute to better embryo implantation.[92]

Additionally, it has been discovered that massage therapy lowers prefeed gastric residual, raises gestational age and birthweight, and decreases prenatal sadness. Preterm delivery does, however, nevertheless occur in certain depressed women.

Massage therapy has been associated with higher weight gain and earlier discharge from the hospital among premature infants. Researchers have compared the effects of massage with other neonatal interventions like exercise and kangaroo care, both of which also contribute to increased body weight and shorter hospital stays.[93–95]

Massage treatment has been demonstrated to alleviate the severe reflux issues that infants with gastroesophageal reflux disease (GERD) have, while also improving the mother-infant feeding interactions and cortisol levels. Massage treatment has been shown to help children with autism spectrum disorder who have trouble sleeping, and to increase oxytocin levels in both the children and the mothers during the massage therapy session.[96, 97]

Many skin conditions, such as ulcers, burn scars, postsurgery scars, and cleft lip scars, have been treated with massage therapy. Research indicates that massage therapy helps enhance symmetry, strength, and range of motion in those with scars on their cleft lips. In a burn scar research, massage therapy reduced scar tissue, pruritis, discomfort, and anxiety as well as sadness.[98, 99]

Research has demonstrated that massage therapy can lessen the severity and limitations caused by pain in a number of illnesses, such as fibromyalgia, heart surgery, and back pain. Its potential to lessen pain and impairment, however, has not been fully quantified, and more study is required to identify the safest and most efficient approaches.[100]

- **Breathing exercises:** Deep breathing exercises (DBE) are paced, nonresisted breathing techniques that have been shown to enhance human health by lowering blood pressure and reducing psychological stress. Before there is widespread participation, it is necessary to address the obstacles that stand in the way of traditional exercise strategies among adults who do not exercise, including low motivation. Common barriers include fear of pain or discomfort, adverse weather conditions, insufficient knowledge, low energy levels, poor health or physical limitations, limited access to equipment or facilities, work commitments or time constraints, and financial considerations.[101]

Studies on the clinical efficacy of DBE have demonstrated an average drop in systolic blood pressure of 6 mm Hg and diastolic blood pressure of 3–6 mm Hg. These results suggest that DBE can lower blood pressure.[102]

For the past 20 years, cardiovascular disease (CVD) has been the primary cause of death in the United States. Individuals with CVD are at an increased risk of developing additional chronic illnesses and early-onset physical disabilities. Improving DBE acceptance on a national or worldwide level and encouraging new and existing participants to stick with DBE over the long term by reducing obstacles are two crucial public health objectives.[101, 103]

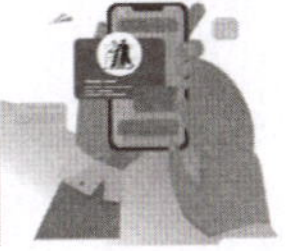

Mind-body interventions are given in Table 19.2.

Table 19.2: Mind-body interventions

Intervention	Description	Benefits	Key findings
Yoga	Combines pranayama (breathing) and asanas (postures)	Enhances respiratory muscle tone, reduces sympathetic activity, strengthens skeletal muscles	Significant improvements in FVC, FEV_1, PEFR, and VO_2 max[81, 82]
Meditation	Practice of mindfulness, reflection, and introspection	Improves cognitive and executive functions, mental and physical health, impacts immune health, genes, and cell longevity	Lowers IL-6 levels, modifies genes, improves PTSD, mood disorders in cancer patients[83–85]
Biofeedback	Techniques to control physiological functions	Relieves chronic pain, exhaustion, insomnia, reduces drug usage	Benefits enhanced with physical therapy, cognitive behavioral therapy, and relaxation methods[86–88]
Mental imagery	Imagining movements mentally	Improves motor performance through central processing systems	Utilizes third-person and first-person perspectives for locomotor motions[89, 90]
Visual and auditory cues	Cues to enhance gait performance	Visual cues increase stride length, auditory cues enhance cadence	Uses metronomes, rhythmic clapping, and musical beats[90, 91]
Massage	Therapeutic manipulation of body tissues	Improves fertility, lowers prefeed gastric residual, decreases prenatal depression, alleviates GERD, helps in autism, improves skin conditions	Increases weight gain, early hospital discharge, reduces pain in various conditions[92–100]
Deep breathing exercise	Paced, nonresisted deep breathing	Lowers blood pressure, reduces psychological stress	Reduces systolic and diastolic blood pressure, improves CVD outcomes[101–103]

COGNITIVE BEHAVIORAL THERAPY

Cognitive restructuring, problem-solving, behavioral self-management, and relaxation training are the main components of the treatment program (CBT). Weekly activity and walking targets, a graded activity plan, and education on the body, mind, and activity level are all included.[104] For instance, chronic back pain is a serious health problem that affects people on both a personal and a societal level. Pain, disability, emotional suffering, and loss of working abilities are all addressed in the curriculum.[107]

Evidence provide effectiveness of cognitive behavioral therapy (CBT) in treating chronic pain in older individuals as investigated through a national telephone survey. The findings indicated that when treating this patient population, only a small percentage of physical therapist's report utilized certain CBT components. Enhancing activity levels (e.g., training patients to pace their activities and encouraging them to participate in enjoyable activities) was the most commonly used CBT treatment. Distraction and visualization are two more CBT procedures that were reported to be utilized sparingly and to have the least interest from the participants.[104, 107]

Although CBT was applied comparatively seldom, participants indicated a significant desire to apply cognitive restructuring to patients suffering from chronic pain. Previous research aimed to increase patient activity levels through the application of cognitive restructuring tools in physical therapy. In another study, only 14% and 16% of participants, respectively, indicated that they were "not interested" in using visualization and distraction tactics. Nonetheless, 57% expressed "great interest" in learning how to teach patients about activity pacing and enjoyable activity scheduling or if they already did so, and 44% showed a comparable inclination toward employing cognitive restructuring.[104–108]

According to literature, the most often mentioned obstacle to putting these techniques into effect was ignorance of them. Another often mentioned potential hurdle, which was shared by the medical profession with relation to all modalities of treatment, was reimbursement concerns. It is necessary to do research on the efficacy and cost-effectiveness of the combined treatment approach, given the concerns raised about time restrictions as a barrier to the integration of CBT into physical therapy practices.[106, 108, 109]

PRINCIPLES OF PROFESSIONAL ETHICS IN PSYCHOPHYSIOTHERAPY

Principles of professional ethics are shown in Figure 19.4.

- **Beneficence:** A deed that is kind, merciful, and compassionate with a strong implied moral obligation to do good to others.[110, 112]

- **Nonmaleficence:** Medical professionals have an obligation to protect their patients. This straightforward idea upholds many moral standards, such as the prohibitions against killing, inflicting pain or suffering, abandoning someone unprotected, inciting hatred, and depriving someone of their fundamental human rights.[110–112]

- **Autonomy:** It implies self-governance, indicating that each person is capable of making their own judgments.[110–112]

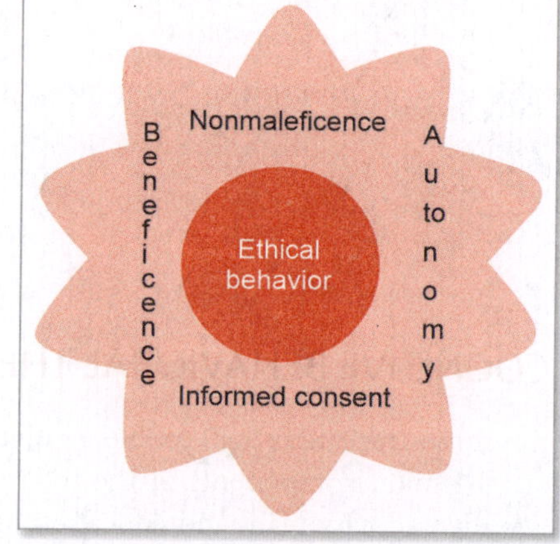

Fig. 19.4: Principles of professional ethics[110–112]

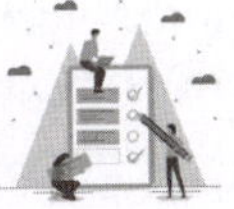
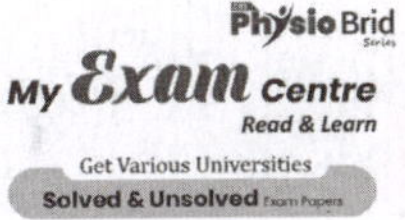

- **Informed consent:** The process by which a physician or other healthcare provider counsels a patient on the advantages, disadvantages, and options for a certain treatment. The patient has to be competent enough to make the decision about whether or not to undergo the intervention or surgery.[112]

PSYCHOLOGICAL PRIMITIVES FOR A PHYSIOTHERAPIST

Figure 19.5 shows the primitives for a physiotherapist.

- **Empathy:** It implies placing oneself in the shoes of the affected. In the medical field, empathy is essential because it allows medical personnel to relate to patients, comprehend their requirements, and administer individualized care. Since functional diagnosis underpins patient-centered physiotherapy, physiotherapists must have empathy for their patients to diagnose and plan treatments that will improve patient outcomes and compliance.[113]

- **Patience:** It is the ability to wait for something. Physiotherapists may need to be patient while working with patients who have chronic illnesses or disabilities that take longer to improve.[113, 114]

- **Positivity:** It has been demonstrated that excellent psychological resources promote both physical and mental health, as well as positive work attitudes and behaviors among healthcare workers.[114]

- **Compassion:** It is the ability to feel another person's misery and the desire to support and enhance that person's well-being to help them solve their situation. Healthcare providers are acknowledged as the central providers of compassion within the healthcare industry. While most healthcare professionals endeavor to demonstrate compassion, patients and their families also hold an expectation of receiving compassionate care.[115]

- **Perseverance:** It is the ability to persist with undertakings in the face of failures. A therapist's consistent efforts can be crucial to rehabilitation.

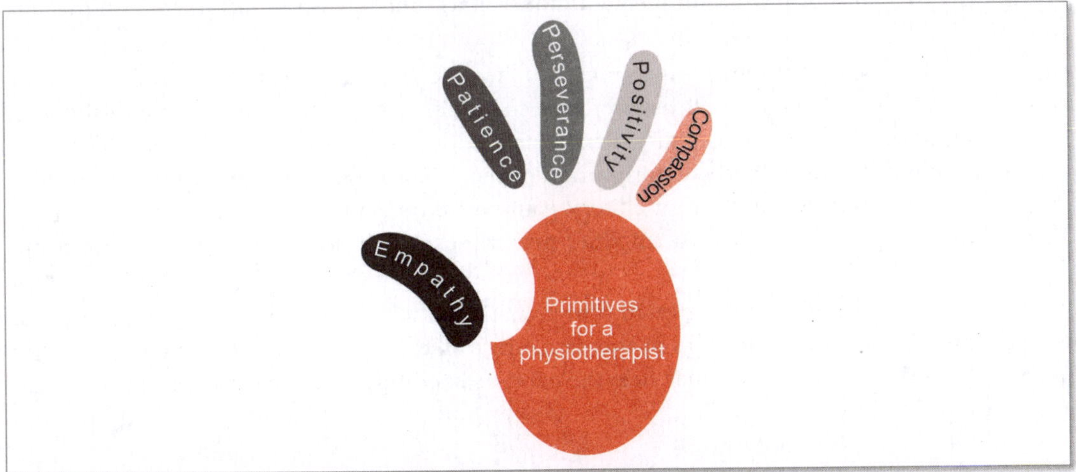

Fig. 19.5: Primitives for a physiotherapist[113–115]

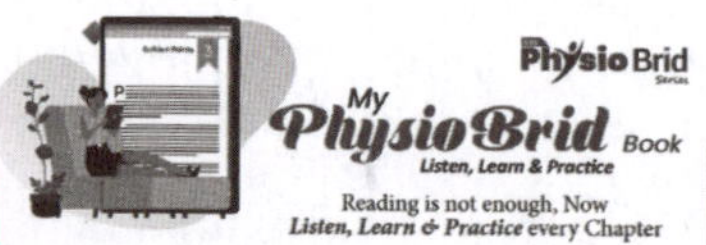

Physio CORNER

We have already discussed how important a therapist's behavior and a patient's outlook are.
Positive thinking patients will eventually find their way out, but it takes skill to deal with people who are in agony and are having mental and physical difficulties. The CBT is one of the most popular forms of therapy.

Cognitive Behavioral Therapy (CBT)
Talk therapy that focuses on altering thought and behavior patterns.[116]

This psychotherapy is popular for treating musculoskeletal pain. In terms of pain, disability, and accompanying mental anguish, chronic back pain is a debilitating health issue for individuals as well as for society at large.[117]

According to the findings of some studies, CBT is an effective treatment for chronic nonspecific back pain, increasing a number of relevant cognitive, behavioral, and physical features. [118]

Studies have investigated how exercise and psychological counseling impact various pain-related conditions, including cancer, fibromyalgia, back pain, knee pain, and chronic fatigue syndrome. These studies involve professionals from different fields who provide both psychological counseling and exercise interventions. The biopsychosocial model of health, which considers biological, psychological, and social factors in understanding health and illness, is being increasingly recognized as applicable to chronic musculoskeletal conditions like knee osteoarthritis.[119–121]

Therefore, emphasis should be placed on an integrated approach to treatment, since data suggests that psychotherapy in addition to physiotherapy can enhance the quality of treatment.

CLINICAL APPLICATION

One of the greatest applications can be seen in cases of fibromyalgia which is a common disorder marked by physical exhaustion, cognitive deterioration, sleep difficulties (especially restless sleep), and persistent widespread pain.[122]

It is unknown where the illness originates, although some things, such as unpleasant experiences, stressful environments or physical or mental traumas, may function as risk factors for fibromyalgia syndrome.[123, 124]

The specific etiology of the illness is unknown; however, unique sleep patterns and differences in neuroendocrine transmitters such as serotonin, substance P, growth hormone, and cortisol point to the autonomic and neuroendocrine systems being controlled as the major reason. The central nervous system (CNS) experiences abnormal neurochemical processing of sensory information due to central sensitization, blunting of inhibitory pain pathways, and changes in neurotransmitters. This reduces the pain threshold and amplifies normal sensory impulses, resulting in continuous discomfort.[125, 126]

Such disorders are frequently treated symptomatically, with pain, depression symptoms, and sleep difficulties being the main areas of attention. Since all of these symptoms are psychological in nature, CBT and exercise therapy may help the patient's condition at the physiological, anatomical, and psychological levels.[127]

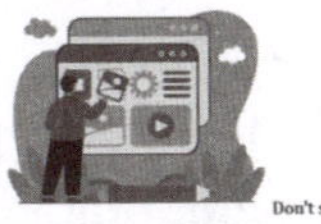
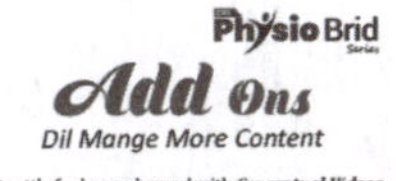

CASE STUDY

Challenges Physiotherapists Face in Supporting Patients with Psychological Distress

We take on people's emotions: A qualitative study of physiotherapists' experiences with patients experiencing psychological distress.

Studies show that it can be difficult for physiotherapists to support patients who are experiencing psychological distress, such as anxiety and depression when they work with them. The study found four interconnected themes: (1) The use of emotional shields to shield oneself from distress, (2) The potential for sympathetic discomfort in physiotherapists, (3) The common and varied experiences with distressed patients, and (4) The emotional tiredness of numerous encounters with distress. These themes emphasize how crucial it is to comprehend how patients' distress, physiotherapists' empathy, and their overall wellness are related. Even though physiotherapists are frequently thought of as physical health specialists, the results indicate that identifying and treating psychological distress in patients is a crucial aspect of physiotherapy practice.[128]

CASE STUDY

Physiotherapists take on Psychological Distress

Psychological distress among patients attending physiotherapy: A survey-based investigation of current practice and opinions of Irish physiotherapists

The purpose of the study was to investigate how the Irish Society of Chartered Physiotherapists (ISCP) currently treats patients who are experiencing psychological discomfort and what views they have on the subject. More than eighty percent of participants stated that they saw patients in psychological distress every week. One of the study's main findings was the absence of mental health education. Numerous physical therapists talked about how important it is to treat underlying psychological problems either in addition to or before treating physical problems. Physiotherapists who received additional training in psychology, mental health or both expressed greater confidence in recognizing signs and symptoms of psychological distress. A significant number of these practitioners routinely included psychological distress assessments as part of their clinical practice.[129]

SUMMARY

- Psychophysiotherapy and the biopsychosocial model are crucial in providing comprehensive care for patients, addressing both emotional and physical aspects of health. The triangle model emphasizes the brain-body association, a comprehensive approach, and an interdisciplinary team working together to provide comprehensive care. Integrating psychology and physiotherapy reduces patient dependency on medications and assistance, helps patients develop knowledge and abilities to take charge of their own health, and enhances overall quality of life.
- The biopsychosocial model underscores the interplay and interconnectedness among biological, psychological, and social factors when examining health and illness. It includes biological factors such as

Contd...

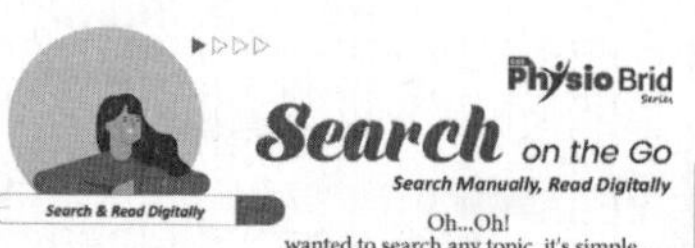

pathology, genetics, physiology, psychological factors like emotions, behavior, and cognition, and social factors like socioeconomic impacts on healthcare access, cultural beliefs, behaviors, and conventions. Personalized healthcare involves creating customized treatment strategies that take into account the individual's distinct social, biological, and psychological characteristics. This approach improves patient outcomes by integrating social and psychological support, reducing social isolation and stress, which can be detrimental to physical health.

- Primary care physicians use the biopsychosocial approach to understand patients' overall health and provide exceptional treatment. Family physicians encourage routine physical screening for social determinants of health and mental health issues. Counselors, psychologists, and psychiatrists use this framework to enhance their understanding of how mental and physical health are interconnected. Physiotherapists, occupational therapists, and other rehabilitation specialists employ this approach to treat injury or illness by incorporating support and social reintegration into the healing process, resulting in both physical recovery and psychological adaptation for patients.

- Pain experts use the biopsychosocial approach to treat chronic pain, addressing not only physical pain but also emotional and social factors that influence pain perception and treatment. Case studies have shown that social circumstances, behavioral aspects, and biological traits all have an impact on health and illness. A multidisciplinary approach is used to manage pain, involving anesthesiologists, psychologists, nurses, physical and occupational therapists, surgeons, neurologists, internists, physiatrists, psychiatrists, social workers, nutritionists, and pharmacists. Individualized treatment plans should combine medical and physical therapies, as well as cognitive behavioral therapy (CBT)-based psychological interventions.

- Psychological stress is a significant issue that can lead to early mortality, medical morbidity, mood disorders, aggressive dyscontrol, hypoimmune dysfunction, anxiety, and structural abnormalities in the central nervous system. To manage stress and improve mental health, individuals can engage in mindfulness workouts, physical activity, and regular exercise.

- Stress management techniques in rehabilitation include aerobic exercises, breathing exercises, and stretching. Aerobic exercise has been shown to lower stress and enhance neurocognitive function, while breathing exercises like alternate nostril breathing (ANB), timed slow breathing, diaphragmatic breathing, and breathing with biofeedback can help treat clinical anxiety and reduce stress in collegiate athletes.

- Medical professionals use various motivational strategies to encourage patients to follow rehabilitation regimens, including forming therapeutic relationships, raising health literacy, setting realistic objectives, tailoring the curriculum, controlling feelings associated with exercise, applying positive reinforcement, avoiding distracting stimuli, and asking for help. Vicarious experiences and visual persuasion can also be used to motivate patients.

- Patients recovering from injury need to engage in physical exercise and functional training. Effective communication is crucial in a doctor-patient relationship; and mental body interventions include yoga, meditation, biofeedback, mental imagery, visual and auditory cues, massage therapy, and deep breathing exercises. However, in order to encourage broad participation, barriers such as low motivation, fear of pain or discomfort, adverse weather conditions, lack of knowledge, energy deficits, poor health or physical limitations, limited access to equipment or facilities, work commitments or time constraints, and financial costs need to be effectively addressed.

REFERENCES

1. Pérez-Álvarez M. Psychology as a Science of Subject and Comportment, beyond the Mind and Behavior. Integr Psychol Behav Sci. 2018;52(1):25–51. Available from: https://doi.org/10.1007/s12124-017-9408-4.

2. Brinkmann S. Psychology as a science of life. Theory Psychol. 2020;30(1):3–17. Available from: https://doi.org/10.1177/0959354319889186.

3. Veras M, Kairy D, Paquet N. What Is Evidence-Based Physiotherapy? Physiother Can. 2016;68(2): 95–8. Available from: https://doi.org/10.3138/ptc.68.2.GEE.

4. In brief: Physical therapy. InformedHealth.org - NCBI Bookshelf. 2022 Jun 24. Available from: https://www.ncbi.nlm.nih.gov/books/NBK561514/.

5. Wei GX, Si G, Tang YY. Editorial: Brain-Mind-Body Practice and Health. Frontiers in Psychology. 2017 Oct 25; 8. Available from: https://doi.org/10.3389/fpsyg.2017.01886.

6. Lo Benjamin WY, Fukuda H, Nishimura Y, Macdonald RI, Farrokhyar F, Thabane L, et al. Pathophysiologic mechanisms of brain-body associations in ruptured brain aneurysms: A systematic review. Surgical Neurology International [Internet]. 2015 [cited 2023 May 8];6(1):136. Available from: https://www.ncbi.nlm.nih.gov/pmc/articles/PMC4544125/.

7. Mendoza LSM, Trujillo-Güiza M, Forero DA, Baez S. Health, psychosocial and cognitive factors associated with anxiety symptoms. Curr Psychol [Internet]. 2024; Available from: http://dx.doi.org/10.1007/s12144-024-05998-3.

8. Quadt L, Esposito G, Critchley HD, Garfinkel SN. Brain-body interactions underlying the association of loneliness with mental and physical health. Neurosci Biobehav Rev [Internet]. 2020;116:283–300. Available from: http://dx.doi.org/10.1016/j.neubiorev.2020.06.015.

9. Jancey J, Barnett L, Smith J, Binns C, Howat P. We need a comprehensive approach to health promotion. Health Promot J Austr. 2016;27(1):1–3. Available from: https://doi.org/10.1071/hev27n1_ed.

10. Wiedermann CJ, Barbieri V, Plagg B, Marino P, Piccoliori G, Engl A. Fortifying the Foundations: A Comprehensive Approach to Enhancing Mental Health Support in Educational Policies Amidst Crises. Healthcare. 2023;11(10):1423. Available from: https://doi.org/10.3390/healthcare11101423.

11. International Journal of Multidisciplinary Research and Analysis. A Comprehensive Healthcare Model: Dimension, Status, and Approach. Int J Multidiscip Res Anal. 2022;5(10):2524–2532. Available from: https://doi.org/10.47191/ijmra/v5-i10-05.

12. Bendowska A, Baum E. The significance of cooperation in interdisciplinary healthcare teams as perceived by Polish medical students. Int J Environ Res Public Health [Internet]. 2023;20(2):954. Available from: http://dx.doi.org/10.3390/ijerph20020954.

13. Hjuler KF, Møller L, Elgaard C, Gaïni L, Iversen L, Hjuler T. On the interdisciplinary treatment and management of patients with immune-mediated inflammatory diseases. A study on patients' personal experiences and perspectives. J Multidiscip Healthc [Internet]. 2024;17:p.2635–46. Available from: http://dx.doi.org/10.2147/jmdh.s432820.

14. Ghebrehiwet T, Ammon M, Burbiel I, Botbol M. Interdisciplinary Team Approach to Clinical Care. In: Springer eBooks. 2016. p. 211–22. Available from: https://doi.org/10.1007/978-3-319-39724-5_16.

15. Yamamoto K. Association between interdisciplinary collaboration and leadership ability in intensive care unit nurses: A cross-sectional study. J Nurs Res [Internet]. 2022;30(2):e202. Available from: http://dx.doi.org/10.1097/jnr.0000000000000483.

Contd...

16. Driver C, Oprescu F, Lovell GP. An exploration of physiotherapists' perceived benefits and barriers towards using psychosocial strategies in their practice. Musculoskelet Care. 2020;18(2):111–21. Available from: https://doi.org/10.1002/msc.1437.

17. Denneny D, Frijdal (nee Klapper) A, Bianchi-Berthouze N, Greenwood J, McLoughlin R, Petersen K, et al. The application of psychologically informed practice: observations of experienced physiotherapists working with people with chronic pain. Physiotherapy [Internet]. 2020;106: 163–73. Available from: http://dx.doi.org/10.1016/j.physio.2019.01.014.

18. Yonatan-Leus R, Abargil M, Cooper-Kazaz R. The combined effect of psychodynamic psychotherapy and pharmacotherapy on healthcare cost. Psychother Res. 2022;32:1–12. Available from: https://doi.org/10.1080/10503307.2022.2032861.

19. Rocks S, Berntson D, Gil-Salmerón A, Kadu M, Ehrenberg N, Stein V, et al. Cost and effects of integrated care: A systematic literature review and meta-analysis. Eur J Health Econ. 2020;21(8):1211–21. Available from: https://doi.org/10.1007/s10198-020-01217-5.

20. Jasemi M, Valizadeh L, Zamanzadeh V, Keogh B. A Concept Analysis of Holistic Care by Hybrid Model. Indian J Palliat Care. 2017;23(1):71–80. Available from: https://doi.org/10.4103/0973-1075.197960.

21. Alvarez E, Garvin A, Germaine N, Guidoni L, Schnurr M. Use of Mental Health Interventions by Physiotherapists to Treat Individuals with Chronic Conditions: A Systematic Scoping Review. Physiother Can. 2022;74(1):35–43. Available from: https://doi.org/10.3138/ptc-2020-0066.

22. Probst M. Physiotherapy and Mental Health. London: IntechOpen; 2017. Available from: https://doi.org/10.5772/67595.

23. Van Dijk H, Köke AJA, Elbers S, Mollema J, Smeets RJEM, Wittink H. Physiotherapists Using the Biopsychosocial Model for Chronic Pain: Barriers and Facilitators-A Scoping Review. Int J Environ Res Public Health. 2023;20(2):1634. Available from: https://doi.org/10.3390/ijerph20021634.

24. Smart KM. The biopsychosocial model of pain in physiotherapy: past, present and future. Phys Ther Rev. 2023;28(2):61–70. Available from: https://doi.org/10.1080/10833196.2023.2177792.

25. Vögele C. Behavioral Medicine. In: Elsevier eBooks. 2015. p. 463–9. Available from: https://doi.org/10.1016/b978-0-08-097086-8.14060-7.

26. Gatchel RJ, Ray CT, Kishino N, Brindle A. The Biopsychosocial Model. In: Gellman MD, Turner JR, editors. The Wiley Encyclopedia of Health Psychology. Hoboken (NJ): John Wiley & Sons, Inc.; 2020. p. 1–8. Available from: https://doi.org/10.1002/9781119057840.ch182.

27. Kusnanto H, Agustian D, Hilmanto D. Biopsychosocial model of illnesses in primary care: A hermeneutic literature review. J Family Med Prim Care. 2018;7(3):497–500. Available from: https://doi.org/10.4103/jfmpc.jfmpc_145_17.

28. Bolton D, Gillett G. The Biopsychosocial Model of Health and Disease. In: Springer eBooks; 2019. Available from: https://doi.org/10.1007/978-3-030-11899-0.

29. Lehman BJ, David DM, Gruber JA. Rethinking the Biopsychosocial Model of health: Understanding Health as a Dynamic System. Social and Personality Psychology Compass. 2017 Aug 3;11(8):1–17.

30. Taukeni SG, editor. Acceleration of the biopsychosocial model in public health. Hershey, PA: IGI Global; 2023.

31. Andermann A, CLEAR Collaboration. Taking action on the social determinants of health in clinical practice: A framework for health professionals. CMAJ. 2016;188(17-18)–E483. Available from: https://doi.org/10.1503/cmaj.160177.

Contd...

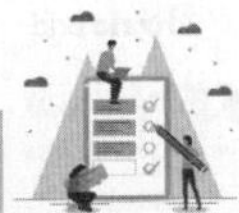 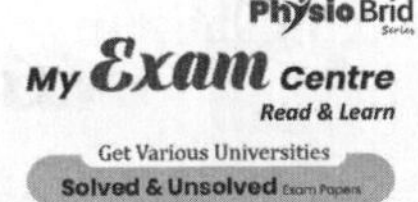

32. Biopsychosocial Model of Health Case Study. NursingAnswers.net. Available from: https://nursinganswers.net/case-studies/the-biopsychosocial-model-of-health.php.

33. Laeeqa Sujee, Munshi S, Christofides N. Moving from theory to practice: Barriers and facilitators to physiotherapy students' use of the biopsychosocial approach in the management of chronic pain. Research Square (Research Square). 2023 Oct 3.

34. Holopainen R, Simpson P, Piirainen A, Karppinen J, Schütze R, Smith A, et al. Physiotherapists' perceptions of learning and implementing a biopsychosocial intervention to treat musculoskeletal pain conditions: A systematic review and metasynthesis of qualitative studies. Pain. 2020 Jan 16;161(6):1150–68.

35. Miki T, Kondo Y, Kurakata H, Takebayashi T, Samukawa M. Effects of a physiotherapist-led approach based on a biopsychosocial model for spinal disorders: protocol for a systematic review. BMJ Open. 2021 Sep;11(9):e055144.

36. Bazira PJ. An overview of the nervous system. Surgery (Oxf). 2021;39(8):451–62. Available from: https://doi.org/10.1016/j.mpsur.2021.06.012.

37. Brain Anatomy and How the Brain Works. Johns Hopkins Medicine. 2021 Jul 14. Available from: https://www.hopkinsmedicine.org/health/conditions-and-diseases/anatomy-of-the-brain.

38. Brain Basics: Know Your Brain. National Institute of Neurological Disorders and Stroke. Available from: https://www.ninds.nih.gov/health-information/public-education/brain-basics/brain-basics-know-your-brain.

39. Khan YS, Lui F. Neuroanatomy, Spinal Cord. StatPearls - NCBI Bookshelf. 2023 Jul 24. Available from: https://www.ncbi.nlm.nih.gov/books/NBK559056/.

40. Ranabir S, Reetu K. Stress and hormones. Indian J Endocrinol Metab. 2011;15(1):18–22. Available from: https://doi.org/10.4103/2230-8210.77573.

41. Shaffer J. Neuroplasticity and Clinical Practice: Building Brain Power for Health. Frontiers in Psychology [Internet]. 2016 Jul 26;7(1118). Available from: https://www.ncbi.nlm.nih.gov/pmc/articles/PMC4960264/.

42. Toussaint L, Nguyen QA, Roettger C, Dixon K, Offenbächer M, Kohls N, et al. Effectiveness of Progressive Muscle Relaxation, Deep Breathing, and Guided Imagery in Promoting Psychological and Physiological States of Relaxation. Taylor-Piliae R, editor. Evidence-Based Complementary and Alternative Medicine [Internet]. 2021 Jul 2;2021(1):1–8. Available from: https://www.ncbi.nlm.nih.gov/pmc/articles/PMC8272667/.

43. Norman SL, Wolpaw JR, Reinkensmeyer DJ. Targeting neuroplasticity to improve motor recovery after stroke: An artificial neural network model. Brain Communications. 2022 Oct 21.

44. Lin TW, Kuo YM. Exercise benefits brain function: The monoamine connection. Brain Sci. 2013;3(1):39–53. Available from: https://doi.org/10.3390/brainsci3010039.

45. Afridi B, Khan H, Akkol EK, Aschner M. Pain Perception and Management: Where do We Stand?. Curr Mol Pharmacol. 2021;14(5):678–88. Available from: https://doi.org/10.2174/1874467213666200611142438.

46. Thompson OJ, Powell-Roach K, Taylor JL, Terry EL, Booker SQ. Pain catastrophizing: A patient-centered approach to assessment. Nurs. 2022;52(4):26–30. Available from: https://doi.org/10.1097/01.NURSE.0000823252.50782.45.

47. Geert Crombez, Veirman E, Dimitri Van Ryckeghem, Scott W, Annick De Paepe. The effect of psychological factors on pain outcomes: lessons learned for the next generation of research. Pain Reports. 2023 Nov 7;8(6):e1112–2.

Contd...

48. Srinivas V, Choubey U, Motwani J, Anamika F, Chennupati C, Garg N, et al. Synergistic strategies: Optimizing outcomes through a multidisciplinary approach to clinical rounds. Proc (Bayl Univ Med Cent). 2023;37(1):144–50. Available from: https://doi.org/10.1080/08998280.2023.2274230.

49. Song MK, Choi SH, Lee DH, Lee KJ, Lee WJ, Kang DH. Effects of Cognitive Behavioral Therapy on Empathy in Patients with Chronic Pain. Psychiatry Investig. 2018;15(3):285–91. Available from: https://doi.org/10.30773/pi.2017.07.03.

50. Bendowska A, Baum E. The Significance of Cooperation in Interdisciplinary Health Care Teams as Perceived by Polish Medical Students. Int J Environ Res Public Health. 2023;20(2):954. Available from: https://doi.org/10.3390/ijerph20020954.

51. James KA, Stromin JI, Steenkamp N, Combrinck MI. Understanding the relationships between physiological and psychosocial stress, cortisol and cognition. Front Endocrinol (Lausanne). 2023;14:1085950. Available from: https://doi.org/10.3389/fendo.2023.1085950.

52. Sharma DK, Government Model Science College. Physiology of stress and its management. Journal of Medicine: Study & Research [Internet]. 2018;1(1):1–5. Available from: http://dx.doi.org/10.24966/msr-5657/100001.

53. McEwen BS. Neurobiological and systemic effects of chronic stress. Chronic Stress (Thousand Oaks) [Internet]. 2017;1:247054701769232. Available from: http://dx.doi.org/10.1177/2470547017692328.

54. Satyjeet F, Naz S, Kumar V, Aung NH, Bansari K, Irfan S, et al. Psychological stress as a risk factor for cardiovascular disease: A case-control study. Cureus [Internet]. 2020 Oct 1;12(10). Available from: https://www.ncbi.nlm.nih.gov/pmc/articles/PMC7603890/.

55. Mahindru A, Patil P, Agrawal V. Role of Physical Activity on Mental Health and Well-Being: A Review. Cureus [Internet]. 2023 Jan 7;15(1). Available from: https://www.ncbi.nlm.nih.gov/pmc/articles/PMC9902068/.

56. Al-Dubai SA, Al-Naggar RA, Alshagga MA, Rampal KG. Stress and coping strategies of students in a medical faculty in Malaysia. Malays J Med Sci. 2011;18(3):57–64.

57. Ganesan, Talwar, Fauzan N, Oon. A study on stress level and coping strategies among undergraduate students. Journal of Cognitive Sciences and Human Development [Internet]. 2018;3(2):37–47. Available from: http://dx.doi.org/10.33736/jcshd.787.2018.

58. Graves BS, Hall ME, Dias-Karch C, Haischer MH, Apter C. Gender differences in perceived stress and coping among college students. Dalby AR, editor. PLOS ONE [Internet]. 2021 Aug 12;16(8):e0255634. Available from: https://www.ncbi.nlm.nih.gov/pmc/articles/PMC8360537/.

59. Chen Y, Peng Y, Xu H, O'Brien WH. Age differences in stress and coping: Problem-focused strategies mediate the relationship between age and positive affect. Int J Aging Hum Dev. 2018;86(4):347–63. Available from: https://doi.org/10.1177/0091415017720890.

60. George SA, John J, Jose J. Effectiveness of aerobic exercise in reducing stress and anxiety among high school level boarding students. Int J Sci Res (IJSR). 2021;10:819–21.

61. Mckune A, Bach C, Semple S, Dyer B. Salivary cortisol and alpha-amylase responses to repeated bouts of downhill running. Am J Hum Biol. 2014;26. Available from: https://doi.org/10.1002/ajhb.22605.

62. Bentley TGK, D'Andrea-Penna G, Rakic M, Arce N, LaFaille M, Berman R, et al. Breathing practices for stress and anxiety reduction: Conceptual framework of implementation guidelines based on a systematic review of the published literature. Brain Sci. 2023;13(12):1612. Available from: https://doi.org/10.3390/brainsci13121612.

Contd...

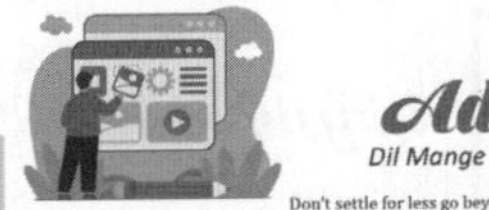

63. Epe J, Stark R, Ott U. Different Effects of Four Yogic Breathing Techniques on Mindfulness, Stress, and Well-being. OBM Integrative and Complementary Medicine. 2021 Jun 29;06(03):1–1.

64. Zaccaro A, Piarulli A, Laurino M, Garbella E, Menicucci D, Neri B, et al. How breath-control can change your life: A systematic review on psycho-physiological correlates of slow breathing. Frontiers in Human Neuroscience. 2018 Sep 7;12(353):1–16.

65. Behm DG, Alizadeh S, Daneshjoo A, Anvar SH, Graham A, Zahiri A, et al. Acute effects of various stretching techniques on range of motion: A systematic review with meta-analysis. Sports Med Open [Internet]. 2023;9(1):107. Available from: http://dx.doi.org/10.1186/s40798-023-00652-x.

66. Harsanyi S, Kupcova I, Danisovic L, Klein M. Selected Biomarkers of Depression: What Are the Effects of Cytokines and Inflammation? International Journal of Molecular Sciences. 2022 Dec 29;24(1):578.

67. Arora S, Bhattacharjee J. Modulation of immune responses in stress by Yoga. International Journal of Yoga. 2008;1(2):45.

68. Linge AD, Bjørkly SK, Jensen C, Hasle B. Bandura's Self-Efficacy Model Used to Explore Participants' Experiences of Health, Lifestyle, and Work After Attending a Vocational Rehabilitation Program with Lifestyle Intervention – A Focus Group Study. Journal of Multidisciplinary Healthcare. 2021 Dec; Volume 14:3533–48.

69. Fernandes JB, Ferreira N, Domingos J, Ferreira R, Amador C, Pardal N, et al. Health Professionals' Motivational Strategies to Enhance Adherence in the Rehabilitation of People with Lower Limb Fractures: Scoping Review. International Journal of Environmental Research and Public Health [Internet]. 2023 Jan 1 [cited 2023 Dec 21];20(22):7050. Available from: https://www.mdpi.com/1660-4601/20/22/7050.

70. Lucini D, Pagani M. Exercise Prescription to Foster Health and Well-Being: A Behavioral Approach to Transform Barriers into Opportunities. International Journal of Environmental Research and Public Health [Internet]. 2021 Jan 22;18(3):968. Available from: https://www.ncbi.nlm.nih.gov/pmc/articles/PMC7908585/.

71. Hafner C, Schneider J, Schindler M, Braillard O. Visual aids in ambulatory clinical practice: Experiences, perceptions and needs of patients and healthcare professionals. Schouten B, editor. PLOS ONE [Internet]. 2022 Feb 2;17(2):e0263041. Available from: https://www.ncbi.nlm.nih.gov/pmc/articles/PMC8809598/.

72. Laurel D, Castagno C, Ciara C, Gil G, Weiss William M. Impact of Traumatic Sports Injury on an Athlete's Psychological Wellbeing, Adherence to Sport and Athletic Identity. Journal of sports medicine and therapy. 2023 Sep 20;8(3):036–46.

73. Yang SX, Cheng S, Su DL. Sports injury and stressor-related disorder in competitive athletes: A systematic review and a new framework. Burns & Trauma. 2022 Jan 1;10.

74. Johnston LH, Carroll D. The psychological impact of injury: Effects of prior sport and exercise involvement. Br J Sports Med. 2000;34(6):436–439.

75. Miller BE, Miller MN, Verhegge R, Linville HH, Pumariega AJ. Alcohol misuse among college athletes: Self-medication for psychiatric symptoms? J Drug Educ. 2002;32(1):41–52. Available from: https://doi.org/10.2190/JDFM-AVAK-G9FV-0MYY.

76. Rice SM, Parker AG, Rosenbaum S, Bailey A, Mawren D, Purcell R. Sport-related concussion and mental health outcomes in elite athletes: A systematic review. Sports Med. 2018;48(2):447–465. Available from: https://doi.org/10.1007/s40279-017-0810-3.

Contd...

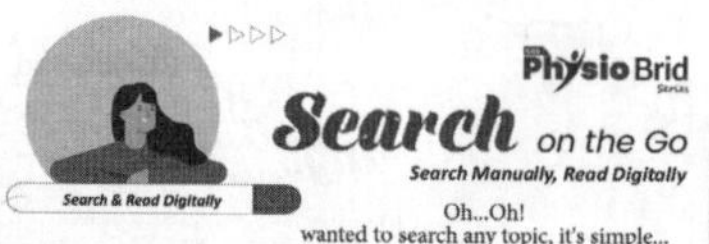

77. Clement D, Arvinen-Barrow M, Fetty T. Psychosocial responses during different phases of sport-injury rehabilitation: A qualitative study. J Athl Train. 2015;50(1):95–104. Available from: https://doi.org/10.4085/1062-6050-49.3.52.

78. Cormier ML, Zizzi SJ. Athletic trainers' skills in identifying and managing athletes experiencing psychological distress. J Athl Train. 2015;50(12):1267–1276. Available from: https://doi.org/10.4085/1062-6050-50.12.02.

79. Bakic-Miric NM, Bakic NM. Successful doctor-patient communication and rapport building as the key skills of medical practice. Med Biol. 2008;15(2):74–79.

80. Gu L, Deng J, Xu H, Zhang S, Gao M, Qu Z, et al. The impact of contract service policy and doctor communication skills on rural patient-doctor trust relationship in the village clinics of three counties. BMC Health Services Research. 2019 Mar 22;19(1).

81. Vedala SR, Mane AB, Paul CN. Pulmonary functions in yogic and sedentary population. Int J Yoga. 2014;7(2):155-159. Available from: https://doi.org/10.4103/0973-6131.133904.

82. Hakked CS, Balakrishnan R, Krishnamurthy MN. Yogic breathing practices improve lung functions of competitive young swimmers. J Ayurveda Integr Med. 2017;8(2):99–104. Available from: https://doi.org/10.1016/j.jaim.2016.12.005.

83. Black DS, Slavich GM. Mindfulness meditation and the immune system: A systematic review of randomized controlled trials. Ann N Y Acad Sci. 2016;1373(1):13–24. Available from: https://doi.org/10.1111/nyas.12998.

84. Lopez G, Chaoul A, Warneke CL, Christie AJ, Powers-James C, Liu W, et al. Self-administered meditation application intervention for cancer patients with psychosocial distress: A pilot study. Integr Cancer Ther [Internet]. 2023;22:15347354221148710. Available from: http://dx.doi.org/10.1177/15347354221148710.

85. Jamil A, Sai Dheeraj Gutlapalli, Ali M, Mrinal J. P. Oble, Shamsun Nahar Sonia, George S, et al. Meditation and Its Mental and Physical Health Benefits in 2023. Cureus [Internet]. 2023 Jun 19;15(6). Available from: https://www.ncbi.nlm.nih.gov/pmc/articles/PMC10355843/.

86. Tosti B, Corrado S, Mancone S, Di Libero T, Rodio A, Andrade A, et al. Integrated use of biofeedback and neurofeedback techniques in treating pathological conditions and improving performance: A narrative review. Front Neurosci. 2024;18:1358481. Available from: https://doi.org/10.3389/fnins.2024.1358481.

87. Liao ED-Y, editor. Smart biofeedback: Perspectives and applications. London, England: IntechOpen; 2020.

88. Kondo K, Noonan KM, Freeman M, Ayers C, Morasco BJ, Kansagara D. Efficacy of biofeedback for medical conditions: An evidence map. J Gen Intern Med. 2019;34(12):2883–2893. Available from: https://doi.org/10.1007/s11606-019-05215-z.

89. Pearson J, Naselaris T, Holmes EA, Kosslyn SM. Mental imagery: Functional mechanisms and clinical applications. Trends Cogn Sci. 2015;19(10):590–602. Available from: https://doi.org/10.1016/j.tics.2015.08.003.

90. Vaz JR, Rand T, Fujan-Hansen J, Mukherjee M, Stergiou N. Auditory and Visual External Cues Have Different Effects on Spatial but Similar Effects on Temporal Measures of Gait Variability. Frontiers in Physiology. 2020 Feb 11;11.

91. Mate KKV. Effects of Visual, Auditory, and Combined Cues on Human Movement and Brain Regions Involved in Perception Action. McGill Journal of Medicine. 2022 Jul 5;20(2).

Contd...

92. Field T. Massage therapy research review. Complementary Therapies in Clinical Practice. 2016 Aug;24:19–31.

93. Choi H, Kim S-J, Oh J, Lee M-N, Kim S, Kang K-A. The effects of massage therapy on physical growth and gastrointestinal function in premature infants: A pilot study: A pilot study. J Child Health Care [Internet]. 2016;20(3):394–404. Available from: http://dx.doi.org/10.1177/1367493515598647.

94. Smith SL, Haley S, Slater H, Moyer-Mileur LJ. Heart rate variability during caregiving and sleep after massage therapy in preterm infants. Early Hum Dev [Internet]. 2013;89(8):525–9. Available from: http://dx.doi.org/10.1016/j.earlhumdev.2013.01.004.

95. Nazari F, Mirzamohamadi M, Yousefi H. The effect of massage therapy on occupational stress of Intensive Care Unit nurses. Iran J Nurs Midwifery Res [Internet]. 2015;20(4):508–15. Available from: http://dx.doi.org/10.4103/1735-9066.161001.

96. Diego MA, Field T, Hernandez-Reif M. Preterm infant weight gain is increased by massage therapy and exercise via different underlying mechanisms. Early Hum Dev [Internet]. 2014;90(3):137–40. Available from: http://dx.doi.org/10.1016/j.earlhumdev.2014.01.009.

97. Neu M, Pan Z, Workman R, Marcheggiani-Howard C, Furuta G, Laudenslager ML. Benefits of massage therapy for infants with symptoms of gastroesophageal reflux disease. Biol Res Nurs [Internet]. 2014;16(4):387–97. Available from: http://dx.doi.org/10.1177/1099800413516187.

98. McKay E. Assessing the effectiveness of massage therapy for bilateral cleft lip reconstruction scars. Int J Ther Massage Bodywork [Internet]. 2014;7(2):3–9. Available from: http://dx.doi.org/10.3822/ijtmb.v7i2.224.

99. Cho YS, Jeon JH, Hong A, Yang HT, Yim H, Cho YS, et al. The effect of burn rehabilitation massage therapy on hypertrophic scar after burn: A randomized controlled trial. Burns [Internet]. 2014;40(8):1513–20. Available from: http://dx.doi.org/10.1016/j.burns.2014.02.005.

100. Franklin NC, Ali MM, Robinson AT, Norkeviciute E, Phillips SA. Massage therapy restores peripheral vascular function after exertion. Arch Phys Med Rehabil [Internet]. 2014;95(6):1127–34. Available from: http://dx.doi.org/10.1016/j.apmr.2014.02.007.

101. Tavoian D, Craighead DH. Deep breathing exercise at work: Potential applications and impact. Front Physiol. 2023;14: 1040091. Available from: https://doi.org/10.3389/fphys.2023.1040091.

102. Gee ME, Bienek A, Campbell NRC, Bancej CM, Robitaille C, Kaczorowski J, et al. Prevalence of, and barriers to, preventive lifestyle behaviors in hypertension (from a national survey of Canadians with hypertension). Am J Cardiol. 2012;109 (4):570–575. Available from: https://doi.org/10.1016/j.amjcard.2011.09.051.

103. Kivimäki M, Steptoe A. Effects of stress on the development and progression of cardiovascular disease. Nat Rev Cardiol. 2018;15(4):215–229. Available from: https://doi.org/10.1038/nrcardio.2017.189.

104. Archer KR, Devin CJ, Vanston SW, Koyama T, Phillips SE, Mathis SL, et al. Cognitive behavioral based physical therapy for patients with chronic pain undergoing lumbar spine surgery: A randomized controlled trial. J Pain. 2016;17(1):76–89. Available from: https://doi.org/10.1016/j.jpain.2015.09.013.

105. Kurnik Mesarič K, Pajek J, Logar Zakrajšek B, Bogataj Š, Kodrič J. Cognitive behavioral therapy for lifestyle changes in patients with obesity and type 2 diabetes: A systematic review and meta-analysis. Sci Rep. 2023;13(1):12793. Available from: https://doi.org/10.1038/s41598-023-40141-5.

Contd...

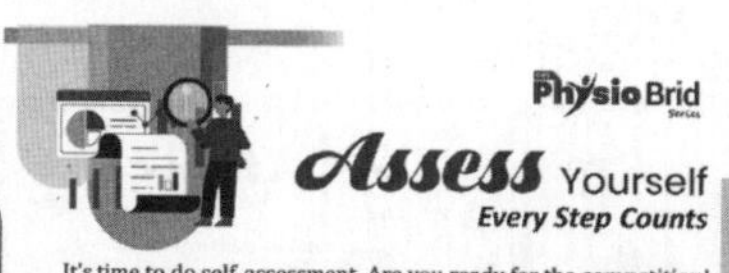

106. Liu TW, Ng GYF, Ng SSM. Effectiveness of a combination of cognitive behavioral therapy and task-oriented balance training in reducing the fear of falling in patients with chronic stroke: study protocol for a randomized controlled trial. Trials. 2018 Mar 7;19(1).

107. Bannink F. Positive CBT in Practice. Positive Psychology Interventions in Practice. 2017;15–28.

108. Onac I, Moldovan A, Ioan. Medication, physiotherapy and cognitive behavior therapy for the treatment of chronic back pain: A clinical trial. Journal of Cognitive and Behavioral Psychotherapies. 2012;12:23–37.

109. Reme S, Sveinsdottir V, Eriksen. Assessing the role of cognitive behavioral therapy in the management of chronic nonspecific back pain. Journal of Pain Research. 2012 Oct;5:371.

110. Adam K, Gibson E, Strong J, Lyle A. Knowledge, skills and professional behaviors needed for occupational therapists and physiotherapists new to work-related practice. Work. 2011;39(3):309–318. Available from: https://doi.org/10.3233/wor-2011-1134.

111. Adam K, Peters S, Chipchase L. Knowledge, skills and professional behaviors required by occupational therapist and physiotherapist beginning practitioners in work-related practice: A systematic review. Aust Occup Ther J. 2013;60(2):76-84. Available from: https://doi.org/10.1111/1440-1630.12006.

112. Varkey B. Principles of Clinical Ethics and Their Application to Practice. Medical Principles and Practice [Internet]. 2021 Feb;30(1):17–28. Available from: https://www.ncbi.nlm.nih.gov/pmc/articles/PMC7923912/.

113. Hernández-Xumet J-E, García-Hernández A-M, Fernández-González J-P, Marrero-González C-M. Beyond scientific and technical training: Assessing the relevance of empathy and assertiveness in future physiotherapists: A cross-sectional study. Health Sci Rep [Internet]. 2023;6(10):e1600. Available from: http://dx.doi.org/10.1002/hsr2.1600.

114. Liu L, Wu H, Sun T. Editorial: Positive Psychology in Healthcare Professionals. Frontiers in Psychology. 2022 Mar 28;13.

115. Sinclair S, Hack TF, Raffin-Bouchal S, McClement S, Stajduhar K, Singh P, et al. What are healthcare providers' understandings and experiences of compassion? The healthcare compassion model: A grounded theory study of healthcare providers in Canada. BMJ Open. 2018 Mar;8(3):e019701.

116. Schultz KR, Brindle SS. Health care providers' perspectives on resilience and positive adjustment within the spinal cord injury population. Rehabil Psychol [Internet]. 2022;67(2):162–9. Available from: http://dx.doi.org/10.1037/rep0000413.

117. Turner J, Sherman K, Anderson M, Balderson B, Cook A, Cherkin D. (481) Catastrophizing, pain self-efficacy, mindfulness, and acceptance: relationships and changes among individuals receiving CBT, MBSR or usual care for chronic back pain. J Pain [Internet]. 2015;16(4):S96. Available from: http://dx.doi.org/10.1016/j.jpain.2015.01.401.

118. Reme S, Sveinsdottir V, Eriksen. Assessing the role of cognitive behavioral therapy in the management of chronic nonspecific back pain. Journal of Pain Research. 2012 Oct;5:371.

119. Reilimo M, Kaila-Kangas L, Shiri R, Laurola M, Miranda H. The effect of pain management group on chronic pain and pain related co-morbidities and symptoms. A stepped-wedge cluster randomized controlled trial. A study protocol. Contemp Clin Trials Commun. 2020;19:100577. Available from: https://doi.org/10.1016/j.conctc.2020.100577.

120. Knoerl R, Lavoie Smith EM, Weisberg J. Chronic Pain and Cognitive Behavioral Therapy. Western Journal of Nursing Research [Internet]. 2015 Nov 24;38(5):596–628. Available from: https://journals.sagepub.com/doi/abs/10.1177/0193945915615869.

Contd...

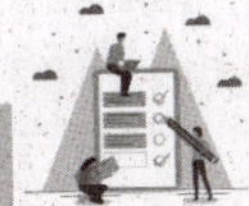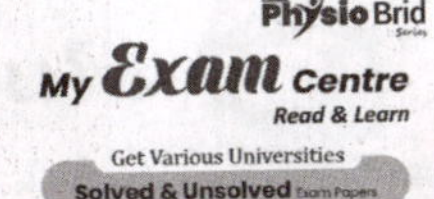

121. Ehde DM, Dillworth TM, Turner JA. Cognitive behavioral therapy for individuals with chronic pain: Efficacy, innovations, and directions for research. Am Psychol. 2014;69(2):153–166. Available from: https://doi.org/10.1037/a0035747.

122. Häuser W, Ablin J, Fitzcharles MA, Littlejohn G, Luciano JV, Usui C, et al. Fibromyalgia. Nature Reviews Disease Primers [Internet]. 2015 Aug 13;1(1). Available from: https://www.nature.com/articles/nrdp201522.

123. Nielsen M, Keefe FJ, Bennell K, Jull GA. Physical Therapist-Delivered Cognitive Behavioral Therapy: A Qualitative Study of Physical Therapists' Perceptions and Experiences. Physical Therapy. 2013 Sep 12;94(2):197–209.

124. Galvez-Sánchez CM, Duschek S, Reyes del Paso GA. Psychological impact of fibromyalgia: Current perspectives. Psychology Research and Behavior Management [Internet]. 2019 Feb; Volume 12(12):117–27. Available from: https://www.dovepress.com/psychological-impact-of-fibromyalgia-current-perspectives-peer-reviewed-fulltext-article-PRBM.

125. Jahan F, Nanji K, Qidwai W, Qasim R. Fibromyalgia Syndrome: An Overview of Pathophysiology, Diagnosis and Management. Oman Medical Journal. 2012 May 16;27(3):192–5.

126. Arrayás-Grajera MJ, Tornero-Quiñones I, Gavilán-Carrera B, Luque-Reca O, Peñacoba-Puente C, Sierra-Robles Á, Carbonell-Baeza A, Estévez-López F. Fibromyalgia: Evidence for deficits in positive psychology resources. A case-control study from the Al-Ándalus project. Int J Environ Res Public Health. 2021;18(22):12021. Available from: https://doi.org/10.3390/ijerph182212021.

127. Rossy LA, Buckelew SP, Dorr N, Hagglund KJ, Thayer JF, McIntosh MJ, et al. A meta-analysis of fibromyalgia treatment interventions. Ann Behav Med [Internet]. 1999;21(2):180–91. Available from: http://dx.doi.org/10.1007/bf02908299.

128. McGrath RL, Parnell T, Verdon S, Pope R. "We take on people's emotions": A qualitative study of physiotherapists' experiences with patients experiencing psychological distress. Physiother Theory Pract. 2024;40 (2):304–326. Available from: https://doi.org/10.1080/09593985.2022.2116964.

129. Lennon O, Ryan C, Helm M, Moore K, Sheridan A, Probst M, et al. Psychological Distress among Patients Attending Physiotherapy: A Survey-Based Investigation of Irish Physiotherapists' Current Practice and Opinions. Physiotherapy Canada [Internet]. 2019 Dec 27;72(3):e20190010. Available from: https://www.ncbi.nlm.nih.gov/pmc/articles/PMC8781485/.

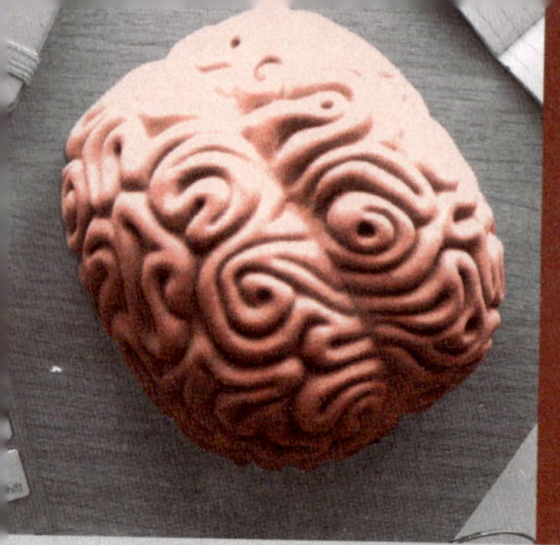

LONG ANSWER QUESTIONS

1. Describe the key principles of the biopsychosocial model in healthcare. How does this model integrate biological, psychological, and social factors to enhance patient care? Provide examples of how each component influences health outcomes.

2. Discuss the role of interdisciplinary teams in psychophysiotherapy. How do different healthcare professionals collaborate to provide comprehensive care?

3. Explain the importance of personalized healthcare in the context of the biopsychosocial model. How can tailored treatment plans that consider individual, social, biological, and psychological backgrounds improve patient outcomes?

4. How does the biopsychosocial approach influence the management of chronic pain? Discuss the multidisciplinary strategies used to address pain, considering the roles of various healthcare professionals and therapeutic interventions mentioned in the text.

5. Analyze the impact of psychological stress on overall health and well-being. What are the physiological and psychological consequences of stress, and how can stress management techniques such as mindfulness, physical activity, and exercise mitigate these effects?

6. Explore the motivational strategies employed by medical professionals to encourage patient adherence to rehabilitation regimens. How do strategies like therapeutic relationships, health literacy enhancement, goal setting, and positive reinforcement contribute to patient motivation and compliance?

7. Discuss the role of communication in the doctor-patient relationship, particularly in the context of psychophysiotherapy. How does effective communication facilitate patient recovery and treatment outcomes?

8. Evaluate the effectiveness of various mind-body interventions such as yoga, meditation, and biofeedback in rehabilitation. How do these interventions improve physical and mental health outcomes for patients?

9. Identify and discuss the barriers that hinder patient participation in rehabilitation programs. How can these barriers, such as lack of motivation, physical disabilities, and logistical challenges, be addressed to promote greater patient engagement?

10. Explain the concept of cognitive behavioral therapy (CBT) and its role in managing chronic pain and improving patient outcomes. How does CBT integrate cognitive restructuring and behavioral techniques to address pain perception and treatment adherence?

SHORT ANSWER QUESTIONS

1. What does the biopsychosocial model emphasize in understanding health and illness?

2. How does integrating psychology and physiotherapy benefit patients?
3. Who employs the biopsychosocial approach to treat injury or illness?
4. Which professionals use the biopsychosocial model to manage chronic pain?
5. What are the effects of psychological stress on the central nervous system?
6. Which techniques are used in stress management for rehabilitation?
7. How do medical professionals motivate patients in rehabilitation?
8. What are examples of mind-body interventions?
9. Why is effective communication crucial in the doctor-patient relationship?
10. What obstacles must be addressed to encourage participation in physical exercise?

MULTIPLE CHOICE QUESTIONS

1. **Which model emphasizes the interconnectedness of biological, psychological, and social factors in understanding health and illness?**
   a. Triangle model
   b. Biopsychosocial model
   c. Comprehensive approach
   d. Interdisciplinary approach

2. **According to the text, what does the triangle model primarily emphasize?**
   a. Physical health over mental health
   b. Interdisciplinary teamwork in healthcare
   c. The impact of thoughts on physical health
   d. Genetic predispositions to illness

3. **How does integrating psychology and physiotherapy benefit patients according to the text?**
   a. It increases dependency on medications
   b. It reduces the need for healthcare costs
   c. It focuses solely on physical symptoms
   d. It limits patient autonomy

4. **Which brain region is responsible for processing sensory data and understanding written and spoken words?**
   a. Frontal lobe
   b. Temporal lobe
   c. Occipital lobe
   d. Parietal lobe

5. **Which system controls involuntary physiological functions like blood pressure and digestion?**
   a. Somatic nervous system
   b. Autonomic nervous system
   c. Central nervous system
   d. Peripheral nervous system

6. **Which hormone is associated with emotional bonding and pain reduction?**
   a. Dopamine
   b. Oxytocin
   c. Cortisol
   d. Endorphins

7. **Which physiological system is primarily impacted by chronic stress, leading to dyslipidemia and increased risk of cardiovascular disease?**
   a. Endocrine system
   b. Respiratory system
   c. Cardiovascular system
   d. Muscular system

8. What psychological impact does stress have on athletes, according to the text?

a. Increased cognitive function
b. Decreased self-awareness
c. Enhanced performance
d. Higher risk of injury

9. Which coping mechanism involves the deliberate mobilization of ideas and behaviors to manage stress?

a. Emotional support
b. Self-distraction
c. Venting
d. Problem-focused coping

10. Which communication trait is most valued by patients in their interactions with healthcare providers?

a. Speaking confidently
b. Using technical jargon
c. Avoiding personal questions
d. Speaking quickly

11. Which mind-body intervention is noted for enhancing lung function and vital capacity through breathing techniques like diaphragmatic breathing?

a. Meditation
b. Biofeedback
c. Yoga
d. Mental imagery

12. Which therapeutic intervention has been shown to alleviate symptoms of gastroesophageal reflux disease (GERD) and improve mother-infant interactions?

a. Meditation
b. Massage
c. Breathing exercises
d. Visual and auditory cues

13. Which cognitive behavioral therapy (CBT) component was reported to be the most commonly used in treating chronic pain in older individuals?

a. Distraction techniques
b. Visualization exercises
c. Cognitive restructuring
d. Activity pacing

14. Which ethical principle in psychophysiotherapy emphasizes the obligation to protect patients from harm?

a. Beneficence
b. Autonomy
c. Nonmaleficence
d. Informed consent

15. Which disorder is frequently treated symptomatically using cognitive behavioral therapy (CBT) and exercise therapy due to its psychological symptoms such as pain, depression, and sleep difficulties?

a. Fibromyalgia
b. Osteoarthritis
c. Chronic fatigue syndrome
d. Cancer

ANSWER KEY

| 1. b | 2. c | 3. b | 4. b | 5. b | 6. b | 7. c | 8. d |
| 9. d | 10. a | 11. c | 12. b | 13. d | 14. c | 15. a | |

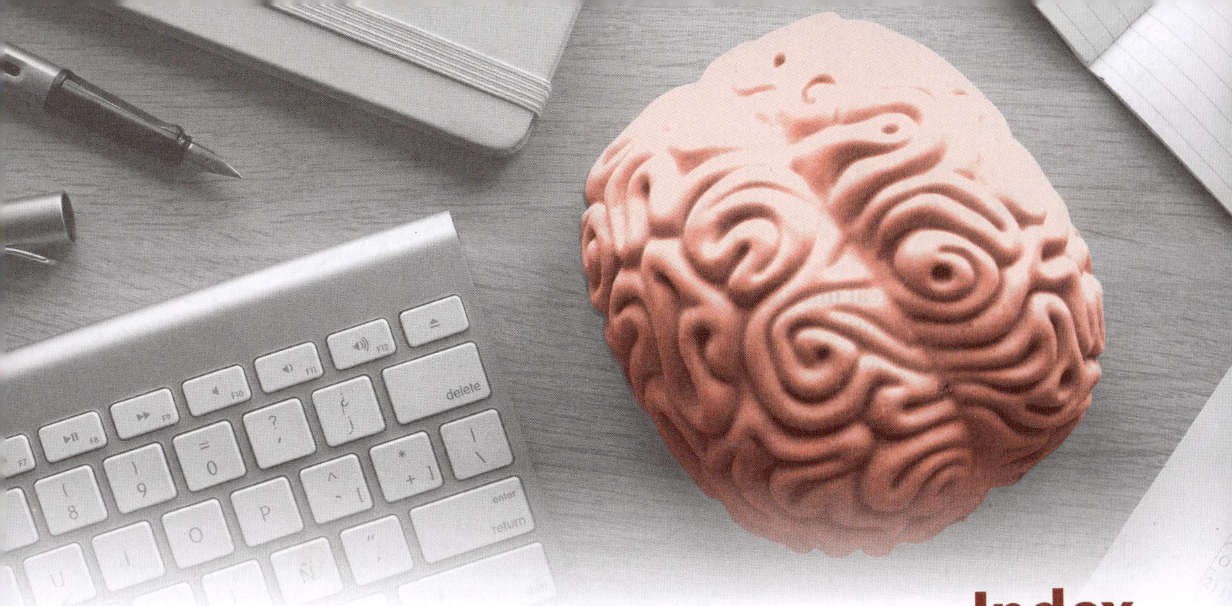

Index

Refer 'f' for figure and 't' for table, respectively.

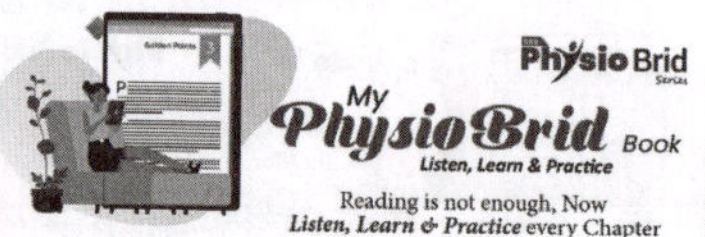

B

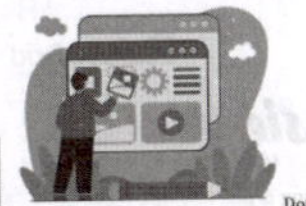

Physio Brid
Series
Add Ons
Dil Mange More Content
Don't settle for less go beyond with *Conceptual Videos,*
Recent Updates, e-Books & Much More...

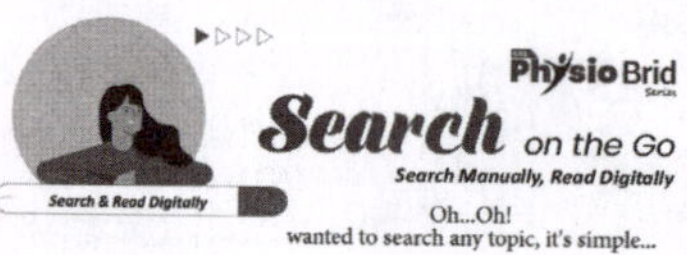

D

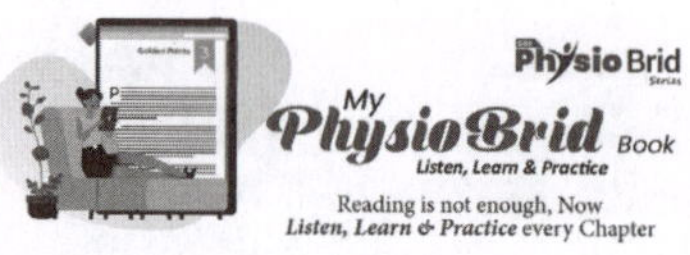

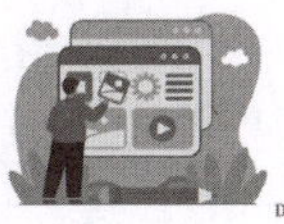

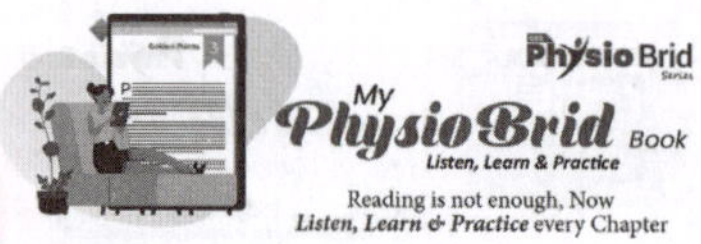
Physio Brid
My
Physio Brid
Book
Listen, Learn & Practice
Reading is not enough, Now
Listen, Learn & Practice every Chapter

Q

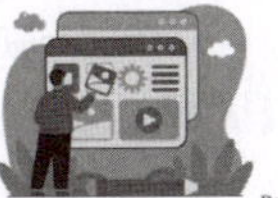

R

Ramelteon *379*

Rapid eye movement (REM) *208*

Rating

    method *282*

    scales for assessing anxiety in geriatric
        population *375t*

Rational

    analysis *169*

    emotive behavior therapy (REBT) *461*

Rationalization *126, 291, 296*

Raven's progressive matrices *175*

Raymond Cattell's trait theory *270*

Realism *255*

Realistic conflict *125*

Realm

    of

        physiotherapy *131*

        psychological defense mechanisms *303*

Recent

    advances in psychology *19*

    developments in AI *182*

Recruitment *394*

Regression *127, 291*

Rehabilitation psychology *360*

Reinforcement *84, 228, 330*

    learning *164*

Relapse *308, 324*

Relationship conflict *124, 125*

Relaxation exercises *452*

Reminiscence therapy *215*

Repetitive transcranial magnetic stimulation
    (rTMS) *368, 387*

Repression *126*

Respective sensations *67f*

Response

    cost *337*

    prompt *339*

Rivermead behavioral memory test
    (RBMT) *211*

Roger's self-theory *280*

Role

    of

        emotions *155*

        in physiotherapy practice *152*

        pediatric psychologists *352*

        physiotherapy in clinical psychology *18*

Rorschach inkblot test *283, 283f*

Rum fits *314*

Russell's two-dimensional circular model *143*

S

Schachter-Singer theory *146*

Schedules of reinforcement *334, 334t*

Schizophrenia *214, 294, 427, 428, 429*

Schools of psychology *7, 20*

Scope/s

    of

        counseling *453*

        industrial psychology *396f*

        psychology *15*

        the industrial psychology *395*

Screening *319*

Seasonal

    adjustment disorder (SAD) *356*

    affective disorder (SAD) *383*

Sedatives *318*

Selective

    attention *66, 68*

    serotonin reuptake inhibitors (SSRIs) *427*

Self-

    actualization *84*

    awareness intelligence *170*

    disclosure *452*

Semantic memory *190, 206*

Sensation *66*

Sense organs *67f, 73*

Sensory

    deceptions *74*

    distortions *74*

    memory *206*

    process to perception *67*

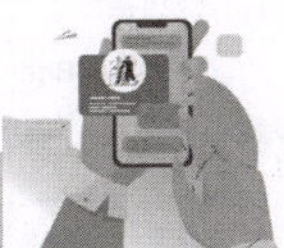